Pediatrics: Pathophysiology, Diagnosis and Treatment

Pediatrics: Pathophysiology, Diagnosis and Treatment

Edited by **Gabriel Tyler**

hayle
medical

New York

Published by Hayle Medical,
30 West, 37th Street, Suite 612,
New York, NY 10018, USA
www.haylemedical.com

Pediatrics: Pathophysiology, Diagnosis and Treatment
Edited by Gabriel Tyler

International Standard Book Number: 978-1-63241-428-1 (Hardback)

Contents

Preface

This book discusses the fundamental as well as modern approaches of pediatrics. Pediatrics is the branch of medicine that aims at providing healthcare for infants, children and adolescents. Subspecialties of pediatrics include pediatric infectious disease, pediatric critical care, neonatology, pediatric neurology, etc. This book aims to equip students and experts with the advanced topics and upcoming concepts in this area. From theories to research to practical applications, case studies related to all contemporary topics of relevance to this field have been included in this book. Those in search of information to further their knowledge in the area of pediatrics will be greatly assisted by this text.

This book is a comprehensive compilation of works of different researchers from varied parts of the world. It includes valuable experiences of the researchers with the sole objective of providing the readers (learners) with a proper knowledge of the concerned field. This book will be beneficial in evoking inspiration and enhancing the knowledge of the interested readers.

In the end, I would like to extend my heartiest thanks to the authors who worked with great determination on their chapters. I also appreciate the publisher's support in the course of the book. I would also like to deeply acknowledge my family who stood by me as a source of inspiration during the project.

Editor

Prevalence of Nocturnal Enuresis and Its Associated Factors in Primary School and Preschool Children of Khorramabad in 2013

Katayoun Bakhtiar,[1] **Yadollah Pournia,**[2] **Farzad Ebrahimzadeh,**[1]
Ali Farhadi,[3] **Fathollah Shafizadeh,**[4] **and Reza Hosseinabadi**[5]

[1] *Department of Public Health, Faculty of Health and Nutrition, Lorestan University of Medical Sciences,*
  Khorramabad 6813833946, Iran
[2] *Faculty of Medicine, Lorestan University of Medical Sciences, Khorramabad 6813833946, Iran*
[3] *Department of Social Medicine, Lorestan University of Medical Sciences, Khorramabad 6813833946, Iran*
[4] *Department of Pediatrics, Lorestan University of Medical Sciences, Khorramabad 6813833946, Iran*
[5] *Social Determinants of Health Research Center, Lorestan University of Medical Sciences, Khorramabad 6813833946, Iran*

Correspondence should be addressed to Reza Hosseinabadi; reza_hosseinabadi@yahoo.com

Academic Editor: Namık Yaşar Özbek

Background. Nocturnal enuresis refers to an inability to control urination during sleep. This study aimed to determine the prevalence of nocturnal enuresis and its associated factors in children in the city of Khorramabad. *Materials and Methods.* In this descriptive-analytic, cross-sectional study, 710 male and female children were divided into two groups with equal numbers. The samples were selected from the schools of Khorramabad using the multistage cluster and stratified random sampling methods based on the diagnostic criteria of DSM-IV. The data was analyzed using the logistic regression. *Results.* The results showed that 8% of the children had nocturnal enuresis, including 5.2% of primary nocturnal enuresis and 2.8% of secondary nocturnal enuresis. The prevalence of nocturnal enuresis in the boys (10.7%) was higher compared with that in the girls (5.4%) ($P = 0.009$). There were statistically significant relationships between nocturnal enuresis and history of nocturnal enuresis in siblings ($P = 0.023$), respiratory infections ($P = 0.036$), deep sleep ($P = 0.007$), corporal punishment at school ($P = 0.036$), anal itching ($P = 0.043$), and history of seizures ($P = 0.043$). *Conclusion.* This study showed that the prevalence of nocturnal enuresis in the boys was higher compared with that in the girls.

1. Introduction

Nocturnal enuresis refers to an inability to control urination and involuntary urination during sleep, which is common among young children [1]. Based on the DSM-IV (diagnostic and statistical manual of mental disorders IV) criteria, enuresis refers to the urination of children over 5 years old in clothes or in bed that happens twice a week for three consecutive months can occur at night, during the day, or a combination of these two, and is also called nocturnal enuresis [2]. Enuresis is classified as primary enuresis (urinary incontinence in a child who has never been dry) and secondary enuresis (urinary incontinence in a child who has been dry for at least 6 months) [3]. Nocturnal

enuresis in children is the second most common disorder after allergic diseases [1]. Nocturnal enuresis can cause a variety of behavioral, psychological, and social problems including embarrassment, blushing, lack of self-esteem, and aggression. Therefore, identifying children at risk and performing therapeutic measures are necessary [1, 3]. Based on the results of various investigations, enuresis has many causes including developmental differences, for example, differences in the growth of the urinary sphincters of a child, various diseases like diabetes, urinary tract infections, and so forth, emotional changes and conflicts such as the birth of a new baby and scholastic or educational stressful conditions, and emotional crises such as parental separation and divorce, family conflicts, and so forth [3–6].

Primary enuresis is often associated with a familial history of delayed urinary bladder control. Secondary enuresis may also be due to urologic and neurological problems, disorders of the spinal cord, and recurrent urinary tract infection [6]. Ninety percent of enuresis cases are primary, and its prevalence usually changes with age [6]. Several studies have been conducted on nocturnal enuresis and its associated factors. The review of the relevant literature showed considerably different prevalence rates for enuresis [3, 4], so that the prevalence rates in different regions and in children older than 5 years old have been reported to be 5–20% [1].

In a study by Unalacak et al. conducted in Turkey, the prevalence of nocturnal enuresis was 8.9%, out of which 7.75% was primary nocturnal enuresis [7]. Also, studies indicated the prevalence rates of 4.7% in China [8] and 18.2% in Australia in which 12.3%, 2.5%, and 3.6% of the children were reported to have mild, moderate, and severe nocturnal enuresis, respectively [9]. In the US, 5–10% of 7-year-old children suffered from nocturnal enuresis while the rate was lower than 5% in children over 10 years old [10]. The prevalence rate of nocturnal enuresis in Ethiopia has been reported to be 5% in small towns, 0.8% in most rural areas, and 9% in big cities [11].

Considering the importance and consequences of nocturnal enuresis and lack of a comprehensive study in this regard in the city of Khorramabad (west of Iran), this study aimed to investigate the prevalence of this disorder and its associated factors in 5–10-year-old children.

2. Materials and Methods

The city of Khorramabad (west of Iran) has two educational areas and 35 public and private schools. Out of this number, 24 schools were selected from the northern, southern, and central areas through the systematic random sampling, so that the distribution of the schools on the map of the city was homogeneous. The method used to select the samples was a combination of the stratified random sampling and the multistage cluster sampling. The educational levels (elementary school and preschool) were considered as two separate strata, and in each stratum, the northern, central, and southern areas of the city were in turn considered as three substrata. In each substratum, different schools were considered as cluster heads and a total of 24 schools were selected via the systematic random sampling from among the schools (cluster heads). Then, in each school, any educational level (grade) was considered as a stratum, one class was selected from each educational level, and the samples were selected from the class through the systematic randomization. The minimum sample size needed to investigate the prevalence of enuresis was calculated to be 708 samples (354 girls and 354 boys), considering similar studies, the significance level of 0.05, and the precision of 0.02. After the samples were selected, their parents attended the schools in coordination with the school principal, completed written informed consents, and completed the questionnaire with the help of the interviewer. The tool applied in this study was a research-made questionnaire

that was prepared based on reviewing the relevant literature and evaluating factors associated with enuresis. The content validation was applied to examine the validity of the questionnaire. To do this, the expert viewpoints of six specialists were considered, including 2 pediatricians, 2 biostatisticians, 1 health education specialist, and 1 child psychologist. To determine the reliability of the questionnaire, the test-retest reliability was applied on a sample size of 30 people with an interval of one week. The reliability was confirmed with a correlation coefficient of more than 0.8 and the significance level of 0.05. Additionally, Kappa's agreement coefficient of 0.8 was applied for the nominal scales for this purpose.

Four interviewers were trained in collecting the data and were calibrated with the researcher with a coefficient of 75%. The questionnaire applied in the study consisted of two parts. The first part contained the demographic and socioeconomic data including age, gender, parental marital status, parental education, parental kinship, parental occupation, family size, birth order, and other variables such as new baby's birth in the family, change of living place, sleep quality, child's corporal punishment by parents, academic failure, and corporal punishment at school. The second part consisted of various kinds of active enuresis (nocturnal enuresis, diurnal enuresis), primary and secondary enuresis, history of active enuresis in other children, history of urinary tract infection and respiratory infection in the child, pinworms, anal itching, seizures, diabetes, hyperactivity, breast feeding, and history of previous treatments for nocturnal enuresis. Primary nocturnal enuresis was considered as bedwetting in a child who had never been dried and secondary nocturnal enuresis was considered as experiencing dryness for more than 6 months. The data was analyzed using the SPSS 16 software. The chi-square test was applied to investigate the relationship between nocturnal enuresis and the variables, and the logistic regression was utilized to model the factors affecting nocturnal enuresis concurrently considering the significance level of 0.05.

3. Results

Out of a total of 710 samples, 355 were male and 355 were female. Moreover, 57 (8%) of the subjects had nocturnal enuresis, and the highest prevalence rate of nocturnal enuresis was found in the 8-year-old age group (11.9%) and the lowest rate in the 10-year-old age group (5.8%). However, no significant relationship was found between the prevalence of nocturnal enuresis and age group ($P > 0.05$). No significant difference was found regarding the decrease in nocturnal enuresis up to the age of 10 ($P > 0.05$) (Table 1). However, the difference between the prevalence rates of nocturnal enuresis in the 5- and 10-year-old age groups was significant ($P < 0.05$). In relation to gender, the prevalence of nocturnal enuresis was 10.7% in the boys and 5.4% in the girls, showing a clearly higher rate in the boys ($P = 0.009$) (Table 1).

Moreover, there were significant differences between the two genders in terms of the frequency of nocturnal enuresis and diurnal enuresis. Eleven boys (3.1%), compared with 3 girls (0.8%), had diurnal enuresis ($P = 0.031$). The frequency

TABLE 1: Prevalence of nocturnal enuresis in primary school children in Khorramabad in terms of age and gender.

Variables	Nocturnal enuresis Number (%)	Total Number (%)	P value
Age			
5	12 (10.2)	118 (100)	
6	7 (5.9)	118 (100)	
7	8 (6.8)	118 (100)	0.435
8	14 (11.9)	118 (100)	
9	9 (7.6)	118 (100)	
10	7 (5.8)	120 (100)	
Gender			
Male	38 (10.7)	355 (100)	0.009
Female	19 (5.4)	355 (100)	

(intensity) of diurnal enuresis in the male children was more than that in the female ones, but no significant difference was found ($P = 0.074$). In addition, concerning the relationship between the frequency of nocturnal enuresis and age, the frequency of nocturnal enuresis in the 5-year-old age group was the highest (5.9%) ($P = 0.061$) (Table 2). Additionally, 5.2% and 2.8% of the children with nocturnal enuresis suffered from primary and secondary enuresis, respectively (based on being dry for 6 months). Moreover, 12 students (10.2%) from the preschool children and 45 students (7.6%) from the primary school children had nocturnal enuresis, showing no significant difference between educational level and nocturnal enuresis ($P > 0.05$) (Table 3). However, the frequency (severity) of nocturnal enuresis in the preschool educational level was significantly higher than that in the primary school educational level ($P < 0.05$).

Concerning the familial history of nocturnal enuresis in parents, no significant difference was found between the children with nocturnal enuresis and those without nocturnal enuresis ($P > 0.05$), while the history of nocturnal enuresis in siblings was significantly associated with nocturnal enuresis in children ($P = 0.023$). This relationship was significant for the prevalence of nocturnal enuresis as well ($P = 0.03$).

Finally, the prevalence of nocturnal enuresis in the children having one sibling (10.5%) was more than that in the children having two or more siblings (6.8%) ($P = 0.07$). Moreover, the prevalence of nocturnal enuresis was higher in the children with maternal education of high school diploma or lower ($P = 0.01$).

The results of the chi-square test showed that a number of 105 children (14.8%) of the samples had a respiratory infection, out of whom 14 children (13.3%) were enuretic, while 605 (85.2%) of the samples had no history of respiratory infection, out of whom 43 cases (7.1%) were enuretic ($P = 0.03$).

The numbers of the subjects with a history of urinary tract infection and seizures were 53 (7.5%) and 25 (3.5%) children, respectively, out of whom 5 (9.4%) and 5 (20%) children, respectively, had nocturnal enuresis as well. However, 52 (7.6%) of the children without a history of seizures and 52 (7.9%) of those with no history of urinary tract infection had nocturnal enuresis ($P > 0.05$).

Thirteen children (1.8%) had congenital problems (back problems, kidney problems, nervous problems, etc.), out of whom 2 children (15.4%) had nocturnal enuresis, while 55 children (7.9%) with no congenital problems suffered from nocturnal enuresis ($P > 0.05$).

According to the reports provided by the parents, 181 of the samples (25.5%) had deep sleep, out of whom 23 samples (12.7%) were enuretic ($P = 0.007$), while 34 children (6.4%) children with no deep sleep were enuretic.

Moreover, 78 children had been punished at school, 11 of whom (14.1%) had nocturnal enuresis ($P = 0.036$), while 46 children (7.3%) of the children who had not been punished at school had nocturnal enuresis.

The investigation of the factors associated with nocturnal enuresis showed no significant relationships between nocturnal enuresis and factors including divorce, history of nocturnal enuresis in one parent or both parents, shared bedroom, breast feeding, child's academic failure, new baby's birth, change in living place, child' age, child's birth order, educational level, maternal age, paternal age, family size, parental death, number of siblings, parental occupation, paternal education, parental kinship, history of pinworm infection, and child's hyperactivity ($P > 0.05$). However, significant relationships were found between nocturnal enuresis and factors including gender, history of nocturnal enuresis in siblings, deep sleep, respiratory infection, seizures, anal itching, and maternal education ($P < 0.05$) (Table 4). Moreover, concerning the relationship between the frequency (intensity) of nocturnal enuresis and the variables discussed, significant relationships were found only for gender, shared bedroom, deep sleep, punishment at school, history of respiratory infections, seizures, anal itching, and dominant right-handedness ($P < 0.05$). Also, diurnal enuresis was significantly associated with deep sleep, overnight nightmare, seizures, and right-handedness in the children ($P < 0.05$). The results of the logistic regression applied to evaluate the factors associated with nocturnal enuresis showed a predictive power of 92.1% for the test in identifying the factors. The results of the applied model in the logistic regression showed that male gender ($P = 0.013$, OR = 2.159, CI: 3.950–1.180), anal itching ($P = 0.000$, OR = 7.041, CI: 20.42–2.427), and seizures ($P = 0.034$, OR = 3.239, CI: 9.576–1.095) were the predictors of nocturnal enuresis in the children. Maternal education, number of siblings, history of nocturnal enuresis in siblings, deep sleep, history of pinworm infection, and respiratory infection were associated with nocturnal enuresis in the children, as detailed in Table 4.

4. Discussion

Nocturnal enuresis is a common developmental problem among school-aged children [5]. This study considered the DSM-IV as the criterion of nocturnal enuresis. The prevalence of nocturnal enuresis in this study was 8%. The studies conducted in Iran reported the prevalence of nocturnal

TABLE 2: Frequency of nocturnal enuresis in the children in terms of age group.

Variable		Frequency (intensity) of nocturnal enuresis				
		4 times or more a week Number (%)	1–3 times a week Number (%)	1-2 times a month Number (%)	No nocturnal enuresis Number (%)	Total Number (%)
Age	5	7	3	2	106	118
		5.9%	2.5%	1.7%	89.8%	100.0%
	6	3	2	2	111	118
		2.5%	1.7%	1.7%	94.1%	100.0%
	7	0	3	5	110	118
		0.0%	2.5%	4.2%	93.2%	100.0%
	8	5	1	8	104	118
		4.2%	8%	6.8%	88.1%	100.0%
	9	0	1	8	109	118
		0.0%	0.8%	6.8%	92.4%	100.0%
	10	3	1	3	113	120
		2.5%	0.8%	2.5%	94.2%	100.0%
	Total	18	11	28	653	710
		2.5%	1.5%	3.9%	92.0%	100.0%

TABLE 3: Relationship between nocturnal enuresis and educational level.

Variables	Nocturnal enuresis Number (%)	Total Number (%)	P value
Educational level			
Preschool	12 (10.2)	118 (100)	0.349
Primary school	45 (7.6)	592 (100)	

enuresis in various regions in Iran to be 8.25%, 8.8%, respectively [3, 12], indicating the fact that there is no significant difference between the prevalence rates of nocturnal enuresis inside the country. However, compared with the rates in the studies conducted in Hong Kong, China, and Thailand [5, 13, 14], the prevalence rate in Iran is higher, but it is lower compared with the studies conducted in Saudi Arabia, Turkey, and Burkina Faso [15–17]. These differences could be attributed to the differences in sample size, sampling method, age range, and definition of nocturnal enuresis based on the DSM-IV or the ICD 10 (internal classification of diseases. 10) criteria. Studies conducted based on the ICD 10 criterion have reported higher rates [15, 17]. In this study, the prevalence of diurnal enuresis was 2.8%, being consistent with the study conducted by Safarinejad in 2007 [18]. In addition, a study by Toktamis et al. reported a 4.2% prevalence rate for diurnal enuresis [19].

The prevalence of diurnal enuresis in this study was significantly higher in the boys than in the girls, which is consistent with the findings of some studies [1, 19], while other studies have reported the rate of this disorder to be higher in girls than in boys [20, 21]. In the present study, the prevalence of nocturnal enuresis decreased with age with no significant relationship, whereas the difference between the prevalence rates at the ages of 5 and 10 was statistically significant. The prevalence of enuresis in this study was 10.2%

at the age of 5 and 5.8% at the age of 10. This finding is compatible with the results of various studies [2, 22, 23]. Özkan et al. reported the prevalence of nocturnal enuresis in the age group of 5-6 years old to be 10.3% and at the age of 11 to be 5.6% [2]. Many studies have reported lower prevalence rates for nocturnal enuresis with age [2, 19, 24], and this difference can be attributed to different selection of age groups, being 5–10 in our study, 5–12, and occasionally 5–16, in several studies [17, 18, 25]. The prevalence of nocturnal enuresis in the boys in our study was 2.15 times higher than that in the girls, being similar with the results obtained from various studies [26–28]. However, some studies, including in China and Thailand, have not reported major differences in this regard [13, 25]. Some studies, including those conducted in Turkey and Sanandaj, have reported higher prevalence of nocturnal enuresis in girls than in boys [3, 16]. In terms of history of nocturnal enuresis in parents, no significant relationship was found between the enuretic and nonenuretic children, while there was a significant relationship between history of nocturnal enuresis in siblings and nocturnal enuresis in the children, confirming the results of other studies regarding the existence of familial history of nocturnal enuresis in enuretic children [15, 29, 30]. The results of a study conducted in Turkey by Gümüş et al. showed positive familial history of nocturnal enuresis in 75% of enuretic children [29]. The relationship between parental education and nocturnal enuresis has been discussed in some references [29, 31]. Several studies have reported lower paternal educational level and higher maternal educational level to be associated with higher prevalence of nocturnal enuresis [31]. In our study, the prevalence of nocturnal enuresis was lower in the children whose mothers had higher educational levels, whereas in Safarinejad's study the prevalence was higher in the children of the mothers with higher educational levels [18]. Other studies have also indicated the relationship between lower parental education and the prevalence of nocturnal enuresis

TABLE 4: Factors associated with nocturnal enuresis based on the logistic regression.

Variables	Enuretic Number (%)	Nonenuretic Number (%)	Total Number (%)	P value	OR	95% CI
Gender						
Male	38 (10.7)	317 (89.3)	355 (100)	0.013	2.159	3.950–1.180
Female	19 (5.4)	336 (94.6)	355 (100)		—	—
Number of siblings						
0 (only child)	9 (1.5)	168 (94.9)	177 (100)		—	—
1	33 (10.5)	280 (89.4)	313 (100)	0.051	2.337	5.185–1.053
2 and more	15 (2.27)	205 (93.1)	220 (100)		1.262	3.065–0.520
Maternal education						
High school diploma and lower	48 (8.9)	486 (91.1)	534 (100)	0.018	564/2	5.609–1.172
Higher than high school diploma	9 (5.2)	167 (94.8)	176		—	—
Enuresis in siblings						
Yes	13 (14)	80 (86)	93 (100)	0.015	2.392	4.836–1.183
No	44 (7.1)	573 (92.9)	617 (100)		—	—
Deep sleep						
Yes	23 (12.7)	158 (87.3)	181 (100)	0.023	1.99	3.599–1.100
No	34 (6.4)	495 (93.6)	529 (100)		—	—
Respiratory infection						
Yes	14 (13.3)	91 (86.7)	105 (100)	0.013	2.381	4.734–1.198
No	43 (7.1)	562 (92.9)	605 (100)		—	—
Seizures						
Yes	5 (20)	20 (80)	25 (100)	0.034	3.239	9.576–1.095
No	52 (7.6)	633 (92.4)	685 (100)		—	—
Pinworm infection						
Yes	4 (5.6)	67 (94.4)	71 (100)	0.053	0.296	1.014–0.086
No	53 (8.3)	586 (91.7)	639 (100)		—	—
Anal itching						
Yes	7 (16.7)	35 (83.3)	42 (100)	<0.001	7.041	20.42–2.427
No	50 (7.5)	618 (92.5)	668 (100)		—	—

[29]. In the present study, no significant relationship was found between paternal educational level and frequency (intensity) of enuresis, which is in accord with the result by Gunes et al.'s study in Turkey [22]. In this study, 15.7% of the children had bedwetting every night, 15.7% 4–6 times a week, 19.2% 1–3 times a week, and 49.1% less than once a week. In Gunes et al., Ozden et al., and Qing et al.'s studies, the prevalence rates for every-night bedwetting were 31%, 33%, and 24.6%, respectively [22, 32, 33]. Concerning the treatment of nocturnal enuresis in this study, 17.45% of the children consumed medicinal plants, 31.57% used chemical treatments, 24.65% used behavioral treatments including limiting fluid intake, and 26.3% expected age increase and spontaneous resolution of nocturnal enuresis. In Ramírez-Backhaus et al.'s study, 17% of the parents did not have any treatments for nocturnal enuresis in their children, and 20% used drug treatments [26]. In the study conducted in Tehran by Safarinejad, 78.6% of the parents applied drug treatments, and this difference can be attributed to cultural differences and more parental sensitivity to the treatment of nocturnal enuresis [18]. The rates of applying treatments in Australia and New Zealand were 4.7% and 28%, respectively [21, 34].

One of the variables discussed in the relevant references is the relationship between paternal occupation and nocturnal enuresis. In our study, no significant relationship was found in this regard, being consistent with the result in Gunes et al.'s study [22]. Rona et al. in their study conducted in Scotland and England concluded that primary enuresis in first children was lower than that in subsequent children [35]. Gunes et al. did not report a significant relationship between birth order and the prevalence of primary enuresis [22]. In this study, the prevalence of nocturnal enuresis in the second children was 2.3 times higher than the rate in the only children. Being an only child seems to be a protective factor [14, 26], while it has been introduced as a risk factor in studies conducted in the US [36]. In our study, the history of urinary tract infection in the children based on parental reports was 9.4%, whereas it was reported to be 3.8% in Safarinejad's study [18], which is much lower than the rate in our study. Some studies have mentioned the ureterovesical reflux due to the contraction of the proximal ureter and the pelvic floor muscles as the cause of urinary tract infection and its relationship with higher prevalence of enuresis [22, 27, 32]. However, there was no relationship between urinary tract infection and enuresis in our study. One of the problems in children with enuresis is deep sleep and difficulty of waking up during the night [37]. This is one of the most important factors associated with the prevalence of enuresis [28]. The findings of our study also indicated a significant relationship between deep sleep and nocturnal enuresis. The results of many studies show that nocturnal enuresis is a developmental problem, while parental dealing with this problem may not be realistic [2, 15, 22, 28]. Some mothers believe that their children are able to control urination during sleep and therefore may punish them. In Özkan et al. and Safarinejad's studies, 12.8% and 26% of the enuretic children had been punished [2, 18]. In our study, 9.2% of the children with nocturnal enuresis had been punished by their parents and 14.1% by school authorities, and there was a significant relationship between corporal punishment at school and nocturnal enuresis. However, the relationship between academic failure and nocturnal enuresis was not significant although Özkan et al. reported a significant relationship between academic failure and nocturnal enuresis [2].

The application of punishment can have adverse outcomes for a child, as the study by Özkan et al. reported that the prevalence of enuresis in the children who had been trained in urination and threatened by their parents was 2.24 times higher than the rate in the children who had received encouragement [2]. In Norgaard et al.'s study, the prevalence of enuresis in the children with inappropriate parental dealing with the problem was 1.74 times higher. Therefore, inappropriate training in urination can be a risk factor of enuresis [38]. In Tai et al.'s study, a relationship was found between enuresis and overnight nightmare, being inconsistent with the results of the present study [28]. In our study, 16.7% of the enuretic children had anal itching, and the rate of nocturnal enuresis in these children was 7.04 times higher. Ghotbi and Kheirabadi in their study reported a significant relationship between anal itching and nocturnal enuresis, which may suggest an association between enuresis and oxyuriasis [3]. It has been, of course, proved that oxyuriasis is not associated with enuresis, and this may be due to the recall bias [18]. In the present study, similar to Özkan et al.'s study, no significant relationship was found between nocturnal enuresis and right-handedness; however, the intensity of nocturnal enuresis was higher in the right-handed children [2]. The prevalence of nocturnal enuresis was relatively low in this study, and this is consistent with other studies conducted in Iran. Cultural and ethnic differences may not be involved in the prevalence enuresis. In addition, the prevalence of nocturnal enuresis and some of its associated factors in our study are different from those in the studies conducted in other countries. Further studies with larger sample sizes, homogenous methods, and similar definitions of enuresis are needed to investigate the differences between the results.

5. Conclusion

The results of this study clearly indicated a higher prevalence rate of nocturnal enuresis in the boys than in the girls.

Moreover, the frequency of nocturnal enuresis in preschool level was higher than that in primary school level. Also, history of nocturnal enuresis in siblings, deep sleep, and punishment of children at school were identified as the risk factors for nocturnal enuresis. Therefore, taking therapeutic measures and training parents in dealing with children are essential to control nocturnal enuresis.

Conflict of Interests

The authors declare that there is no conflict of interests regarding the publication of this paper.

References

[1] E. Gür, P. Turhan, G. Can et al., "Enuresis: prevalence, risk factors and urinary pathology among school children in Istanbul, Turkey," *Pediatrics International*, vol. 46, no. 1, pp. 58–63, 2004.

[2] S. Özkan, E. Durukan, E. Iseri, S. Gürocak, I. Maral, and M. A. Bumin, "Prevalence and risk factors of monosymptomatic nocturnal enuresis in Turkish children," *Indian Journal of Urology*, vol. 26, no. 2, pp. 200–205, 2010.

[3] N. Ghotbi and G. H. Kheirabadi, "Prevalence of nocturia and its associated factors in primary school children in Sanandaj in 2002," *Journal of Kurdistan University of Medical Sciences*, vol. 5, no. 20, pp. 30–33, 2001.

[4] M. Jamali and G. H. Rafiee, "A comparison between the results of treatment with imipramine and oxybutynin in non-symptomatic 6–12 children with enuresis," *Journal of Rafsanjan University of Medical Sciences*, vol. 3, no. 2, pp. 113–117, 2004.

[5] C. K. Yeung, "Nocturnal enuresis in Hong Kong: different Chinese phenotypes," *Scandinavian Journal of Urology and Nephrology*, vol. 183, pp. 17–21, 1996.

[6] E. R. Behrman, M. R. Kliegman, and B. H. Jenson, *Nelson Textbook of Pediatrics*, Saunders, Philadelphia, Pa, USA, 18th edition, 2007.

[7] M. Unalacak, A. Söğüt, E. Aktunç, N. Demircan, and R. Altin, "E nuresis noctural prevalence and risk factors amog school age children in northwest turkey," *European Journal of General Medicine*, vol. 1, no. 3, pp. 21–25, 2004.

[8] J. G. Wen, Q. W. Wang, Y. Chen, J. J. Wen, and K. Liu, "An epidemiological study of primary nocturnal enuresis in Chinese children and adolescents," *European Urology*, vol. 49, no. 6, pp. 1107–1113, 2006.

[9] P. Sureshkumar, M. Jones, P. H. Y. Caldwell, and J. C. Craig, "Risk factors for nocturnal enuresis in school-age children," *The Journal of Urology*, vol. 182, no. 6, pp. 2893–2899, 2009.

[10] K. Dehghani, Z. Pour Movahed, H. Dehghani et al., "Factors associated with enuresis in 6–12 year-old children," *Shahed University Research Journal*, vol. 16, no. 79, pp. 33–38, 1998.

[11] B. Hägglöf, D. Kebede, A. Alem, and M. Desta, "Socio-demographic and psychopathologic correlates of enuresis in urban Ethiopian children," *Acta Paediatrica*, vol. 96, no. 4, pp. 556–560, 2007.

[12] A. Karbasi, M. Golestan, and R. Fallah, "Nocturnal enuresis in children at the age of six and its associated factors," *Ofogh-e Danesh*, vol. 15, no. 4, pp. 63–70, 2009.

[13] X. Liu, Z. Sun, M. Uchiyama, Y. Li, and M. Okawa, "Attaining nocturnal urinary control, nocturnal enuresis, and behavioral problems in chinese children aged 6 through 16 years," *Journal*

of the American Academy of Child and Adolescent Psychiatry, vol. 39, no. 12, pp. 1557–1564, 2000.

[14] T. Hansakunachai, N. Ruangdaraganon, U. Udomsubpayakul, T. Sombuntham, and N. Kotchabhakdi, "Epidemiology of enuresis among school-age children in Thailand," *Journal of Developmental and Behavioral Pediatrics*, vol. 26, no. 5, pp. 356–360, 2005.

[15] B. B. Kalo and H. Bella, "Enuresis: prevalence and associated factors among primary school children in Saudi Arabia," *Acta Paediatrica*, vol. 85, no. 10, pp. 1217–1222, 1996.

[16] T. Serel, G. Akhan, H. R. Koyuncuoğlu et al., "Epidemiology of enuresis in Turkish children," *Scandinavian Journal of Urology and Nephrology*, vol. 31, no. 6, pp. 537–539, 1997.

[17] A. Ouédraogo, M. Kere, T. Ouédraogo, and F. Jesu, "Epidemiology of enuresis among children and teenagers, 5 to 16-years old, in Ouagadougou (Burkina Faso)," *Archives de Pediatrie*, vol. 4, no. 10, pp. 947–951, 1997.

[18] M. R. Safarinejad, "Prevalence of nocturnal enuresis, risk factors, associated familial factors and urinary pathology among school children in Iran," *Journal of Pediatric Urology*, vol. 3, no. 6, pp. 443–452, 2007.

[19] A. Toktamis, Y. Demirel, K. U. Ozkan, M. Garipardiç, A. Gözüküçük, and N. Nur, "Prevalence and associated factors of day wetting and combined day and night wetting," *Urologia Internationalis*, vol. 81, no. 1, pp. 54–59, 2008.

[20] "Recommendations of the International Scientific Committee: conservative management of urinary incontinence in childhood," in *Proceedings of the 2nd International Consultation on Incontinence*, Paris, France, 2002, http://www.ics.com/documents.

[21] M. R. Jarvelin, L. Vikevainen-Tervonen, I. Moilanen, and N.-P. Huttunen, "Enuresis in seven-year-old children," *Acta Paediatrica Scandinavica*, vol. 77, no. 1, pp. 148–153, 1988.

[22] A. Gunes, G. Gunes, Y. Acik, and A. Akilli, "The epidemiology and factors associated with nocturnal enuresis among boarding and daytime school children in southeast of Turkey: a cross sectional study," *BMC Public Health*, vol. 9, article 357, 2009.

[23] C. K. Yeung, B. Sreedhar, J. D. Y. Sihoe, F. K. Y. Sit, and J. Lau, "Differences in characteristics of nocturnal enuresis between children and adolescents: a critical appraisal from a large epidemiological study," *The British Journal of Urology International*, vol. 97, no. 5, pp. 1069–1073, 2006.

[24] F. C. Verhulst, J. H. van der Lee, G. W. Akkerhuis, J. A. Sanders-Woudstra, F. C. Timmer, and I. D. Donkhorst, "The prevalence of nocturnal enuresis: do DSM III criteria need to be changed? A brief research report," *Journal of Child Psychology and Psychiatry*, vol. 26, no. 6, pp. 989–993, 1985.

[25] V. Piyasil and J. Udomsup, "Enuresis in children 5–15 years at Queen Sirikit National Institute of Child Health," *Journal of the Medical Association of Thailand*, vol. 85, no. 1, pp. 11–16, 2002.

[26] M. Ramírez-Backhaus, E. M. Agullo, S. A. Guzman et al., "Prevalence of nocturnal enuresis in the Valencian Community. Pediatric section of the National Incontinence Survey. the EPICC Study," *Actas Urologicas Espanolas*, vol. 33, no. 9, pp. 1011–1018, 2009.

[27] M. Kajiwara, K. Inoue, M. Kato, A. Usui, M. Kurihara, and T. Usui, "Nocturnal enuresis and overactive bladder in children: an epidemiological study," *International Journal of Urology*, vol. 13, no. 1, pp. 36–41, 2006.

[28] H.-L. Tai, Y.-J. Chang, S. C.-C. Chang, G.-D. Chen, C.-P. Chang, and M.-C. Chou, "The epidemiology and factors associated with nocturnal enuresis and its severity in primary school children in Taiwan," *Acta Paediatrica*, vol. 96, no. 2, pp. 242–245, 2007.

[29] B. Gümüş, N. Vurgun, M. Lekili, A. Işcan, T. Müezzinoğlu, and C. Büyüksu, "Prevalence of nocturnal enuresis and accompanying factors in children aged 7–11 years in Turkey," *Acta Paediatrica*, vol. 88, no. 12, pp. 1369–1372, 1999.

[30] Y. Kanaheswari, "Epidemiology of childhood nocturnal enuresis in Malaysia," *Journal of Paediatrics and Child Health*, vol. 39, no. 2, pp. 118–123, 2003.

[31] T.-W. Cher, G.-J. Lin, and K.-H. Hsu, "Prevalence of nocturnal enuresis and associated familial factors in primary school children in Taiwan," *The Journal of Urology*, vol. 168, no. 3, pp. 1142–1146, 2002.

[32] C. Ozden, O. L. Ozdal, S. Altinova, I. Oguzulgen, G. Urgancioglu, and A. Memis, "Prevalence and associated factors of enuresis in Turkish children," *The International Brazilian Journal of Urology*, vol. 33, no. 2, pp. 216–222, 2007.

[33] W. W. Qing, G. W. Jian, K. S. Dong et al., "Bed-wetting in Chinese children: epidemiology and predictive factors," *Neurourology and Urodynamics*, vol. 26, no. 4, pp. 512–517, 2007.

[34] J. B. Devlin, "Prevalence and risk factors for childhood nocturnal enuresis," *Archives of Disease in Childhood*, vol. 84, pp. 118–120, 1992.

[35] R. J. Rona, L. Li, and S. Chinn, "Determinants of nocturnal enuresis in England and Scotland in the '90s," *Developmental Medicine and Child Neurology*, vol. 39, no. 10, pp. 677–681, 1997.

[36] R. S. Byrd, M. Weitzman, N. E. Lanphear, and P. Auinger, "Bed-wetting in US children: epidemiology and related behavior problems," *Pediatrics*, vol. 98, no. 3, pp. 414–419, 1996.

[37] S. Wille, "Nocturnal enuresis: sleep disturbance and behavioural patterns," *Acta Paediatrica*, vol. 83, no. 7, pp. 772–774, 1994.

[38] J. P. Norgaard, S. Rittig, and J. C. Djurhuus, "Nocturnal enuresis: an approach to treatment based on pathogenesis," *Journal of Pediatrics*, vol. 114, no. 4, pp. 705–710, 1989.

Do Maternal Quality of Life and Breastfeeding Difficulties Influence the Continuation of Exclusive Breastfeeding?

Forough Mortazavi,[1] Seyed Abbas Mousavi,[2] Reza Chaman,[3] and Ahmad Khosravi[4]

[1] *Department of Midwifery, Faculty of Nursing and Midwifery, Sabzevar University of Medical Sciences, Sabzevar 9613873136, Iran*
[2] *Research Center of Psychiatry, Golestan University of Medical Sciences, Golestan 49189 36316, Iran*
[3] *Department of Community Medicine, School of Medicine, Yasuj University of Medical Sciences, Yasuj 7591741417, Iran*
[4] *Center for Health Related Social and Behavioral Sciences Research, Shahroud University of Medical Sciences, Shahroud 3613773955, Iran*

Correspondence should be addressed to Forough Mortazavi; frmortazavi@yahoo.com

Academic Editor: Namık Yaşar Özbek

Objectives. This study was conducted to determine whether maternal quality of life (QOL) and breastfeeding difficulties influence the continuation of exclusive breastfeeding (EBF). *Methods.* In a survey, 358 consecutive pregnant women filled out a quality of life questionnaire in the third trimester of pregnancy and the breastfeeding experience scale at 4 weeks postpartum. We assessed breastfeeding practices every month up to 6 months postpartum. *Results.* Only 11.8% of women continued EBF at six months. Mothers who continued EBF at 2 and 4 months postpartum had better QOL in late pregnancy than mothers who discontinued it ($P < 0.05$). There were no significant differences between the two groups in QOL scores at 6 months postpartum. Mothers who continued EBF at 2 months postpartum experienced less breastfeeding difficultties during one month postpartum than mothers who discontinued it ($P < 0.05$). *Conclusion.* In attempts to promote EBF, mothers with poor QOL or breastfeeding difficulties in early postpartum should be identified and helped.

1. Introduction

There is extensive evidence for short-term and long-term health benefits of breastfeeding for mothers, such as reduced risk of breast and ovarian cancers, and for babies, such as decreased gastroenteritis, respiratory infection, early childhood caries, and diabetes mellitus [1, 2]. The benefits of breastfeeding are maximized when the baby is fed with breast milk exclusively [3]. The World Health Organization recommends that all infants should be fed exclusively on breast milk from birth to six months of age [4].

For many women, breastfeeding is a satisfying and enjoyable experience and they breastfeed successfully despite experiencing breastfeeding difficulties. However, for some women coping with common breastfeeding problems and the recurrent demands of the baby in early postpartum is a physically and emotionally exhausting task [5]. Furthermore, they may have feelings of guilt for not being able to satisfy the baby's needs and harbor doubts about the continuation of breastfeeding, or may even discontinue it [6]. Also, during pregnancy and the first weeks of postpartum, the physical and psychological health of the mother goes through considerable changes. Most mothers experience symptoms, which may influence the mother's physical and emotional health [7]. A previous study has found that maternal depressive symptoms in early postpartum were related to breastfeeding experience [8]. Results of another study revealed that the mother's breastfeeding experience is affected by multiple factors, such as psychological and physical health, sociodemographic characteristics, quality of marital relationship, and living condition [9]. Quality of life (QOL) is a broad ranging concept that includes all the mentioned aspects [10]. Despite the potential role of maternal quality of life (QOL) in the breastfeeding experience, there is limited scientific evidence about the relationship between QOL and breastfeeding continuation. A Brazilian study reported that QOL was correlated with breastfeeding self-efficacy in postpartum [11]. In a cross-sectional study in Taiwan, QOL was related to breastfeeding continuation [12].

The Iranian government has successfully promoted breastfeeding through policy change. In 2007, the rate of breastfeeding in the country at first 2 years of age was reported at 57% [13]. Although Iran has a high rate of breastfeeding initiation and continuation, its rate of exclusive breastfeeding (EBF) is decreasing. The rates of EBF at sixth months of age were 44% in 2000 and 23% in 2010 [14]. Studies conducted in Iran have reported that difficulties such as sore nipples, latching-on problems, and the mother's perception of having insufficient milk or her perception of insufficient infant weight gain were the reasons for the discontinuation of breastfeeding [15, 16].

The present study aims to investigate the relationships between QOL and breastfeeding difficulties and the continuation of EBF in a sample of mothers from northeast of Iran. The use of WHOQOL-BREF, which covers four domains of QOL (somatic, psychological, social, and environmental) allowed us to overcome a shortcoming of previous studies, which have generally focused on somatic and psychological domains. In addition, previous studies have investigated breastfeeding difficulties using questionnaires, which allow only yes or no responses or assess difficulties separately. In the present study, we assessed breastfeeding difficulties using BES, which was developed to measure common breastfeeding difficulties in the form of a continuous variable in the postpartum and to assess the total breastfeeding difficulties. Moreover, the BES includes multiple factors related to infant and mother, which allowed us to measure difficulties more multidimensionally. To the authors' best knowledge, this is the first study to explore the relationship between maternal QOL and breastfeeding difficulties and the continuation of EBF using these questionnaires.

2. Methods

2.1. Study Design and Participants. This survey was started in May 2011 in Shahroud, a city in northeast Iran. We selected 370 consecutive women, who attended 10 urban health clinics, affiliated to Shahroud University of Medical Sciences, for prenatal care and met the inclusion criteria over a period of six months. We chose health clinics as our research environment because 94% of pregnant women in Iran have at least 4 visits to health clinics during pregnancy [16]. Three hundred and fifty eight of the women agreed to participate in the study and gave informed consent, of which 347 were followed up until 6 months postpartum. Midwives at the health clinics were responsible for distributing and collecting questionnaires and assessing infant feeding methods.The inclusion criteria were gestational age of at least 28 weeks and no serious medical condition that prevented breastfeeding. The exclusion criteria were fetal death, infant death, infant major abnormalities and serious medical condition that prevented breastfeeding, and twin

pregnancy. The participants completed the WHOQOL-BREF in the third trimester of pregnancy. Women completed the BES at 4 weeks postpartum. Shahroud University of Medical Center Institutional Review Board approved this study. All procedures followed were in accordance with the ethical standards of the Ethics Committee of the Shahroud University of Medical Sciences (approval number 900.02).

2.2. Instruments

2.2.1. Sociodemographic and Obstetrical Questionnaire. Women completed a questionnaire consisting of sociodemograph-ic information (age, education, income, and occupation) at the first visit. They completed another questionnaire consisting of obstetrical information (parity, pregnancy wantedness, mode of delivery, BMI, pregnancy weight gain, weight at last prenatal visit, and previous breastfeeding experience) at the 2 weeks postpartum.

2.3. Infant Feeding Checklist. Midwives assessed the infant feeding method at 2 and 4 weeks postpartum and then every month up to 6 months by asking mother to list all fluids and foods consumed by the infant (including breast milk, formula, other fluids, semisolids, and solids) during the month previous to the face-to-face interview using a check list. EBF were defined according to WHO definitions [4]. The 2nd, 4th, 8th, 16th, and 24th weeks of postpartum coincide with women's scheduled clinic visits. Midwives made phone calls at 12th and 20th weeks postpartum to assess the infant feeding method.

2.4. WHOQOL-BREF. The WHOQOL-BREF was developed by the World Health Organization [10]. It contains 24 questions divided into 4 domains: physical (7 questions), psychological (6 questions), social relationships (3 questions), and environment (8 questions). There are also two more questions: question 1 asks about an individual's overall perception of quality of life and question 2 asks about an individual's overall perception of his or her health. The items are rated on a 5-point Likert scale. We transformed the raw domain scores to a 0–100 scale. In addition, we calculated the mean score of all 26 questions and then transformed the global score of QOL to a 0–100 scale. The validity and reliability of the Iranian version of WHOQOL-BREF have been supported in a previous study [17]. The validity of the questionnaire among women in the postpartum period has also been supported by previous studies [18, 19].

2.5. Breastfeeding Experience Scale. The breastfeeding experience scale (BES) is a questionnaire consisting of 30-items, which measure breastfeeding methods, experiences, and outcomes. We only used the first 18 questions of this 30-item scale which rate the severity of common breastfeeding difficulties in the early postpartum period using a 5-point Likert scale (1 = not at all and 5 = unbearable). The scale assesses if these problems ever occurred. Items are as follows: sore nipples, cracked nipples, leaking breasts, breast engorgement, breast infection, baby having sucking difficulty, baby having difficulty in latching on, baby reluctant to nurse due to sleepiness, baby reluctant to nurse due to fussiness, baby nursing too frequently, feeling very tired, feeling tense and overwhelmed, worry about not having enough milk, worry that baby was not getting enough milk, difficulty positioning baby, worry about baby's weight gain, feeling embarrassed when nursing, and difficulty combining work and breastfeeding. Responses are then summed up to obtain a total breastfeeding difficulties score (range of 18–90), with a higher score representing increased problem severity. Content validity and internal consistency of this scale (alpha coefficient 0.76) have been reported and supported in a previous study [20]. In our study, the alpha coefficient was 0.82 at 4 weeks postpartum. We translated the instrument into Persian and a PhD in English language back-translated the instrument into English. We compared the back-translated version with the original instrument and found no discrepancy in items' meaning. Then a panel of experts in obstetrics and pediatrics assessed the instrument. We changed no item.

2.6. Breastfeeding Intention. Intention to breastfeed was assessed by a question using a 5-point numerical rating scale (1 = definitely breastfeed and 6 = definitely not breastfeed)

2.7. Statistical Analysis. Statistical analyses were performed using Spss 18 (SPSS Inc., Chicago, IL, USA). The results are reported as means and standard deviations for continuous variables and as frequencies and percentages for categorical variables. Differences between exclusive and nonexclusive breastfeeding groups were assessed using t-tests for continuous variables and chi-square test for categorical variables. The significance level of tests was set at 0.05.

3. Results

3.1. Women's Characteristics. A total of 358 women participate in the study of which 347 were followed up until 6 months postpartum. Mean age of women was 26.17 ± 4.42. Median monthly household income was 4 million RlS. The educational levels of women were primary school 11%, secondary school 61%, and university 28%. None of them smoked or had a history of smoking or alcohol dependence. All were married. About 28% of women described their previous breastfeeding experience as excellent or good and 4.5% as moderate. Table 1 shows women's characteristics based on breastfeeding method at 2 and 4 months postpartum. The relative risk of exclusive breastfeeding discontinuation at 2 months postpartum was 1.4 times higher for women who had no breastfeeding experience than women who had previous breastfeeding experience. Table 2 shows the frequency of different breastfeeding methods at 2, 4, and 6 months postpartum. The value of Alpha Cronbach coefficient for the whole WHOQOL-BREF questionnaire was 0.92.

3.2. QOL. The two first independent questions of WHO-QOL-BREF assess woman's overall perception of quality of life and her health, respectively. 27% of women evaluated their overall quality of life as "very good," 54% as "good," 18%

as "not good, not bad," 8% as "bad," and 0.3% as "very bad." Also, 29% of women evaluated their overall health as "very good," 52% as "good," 16% as "not good not bad," 1.7% as "bad," and 1.7% as "very bad."

3.3. Breastfeeding Difficulties. The mean total score of the breastfeeding difficulties scale (i.e., the score for the first 18 items of BES) was 31.4 ± 8.5 with range of 18–74. The value of Alpha Cronbach coefficient for the breastfeeding difficulties scale was 0.83. Common difficulties experienced by women were baby's frequent demand for breastfeeding (81.6%), leaking breasts (78.2%), difficulty combining work and breastfeeding (69%), feeling exhausted (59%), and worry about having enough milk (52%). The mean scores of the breastfeeding difficulties questionnaire for primigravidas and multigravidas were 32.32 ± 9.7 and 30.1 ± 6.4, respectively ($P = 0.012$).

3.4. QOL and Breastfeeding Difficulties and the Continuation of Exclusive Breastfeeding. Table 3 shows the scores of QOL and breastfeeding difficulties for women with exclusive and nonexclusive breastfeeding at 2 and 4 months postpartum. There were no significant differences between the two groups in QOL and breastfeeding difficulties scores at 6 months postpartum.

4. Discussion

In this study, we examined the relationship between QOL and breastfeeding difficulties during 4 weeks postpartum and the continuation of EBF in women visiting urban health clinics in Shahroud, Iran. Our results indicate that mothers who continued EBF at 2 and 4 months postpartum had better QOL in late pregnancy than mothers who discontinued EBF. These findings are comparable with a Brazilian research, which found a correlation between breastfeeding self-efficacy and maternal QOL [11]. It is possible that maternal QOL improved after childbirth gradually due to improvement in mother's physical and emotional health. Two months postpartum is the period in which physiological changes resulting from pregnancy recede and the body returns to its normal condition. Also, during the same period the postpartum mood fluctuations disappear. However, mothers with low QOL in late pregnancy may undergo the transitional period more slowly than mothers with higher QOL. This difference may account for the failure to continue EBF in mothers with a low QOL. On the other hand, the rate of complementary breastfeeding at 4 and 6 months postpartum were 3.2% and 45.8%, respectively. This means that more than 40% of mothers discontinue EBF during 5th and 6th months postpartum. This may be due to traditional beliefs about infant feeding with its emphasis on introducing semisolid foods after 4 months postpartum rather than a low QOL. This may account for the similarity of 2 groups in the QOL scores at 6 months postpartum. In other words, since the introduction of solid and semisolid foods was a common practice during the fifth and sixth months postpartum in this study, antepartum QOL could not affect the continuation

TABLE 1: Women's characteristics based on breastfeeding practices.

Variable	2 months postpartum			4 months postpartum		
	EBF[†]	Non-EBF		EBF	Non-EBF	
	N (%) or M ± SD		P	N (%) or M ± SD		P
Age	26.3 ± 4.6	26.2 ± 4.3	0.870	26.7 ± 4.8	26.1 ± 4.3	0.297
Education	10.7 ± 4.2	11.7 ± 3.5	0.031[*]	10.6 ± 4.2	11.6 ± 3.6	0.063
Income	431 ± 165	423 ± 146	0.688	430 ± 170	424 ± 146	0.785
BMI	23.4 ± 3.7	24.4 ± 4.6	0.129	23.5 ± 3.6	24.3 ± 4.5	0.264
Occupation						
Yes	12 (37.5)	20 (62.5)	0.291	9 (28.1)	23 (71.9)	0.502
No	90 (28.6)	225 (71.4)		72 (22.9)	243 (77.1)	
Mode of delivery						
Cesarean	54 (30.3)	124 (69.7)	0.719	47 (26.4)	131 (73.6)	0.176
Vaginal delivery	48 (28.6)	120 (71.4)		34 (20.2)	134 (9.8)	
Parity						
Primiparity	52 (25.7)	150 (74.3)	0.078	40 (19.8)	162 (80.2)	0.066
Multiparity	49 (34.5)	96 (65.5)		41 (28.3)	104 (71.7)	
Desirability of pregnancy						
Yes	88 (28.9)	217 (71.1)	0.706	69 (22.6)	236 (77.4)	0.549
No	13 (31.7)	28 (68.3)		11 (26.8)	30 (73.2)	
Health						
Healthy	98 (30.1)	228 (69.9)	0.602	79 (24.2)	247 (75.8)	0.263
Patient	4 (22.2)	14 (77.8)		2 (11.1)	16 (88.9)	
Postpartum rehospitalization						
Yes	7 (35)	13 (65)	0.589	6 (30)	14 (70)	0.322
No	95 (29.3)	229 (70.7)		75 (23.1)	249 (76.9)	
Previous breastfeeding experience						
Yes	47 (36.7)	81 (63.3)	0.022[*]	38 (29.7)	90 (70.3)	0.033[*]
No	55 (25.1)	164 (74.9)		43 (19.6)	176 (80.4)	

[*]$P < 0.05$; t-test; chi-square test; Fisher's exact test; [†]exclusive breastfeeding.

TABLE 2: Frequency of different breastfeeding practices.

Breastfeeding methods	2 months postpartum	4 months postpartum	6 months postpartum
Exclusive breastfeeding[†]	100 (28.8%)	80 (23.0%)	41 (11.8%)
Predominant breastfeeding[‡]	211 (60.8%)	218 (62.8%)	97 (28%)
Partial feeding[δ]	34 (9.8%)	33 (9.5%)	40 (11.5%)
Complementary feeding[§]	—	11 (3.2%)	159 (45.8%)
Formula feeding	2 (0.6%)	5 (1.4%)	10 (2.9%)

[†]Breast milk; [‡]breast milk and water based fluid; [δ]breast milk and nonhuman milk or formula; [§]breast milk and any solid or semisolid foods or liquid.

of EBF at 6 months. In addition, mothers who continued EBF at 2 months postpartum experienced lower breastfeeding difficulties during first month postpartum than mothers who discontinued it. There were no significant differences between the 2 groups in breastfeeding difficulties scores at 4 and 6 months postpartum. Breastfeeding difficulties are common and transient during early postpartum [21]. Results of a previous study revealed that breastfeeding difficulty and severity decrease from 3 days to 9 weeks postpartum [22]. Therefore, the breastfeeding difficulty at 4 weeks postpartum may not account for EBF discontinuation at 4 and 6 months postpartum. Previous qualitative research indicated that obstacles or problems, such as perceptions of insufficient milk supply,

nipple/breast pain, difficulty combining work and breastfeeding, problems with pumping, and feeling overwhelmed and frustrated, led adolescent mothers to weaning [23]. In our study, baby nursing too frequently, leaking breasts, difficulty combining housekeeping and breastfeeding, feeling very tired or fatigued, and worry about having enough milk were the most frequent major breastfeeding difficulties identified by women. In a study, painful nipples/breasts, low milk supply, and latching difficulties were the three most frequent major breastfeeding problems identified by women [24].

In this study, the rates of EBF were 28.8%, 23%, and 11.8% at 2, 4, and 6 months postpartum, respectively. The sampling site represents its own local characteristics and could not

TABLE 3: Means and standard deviations of the quality of life score, breastfeeding difficulties score, and intention to breastfeeding based on breastfeeding practices.

2 months postpartum	Exclusive breastfeeding ($N = 100$) M ± Sd	Nonexclusive breastfeeding ($N = 247$) M ± Sd	P value
Domains of quality of life			
Physical	66.7 ± 17.3	61 ± 16.9	0.005**
Mental	66.3 ± 18.5	62.3 ± 15.7	0.040*
Social	67.7 ± 20.7	65.5 ± 20.5	0.366
Environmental	69.7 ± 14.9	68.4 ± 14.6	0.450
Global	68.5 ± 14.8	65.2 ± 13.1	0.042*
Breastfeeding difficulties score	29.71 ± 7.3	8.9 ± 32.12	0.017*
Intention to breastfeeding	5.8 ± 0.6	5.7 ± 0.7	0.714
4 months postpartum	Exclusive breastfeeding ($N = 80$)	Nonexclusive breastfeeding ($N = 267$)	
Domains of quality of life			
Physical	67.2 ± 17.4	61.3 ± 17.5	0.001**
Mental	66.8 ± 18.9	62.5 ± 15.7	0.013*
Social	67.5 ± 21.9	66.1 ± 20.1	0.604
Environmental	69.0 ± 14.9	68.8 ± 14.6	0.720
Global	68.4 ± 15.1	65.5 ± 11.2	0.025*
Breastfeeding difficulties score	29.9 ± 7.1	31.9 ± 8.9	0.063
Intention to breastfeeding	5.8 ± 0.6	5.7 ± 0.7	0.323

*$P < 0.05$; **$P < 0.01$; t-test.

represent national status. In fact, previous studies in Iran have variously reported the rate of EBF at 6 months at 27.7%, 52.6%, and 33.1% [13, 16, 25]. The differences may be due to the different approaches to data collection methods and study design. Our study was longitudinal and we asked mothers to recall what their babies had eaten during last month while the cited cross-sectional studies had used the 24 hours recall method to collect the data related to infant feeding. Therefore, we could identify four breastfeeding groups (exclusive, predominant, partial, and complementary), while other studies mentioned three groups (exclusive, partial, and complementary).

In relation to women's QOL, the majority of women in this study (81%) described their QOL as "good" or "very good" according to the first independent question of WHOQOL-BREF and 81% were "satisfied" with their health status according to the second independent question of the WHOQOL-BREF. Results of a Brazilian study on maternal postpartum QOL indicated that 70.8% of mothers rated their overall QOL as "very good" or "good" [11].

We could find a negative relationship between educational attainment and EBF. In a previous study conducted in Peru, maternal education was negatively associated with EBF at 3 months [26], while in a study on Icelandic women, educational attainment was an important factor in EBF continuation [27].

As expected, multiparous women had less breastfeeding difficulties. This is due to their previous experience in breastfeeding. Eighty percent of multiparous women described their breastfeeding experience as good or excellent.

This study increased our knowledge about maternal QOL and breastfeeding difficulties in Shahroud and contributed to our understanding of the relationship between QOL and breastfeeding difficulties and the continuation of exclusive breastfeeding. We recommend that further studies be designed to assess the relationship between QOL, breastfeeding difficulties and breastfeeding discontinuation. Since 62.8% of our sample adopted predominant breastfeeding up to 2 months postpartum, and breastfeeding intention was not different in EBF and non-EBF groups, we recommend that qualitative research be designed to investigate the other reasons of discontinuation of EBF in early postpartum.

In this study, the QOL questionnaire was conducted only in the third trimester of pregnancy, so it is possible that childbirth and breastfeeding improved mother's perception of wellbeing and the QOL. We recommend that further studies be designed to assess the trajectory of changes in the maternal QOL during the first six months postpartum and its influence on breastfeeding practices and duration.

5. Limitations

The sample in this study was representative of low risk Iranian women visiting public health clinics to receive prenatal care in Shahroud. Only 32 women did not choose to participate in our study due to lack of time to fill out the questionnaire. Limitation of our study includes potential for recall bias. We acknowledge that the method used to assess breastfeeding outcomes may lead to misclassifications. Since the 24-hour recall method overestimates EBF rates, we chose a longer recall time (the month recall). Also, we asked mothers to recall breastfeeding difficulties during 4 weeks postpartum, so recall bias is possible.

6. Conclusion

Breastfeeding difficulties and QOL could affect the continuation of exclusive breastfeeding. To promote EBF, mothers with low QOL or breastfeeding difficulties should be supported during the early postpartum.

Conflict of Interests

The authors declare that there is no conflict of interests regarding the publication of this paper.

Authors' Contribution

Forough Mortazavi was the main investigator and wrote the proposal, collected the data, wrote the first draft, and contributed to the statistical analysis. Seyed Abbas Mousavi contributed to the study design. Reza Chaman contributed to the interpretation of the findings. Ahmad Khosravi revised the final draft.

Acknowledgments

The authors wish to thank Professor Wambach who kindly guide them to use the breastfeeding experience scale. This essay is part of a PhD degree thesis on the relationship between maternal QOL and breastfeeding duration and was partially financed by Research Management of Shahroud University of Medical Sciences.

References

[1] S. Ip, M. Chung, G. Raman et al., "Breastfeeding and maternal and infant health outcomes in developed countries," *Evidence Report/Technology Assessment*, no. 153, pp. 1–186, 2007.

[2] L. R. Salone, W. F. Vann Jr., and D. L. Dee, "Breastfeeding: an overview of oral and general health benefits," *The Journal of the American Dental Association*, vol. 144, pp. 143–151, 2013.

[3] M. Kramer and R. Kakuma, *The Optimal Duration of Exclusive Breastfeeding a Systematic Review*, Department of Nutrition for Health and Development, Department of Child and Adolescent Health and Development, World Health Organization, 2002.

[4] World Health Organization, "Infant and young child nutrition, global strategy for infant and young child feeding," Tech. Rep. EB 109/12, 2002.

[5] V. Schmied and L. Barclay, "Connection and pleasure, disruption and distress: women's experience of breastfeeding," *Journal of Human Lactation*, vol. 15, no. 4, pp. 325–334, 1999.

[6] J. N. Mozingo, M. W. Davis, P. G. Droppleman, and A. Merideth, "It wasn't working: women's experiences with short-term breastfeeding," *MCN The American Journal of Maternal Child Nursing*, vol. 25, no. 3, pp. 120–126, 2000.

[7] O. Vesga-López, C. Blanco, K. Keyes, M. Olfson, B. F. Grant, and D. S. Hasin, "Psychiatric disorders in pregnant and postpartum

women in the United States," *Archives of General Psychiatry*, vol. 65, no. 7, pp. 805–815, 2008.

[8] C.-L. Dennis and K. McQueen, "Does maternal postpartum depressive symptomatology influence infant feeding outcomes?" *Acta Paediatrica*, vol. 96, no. 4, pp. 590–594, 2007.

[9] P. Hoddinott and R. Pill, "Qualitative study of decisions about infant feeding among women in east end of London," *British Medical Journal*, vol. 318, no. 7175, pp. 30–34, 1999.

[10] "World health organization: program on mental health. WHOQOL-BREF introduction, administration, scoring and generic version of the assessment," World health organization, 1996, http://www.who.int/mental_health/media/en/76.pdf.

[11] C. Zubaran and K. Foresti, "The correlation between breastfeeding and maternal quality of life in southern Brazil," *Breastfeeding Medicine*, vol. 6, no. 1, pp. 25–30, 2011.

[12] Y.-C. Chen, W.-C. Chie, S.-C. Kuo, Y.-H. Lin, S.-J. Lin, and P.-C. Chen, "The association between infant feeding pattern and mother's quality of life in Taiwan," *Quality of Life Research*, vol. 16, no. 8, pp. 1281–1288, 2007.

[13] B. Olang, K. Farivar, A. Heidarzadeh, B. Strandvik, and A. Yngve, "Breastfeeding in Iran: prevalence, duration and current recommendations," *International Breastfeeding Journal*, vol. 4, article 8, 2009.

[14] UNICEF, "Iran Islamic Republic of Statistics," 2011, http://www.unicef.org/infobycountry/iran_statistics.html.

[15] S. Mehrparvar and M. Varaeneen, "Investigation of decreasing causes of exclusive breastfeeding in children below six months old, in Kerman City during 2008-2009," *Journal of Fasa University of Medical Sciences*, vol. 1, pp. 45–51, 2011.

[16] L. Rahmatnejad and F. Bastani, "Reasons of exclusive breastfeeding discontinuation among primiparas," *Iran Journal of Nursing*, vol. 24, pp. 42–53, 2011.

[17] S. Nedjat, A. Montazeri, K. Holakouie, K. Mohammad, and R. Majdzadeh, "Psychometric properties of the Iranian interview-administered version of the World Health Organization's Quality of Life Questionnaire (WHOQOL-BREF): a population-based study," *BMC Health Services Research*, vol. 8, article 61, 2008.

[18] C. Zubaran, K. Foresti, M. V. Schumacher, L. C. Muller, and A. L. Amoretti, "An assessment of maternal quality of life in the postpartum period in southern Brazil: a comparison of two questionnaires," *Clinics*, vol. 64, no. 8, pp. 751–756, 2009.

[19] J. Webster, C. Nicholas, C. Velacott, N. Cridland, and L. Fawcett, "Validation of the WHOQOL-BREF among women following childbirth," *Australian and New Zealand Journal of Obstetrics and Gynaecology*, vol. 50, no. 2, pp. 132–137, 2010.

[20] K. A. Wambach, "Breastfeeding intention and outcome: a test of the theory of planned behavior," *Research in Nursing and Health*, vol. 20, no. 1, pp. 51–59, 1997.

[21] K. H. Chaput, *The Effect of Breastfeeding Difficulty and Associated Factors on Postpartum Depression*, Department of Comunity Health Sciences. University of Galgary, Galgary, Canada, 2013.

[22] K. A. Wambach, "Maternal fatigue in breastfeeding primiparae during the first nine weeks postpartum," *Journal of Human Lactation*, vol. 14, no. 3, pp. 219–229, 1998.

[23] K. A. Wambach and S. M. Cohen, "Breastfeeding experiences of urban adolescent mothers," *Journal of Pediatric Nursing*, vol. 24, no. 4, pp. 244–254, 2009.

[24] C. Lamontagne, A.-M. Hamelin, and M. St-Pierre, "The breastfeeding experience of women with major difficulties who use

the services of a breastfeeding clinic: a descriptive study," *International Breastfeeding Journal*, vol. 3, article 17, 2008.

[25] H. Almasi, H. Saberi, and A. Moravveji, "The pattern of exclusive breast feeding in neonates under healthcares in health clinics of Kashan city during 2006," *Feyz Journal of Kashan University of Medical Sciences*, vol. 14, pp. 163–168, 2010.

[26] S. L. Matias, L. A. Nommsen-Rivers, and K. G. Dewey, "Determinants of exclusive breastfeeding in a cohort of primiparous periurban peruvian mothers," *Journal of Human Lactation*, vol. 28, no. 1, pp. 45–54, 2012.

[27] M. Thome, E. M. Alder, and A. Ramel, "A population-based study of exclusive breastfeeding in Icelandic women: is there a relationship with depressive symptoms and parenting stress?" *International Journal of Nursing Studies*, vol. 43, no. 1, pp. 11–20, 2006.

3

2-Year BMI Changes of Children Referred for Multidisciplinary Weight Management

**Jennifer K. Cheng,[1] Xiaozhong Wen,[2] Kristen D. Coletti,[1]
Joanne E. Cox,[1] and Elsie M. Taveras[3,4]**

[1] *Division of General Pediatrics, Department of Medicine, Boston Children's Hospital, Boston, MA 02115, USA*
[2] *Division of Behavioral Medicine, Department of Pediatrics, School of Medicine and Biomedical Sciences,
   State University of New York at Buffalo, Buffalo, NY 14214, USA*
[3] *Obesity Prevention Program, Department of Population Medicine, Harvard Medical School and Harvard Pilgrim Health Care
   Institute, Boston, MA 02215, USA*
[4] *Division of General Pediatrics, Massachusetts General Hospital, Boston, MA 02114, USA*

Correspondence should be addressed to Jennifer K. Cheng; jennifer.cheng@childrens.harvard.edu

Academic Editor: Samuel Menahem

Objective. To examine body mass index (BMI) changes among pediatric multidisciplinary weight management participants and nonparticipants. *Design.* In this retrospective database analysis, we used multivariable mixed effect models to compare 2-year BMI z-score trajectories among 583 eligible overweight or obese children referred to the One Step Ahead program at the Boston Children's Primary Care Center between 2003 and 2009. *Results.* Of the referred children, 338 (58%) attended the program; 245 (42%) did not participate and were instead followed by their primary care providers within the group practice. The mean BMI z-score of program participants decreased modestly over a 2-year period and was lower than that of nonparticipants. The group-level difference in the rate of change in BMI z-score between participants and nonparticipants was statistically significant for 0–6 months ($P = 0.001$) and 19–24 months ($P = 0.008$); it was marginally significant for 13–18 months ($P = 0.051$) after referral. Younger participants (<5 years) had better outcomes across all time periods examined. *Conclusion.* Children attending a multidisciplinary program experienced greater BMI z-score reductions compared with usual primary care in a real world practice; younger participants had significantly better outcomes. Future research should consider early intervention and cost-effectiveness analyses.

1. Introduction

Pediatric obesity is a serious health condition, conferring both immediate and long-term health risks [1–3]. Multidisciplinary approaches in diverse sectors, including pediatric primary care, have been proposed to reduce the high prevalence of childhood obesity [4].

Multi-disciplinary clinical programs require a considerable investment of time and resources, but limited data exists on long-term weight outcomes of children participating in such programs, and few studies have examined real-world pediatric weight management of different intensity.

The purpose of this study was to examine changes in body mass index (BMI) among children who were referred to a multi-disciplinary weight management program. We were particularly interested in learning whether there were differences in weight outcomes among program participants as compared with nonparticipants who continued to be followed by their primary care providers within the group practice over a 2-year period following referral. We designated program participants as the "intervention group" and non-participants as the "comparison group" for the purpose of this study, although we recognized that this analysis was based on observational rather than experimental data.

2. Methods

2.1. Setting and Study Design. The One Step Ahead (OSA) program was developed in 2003 specifically to provide stepped-up care for the growing numbers of children with increasing obesity severity within the Boston Children's Primary Care Center (CHPCC). The CHPCC practice comprises over 80 healthcare providers annually serving more than 14,000 children from mostly economically challenged neighborhoods in Boston, MA. Approximately 44% of children seen for well-child care are overweight or obese; 65% are insured through Medicaid.

In this retrospective observational study, we used the clinically derived OSA database to compare BMI z-score changes among program participants (intervention group) versus non-participating children who were followed by primary care providers within the group practice (comparison). The study protocol was approved by the human subjects committee of Boston Children's Hospital.

2.2. Study Population. The study population comprised overweight (BMI $\geq$ 85th and <95th sex- and age-specific percentile based on Centers for Disease Prevention and Control 2000 Growth Charts) or obese (>95th percentile) children aged 2–18 years who were referred from the CHPCC to the OSA program between 2003 and 2009. The *intervention group* comprised children who attended the OSA program and had completed at least 2 visits of any type where BMI was measured in the 2-year period following referral. The *comparison group* comprised referred children who did not keep their OSA appointments, but had nonetheless completed at least 2 primary care visits where BMI was measured over the same 2-year period.

2.3. Intervention. The OSA team includes medical providers, a nurse educator, registered dietitians, a behavioral psychologist, a social worker, and a physical activity coordinator. The goal of the program is to achieve weight maintenance or loss among children as they continue growing in height. The OSA program utilizes the social ecological model as a framework for its services and considers individual, interpersonal, community, and societal levels of influences on the child's behavior change. Motivational interviewing [5, 6] techniques are used to assess families' readiness to change, help families set achievable healthful lifestyle goals, and navigate potential obstacles.

Dieticians provide family-centered nutrition education and teach families practical skills including meal planning, label reading, and culturally appropriate healthful cooking techniques. A physical activity coordinator matches families with free or low-cost neighborhood exercise programs. A behavioral psychologist evaluates families for maladaptive behaviors and provides supportive mental health services including individual and family counseling to bolster self-esteem and resiliency. A medical social worker frequently assists families with acute social support needs including housing, transportation, utilities, and food assistance. In general, visits are scheduled at monthly intervals for at least

the first 3 visits and for a total of 6 visits over the course of 12 months; however, actual visit intervals and total program duration are quite variable due to the highly individualized nature of the program. The OSA program staff calls the families of children who do not keep their OSA appointments to help them reschedule missed visits and emails referring providers to inform them about the missed visit. Approximately 40% of families are reached by phone and the most common reasons given for missing their scheduled OSA visits include forgetting about the appointment, transportation issues, and scheduling conflicts with work, school or other competing priorities. Many of the families served by the OSA clinic struggle with social stressors including unemployment, food, or home insecurity, and may have difficulty affording basic needs such as clothing, electricity, or telephone service.

Children who were referred but did not keep any OSA appointments were seen by their primary care providers for routine well child-care annually or more frequently for problem-focused visits (e.g., for weight related or other issues). CHPCC well care visit content is based on the *Bright-Futures Guidelines for Health Supervision* [7], but no practice-wide standards existed at the time of this study for obesity assessment, education or follow-up intervals. CHPCC providers manage obese children using general patient education, materials. Among 245 referred children who did not attend the OSA program, 17.3% had weight monitoring visits in addition to well child-care visits with their primary care providers.

2.4. Outcomes. At each visit, clinical assistants measured the child's weight and height. We calculated BMI as "weight in kg/height in meters^2" and then used the Centers for Disease Prevention and Control (CDC) 2000 Growth Charts [8] to calculate gender- and age-specific BMI z-score. Change in BMI z-score at each postreferral visit was calculated as current BMI z-score minus baseline BMI z-score at referral. The primary outcome was the rate of change in BMI z-score (defined as "difference in BMI z-score/time interval") per month during each of 4 time periods within 24 months after referral: referral-6 months, 7–12 months, 13–18 months, and 19–24 months.

Covariates of interest included gender, age at referral, race/ethnicity (Black, White, Hispanics, and other), language (English, Spanish, and other), and baseline BMI z-score at referral.

2.5. Statistical Analysis. To examine group differences in baseline characteristics, we performed Chi-square tests for categorical variables (e.g., gender) and t-tests for continuous variables (e.g., age).

Because each child in the analytic sample had multiple visits and childhood BMI usually tracks with age, we used mixed effect models to examine the rate of change in BMI z-score after referral. In our sample, an autoregressive correlation structure was chosen for different visits of the same child in the final model, because this structure was associated with a lower Akaike Information Criterion than several other candidate correlation structures. Briefly, an auto-regressive correlation structure indicates that two BMI z-scores observed at two closer visits for a particular child tend to be more correlated than two BMI z-scores observed at farther apart visits. Specifically, we specified a random effect for the intercept reflecting between-subject variation in baseline BMI z-score at referral, and specified a fixed effect for intervention, time after referral and potential interaction between intervention and time after referral. We used piece-wise linear methods to allow for nonlinear trends of change in BMI z-score. Specifically, we first divided the 2 years of followup into the four 6-month periods (i.e., referral-6 months, 7–12 months, 13–18 months, and 19–24 months) and then considered a linear trend within each period. Accordingly, we fit a series of hierarchical models with main effects of intervention and time; 2-way interaction between Intervention and time; and 3-way interactions between intervention, time, and the 4 time periods. For the purpose of visualization, we used the smoothing function in Microsoft Excel to connect the 4 time periods smoothly and then to compare the group-level mean BMI z-score trajectories between the intervention and comparison groups (Figure 2).

All regression models were adjusted for potential confounders: the child's gender, age at referral, race/ethnicity, primary language, and BMI z-score at referral. We also tested for potential interactions between intervention group and demographic characteristics by performing stratified analyses by the child's gender, race/ethnicity, age at referral, and primary language.

We conducted all analyses in SAS 9.2 (SAS Institute Inc., Cary, NC).

3. Results

3.1. Comparison of Baseline Characteristics. Table 1 shows the characteristics of the multi-disciplinary intervention (OSA, $N = 338$) and comparison ($N = 245$) groups. The mean (standard deviation or SD) age of patients at the time of referral to the OSA program was 8.7 (2.6) years, mean BMI z-score was 2.3 (0.5) units, and the prevalence of obesity was 93.5%. The two groups did not differ by gender, age, race, BMI, or prevalence of obesity. However, children in the intervention group had a slightly higher mean BMI z-score (2.3 versus 2.2), more visits within 2 years after referral (mean number of visits, 5.5 [3.2] versus 2.5 [1.2]), and were more likely to speak Spanish as a primary language (21.0% versus 14.3%). Most of the OSA team providers including all physicians also speak Spanish.

3.2. Distribution of Visits. Figure 1 shows the distribution of visits for the 2 groups. There were a total of 1,855 visits for the intervention group and 615 visits for the comparison group. For both groups, the visits after referral dispersed between 2 months and 24 months. The visit frequency decreased over time in the OSA group. The mean time for follow-up visits was similar between the two groups (8.4 versus 8.1 months after referral). As shown in Table 1, 855 (26%) children in the OSA group and 43 (17.6%) children in the comparison

group were followed to 2 years (22–24 months). The mean follow-up time was slightly longer for the OSA group than the comparison group (14.8 (SD, 7.2) versus 13.3 (SD, 7.7) months after referral; $P = 0.01$).

3.3. Change in BMI z-Score after Referral. Figure 2 shows change in BMI z-score at 6, 12, 18, and 24 months after referral. For the intervention group, the mean BMI z-score decreased more steeply during the first 6 months and continuously during the 2-year period. In contrast, the mean BMI z-score for the comparison group increased during the first 6-postreferral months then decreased to 18 months, after which it leveled off.

Table 2 shows the estimated rates of change in BMI z-score (units per month) for the 4 time periods. From 0 to 6 months, BMI z-score decreased for the intervention group at the rate of −0.013 units/month (95% confidence interval or CI, −0.017 to −0.009)) but increased for the comparison group (0.004 units/month (95% CI, −0.005 to 0.013)). The BMI z-score continued to decrease more steeply for the intervention group than the comparison group from 7 to 12 months (−0.008 versus −0.005), 13 to 18 months (−0.008 versus −0.005), and 19 to 24 months (−0.008 versus −0.004). The group difference (interventional versus comparison) in the rate of change in BMI z-score was statistically significant for 0–6 months ($P = 0.001$) and 19–24 months ($P = 0.008$); it was marginally significant for 13–18 months ($P = 0.051$). Among OSA participants, there were no significant racial/ethnic differences except non-Hispanic Black children who had a smaller decrease in BMI z-score than all other groups during the 0 to 6-month period (−0.007 versus −0.017, $P = 0.009$). There were also no significant group-differences in the rate of change in BMI z-score based on gender. Among OSA participants, children younger than 5 years had significantly greater decreases in BMI z-score than older children during all time periods (0 to 6 months: −0.067 versus −0.005, $P = 0.001$; 7 to 12 months: −0.032 versus −0.003, $P = 0.001$; 13 to 18 months, −0.024 versus −0.004, $P = 0.001$; 19 to 24 months, −0.024 versus −0.004, P value = 0.001).

4. Discussion

In this study, we found that a group of racial ethnically diverse children attending a multi-disciplinary weight management program experienced reductions in BMI z-score over a 2-year follow-up period. These BMI reductions were of greater magnitude than those of non-participants but were overall modest. Among OSA program participants, younger children experienced significantly greater reductions in BMI z-score than older children, but we did not observe gender or racial/ethnic differences. Our findings add to the scarce evidence on the effectiveness of real-world pediatric weight management among overweight children of diverse races/ethnicities and low family socioeconomic status.

The reasons for the modest reduction in BMI z-score seen among OSA participants are likely multifactorial. A large proportion of our families have endorsed challenging ongoing psychosocial stressors including limited financial

TABLE 1: Characteristics and visit frequency of analytic samples for the OSA and comparison groups.

	OSA	Comparison	P value
Child level			
Total number of children	338	245	
Gender, %			
Boys	46.5	49.0	0.55
Girls	53.6	51.0	
Age at referral, %			
2–5 y	11.0	13.9	
6–8 y	35.5	25.3	
9–10 y	27.2	33.1	
11–18 y	26.3	27.8	
Mean (SD)	8.7 (2.6)	8.8 (2.8)	0.47
Race, %			
White	5.6	3.3	
Black	51.8	61.6	0.10
Hispanic	24.0	18.8	
Others	18.6	16.3	
Language, %			
English	74.3	84.1	
Spanish	21.0	14.3	0.01
Others	4.7	1.6	
Prevalence of obesity at baseline, %	93.5	91.0	0.27
Baseline BMI, mean (SD)	26.5 (3.9)	26.2 (4.6)	0.37
Baseline BMI z-score, mean (SD)	2.3 (0.5)	2.2 (0.5)	0.03
Number of all-type visits, mean (SD)	5.5 (3.2)	2.5 (1.2)	<0.001
Number of OSA visits, mean (SD)	2.7 (1.9)	N/A	—
Duration of OSA intervention in months, mean (SD)	9.5 (6.9)	N/A	—
Time after referral at the last visit (months)			
0–6 months	21.2	19.2	
7–12 months	11.0	11.8	
13–15 months	24.9	15.4	
16–18 months	11.4	11.0	
19–21 months	13.9	16.6	
22–24 months	17.6	26.0	
Mean (SD)	14.8 (7.2)	13.3 (7.7)	0.01
Visit level			
Total number of visits	1855	615	
Time after referral in months, mean (SD)	8.4 (7.0)	8.1 (8.0)	0.49

TABLE 2: Rate of change in BMI z-score (units per month) after referral for OSA and comparison groups.

Time period	Mean rate of change in BMI z-score (95% CI)[*]			P value
	OSA group	Comparison group	Mean difference (OSA-comparison)	
Referral-6 m	−0.013 (−0.017, −0.009)	0.004 (−0.005, 0.013)	−0.017 (−0.027, −0.007)	0.001
7–12 m	−0.008 (−0.011, −0.006)	−0.005 (−0.008, −0.003)	−0.003 (−0.007, 0.001)	0.093
13–18 m	−0.008 (−0.010, −0.006)	−0.005 (−0.007, −0.003)	−0.003 (−0.006, 0.000)	0.051
19–24 m	−0.008 (−0.010, −0.006)	−0.004 (−0.006, −0.002)	−0.004 (−0.006, −0.001)	0.008

[*] Adjusted for the child's gender, age at referral, race/ethnicity, spoken language, and BMI z-score at referral.

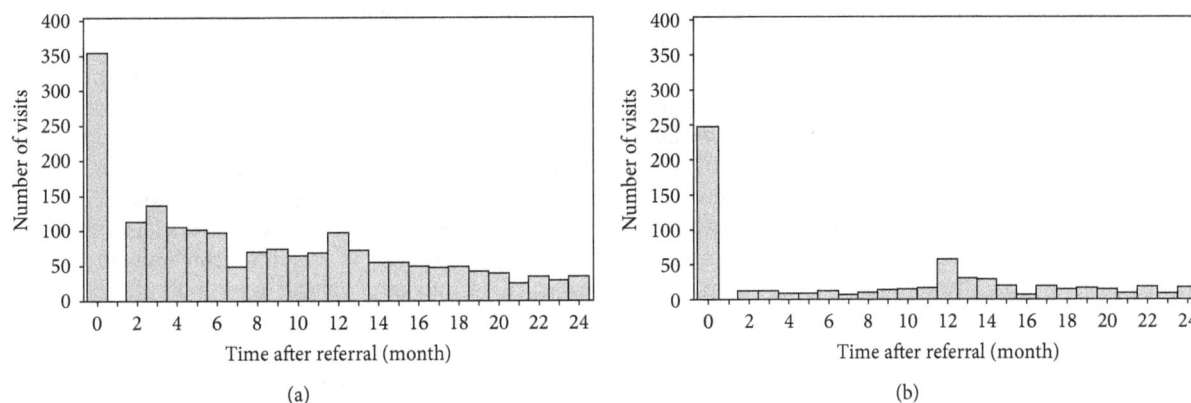

FIGURE 1: Distribution of time at visits for OSA and comparison groups: (a) OSA group (1,855 visits by 338 children); (b) comparison group (615 visits by 245 children).

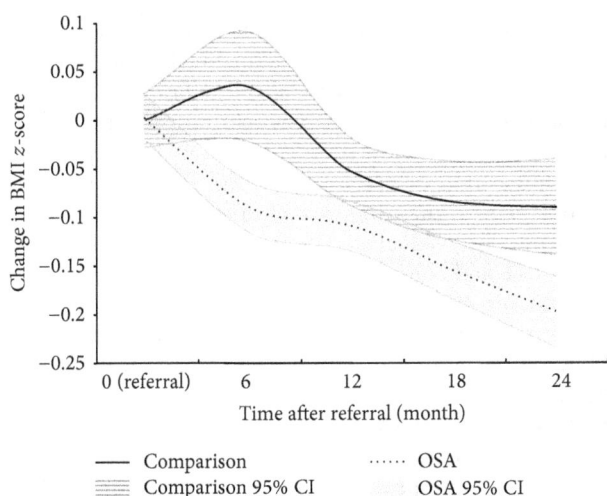

FIGURE 2: Change in BMI z-score after referral for OSA and comparison groups.

resources to purchase healthful items or enroll children in organized physical activity programs, food or housing insecurity, competing priorities, simultaneous exacerbations of chronic illness in a family member, and difficulty sustaining motivation over time as significant barriers to maintaining a healthy weight. In addition, a number of biological adaptations including changes in the circulating levels of several peripheral hormones involved in the homeostatic regulation of body weight likely contribute to weight gain recidivism. Sumithran et al. found that circulating levels of leptin, peptide YY, cholecystokinin, insulin, ghrelin, gastric inhibitory polypeptide, and pancreatic polypeptide, as well as subjective feelings of hunger, do not revert to the preweight loss levels even one year after initial weight reduction [9]. While the BMI changes we observed were modest, a necessary level (threshold) of pediatric BMI change associated with health benefits among children has not been established. Adult studies have shown that even modest weight loss (5–10%) is

associated with cardiovascular benefits [10]. Among children, some experts have suggested that even BMI stabilization/maintenance might be considered to be a successful endpoint [11], especially given the almost linear increase in BMI after adiposity rebound at age 5-6 y experienced by most children [12]. In addition, psychological benefits associated with even modest weight loss (and the lifestyle changes accompanying such weight loss) among children include a sense of mastery and improved self-esteem[13].

While children and their parents choosing to attend our weight management programs might inherently possess higher motivation relative to nonattendees, our findings provide invaluable insight as a reflection of "real-world" clinical practice as randomization is not always practical in service priority settings. The One Step Ahead program was developed specifically to meet demands for readily accessible, culturally sensitive, multidisciplinary weight management services for the growing numbers of obese children in our safety-net practice serving families predominantly from low-income, racial ethnically diverse Boston neighborhoods. Embedded within a busy academic primary care practice of more than 80 pediatricians in cohabitation with several other clinical programs, OSA program research capacity is limited by space, scheduling, staffing, and budgetary constraints and subsumed by the impetus to deliver patient-centered care in a medical home practice model. Our approach represents a realistic, culturally appropriate weight management intervention targeting a predominantly low-income Hispanic or African-American population and may inform many similar programs where randomization may not be feasible, acceptable, or sustainable on a long-term basis.

Limited evidence has suggested the greater effectiveness of medium- to high-intensity behavioral interventions, compared with low-intensity interventions conducted in primary care settings [14]. The Expert Committee Recommendations for Childhood Obesity Management [15] propose a staged approach to obesity treatment. Stage 1, "Prevention Plus," comprises brief counseling regarding key healthful lifestyle behaviors that can be delivered in primary care office settings; Stage 2, "Structured Weight Management," delivers similar messages through the added structure of a dietician or other trained professional such as an exercise counselor. Stage 3, "Comprehensive Multidisciplinary Intervention," is a structured program in behavior modification that includes goal setting and contingency management facilitated by a team approach. Stage 4, "Tertiary Care Intervention" includes the use of medications and bariatric surgery as potential treatment modalities and is reserved for children who are refractory to more conservative treatment at the lower stages. Children in the One Step Ahead program can be considered Stage 3 treatment recipients, while those in the comparison group (referred but did participate and were followed by primary care physicians) can be considered Stage 1 treatment recipients. The steadier and greater reduction in BMI z-score seen with children enrolled in our "Stage 3" intervention compared with children in the comparison "Stage 1" strategy appears to support the premise of higher effectiveness for more intensive approaches. If more intensive treatment more effectively reduces BMI, a staged treatment approach per the Expert Committee Guidelines seems sensible. However, we do not contend that greater decreases in BMI alone result in better outcomes in the pediatric population. It may also be important to account for the impact of nonweight outcomes on child and family well being. In the era of Accountable Care Organizations [16], for the greater resources necessary per unit increased BMI effect, whether children should be treated with Stage 3 and Stage 4 interventions at all requires further study to first define and then maximize core health outcomes for the resources expended.

Careful examination of the BMI z-score trajectory over time can offer additional insights regarding why our intervention works and how to improve it in future. First, the overall decline in BMI z-scores observed over the 2-year study period among intervention participants suggests that weight management may be maintained over time, although the effect size may decrease. This is encouraging given the recidivism of weight gain due to compensatory metabolic processes that resist the maintenance of the altered body weight [17]. The rise in BMI z-scores during the initial 0–6-month period among comparison children may be related to delayed followup by providers who had referred the patients to OSA, only to find later that the families had not participated. Secondly, the greatest difference in the change in BMI z-score between intervention (decrease) and comparison (increase) children occurred in the 0–6 months period. This difference may be related to higher initial self-motivation and vigilance, more intensive intervention within the earlier periods, or higher-impact behavioral changes that represent "low-lying fruit," where later improvements may be more incremental and require greater efforts. These findings are consistent with previous work showing greater intervention impact on weight outcomes in the early periods of weight management [18]. Interestingly, BMI z-scores for the comparison group also decreased following the initial rise, although being at a lesser rate than for the intervention group, suggesting that the Stage 1 strategy by primary care providers in our CHPCC is also somewhat effective. Therefore, closer followup by primary care providers is needed to ensure that referral or primary provider care occurs. Standardized time intervals for followup of obese children could potentially improve outcomes.

Among children who attended our multidisciplinary program, we found that younger age was associated with better weight outcomes, which is consistent with a growing body of evidence linking earlier intervention with better long-term weight outcomes. For example, in two long-term follow-up studies of randomized trials, Brotman et al. found that children at risk for behavioral problems who received a family intervention to promote effective parenting at age 4 y had lower BMI and improved health behaviors in preadolescence [19]. Reinehr et al. found that younger age (<8 years) predicted the best long-term weight outcomes among obese children enrolled in a year-long lifestyle intervention [20]. These findings collectively support the premise that early prevention may optimize weight outcomes in high-risk children, with important implications for future childhood obesity interventions.

4.1. Limitations. Our study is limited by its retrospective observational design, which did not allow for the allocation of subjects in a randomized-controlled fashion to control unmeasured confounders such as self-motivation of changing lifestyle. However, a stratified data analysis by gender, race/ethnicity, and primary language did not yield substantial differences in estimated intervention effects, so it is unlikely that any unobserved allocation imbalances of baseline characteristics could completely explained the significant group differences in BMI z-score we observed. Other limitations include selection bias due to eligibility criteria or loss to follow up since families with higher initial self-motivation and vigilance were more likely to accept and/or continue the intervention; variations in intervention activities, intensity, and length; and residual confounding by family socioeconomics. Finally, the primary-care embedded within a tertiary hospital setting model may limit its generalizability.

5. Conclusion

In this study, a group of racial-ethnically diverse overweight children attending a multidisciplinary weight management program demonstrated sustained but modest BMI z-score reductions over a 2-year period. Younger children (<5 years) had significantly better weight outcomes compared with older children. Our findings suggest that multi-disciplinary programs might be considered as a treatment option within the spectrum of pediatric obesity management in health care settings and also that interventions targeting younger children might have greater impact. It is our next step to refine our intervention strategies to further increase their effectiveness. Finally, future studies ought to evaluate the promise of early intervention and also consider cost-effectiveness analyses.

Conflict of Interests

The authors have no conflict of interests and financial relationships relevant to this paper to disclose.

Authors' Contribution

Drs. Cheng and Wen share first coauthorship for their work on this paper; they had full access to the data in the study and jointly assume responsibility for the integrity of the data and the accuracy of the data analysis. Each of the authors substantially participated in the concept and design, analysis and interpretation of data, and drafting/revising of the paper. The study concept and design were made by Cheng JK, Wen X, and Taveras EM. The data acquisition was conducted by Cheng JK and Coletti KD. The data analysis and interpretation were done by Cheng JK, Wen X, Coletti KD, Cox JE, and Taveras EM. The drafting of this paper was conducted by Cheng JK and Wen X. The critical paper review for important intellectual content was done by Cox JE and Taveras EM. The statistical analysis was conducted by Wen X. The administrative, technical, or material support was done by Coletti KD. Cheng JK and Taveras EM were responsible for the study supervision.

Funding

The work is funded in part by the National Institute on Minority Health and Health Disparities (Grant no. R01MD00396).

Acknowledgments

The authors thank Peter Forbes, Ph.D. and Henry Feldman, Ph.D., for their advice and assistance. The authors also acknowledge the children who collectively provided the data for this study.

References

[1] L. J. Aronne, "Epidemiology, morbidity, and treatment of overweight and obesity," *Journal of Clinical Psychiatry*, vol. 62, supplement 23, pp. 13–22, 2001.

[2] S. R. Daniels, D. K. Arnett, R. H. Eckel et al., "Overweight in children and adolescents: pathophysiology, consequences, prevention, and treatment," *Circulation*, vol. 111, no. 15, pp. 1999–2012, 2005.

[3] A. Must, J. Spadano, E. H. Coakley, A. E. Field, G. Colditz, and W. H. Dietz, "The disease burden associated with overweight and obesity," *Journal of the American Medical Association*, vol. 282, no. 16, pp. 1523–1529, 1999.

[4] I. Eneli, V. Norwood, S. Hampl et al., "Perspectives on obesity programs at children's hospitals: insights from senior program administrators," *Pediatrics*, vol. 128, supplement 2, pp. S86–S90, 2011.

[5] W. R. Miller and S. Rollnick, *Motivational Interviewing: Preparing People for Change*, Guilford Press, New York, NY, USA, 2nd edition, 2002.

[6] S. Rollnick, C. C. Butler, P. Kinnersley, J. Gregory, and B. Mash, "Motivational interviewing," *British Medical Journal*, vol. 340, article c1900, 2010.

[7] J. Hagan, J. Shaw, and P. Duncan, *Bright Futures Guidelines for Health Supervision of Infants, Children, and Adolescents*, 3rd edition, 2008.

[8] R. J. Kuczmarski, C. L. Ogden, L. M. Grummer-Strawn et al., "CDC growth charts: United States," *Advance Data*, no. 314, pp. 1–27, 2000.

[9] P. Sumithran, L. A. Prendergast, E. Delbridge et al., "Long-term persistence of hormonal adaptations to weight loss," *The New England Journal of Medicine*, vol. 365, no. 17, pp. 1597–1604, 2011.

[10] R. R. Wing, W. Lang, T. A. Wadden et al., "Benefits of modest weight loss in improving cardiovascular risk factors in overweight and obese individuals with type 2 diabetes," *Diabetes care*, vol. 34, no. 7, pp. 1481–1486, 2011.

[11] E. P. Whitlock, E. A. O'Connor, S. B. Williams, T. L. Beil, and K. W. Lutz, "Effectiveness of weight management interventions in children: a targeted systematic review for the USPSTF," *Pediatrics*, vol. 125, no. 2, pp. e396–e418, 2010.

[12] E. A. Whitlock, E. P. O'Connor, S. B. Williams, T. L. Beil, and K. W. Lutz, "Effectiveness of weight management programs in children and adolescents," *Evidence Report/Technology Assessment*, no. 170, pp. 1–308, 2008.

[13] M. Morano, D. Colella, I. Rutigliano, P. Fiore, M. Pettoello-Mantovani, and A. Campanozzi, "Changes in actual and perceived physical abilities in clinically obese children: a 9-month multi-component intervention study," *PLoS One*, vol. 7, no. 12, Article ID e50782, 2012.

[14] R. C. Whitaker, M. S. Pepe, J. A. Wright, K. D. Seidel, and W. H. Dietz, "Early adiposity rebound and the risk of adult obesity," *Pediatrics*, vol. 101, no. 3, p. E5, 1998.

[15] S. E. Barlow, "Expert committee recommendations regarding the prevention, assessment, and treatment of child and adolescent overweight and obesity: summary report," *Pediatrics*, vol. 120, supplement 4, pp. S164–S192, 2007.

[16] K. H. Lowell and J. Bertko, "The accountable care organization (ACO) model: building blocks for success," *Journal of Ambulatory Care Management*, vol. 33, no. 1, pp. 81–88, 2010.

[17] J. Reinholz, O. Skopp, C. Breitenstein, I. Bohr, H. Winterhoff, and S. Knecht, "Compensatory weight gain due to dopaminergic hypofunction: new evidence and own incidental observations," *Nutrition and Metabolism*, vol. 5, no. 1, article 35, 2008.

[18] C. G. Ulen, M. M. Huizinga, B. Beech, and T. A. Elasy, "Weight regain prevention," *Clinical Diabetes*, vol. 26, no. 3, pp. 100–113, 2008.

[19] L. M. Brotman, S. Dawson-McClure, K.-Y. Huang et al., "Early childhood family intervention and long-term obesity prevention among high-risk minority youth," *Pediatrics*, vol. 129, no. 3, pp. e621–e628, 2012.

[20] T. Reinehr, M. Kleber, N. Lass, and A. M. Toschke, "Body mass index patterns over 5 y in obese children motivated to participate in a 1-y lifestyle intervention: age as a predictor of long-term success," *American Journal of Clinical Nutrition*, vol. 91, no. 5, pp. 1165–1171, 2010.

Abnormal Blood Glucose as a Prognostic Factor for Adverse Clinical Outcome in Children Admitted to the Paediatric Emergency Unit at Komfo Anokye Teaching Hospital, Kumasi, Ghana

Emmanuel Ameyaw,[1] Kwame Amponsah-Achiano,[2] Peter Yamoah,[1] and Jean-Pierre Chanoine[3]

[1]*Komfo Anokye Teaching Hospital, P.O. Box 1934, Kumasi, Ghana*
[2]*Disease Control Unit, Ghana Health Service, Accra, Ghana*
[3]*Endocrinology and Diabetes Unit, British Columbia Children's Hospital, Room K4-212, 4480 Oak Street, Vancouver, BC, Canada V6H 3V4*

Correspondence should be addressed to Emmanuel Ameyaw; ekameyaw@yahoo.com

Academic Editor: Stefan Burdach

Dysglycaemia (hyper- or hypoglycaemia) in critically ill children has been associated with poor outcome. We compared the clinical outcomes in children admitted to Pediatric Emergency Unit (PEU) at Komfo Anokye Teaching Hospital (KATH) for acute medical conditions and presenting with euglycaemia or dysglycaemia. This is a prospective case matching cohort study. Eight hundred subjects aged between 3 and 144 months were screened out of whom 430 (215 with euglycaemia and 215 with dysglycaemia) were enrolled. The median age was 24 months (range: 3–144 months). In the dysglycaemia group, 28 (13%) subjects had hypoglycemia and 187 (87%) had hyperglycemia. Overall, there were 128 complications in 116 subjects. The number of subjects with complications was significantly higher in dysglycaemia group ($n = 99$, 46%) compared to euglycaemia group ($n = 17$, 8%) ($P < 0.001$). Forty subjects died out of whom 30 had dysglycaemia ($P = 0.001$). Subjects with dysglycaemia were 3 times (95% CI: 1.5–6.0) more likely to die and 4.8 times (95% CI: 3.1–7.5) more likely to develop complications ($P = 0.001$). Dysglycaemia is associated with increased morbidity and mortality in children with acute medical conditions and should lead to intensive management of the underlying condition.

1. Introduction

In children, the response to the stress of an acute illness can present as abnormal blood glucose [1–6]. Bhisitkul et al. [3] found that 3.8% of children and adolescents presenting to the emergency room in Norfolk (VA) had hyperglycaemia. Hyperglycaemia was not associated with a specific diagnosis category but reflected a greater severity of the underlying condition. In contrast, Elusiyan et al. [4] observed that 6.4% of pediatric subjects admitted to a hospital in Nigeria had hypoglycaemia. Similarly, hypoglycaemia was observed across a large range of conditions and was associated with increased mortality. Overall, hypoglycaemia as well as hyperglycaemia [1–5] and, in addition, increased glucose variability [7] have been found to be associated with increased morbidity and mortality rates in acutely ill children in a variety of settings.

There is presently no data on abnormal blood glucose concentrations as well as on their potential relationship with patient outcome, in children with acute illnesses admitted to the Pediatric Emergency Unit (PEU) at KATH. We hypothesized that both hypoglycaemia and hyperglycaemia (referred to as dysglycemia in this paper) would be observed in children presenting to PEU and would be associated with unfavourable outcome. Using a prospective, case match design, the objectives of this study were (1) to describe and compare the characteristics of subjects as a function of their baseline blood glucose concentration and (2) to assess dysglycaemia as a prognostic factor for adverse clinical outcome in children admitted to PEU at KATH, Kumasi, Ghana.

The long term goal of our project is to learn from the results of this study to help develop and implement appropriate policies and treatment protocols and, ultimately, to better manage children at risk of complications. This could decrease morbidity and mortality and, ultimately, increase treatment efficiency and decrease treatment costs.

2. Material and Methods

2.1. Study Population. The study was conducted on consecutive subjects presenting over a four-month period to PEU, between December, 2010, and March, 2011. All children admitted with acute illness were eligible to participate in this prospective study. Inclusion criteria were admission to PEU with acute illness and age between 3 months and 12 years. Exclusion criteria were known history of diabetes mellitus; infusion of dextrose containing fluids up to 2 hours prior to admission; and intake of steroids within 72 hours of admission.

2.2. Study Site. The study was conducted at the PEU of the Department of Child Health, KATH, Kumasi. KATH is a 1200-bed capacity tertiary hospital which serves the Kumasi Metropolis and the surrounding towns and villages and also serves as a referral center for the middle belt and the northern part of Ghana. It has a polyclinic department which takes care of the outpatient cases. The paediatric unit of the polyclinic accepts children from birth to 12 years of age. Children who are critically ill are admitted from the polyclinic to the wards through the PEU. Both the polyclinic and the wards run a 24-hour duty every day. The number of admissions to PEU is between 15 and 30 patients everyday (unpublished data). Patients admitted to PEU are monitored till they are stable and then they are transferred to the wards for further treatment till they are well enough to be discharged.

2.3. Study Procedure. Data were collected daily between 8 a.m. and 8 p.m. All subjects admitted to PEU with acute illnesses had their blood glucose checked with One Touch Ultra2 glucometer (Lifescan Company, Milpitas, CA, USA). The range of the glucose concentrations measured with One Touch Ultra2 glucometer is 0.6–33.3 mmol/L (10–600 mg/dL). Glucometers were calibrated at the KATH Biochemistry Laboratory for every twentieth patient. A difference of less than 10% between that measure by glucometer and that by the biochemistry laboratory was regarded as acceptable [8]. Hyperglycaemia and hypoglycaemia were defined as blood glucose greater than 8.3 mmol/L (150 mg/dL) and less than 2.5 mmol/L (45 mg/dL), respectively [1–4].

A subject with acute illness and abnormal blood glucose (dysglycaemia group) was matched to the next patient with

normal blood glucose (euglycaemia group) but with the same diagnosis category (Table 3) and age group (age from 3 months to <2 years, 2 to <5 years, and 5 to 12 years) in order to better compare the characteristics of the conditions associated with dysglycemia. They were followed up till discharge or death. On discharge, their folders were collected and case record form was completed for final diagnosis and complications developed including death. Subjects in whom hyperglycemia did not resolve or worsened after initiating specific treatment of the primary condition were treated with regular insulin and monitored closely [9]. In contrast, those with hypoglycaemia were managed immediately according to our local protocol. Our hospital protocol calls for an initial bolus intravenous (iv), intraosseous (io), or rectal dextrose or intramuscular (im) glucagon followed by i.v. 10% dextrose at maintenance. Feeding is resumed as soon as possible. Necessary supportive management was given to each patient.

2.4. Data Collection and Analysis. Data were collected on CRF which was designed to capture demographic (age, sex) and clinical data and outcome. Data were entered onto a predesigned electronic CRF using Epi-Info version 3.5.1. and transferred to Stata version 10 (StataCorp, TX, USA), for analysis. Descriptive analysis of baseline characteristics was compared in both groups. Exposure-outcome relationship was explored using univariate, bivariate, stratified, and multivariate analysis as appropriate. Risks of adverse outcomes in both groups were calculated and compared using risk ratios with 95% confidence intervals. Student's t-test was used to assess differences in the means of continuous variables and significant levels were assessed using P value of <0.05.

2.5. Ethical Considerations. A written informed consent form (ICF) detailing the study purpose, benefit, and possible risks to participants and their caregivers was provided. Authorization to conduct the study was obtained from the Head of Department of Child Health and the Medical Director of KATH. Ethical clearance was obtained from the Committee on Human Research Publication and Ethics of the Kwame Nkrumah University of Science and Technology, Kumasi, Ghana. Written informed consent was received from the parents/caregivers of the patients. Assent was sought from patients older than 8 years.

3. Results

Over the course of 4 months, 215 subjects with dysglycaemia were recruited and matched for age group and diagnosis category with 215 euglycaemic subjects. In total, 800 subjects were screened (546 euglycemic, 34 hypoglycaemic, and 220 hyperglycaemic).

Tables 1 and 2 describe the demographic and clinical characteristics of the 430 subjects with euglycaemia and with dysglycaemia. The median age of the subjects was 24 months (range: 3–144 months). The proportion of males and females was similar (60% boys in the euglycemic group and 55% boys in the dysglycaemia group). In the dysglycaemia group, 28 (13%) out of 215 subjects had hypoglycemia and

TABLE 1: Demographic characteristics.

| Age (months) | Euglycaemia n (%) | Dysglycaemia n (%) | | |
		All	Hypoglycemia	Hyperglycemia
3.0–23.9	101 (47)	101 (47)	17 (61)	84 (45)
24.0–59.9	58 (27)	58 (27)	5 (18)	53 (28)
60.0–144.0	56 (26)	56 (26)	6 (21)	50 (27)
All ages	215	215	28	187

Data are given as n (% of the patients with euglycemia or with dysglycemia (all, hypoglycemia and hyperglycemia)).

TABLE 2: Clinical features of children presenting with acute medical conditions at PEU (n = 430).

Symptom*	Frequency n	Percent (%)
Fever	377	88
Vomiting	289	67
Diarrhea	125	29
Poor feeding	227	53
Convulsion	110	26
Cough	148	35
Rhinorrhoea	77	18
Other symptoms**	230	54
Clinical signs		
Flaring	84	20
Intercostal recessions	57	13
Other clinical signs***	41	10

* Subjects can present with one or more symptoms or clinical signs.
** "Other symptoms" included chills, bodily pains, repeated convulsions, earache, ear discharge, painful throat, dysuria, headache, and abdominal pain.
*** "Other clinical signs" included inflamed tonsils, pallor, abdominal tenderness, and inflamed eardrum.

TABLE 3: Categories of diagnosis in children presenting with acute medical conditions at PEU (n = 430).

Diagnosis	Frequency (n)	Percent (%)
Severe malaria	162	38
Severe malaria with acute disease	22	5
Assumed severe malaria	50	12
Septicaemia	40	9
Enteric fever	14	3
Meningitis	16	4
Diarrhea and vomiting	46	11
Acute respiratory disease	46	11
Sickle cell disease with acute disease	28	6
Others	6	1

Malaria with acute disease: malaria with one of the following: septicaemia, enteric fever, meningitis, or pneumonia.
Acute respiratory disease: acute asthma attack, pneumonia, or bronchiolitis.
Assumed severe malaria: patient with acute illness treated as severe malaria but not malaria parasites on blood film and negative blood, urine, and/or cerebrospinal fluid cultures. These patients improved on an antimalaria treatment.
Sickle cell disease (SCD) with acute disease: SCD with one of the following, severe malaria, severe anaemia, acute haemolysis, acute chest syndrome, septicaemia, and vasooclusive crisis.
Others: urinary tract infection, tonsillitis, and otitis media.

187 (87%) had hyperglycemia. Table 3 describes the medical conditions observed in the 430 subjects enrolled in the study. In keeping with the case-matching design of the study, the age distribution and the diagnosis categories were identical in euglycaemic and dysglycaemic subjects.

Table 4 describes the complications of the subjects at admission. Overall, there were 128 complications in 116 subjects. The number of subjects with complications was significantly higher in the dysglycaemia group (n = 99; 46%) compared to the euglycaemia group (n = 17; 8%) (P < 0.001). In the dysglycemia group, the proportion of subjects with complications was similar for hypoglycemia (13/28 subjects = 46%) and hyperglycemia (86/187 = 46%).

Table 5 shows the outcome at discharge of the subjects. The majority of the subjects (n = 382, 88%) had no complications at discharge and 8 (2%) were discharged with one or more complications. Six of them were in the dysglycemia group (hyperglycemia) (P < 0.001). Those who were discharged with complications were followed up till resolution. At the end of the study, 40 subjects had died. Death was statistically more common in subjects with dysglycaemia (n = 30) at admission than in euglycaemic subjects (n = 10) (Chi square test with Yates correction, P < 0.003). Among the 30 subjects with dysglycemia who died, 20 presented with

hyperglycemia (=11% of the subjects with hyperglycemia) and 10 with hypoglycemia (=36% of the subjects with hypoglycemia) (Chi square test with Yates correction, P = 0.001). The risk of dying or of developing complications for subjects with dysglycaemia was, respectively, 3 times (95% CI: 1.5–6.0) and 4.8 times higher (95% CI: 3.1–7.5) than for euglycaemic subjects (P < 0.001).

4. Discussion

The results of our study show that both hypoglycemia and hyperglycemia reflect increased severity of an acute medical condition in children presenting to the Emergency Room at KATH.

These figures are similar to findings in other studies. Elusiyan et al. [4] found out that presence of hypoglycaemia at admission was associated with death and dying within 24 hours of admission. Moreover, Osier et al. [5] in Kenya found out that mortality for children with abnormal blood glucose was 34.2% compared to 7.6% in euglycaemic children

TABLE 4: Complications among the participants.

	All	Euglycaemia n (%)	Dysglycaemia n (%)		
			All	Hypoglycemia	Hyperglycemia
DIC	9 (2)	1 (0.5)	8 (4)[#]	3 (11)	5 (3)
ARF	17 (4)	2 (1)	15 (7)[#]	4 (14)	11 (6)
Shock	39 (9)	4 (2)	35 (16)[#]	6 (21)	29 (16)
Hepatitis	8 (2)	2 (1)	6 (2)	0 (0)	6 (3)
IVH	28 (7)	6 (3)	22 (10)[#]	0 (0)	22 (12)
Other complications*	27 (7)	2 (2)	25 (11)[#]	3 (11)	22 (12)

DIC: disseminated intravascular coagulation; ARF: acute respiratory failure; IVH: intraventricular hemorrhage.
*"Other complications" include cortical blindness, hemiparesis, haemoglobinuria, heart failure, hypoglycaemia, intestinal perforation, and repeated convulsions.
[#]$P < 0.05$ compared to corresponding group with euglycemia.
Data are given as n (%). % reflects the percentage of complications in all subjects ($n = 430$), in subjects with euglycemia ($n = 215$) and in subjects with dysglycemia (all ($n = 215$), hypoglycemia ($n = 28$), or hyperglycemia ($n = 187$)). There were 128 complications in 116 subjects.

TABLE 5: Outcome at discharge.

Outcome	All n (%)	Euglycaemia n (%)	Dysglycaemia n (%)		
			All	Hypoglycemia	Hyperglycemia
Discharge without complications	382 (89)	203 (94)	177 (83)	18 (64)	159 (85)
Discharge with complications	8 (2)	2 (1)	6 (3)	0 (0)	6 (4)
Death	40 (9)	10 (5)	30 (14)	10 (36)	20 (11)
All	430 (100)	215 (100)	215 (100)	28 (100)	187 (100)

admitted to an emergency ward. Furthermore, Dungan et al. [9] demonstrated that mortality in hyperglycaemic children was about twice as much as that in euglycaemic children even though the correlation between blood sugar and mortality could not be established. Additionally, a study in Mozambique revealed that mortality in children with acute medical disease was 16.3% in children with hypoglycaemia compared to 3.2% in those who were normoglycaemic [10].

Accordingly, we found out that subjects with dysglycaemia were 3 times more likely to die and 4.8 times more likely to have complications than those with euglycemia. Solomon et al. [11] found a relative risk of 5.8 for mortality in children with acute medical conditions and hypoglycaemia in Mozambique. The relative risk of dying of hypoglycaemia in the Mozambique study was about twice that of this study. Whilst the sample sizes of the Mozambique study (603 children) and our study were similar, the different results may be explained by differences in the selection of the study participants. Overall, the value of dysglycemia as a prognostic factor for mortality and morbidity seems well established.

In our study, the commonest disease found to be associated with dysglycaemia was severe malaria. This is not surprising as malaria is a common infection in most parts of Africa, including Ghana. The other common disease conditions we encountered were diarrhea and vomiting, acute respiratory diseases, and septicaemia. Various diseases have been established in other studies to be associated with abnormal blood glucose including severe malaria [12–15], gastroenteritis [16], septicaemia [17, 18], pneumonia [19], and acute febrile seizures [2]. Elusiyan et al. [4] in Nigeria found that hypoglycaemia was associated with severe malaria,

septicaemia, pneumonia, and protein energy malnutrition among children admitted to a paediatric emergency ward.

Looking more in depth at malaria, the most common condition identified in this study, the link between dysglycaemia and severity of the disease is not completely understood. In a mostly pediatric population, Eltahir et al. [20] observed hyperglycemia in severe cerebral malaria which was secondary to an increase in insulin resistance and, possibly, to a decrease in insulin production. On the other hand, hypoglycemia is also commonly reported in children with severe malaria, more so in Africa than in other continents [21]. The reason is unclear and may reflect differences in nutritional status, infection itself, genetic predisposition, or preadmission use of quinine. Indeed, quinine, which is commonly used for treatment of severe malaria in many parts of Africa, including Ghana, has been suggested to affect insulin secretion. Abdallah et al. [22] observed hypoglycemia in 12% of adult subjects receiving intravenous quinine for severe malaria. However, Kawo et al. [23] did not observe significant changes in blood glucose in subjects with falciparum malaria receiving intravenous administration of quinine.

Putting together, these data suggest that early recognition of dysglycaemia in subjects with acute illness should prompt the health professional to adopt a more aggressive management approach.

Several issues remain to be clarified. First, there is a need for a better definition of the severity of hypoglycemia with regard to the increased risk of morbidity and mortality [24]. Second, whether correction of dysglycemia in addition to aggressive management of the underlying condition is beneficial to the subject remains unclear. However, administration of glucose is recommended by the WHO [25] and advocated by some authors [11, 12, 26]. A recent review on the effect of acute hypoglycemia management in children suggests that the evidence remains insufficient and that longer term studies are needed [27]. Similarly, two recent reviews did not find that, although good glycemic control may improve outcome [28, 29], the role of hyperglycemia management in critically ill children was clearly demonstrated [30].

A strength of our study is the prospective, case matched cohort design. Previous studies that compared the health outcomes according to glycaemia at admission did include all patients without attempt to matching. As dysglycaemia is much less common than euglycaemia, this resulted in groups of very different sizes and etiologies [4, 5]. While the latter design allows for a description of the epidemiology of subjects with dysglycemia, our design is stronger when it comes to comparing the outcomes.

5. Conclusion

Abnormal blood glucose (dysglycaemia) is associated with increased morbidity and mortality in children with acute medical conditions on admission. Fatal outcome was more common in those who are hypoglycemic at admission. We suggest that all children with acute medical condition should be screened for dysglycaemia at admission and that abnormal blood glucose should promote aggressive management of the underlying condition. The role of hypo- or hyperglycemia management in the overall treatment plan remains unclear.

Conflict of Interests

The authors declare that there is no conflict of interests regarding the publication of this paper.

Acknowledgments

The European Society for Pediatric Endocrinology (ESPE) supported the project. The authors are grateful to Mrs. Georgina Yeboah, the Head of the Human Resource Unit, KATH, for helping them with 2 national service personnel to help in data collection. They are profoundly thankful to these national service members Benjamin Adomako and Bernard Ohene-Amoah for their invaluable work.

References

[1] D. M. Bhisitkul, A. I. Vinik, A. L. Morrow et al., "Prediabetic markers in children with stress hyperglycemia," Archives of Pediatrics and Adolescent Medicine, vol. 150, no. 9, pp. 936–941, 1996.

[2] G. Valerio, A. Franzese, E. Carlin, P. Pecile, R. Perini, and A. Tenore, "High prevalence of stress hyperglycaemia in children with febrile seizures and traumatic injuries," Acta Paediatrica, International Journal of Paediatrics, vol. 90, no. 6, pp. 618–622, 2001.

[3] D. M. Bhisitkul, A. L. Morrow, A. I. Vinik, J. Shults, J. C. Layland, and R. Rohn, "Prevalence of stress hyperglycemia among patients attending a pediatric emergency department," Journal of Pediatrics, vol. 124, no. 4, pp. 547–551, 1994.

[4] J. B. E. Elusiyan, E. A. Adejuyigbe, and O. O. Adeodu, "Hypoglycaemia in a Nigerian paediatric emergency ward," Journal of Tropical Pediatrics, vol. 52, no. 2, pp. 96–102, 2006.

[5] F. H. A. Osier, J. A. Berkley, A. Ross, F. Sanderson, S. Mohammed, and C. R. J. C. Newton, "Abnormal blood glucose concentrations on admission to a rural Kenyan district hospital: Prevalence and outcome," Archives of Disease in Childhood, vol. 88, no. 7, pp. 621–625, 2003.

[6] D. Kwiatkowski, A. V. S. Hill, I. Sambou et al., "TNF concentration in fatal cerebral, non-fatal cerebral, and uncomplicated Plasmodium falciparum malaria," The Lancet, vol. 336, no. 8725, pp. 1201–1204, 1990.

[7] K. A. Wintergerst, B. Buckingham, L. Gandrud, B. J. Wong, S. Kache, and D. M. Wilson, "Association of hypoglycemia, hyperglycemia, and glucose variability with morbidity and death in the pediatric intensive care unit," Pediatrics, vol. 118, no. 1, pp. 173–179, 2006.

[8] D. R. Langdon, C. A. Stanley, and M. A. Sperling, "Hypoglycemia in the infant and child," in Pediatric Endocrinology, M. A. Sperling, Ed., pp. 422–443, Saunders Elsevier, Philadelphia, Pa, USA, 3rd edition, 2008.

[9] K. M. Dungan, S. S. Braithwaite, and J.-C. Preiser, "Stress hyperglycaemia," The Lancet, vol. 373, no. 9677, pp. 1798–1807, 2009.

[10] P. Gupta, G. Natarajan, and K. N. Agarwal, "Transient hyperglycemia in acute childhood illnesses: to attend or ignore?" Indian Journal of Pediatrics, vol. 64, no. 2, pp. 205–210, 1997.

[11] T. Solomon, J. M. Felix, M. Samuel et al., "Hypoglycaemia in paediatric admissions in Mozambique," The Lancet, vol. 343, no. 8890, pp. 149–150, 1994.

[12] M. English, S. Wale, G. Binns, I. Mwangi, H. Sauerwein, and K. Marsh, "Hypoglycaemia on and after admission in Kenyan children with severe malaria," QJM, vol. 91, no. 3, pp. 191–197, 1998.

[13] H. V. Thien, P. A. Kager, and H. P. Sauerwein, "Hypoglycemia in falciparum malaria: is fasting an unrecognized and insufficiently emphasized risk factor?" Trends in Parasitology, vol. 22, no. 9, pp. 410–415, 2006.

[14] W. Zijlmans, A. van Kempen, M. Ackermans, J. de Metz, P. Kager, and H. Sauerwein, "Glucose kinetics during fasting in young children with severe and non-severe malaria in suriname," The American Journal of Tropical Medicine and Hygiene, vol. 79, no. 4, pp. 605–612, 2008.

[15] D. Waller, S. Krishna, J. Crawley et al., "Clinical features and outcome of severe malaria in Gambian children," Clinical Infectious Diseases, vol. 21, no. 3, pp. 577–587, 1995.

[16] J. V. Bjerre, "Stress hyperglycemia in a child with severe acute gastroenteritis," Ugeskrift for Laeger, vol. 164, no. 47, pp. 5524–5525, 2002.

[17] F. de Groof, K. F. M. Joosten, J. A. M. J. L. Janssen et al., "Acute stress response in children with meningococcal sepsis: important differences in the growth hormone/insulin-like growth factor I axis between nonsurvivors and survivors," The Journal of Clinical Endocrinology and Metabolism, vol. 87, no. 7, pp. 3118–3124, 2002.

[18] D. A. van Waardenburg, T. C. Jansen, G. D. Vos, and W. A. Buurman, "Hyperglycemia in children with meningococcal sepsis and septic shock: the relation between plasma levels of insulin and inflammatory mediators," The Journal of Clinical

Endocrinology & Metabolism, vol. 91, no. 10, pp. 3916–3921, 2006.

[19] M. Don, G. Valerio, M. Korppi, and M. Canciani, "Hyper- and hypoglycemia in children with community-acquired pneumonia," *Journal of Pediatric Endocrinology and Metabolism*, vol. 21, no. 7, pp. 657–664, 2008.

[20] E. M. Eltahir, G. ElGhazali, T. M. E. A-Elgadir, I. E. A-Elbasit, M. I. Elbashir, and H. A. Giha, "Raised plasma insulin level and homeostasis model assessment (HOMA) score in cerebral malaria: evidence for insulin resistance and marker of virulence," *Acta Biochimica Polonica*, vol. 57, no. 4, pp. 513–520, 2010.

[21] L. Manning, M. Laman, W. A. Davis, and T. M. E. Davis, "Clinical features and outcome in children with severe *Plasmodium falciparum* malaria: a meta-analysis," *PLoS ONE*, vol. 9, no. 2, Article ID e86737, 2014.

[22] T. M. Abdallah, K. A. Elmardi, A. H. Elhassan et al., "Comparison of artesunate and quinine in the treatment of severe *Plasmodium falciparum* malaria at Kassala hospital, Sudan," *Journal of Infection in Developing Countries*, vol. 8, no. 5, pp. 611–615, 2014.

[23] N. G. Kawo, A. E. Msengi, A. B. M. Swai, H. Orskov, K. G. M. M. Alberti, and D. G. McLarty, "The metabolic effects of quinine in children with severe and complicated *Plasmodium falciparum* malaria in Dar es Salaam," *Transactions of the Royal Society of Tropical Medicine and Hygiene*, vol. 85, no. 6, pp. 711–713, 1991.

[24] M. L. Willcox, M. Forster, M. I. Dicko, B. Graz, R. Mayon-White, and H. Barennes, "Blood glucose and prognosis in children with presumed severe malaria: is there a threshold for "hypoglycaemia"?" *Tropical Medicine & International Health*, vol. 15, no. 2, pp. 232–240, 2010.

[25] http://www.who.int/elena/titles/hypoglycaemia_sam/en/index.html.

[26] E. Sambany, E. Pussard, C. Rajaonarivo, H. Raobijaona, and H. Barennes, "Childhood dysglycemia: prevalence and outcome in a referral hospital," *PLoS ONE*, vol. 8, no. 5, Article ID e65193, 2013.

[27] R. Achoki, N. Opiyo, and M. English, "Mini-review: management of hypoglycaemia in children aged 0–59 months," *Journal of Tropical Pediatrics*, vol. 56, no. 4, Article ID fmp109, pp. 227–234, 2009.

[28] P. E. Marik and M. Raghavan, "Stress-hyperglycemia, insulin and immunomodulation in sepsis," *Intensive Care Medicine*, vol. 30, no. 5, pp. 748–756, 2004.

[29] G. van den Berghe and D. Mesotten, "Paediatric endocrinology: tight glycaemic control in critically ill children," *Nature Reviews Endocrinology*, vol. 10, no. 4, pp. 196–197, 2014.

[30] S. M. Ng and S. Balmuri, "Review of insulin treatment in stress-related hyperglycaemia in children without preexisting diabetes," *Acta Paediatrica*, vol. 103, no. 1, pp. 6–9, 2014.

Comparative Effect of Massage Therapy versus Kangaroo Mother Care on Body Weight and Length of Hospital Stay in Low Birth Weight Preterm Infants

Priya Singh Rangey and Megha Sheth

S.B.B. College of Physiotherapy, V.S. Hospital Campus, Ellisbridge, Ahmedabad, Gujarat 380006, India

Correspondence should be addressed to Priya Singh Rangey; priya_singh9192@yahoo.in

Academic Editor: R. W. Jennings

Background. Massage therapy (MT) and kangaroo mother care (KMC) are both effective in increasing the weight and reducing length of hospital stay in low birth weight preterm infants but they have not been compared. *Aim*. Comparison of effectiveness of MT and KMC on body weight and length of hospital stay in low birth weight preterm (LBWPT) infants. *Method*. 30 LBWPT infants using convenience sampling from Neonatal Intensive Care Unit, V.S. hospital, were randomly divided into 2 equal groups. Group 1 received MT and Group 2 received KMC for 15 minutes, thrice daily for 5 days. Medically stable babies with gestational age < 37 weeks and birth weight < 2500 g were included. Those on ventilators and with congenital, orthopedic, or genetic abnormality were excluded. Outcome measures, body weight and length of hospital stay, were taken before intervention day 1 and after intervention day 5. Level of significance was 5%. *Result*. Data was analyzed using SPSS16. Both MT and KMC were found to be effective in improving body weight ($P = 0.001$, $P = 0.001$). Both were found to be equally effective for improving body weight ($P = 0.328$) and reducing length of hospital stay ($P = 0.868$). *Conclusion*. MT and KMC were found to be equally effective in improving body weight and reducing length of hospital stay. *Limitation*. Long term follow-up was not taken.

1. Introduction

Preterm birth is defined as childbirth occurring at less than 37 completed weeks or 259 days of gestation [1].

Low birth weight (LBW), defined as weight at birth of less than 2500 grams irrespective of gestational age, has an adverse effect on child survival and development and may even be an important risk factor for adult diseases [2].

Newborn deaths currently account for approximately 40% of all deaths of children under five years of age in developing countries—the three major causes being birth asphyxia, infections, and complications due to prematurity and LBW [3]. Birth weight is a significant determinant of newborn survival. LBW is an underlying factor in 60–80% of all neonatal deaths. LBW infants are approximately 20 times more likely to die, compared with heavier babies [4].

Children who are born prematurely have higher rates of cerebral palsy, sensory deficits, learning disabilities, and respiratory illnesses compared with children born at term. The morbidity associated with preterm birth often extends to later life, resulting in enormous physical, psychological, and economic costs [5].

Researchers have provided hospitalized preterm infants with various forms of supplemental stimulation in an effort to enrich the environment of the neonatal intensive care unit (NICU) or to accelerate development [6, 7]. Two of the most widely studied interventions have been massage therapy and kangaroo mother care. In developing countries, financial and human resources for neonatal care are limited and hospital wards for LBW infants are often overcrowded [8]. KMC and MT are cost effective approaches that can be used by one and all irrespective of their financial status.

Massage is referred to as "a methodological touch intended to stimulate the baby." A number of studies have shown the positive effects of massage therapy in preterm infants. These positive effects include weight gain, improved

Comparative Effect of Massage Therapy versus Kangaroo Mother Care on Body Weight and Length...

29

TABLE 1: Comparison of means of body weight in Groups A and B.

Parameter	Group	Pre	Post	Z value	P value	Significance
Body weight (kgs)	A	1.53 ± 0.26	1.57 ± 0.25	-3.412	0.001	Yes
	B	1.46 ± 0.23	1.51 ± 0.22	-3.353	0.001	Yes

TABLE 2: Comparison of difference of means of Groups A and B for body weight and length of hospital stay.

Parameter	Group A	Group B	U value	P value	Significance
Body weight (gms)	45.3 ± 22.08	41.0 ± 29.83	89	0.328	No
Length of hospital stay (days)	22.13 ± 4.31	21.87 ± 3.33	108.5	0.868	No

sleep/wake states, decreased stress, early discharge from the NICU, improved skin integrity, increased development of the sympathetic nervous system, and enhanced parent-infant bonding [9].

In 1978, Rey and Martinez proposed and developed Kangaroo mother care (KMC) at Instituto Materno Infantil in Santa Fe de Bogotá, Colombia, as an alternative to the conventional contemporary method of care for LBW infants. The term KMC is derived from similarities to marsupial care-giving. The mothers are used as "incubators" and as the main source of food and stimulation for LBW infants while they mature enough to face extrauterine life in similar conditions as those born at term [10]. Kangaroo mother care is defined as "Early, prolonged and continuous skin-to-skin contact between the mother and low birth weight infant both in the hospital and after discharge with exclusive breastfeeding and proper follow-up" [10]. Kangaroo mother care regularizes heart rate and respirations, deepens sleep and alert inactivity, reduces crying, prevents infections, shortens the neonatal hospital stay, enhances weight gain, improves physical growth and breastfeeding rates, decreases pain from heel prick procedure, and lessens maternal depression [8, 11–14].

Massage therapy (MT) and kangaroo mother care (KMC) are both effective in increasing the weight in low birth weight preterm infants and reducing the hospital stay. But still, they have not been compared to know which is more effective.

2. Aims and Objectives

The aims and objectives of this study are to compare the effectiveness of massage therapy and kangaroo mother care on weight gain and length of hospital stay in low birth weight preterm infants.

3. Materials and Methods

A quasi-experimental study was conducted with a convenience sample of 30 subjects at the NICU of V. S. Hospital in 2013. Infants born at gestational age of <37 weeks, having low birth weight, and medically stable were included and those who were medically unstable, had any congenital, orthopedic, or genetic abnormality, or were ventilated were excluded. Informed consent was taken from the parents. The infants were randomly divided in 2 groups with 15 infants in each

group. Group 1 received 15 minutes of MT thrice daily for 5 days. Group 2 received at least 15 minutes of KMC thrice daily and it was continued later on as well by the mother with the physiotherapist in the NICU for 5 days. Body weight was taken before intervention on day 1 and after intervention on day 5, whereas length of hospital stay was calculated from the day of birth to discharge. Level of significance was kept at 5%.

MT was given according to the Field massage therapy protocol. Infants were massaged for 15 minutes, 3 times each day, at least 1 hour after being fed. Each massage session consisted of 5 minutes of tactile stimulation, 5 minutes of kinesthetic stimulation, and another 5 minutes of tactile stimulation. During the tactile stimulation the infant was placed in a prone (face down) position and given moderate pressure stroking with the bottom of the fingers of both hands. During the kinesthetic stimulation, the infant was placed in a supine (on back) position and led through passive flexion/extension actions [6]. For massage therapy, coconut oil was used as it has been found to be better than mineral oil [15].

During KMC the infant, wearing only a nappy (diaper), was placed between the mother's uncovered breasts. The mother was seated on a standard rocking chair, tilted at an angle of approximately 60°.

4. Results

Data was analyzed using SPSS version 16. Wilcoxon test was applied to determine whether there was significant difference within the groups. Mann Whitney-U test was applied to determine whether there was any significant difference between both groups or not. Both MT and KMC, respectively, were found to be effective in improving body weight ($P = 0.001$, $P = 0.001$) as shown in Table 1. However, both were found to be equally effective for improving body weight ($P = 0.328$) and reducing hospital stay ($P = 0.868$) as shown in Table 2.

5. Discussion

These findings show that MT and KMC promote weight gain and reduce hospital stay. There was an increase in body weight in the MT group similar to the findings of Dieter et al. who in 2003 studied that massage therapy leads to weight gain [16]. Dieter et al. in 2003 examined the effects of 5 days of massage therapy on the weight gain and sleep/wake behavior of hospitalized stable preterm infants and concluded that even 5 days of massage therapy were effective in improving weight and reducing sleep instead of 10 days that were practiced earlier [16].

It has been noticed that the neonates who gained more weight in the previous studies neither ingested more calories, nor spent more time sleeping, which might have allowed them more time to digest. In response to these findings Diego et al. in 2008 explored a theory that moderate pressure massage stimulates vagal activity (the activation of the vagal nerve is an index of parasympathetic nervous system activation), which leads to an increase in the release of digestive hormones and an increase in gastric motility.

Massage has also been shown to help neonates decrease stress behaviors and activities. The pacifying effect that massage has on preterm infants could benefit their health and reduce their length of time in the NICU. It may also desensitize the neonates to the stressful environment of the NICU by prolonging the time of parasympathetic activity (the resting, steady state, or nonstressed state of the autonomic nervous system). This in turn relates to increased vagal activity, which, as discussed earlier, leads to weight gain [17].

There was also a reduction in the length of hospital stay. The same findings were observed by Mendes and Procianoy in 2008. They studied the effect of maternal massage therapy on hospital stay in very low birth weight infants who were already submitted to skin-to-skin care and concluded that maternal massage therapy in very low birth weight infants decreases the length of hospital stay and the incidence of late-onset neonatal sepsis [18]. This reduction might be attributed to the improvement in body weight of the infant, improved sleep-wake states, improved immunity, and reduced stress behaviors and activity after massage therapy.

In the KMC group there was an increase in body weight and reduction in hospital stay. Roberts et al. in 2000 compared KMC with conventional cuddling care and found that KMC led to an improvement in body weight but it was equal to the weight gain observed in the conventional cuddling group [19]. They also observed that KMC leads to a reduction in the length of hospital stay. Cattaneo et al. also concluded that KMC infants have a higher mean daily weight gain and are discharged earlier compared to infants receiving conventional methods of care [20].

The weight gain in the KMC group might be due to improved breastfeeding rates, improved vagal tone, improved sleep cycles, and improved metabolic rates. Similarly the reduction in the hospital stay may be attributed to an overall decline in the infection rates and illnesses. Also, improved mother-infant bonding leads to a better health condition.

6. Conclusion

MT and KMC are both equally effective in improving weight and reducing hospital stay. MT and KMC can be used interchangeably as both are equally effective. In settings where professionals are not available to apply MT, KMC can be used in place of massage. KMC is also more community friendly as it does not require any special set-up or training. It

can be given at any time according to the mother's wish. Also, the procedure can be performed by any other family member in absence of the mother.

Limitations. There are several factors that can have an effect on the outcome measures used in this study. Here, such factors like feeding amount and urine and stool output for body weight, basal metabolic rate, measures, and so forth were not monitored. Also, there are several measures to monitor the vagal activity like electroencephalography, electrogastrography, and so forth. But these measures are beyond the scope of physiotherapy. But still, they should also be monitored.

Ethical Approval

Ethical approval was taken from the Institutional Ethics Committee of S.B.B College of Physiotherapy, V.S General Hospital, Ahmedabad, Gujarat.

Conflict of Interests

The authors declare that they have no conflict of interests regarding the publication of this paper.

Acknowledgments

The authors thank the neonates and their parents who participated in this study. They would also like to thank their colleagues and staff members and all those who supported this study. Special and heart-warming thanks are due to Dr. Neeta Vyas and Dr. Shraddha Diwan for their invaluable help and support in this study.

References

[1] *International Classification of Diseases and Related Health Problems. 10th Revision*, World Health Organization, Geneva, Switzerland, 1992.

[2] D. J. P. Barker, "The fetal and infant origins of disease," *European Journal of Clinical Investigation*, vol. 25, no. 7, pp. 457–463, 1995.

[3] J. Standley, "Kangaroo mother care implementation guide. Washington (District of Columbia): Maternal and Child Health Integrated Program," 2011, http://www.mchip.net/sites/default/files/MCHIP%20KMC%20Guide.pdf.

[4] M. S. Kramer, "Intrauterine growth and gestational duration determinants," *Pediatrics*, vol. 80, no. 4, pp. 502–511, 1987.

[5] S. Petrou, "The economic consequences of preterm birth during the first 10 years of life," *BJOG: An International Journal of Obstetrics and Gynaecology*, vol. 112, no. 1, pp. 10–15, 2005.

[6] J. N. I. Dieter and E. K. Emory, "Supplemental stimulation of premature infants: a treatment model," *Journal of Pediatric Psychology*, vol. 22, pp. 281–295, 1997.

[7] R. Feldman and A. I. Eidelman, "Intervention programs for premature infants: how and do they affect development?" *Clinics in Perinatology*, vol. 25, no. 3, pp. 613–626, 1998.

[8] A. Conde-Agudelo, J. M. Belizán, and J. L. Diaz-Rossello, "Kangaroo mother care to reduce morbidity and mortality in low birthweight infants (Review)," *The Cochrane Library*, vol. 3, 2011.

[9] Leonard J, "Exploring neonatal touch," *The Wesleyan Journal of Psychology*, vol. 3, pp. 39–47, 2008.

[10] E. Rey and H. Martinez, *Manejo Racional del Nino Prematuro*, Universidad Nacional, Cursod eMedicina Fetal, Bogota, Colombia, 1983.

[11] J. E. Lawn, J. Mwansa-Kambafwile, B. L. Horta, F. C. Barros, and S. Cousens, "'Kangaroo mother care' to prevent neonatal deaths due to preterm birth complications," *International Journal of Epidemiology*, vol. 39, pp. i144–154, 2010.

[12] G. C. Anderson, "Current knowledge about skin-to-skin (kangaroo) care for preterm infants," *Journal of Perinatology*, vol. 11, no. 3, pp. 216–226, 1991.

[13] S. Nimbalkar, N. Chaudhary, K. Gadhavi, and A. Phatak, "Kangaroo mother care in reducing pain in preterm neonates on heel prick," *The Indian Journal of Pediatrics*, vol. 80, no. 1, pp. 6–10, 2013.

[14] A. Alencar, L. Arraes, E. de Albuquerque, and J. Alves, "Effect of kangaroo mother care on postpartum depression," *Journal of Tropical Pediatrics*, vol. 55, no. 1, pp. 36–38, 2009.

[15] K. Sankaranarayanan, J. A. Mondkar, M. M. Chauhan, B. M. Mascarenhas, A. R. Mainkar, and R. Y. Salvi, "Oil massage in neonates: an open randomized controlled study of coconut versus mineral oil," *Indian Pediatrics*, vol. 42, no. 9, pp. 877–884, 2005.

[16] J. N. I. Dieter, T. Field, M. Hernandez-Reif, E. K. Emory, and M. Redzepi, "Stable preterm infants gain more weight and sleep less after five days of massage therapy," *Journal of Pediatric Psychology*, vol. 28, no. 6, pp. 403–411, 2003.

[17] M. A. Diego, T. Field, and M. Hernandez-Reif, "Temperature increases in preterm infants during massage therapy," *Infant Behavior and Development*, vol. 31, no. 1, pp. 149–152, 2008.

[18] E. W. Mendes and R. S. Procianoy, "Massage therapy reduces hospital stay and occurrence of late-onset sepsis in very preterm neonates," *Journal of Perinatology*, vol. 28, no. 12, pp. 815–820, 2008.

[19] K. L. Roberts, C. Paynter, and B. McEwan, "A comparison of kangaroo mother care and conventional cuddling care," *Neonatal Network*, vol. 19, no. 4, pp. 31–35, 2000.

[20] A. Cattaneo, R. Davanzo, B. Worku et al., "Kangaroo mother care for low birthweight infants: a randomized controlled trial in different settings," *Acta Paediatrica*, vol. 87, no. 9, pp. 976–985, 1998.

6

Computer Game Use and Television Viewing Increased Risk for Overweight among Low Activity Girls: Fourth Thai National Health Examination Survey 2008-2009

Ladda Mo-suwan,[1] **Jiraluck Nontarak,**[2]
Wichai Aekplakorn,[2,3] **and Warapone Satheannoppakao**[4]

[1] *Department of Pediatrics, Faculty of Medicine, Prince of Songkla University, Songkhla 90110, Thailand*
[2] *Office of National Health Examination Survey, Health System Research Institute, Bangkok 11000, Thailand*
[3] *Department of Community Medicine, Faculty of Medicine Ramathibodi Hospital, Mahidol University, Bangkok 10400, Thailand*
[4] *Faculty of Public Health, Mahidol University, Bangkok 10400, Thailand*

Correspondence should be addressed to Ladda Mo-suwan; ladda.m@psu.ac.th

Academic Editor: Alessandro Mussa

Studies of the relationship between sedentary behaviors and overweight among children and adolescents show mixed results. The fourth Thai National Health Examination Survey data collected between 2008 and 2009 were used to explore this association in 5,999 children aged 6 to 14 years. The prevalence of overweight defined by the age- and gender-specific body mass index cut-points of the International Obesity Task Force was 16%. Using multiple logistic regression, computer game use for more than 1 hour a day was found to be associated with an increased risk of overweight (adjusted odds ratio (AOR) = 1.4; 95% confidence interval: 1.02–1.93). The effect of computer game use and TV viewing on the risk for overweight was significantly pronounced among girls who spent ≤3 days/week in 60 minutes of moderate-intensity physical activity (AOR = 1.99 and 1.72, resp.). On the contrary, these sedentary behaviors did not exert significant risk for overweight among boys. The moderating effect on risk of overweight by physical inactivity and media use should be taken into consideration in designing the interventions for overweight control in children and adolescents. Tracking societal changes is essential for identification of potential areas for targeted interventions.

1. Introduction

Childhood obesity has emerged as a significant health problem in a transitional society. Rapidly changing dietary practices and a sedentary lifestyle have led to a high prevalence of childhood overweight and obesity among school-aged children (defined by the International Obesity Task Force cut-points) in developing countries between 2004 and 2010: 41.8% in Mexico, 22.1% in Brazil, 13.3–22.3% in South Africa, 27.9% in Argentina, and 2.8–28% in India [1]. In Thailand, data from the two national surveys demonstrated an increase of the obesity prevalence among the 6- to 12-year-old children from 5.8% in 1997 to 6.7% in 2001 by using the weight-for-height criteria of a local reference [2]. This rising trend coincided with an increase of type 2 diabetes among Thai

diabetic pediatric patients from 5% between 1986 and 1995 to 17.9% between 1996 and 1999 [3].

Increased energy content in diet, decreased levels of physical activity, and increased sedentary lifestyles as well as a number of cultural and environmental factors have been identified as the causes of obesity in children [4–6]. In the Thai context, determinants of overweight and obesity among children in previous reports included having obese parents, being in a family with a high income, maternal overweight prior to pregnancy, high birth weight, being the only child, large amounts of food consumed by children, having a lesser amount of exercise than peers, and TV viewing time more than 2 hours per day [7–10].

Changes in several social and environmental factors have been suggested as causes of the "obesity epidemic" among children, for example, reduced physical education at school, increased homework loads, school vending machines, TV, larger food portion sizes, fast-food restaurants, video games, and many others [11]. Time spent in seated sedentary behaviors (SB) (e.g., electronic media use) reduces time allocation for physical activity (PA) and hence increases risk of overweight and obesity. Moreover, snack and sugar-sweetened beverage consumption while watching TV further augments the positive energy balance. Children worldwide have increasing access to electronic media, such as TV, computer/video games, cell phones, and the internet in daily life. In Thailand, the number of internet cafés which provide online game service increased 1.8 times over 2 years from 2008 to 2010 [12]. The fourth National Health Examination Survey in Thailand revealed that 5% of the 6 to 9 year olds and 12% of the 10 to 14 year olds engaged in computer games more than 1 hour each day, while 57.1% and 73.1%, respectively, watched TV more than 2 hours/day during the weekdays [13]. A report from the Child and Adolescent Mental Health Center in Bangkok demonstrated an increase in the game addiction rate from 5% in 2005 to 9% in 2009 [12]. In regard to media use, an association of sedentary behavior, primarily through TV viewing, with body mass index (BMI) and obesity has been well documented [14, 15], while the relationship of seated computer game use with obesity was unclear. Most of the studies investigated total screen time including TV viewing, working on a computer, and playing video games [15, 16]. A limited number of studies that looked at computer games independently had mixed results [16–19].

In order to gain an understanding of the current rising prevalence of childhood overweight, we used recent data from the fourth National Health Examination Survey (NHES IV) to investigate the associations of SB (i.e., time spent at computer gaming and television viewing) with overweight among children aged 6 to 14 years in Thailand. In addition, we examined whether the effect of screen time on overweight varied by physical activity status and gender.

2. Subjects and Methods

2.1. Design. The National Health Examination Surveys have been conducted every 5 years since 1991. The fourth National Health Examination Survey (NHES IV) 2008-2009 conducted by the National Health Examination Survey Office was designed to represent the noninstitutionalized Thai population using a multistage stratified sampling based on 2008 Thai population registers [20]. For the first stage, 5 provinces were randomly sampled by proportion to size (PPS) from each of the 4 regions, except Bangkok. In the second stage, 3 to 5 districts were selected by PPS from each province. In the third stage, in each province, 13-14 electoral units (EUs) or villages were selected by PPS from each of the urban and rural areas. In the final stage, for each EU/village, 8 to 10 males and 8 to 10 females were selected by systematic random sampling from population registers from each of the six broad age and gender groups (1–14-, 15–59-, and ≥60-year-old males/females). In Bangkok, 5 to 6 EUs were randomly

selected by PPS from each of the 12 districts. The final stage was identical to the methods used in other provinces.

2.2. Subjects. The NHES IV enrolled 29,485 subjects aged 1 to 60+ years. The final sample size of the 1- to 14-year-old subjects was 9,035 individuals (response rate of 92.8%). The response rate for boys and girls was 92.4% and 93.1%, respectively. This report presents an analysis of the data from the school-aged population: 5,999 children aged 6 to 14 years.

2.3. Data Collection. Subjects were weighed in light clothes using a Tanita scale and recorded to the nearest 0.1 kg. Standing heights were measured by trained research assistants using a locally made stadiometer and recorded to the nearest 0.1 cm.

Demographic and socioeconomic data were obtained by interviewing the parents. Information regarding dietary intake and physical and sedentary activities was taken by interviewing the parents of children under 10 years of age and the subjects themselves for those aged 10 years and older. The questions for media use were "How many hours a day during the past month did you watch television?" and "How many hours a day during the past month did you play computer games?" For physical activity, the question was "How many days during the past week did you have physical activity that increased your breathing rate and heart rate for at least 60 minutes?"

2.4. Statistical Analysis. Overweight was defined using the age- and gender-specific BMI cut-points of the International Obesity Task Force [21]. For media use, TV time was categorized into 2 hours/day or less and more than 2 hours/day according to the American Academy of Pediatrics recommendation [22] and time spent in playing computer games was classified into 1 hour/day or less and more than 1 hour/day. Exercise of moderate intensity was grouped into having 60 minutes for 3 days/week or more and less than 3 days/week. Since gender difference has been noted in the studies of obesity especially in relation to physical activity behaviors [15, 23], the analysis was thus computed separately for boys and girls. Distribution of all study variables was explored by descriptive statistics. Logistic regressions were computed to examine the association of media use and physical activity level with overweight. Consumption of high energy snacks (examples given were potato crisps and rice-shrimp crisps), which was highly associated with overweight in both male and female subjects, was selected as a covariate in the logistic regression analysis. In addition, family income, which was reported to be associated with overweight in Thai children, [7] was also included in the regression models. The analyses were performed using STATA 11.0 [24].

2.5. Ethical Clearance. The National Ethical Review Committee for Research in Human Subjects, Ministry of Public Health, approved the study. The sampled families were informed of the data collection process and verbal permission was obtained.

TABLE 1: Subject characteristics.

Characteristics	Total $N = 5{,}998$	Boys $n = 2{,}972$	Girls $n = 3{,}026$
Overweight (%, 95% CI)	16.0 (14.6–17.4)	16.7 (15.0–18.5)	15.2 (13.7–16.9)
Watching TV (%, 95% CI)	$N = 5{,}778$	$n = 2{,}854$	$n = 2{,}924$
More than 2 h/d	89.3 (88.1–90.3)	88.2 (86.8–89.5)	90.4 (88.8–91.8)
Computer game use (%, 95% CI)	$N = 5{,}777$	$n = 2{,}855$	$n = 2{,}922$
More than 1 h/d	5.2 (4.4–6.2)	7.1 (6.0–8.5)[#]	3.2 (2.5–4.1)[#]
Having 60 minutes of moderate-intensity physical activity (%, 95% CI)	$N = 5{,}925$	$n = 2{,}934$	$n = 2{,}991$
More than 3 d/wk	41.6 (38.4–44.9)	48.6 (44.6–52.7)[#]	34.4 (31.8–37.1)[#]
Frequency of high energy snack consumption (%, 95% CI)	$N = 5{,}985$	$n = 2{,}964$	$n = 3{,}021$
1 time/d or more	4.2 (3.5–4.9)	3.7 (2.9–4.7)	4.6 (4.0–5.3)
Family income (%, 95% CI)	$N = 5{,}374$	$n = 2{,}671$	$n = 2{,}703$
15,000 B/month or more	24.4 (21.5–27.5)	25.4 (22.5–28.6)	23.3 (20.1–26.8)

CI: confidence interval; [#]$P < 0.001$.

TABLE 2: Odds ratio for the associations of computer game use and television viewing with overweight by gender.

Variables	All		Boys		Girls	
	Unadjusted OR (95% CI)	Adjusted OR* (95% CI)	Unadjusted OR (95% CI)	Adjusted OR* (95% CI)	Unadjusted OR (95% CI)	Adjusted OR* (95% CI)
Computer game use						
1 h/d or less	1	1	1	1	1	1
More than 1 h/d	1.53 (1.13–2.06)	1.40 (1.02–1.93)	1.50 (1.11–2.03)	1.27 (0.92–1.76)	1.50 (0.91–2.45)	1.54 (0.95–2.49)
Watching TV						
2 h/d or less	1	1	1	1	1	1
More than 2 h/d	1.09 (0.88–1.35)	1.11 (0.89–1.39)	0.86 (0.66–1.12)	0.89 (0.68–1.16)	1.64 (1.17–2.30)	1.67 (1.17–2.40)
Having 60 minutes of moderate-intensity physical activity						
3 d/wk or less	1	1	1	1	1	1
More than 3 d/wk	0.71 (0.64–0.80)	0.75 (0.66–0.84)	0.78 (0.64–0.95)	0.85 (0.69–1.03)	0.60 (0.50–0.72)	0.62 (0.51–0.76)

CI: confidence interval. *Adjusted for high energy snack consumption and family income.

3. Results

Table 1 describes overweight prevalence, media use, physical activity, consumption of high energy snack, and family income characteristics of the subjects. Prevalence of overweight using age- and gender-specific BMI cut-points of the International Obesity Task Force [21] was 15.2% for girls versus 16.7% for boys. Most subjects watched TV more than 2 hours/day. On the other hand, only 5.2% engaged in computer games more than 1 hour/day; male subjects played computer games twice as much as the females ($P < 0.001$). Male subjects also engaged in moderate-intensity physical activity significantly more than the females ($P < 0.001$). No gender difference was noted in the frequency of having high energy snacks and family income levels.

The associations of media use and physical activity with overweight are shown in Table 2. From the multiple logistic regression analysis, computer game use and physical activity behavior had a significant effect on the likelihood of overweight among the 6- to 14-year-old subjects.

With the 1 hour/day or less as the referent group, use of computer games more than 1 hour/day increased the likelihood of overweight (adjusted odds ratio (AOR) = 1.40; 95% confidence interval (CI): 1.02–1.93), whereas children who engaged in 60 minutes of moderate-intensity physical activity for more than 3 days/week were less likely to be overweight (AOR = 0.75; 95% CI: 0.66–0.84). The subgroup analysis by gender shows different risks between boys and girls. Watching TV more than 2 hours/day significantly increased the risk for overweight (AOR = 1.67; 95% CI: 1.17–2.40), while engagement in moderate-intensity physical activity significantly decreased the risk among girls (AOR = 0.62; 95% CI: 0.51–0.76). For boys, associations of computer game use and engagement in moderate-intensity PA with overweight were no longer significant after adjustment for high energy snack consumption and family income.

The relationship between media use and overweight was further explored by a subgroup analysis according to the PA level (Table 3). The effect of media use was significant only among the girls with a lower level of PA. Female subjects

TABLE 3: Adjusted odds ratio for associations of computer game use and television viewing with overweight by physical activity levels and gender*.

	Having 60 minutes of moderate intensity physical activity	
	3 days per week or less Adjusted odds ratio (95% CI)	More than 3 days per week Adjusted odds ratio (95% CI)
Boy		
Computer game use		
1 h/d or less	1	1
More than 1 h/d	1.11 (0.70–1.74)	1.36 (0.80–2.31)
Watching TV		
2 h/d or less	1	1
More than 2 h/d	0.93 (0.66–1.32)	0.82 (0.47–1.45)
Girl		
Computer game use		
1 h/d or less	1	1
More than 1 h/d	1.99 (1.15–3.47)	0.77 (0.33–1.80)
Watching TV		
2 h/d or less	1	1
More than 2 h/d	1.72 (1.09–2.74)	1.54 (0.81–2.90)

CI: confidence interval. *Adjusted for high energy snack consumption and family income.

who spent ≤3 days/week in 60 minutes of moderate-intensity PA had a greater risk for overweight if they spent more than 2 hours/day viewing TV (AOR = 1.72; 95% CI: 1.09–2.74 versus 2 hours/day or less) or more than 1 hour/day playing computer games (AOR = 1.99; 95% CI: 1.15–3.47 versus 1 hour/day or less), while those having more than 3 days/week of moderate-intensity PA and engagement in either TV viewing or computer gaming did not pose significant risks. For boys, media use did not exert significant risk for overweight in either group of PA.

4. Discussion

By using the data from the recent National Health Examination Survey, we found that computer game use for more than 1 hour a day was associated with an increased risk for overweight while engagement in moderate-intensity PA significantly decreased the likelihood of overweight among the 6- to 14-year-old female subjects. Further analysis showed that the effect of computer game use and TV viewing on the risk for overweight was significant among girls, but not boys, who spent ≤3 days/week in 60 minutes of moderate-intensity PA.

The association between the level of PA and weight status has been shown to be nonuniform in the recent systematic review of cross-sectional studies [15]. Like ours, most of the reports that found significant negative associations, the outcomes were different for boys and girls. Gender differences in health behaviors relating to obesity have been documented in other studies [23, 25, 26]. These results may be due to the differences in physiological responses or gender role expectation in the society for boys and girls [27–29]. On the other hand, child weight status itself may influence the intensity and frequency of PA and this may give rise to

the mixed findings of their associations [15]. Moreover, the self-report of PA which was used in most surveys may affect the accuracy and lead to inconsistent results.

The positive association between sedentary behaviors, namely, TV viewing or playing video/computer games, and child weight status found in this study is consistent with the majority of previous studies in the recent systematic review [15]. Research on the association between screen time and overweight/obesity in children mostly used total screen time (i.e., combining TV viewing, video/computer game use, and non-leisure computer use). Nowadays, the media such as computer games and the internet substantially occupies children's pastime. An investigation of the independent effect of this electronic media use on overweight/obesity in children will have public health importance. Like studies of physical activity, research assessing the effect of video/computer game use on the weight status of children showed mixed results. A meta-analysis by Marshall et al. [16] and three other recent studies [30–32] among children and adolescents found no association, while a positive relationship between electronic game use and weight status were found to be curvilinear with a difference in ages in a study of US children using 24-hour time-use diaries to record the amount of video game use [19]. Children under the age of 8 with higher weight status played moderate amounts of electronic games, while children with lower weight status played either very little or a lot of electronic games. This study also found that girls, but not boys, with higher weight status played more video games. Video game use was also found to be associated with an increased cardiometabolic risk score, blood pressure, and lipids [17, 18]. As children usually engage in multiple SB, an effect of each activity on child weight status should be disentangled to provide evidence for development of effective interventions to promote healthy behaviors for obesity control.

We found physical activity to be a moderator of the relation between sedentary activities (i.e., TV viewing time and computer game time) and overweight. Girls who had 60 minutes of moderate-intensity PA ≤ 3 days/week were more likely to be at risk for overweight if they watched TV > 2 hours/day or played computer games > 1 hour/day than those who had such level of PA > 3 days/week. This moderating effect was not observed in boys. In a study of 9,278 Taiwanese adolescents, Yen et al. demonstrated that the relationship between increased BMI and a high level of TV viewing was found only in adolescents who exercised less than 1 hour/day, but not in those who exercised 1 hour/day or more [33]. These findings indicated that adequate exercise may be protective for children who spend a lot of time on sedentary activities from increased adiposity, particularly among girls. These moderators, namely, age, gender, and PA, should be taken into account in developing interventions for children and adolescents. However, in the present study, it is not clear whether the findings of differences in the associations by gender are due to a variation in energy expenditures pattern during TV watching or in the type of computer game use between boys and girls. The reasons behind this discrepancy need further investigation.

Our study has some limitations. As is the nature of surveys, one could not interpret the findings as causal. The PA and SB were collected by questionnaires. Given the publicized untoward effect of TV viewing and computer game use, the bias may be likely towards underreporting. Nevertheless, this study has its strength as a national representative study with a relatively large sample size. The findings could reflect the behavioral pattern of Thai children and a meaningful relationship of these behaviors to child overweight problem.

5. Conclusions

The lives of children nowadays have been considerably affected by societal changes and media technologies. We found that computer game use for more than 1 hour a day and TV viewing for more than 2 hours a day increased the risk for overweight among girls who had a low PA level. These findings are helpful for developing effective interventions to promote healthy behaviors for the control of obesity. As computers are being used in schools and at home for educating children at a younger age, the risk of this electronic media should be communicated to the families and the public as well. Parents should be informed to discipline the use of a computer in order to control sedentary time. Tracking societal changes on lifestyles should be carried out regularly to identify potential areas for targeted interventions.

Conflict of Interests

The authors declare no conflict of interests regarding the publication of this paper.

Acknowledgments

The Thai National Health Examination Survey IV was supported financially by the Bureau of Policy and Strategy, Ministry of Public Health, Thai Health Promotion Foundation, National Health Security Office, and the Health System Research Institute. The authors are thankful to the studied families and children and the NHES IV study group (National Health Examination Survey Office: Wichai Aekplakorn, Rungkarn Inthawong, Jiraluck Nonthaluck, Supornsak Tipsukum, and Yawarat Porrapakkham; Northern Region: Suwat Chariyalertsak, Kanittha Thaikla (Chiang Mai University), Wongsa Laohasiriwong, Wanlop Jaidee, Sutthinan Srathonghon, Ratana Phanphanit, Jiraporn Suwanteerangkul, and Kriangkai Srithanaviboonchai; North Eastern Region: Pattapong Kessomboon, Somdej Pinitsoontorn, Piyathida Kuhirunyaratn, Sauwanan Bumrurraj, Amornrat Rattanasiri, Suchada Paileeklee, Bangornsri Jindawong, Napaporn Krusun, and Weerapong Seeupalat (Khon Kaen University); Southern Region: Virasakdi Chongsuvivatwong, Rassamee Sangthong, and Mafausis Dueravee; Central Region: Surasak Taneepanichskul, Somrat Lertmaharit, Vilai Chinveschakitvanich, Onuma Zongram, Nuchanad Hounnaklang, and Sukarin Wimuktayon (Chulalongkorn University); Bangkok Region: Panwadee Putwatana, Chalermsri Nuntawan, and Karn Chaladthanyagid (Mahidol University)). They also thank the following persons for their contributions in the designing of the questionnaire: Dr. Nichara Ruangdaragaonon, Dr. Pasuree Sangsupavanich, Dr. Mandhana Pradipasen, Miss Sujit Saleepan, Dr. Uraiporn Chittchang, Dr. Pattanee Winichagoon, and Dr. Sangsom Sinawat.

References

[1] N. Gupta, K. Goel, P. Shah, and A. Misra, "Childhood obesity in developing countries: epidemiology, determinants, and prevention," *Endocrine Reviews*, vol. 33, no. 1, pp. 48–70, 2012.

[2] W. Aekplakorn and L. Mo-suwan, "Prevalence of obesity in Thailand," *Obesity Reviews*, vol. 10, no. 6, pp. 589–592, 2009.

[3] S. Likitmaskul, P. Kiattisathavee, K. Chaichanwatanakul, L. Punnakanta, K. Angsusingha, and C. Tuchinda, "Increasing prevalence of type 2 diabetes mellitus in Thai children and adolescents associated with increasing prevalence of obesity," *Journal of Pediatric Endocrinology and Metabolism*, vol. 16, no. 1, pp. 71–77, 2003.

[4] J. C. Eisenmann, "Insight into the causes of the recent secular trend in pediatric obesity: common sense does not always prevail for complex, multi-factorial phenotypes," *Preventive Medicine*, vol. 42, no. 5, pp. 329–335, 2006.

[5] C. Maffeis, "Aetiology of overweight and obesity in children and adolescents," *European Journal of Pediatrics*, vol. 159, supplement 1, pp. S35–S44, 2000.

[6] A. W. Taylor, H. Winefield, L. Kettler, R. Roberts, and T. K. Gill, "A population study of 5 to 15 year olds: full time maternal employment not associated with high BMI. The importance of screen-based activity, reading for pleasure and sleep duration in children's BMI," *Maternal and Child Health Journal*, vol. 16, no. 3, pp. 587–599, 2012.

[7] L. Mo-suwan and A. Geater, "Risk factors for childhood obesity in a transitional society in Thailand," *International Journal of Obesity*, vol. 20, no. 8, pp. 697–703, 1996.

[8] L. Mo-suwan, P. Tongkumchum, and A. Puetpaiboon, "Determinants of overweight tracking from childhood to adolescence: a 5 y follow-up study of Hat Yai schoolchildren," *International Journal of Obesity*, vol. 24, no. 12, pp. 1642–1647, 2000.

[9] U. Yamborisut, V. Kosulwat, U. Chittchang, W. Wimonpeera-pattana, and U. Suthutvoravut, "Factors associated with dual form of malnutrition in school children in Nakhon Pathom and Bangkok," *Journal of the Medical Association of Thailand*, vol. 89, no. 7, pp. 1012–1023, 2006.

[10] N. Ruangdaraganon, N. Kotchabhakdi, U. Udomsubpayakul, C. Kunanusont, and P. Suriyawongpaisal, "The association between television viewing and childhood obesity: a national survey in Thailand," *Journal of the Medical Association of Thailand*, vol. 85, supplement 4, pp. S1075–S1080, 2002.

[11] R. Sturm, "Childhood obesity—what we can learn from existing data on societal trends, part 1," *Preventing Chronic Disease*, vol. 2, no. 1, 2005.

[12] Thailand's Ministry of Culture, "Situational analysis of game addiction in Thai children," 2012, http://www.healthygamer.net/sites/default/files/scribd/game_addiction_2012.pdf.

[13] L. Mo-suwan, "Health behaviors," in *Report of the Fourth National Health Examination Survey 2008-2009: Child Health*, W. Aekplakorn, Ed., pp. 27–47, The Thai National Health Examination Survey, 2011.

[14] M. S. Tremblay, A. G. LeBlanc, M. E. Kho et al., "Systematic review of sedentary behaviour and health indicators in school-aged children and youth," *International Journal of Behavioral Nutrition and Physical Activity*, vol. 8, article 98, 2011.

[15] H. Prentice-Dunn and S. Prentice-Dunn, "Physical activity, sedentary behavior, and childhood obesity: a review of cross-sectional studies," *Psychology, Health & Medicine*, vol. 17, no. 3, pp. 255–273, 2012.

[16] S. J. Marshall, S. J. H. Biddle, T. Gorely, N. Cameron, and I. Murdey, "Relationships between media use, body fatness and physical activity in children and youth: a meta-analysis," *International Journal of Obesity*, vol. 28, no. 11, pp. 1238–1246, 2004.

[17] G. S. Goldfield, G. P. Kenny, S. Hadjiyannakis et al., "Video game playing is independently associated with blood pressure and lipids in overweight and obese adolescents," *PLoS ONE*, vol. 6, no. 11, article e26643, 2011.

[18] T. J. Saunders, M. S. Tremblay, M. E. Mathieu et al., "Associations of sedentary behavior, sedentary bouts and breaks in sedentary time with cardiometabolic risk in children with a family history of obesity," *PLoS ONE*, vol. 8, no. 11, article e79143, 2013.

[19] E. A. Vandewater, M. S. Shim, and A. G. Caplovitz, "Linking obesity and activity level with children's television and video game use," *Journal of Adolescence*, vol. 27, no. 1, pp. 71–85, 2004.

[20] W. Aekplakorn, S. Chariyalertsak, P. Kessomboon et al., "Prevalence and management of diabetes and metabolic risk factors in Thai adults: the Thai National Health Examination Survey IV, 2009," *Diabetes Care*, vol. 34, no. 9, pp. 1980–1985, 2011.

[21] T. J. Cole, M. C. Bellizzi, K. M. Flegal, and W. H. Dietz, "Establishing a standard definition for child overweight and obesity worldwide: international survey," *British Medical Journal*, vol. 320, no. 7244, pp. 1240–1245, 2000.

[22] American Academy of Pediatrics, Committee on Public Education, "American Academy of Pediatrics: Children, adolescents, and television," *Pediatrics*, vol. 107, no. 2, pp. 423–426, 2001.

[23] A. Simen-Kapeu and P. J. Veugelers, "Should public health interventions aimed at reducing childhood overweight and obesity be gender-focused?" *BMC Public Health*, vol. 10, article 340, 2010.

[24] StataCorp, *Stata Statistical Software: Release 10*, StataCorp, College Station, Tex, USA, 2007.

[25] M. Ferrante, M. Fiore, G. E. Sciacca et al., "The role of weight status, gender and self-esteem in following a diet among middle-school children in Sicily (Italy)," *BMC Public Health*, vol. 10, article 241, 2010.

[26] M. Govindan, R. Gurm, S. Mohan et al., "Gender differences in physiologic markers and health behaviors associated with childhood obesity," *Pediatrics*, vol. 132, no. 3, pp. 468–474, 2013.

[27] C. E. Bird and P. P. Rieker, "Gender matters: an integrated model for understanding men's and women's health," *Social Science & Medicine*, vol. 48, no. 6, pp. 745–755, 1999.

[28] N. Krieger, "Genders, sexes, and health: what are the connections—and why does it matter?" *International Journal of Epidemiology*, vol. 32, no. 4, pp. 652–657, 2003.

[29] Y. F. Chiu, L. M. Chuang, H. Y. Kao et al., "Sex-specific genetic architecture of human fatness in Chinese: the SAPPHIRe Study," *Human Genetics*, vol. 128, no. 5, pp. 501–513, 2010.

[30] C. M. Arango, D. C. Parra, L. F. Gómez, L. Lema, F. Lobelo, and U. Ekelund, "Screen time, cardiorespiratory fitness and adiposity among school-age children from Monteria, Colombia," *Journal of Science and Medicine in Sport*, 2013.

[31] D. S. Bickham, E. A. Blood, C. E. Walls, L. A. Shrier, and M. Rich, "Characteristics of screen media use associated with higher BMI in young adolescents," *Pediatrics*, vol. 131, no. 5, pp. 935–941, 2013.

[32] S. B. Sisson, S. T. Broyles, B. L. Baker, and P. T. Katzmarzyk, "Television, reading, and computer time: correlates of school-day leisure-time sedentary behavior and relationship with overweight in children in the U.S.," *Journal of Physical Activity & Health*, vol. 8, supplement 2, pp. S188–S197, 2011.

[33] C. F. Yen, R. C. Hsiao, C. H. Ko et al., "The relationships between body mass index and television viewing, internet use and cellular phone use: the moderating effects of socio-demographic characteristics and exercise," *International Journal of Eating Disorders*, vol. 43, no. 6, pp. 565–571, 2010.

7

Factors Associated with Acute Malnutrition among Children Admitted to a Diarrhoea Treatment Facility in Bangladesh

Connor Fuchs,[1] Tania Sultana,[2] Tahmeed Ahmed,[2] and M. Iqbal Hossain[2]

[1] *University of Arkansas, Fayetteville, AR, USA*
[2] *Centre for Nutrition and Food Security, and Nutrition Unit, Dhaka Hospital, icddr,b, Mohakhali, Dhaka 1212, Bangladesh*

Correspondence should be addressed to M. Iqbal Hossain; ihossain@icddrb.org

Academic Editor: Samuel Menahem

To assess the risk factors for acute malnutrition (weight-for-height z-score (WHZ) < −2), a case-control study was conducted during June–September 2012 in 449 children aged 6–59 months (178 with WHZ < −2 and 271 comparing children with WHZ ≥ −2 and no edema) admitted to the Dhaka Hospital of icddr,b in Bangladesh. The overall mean ± SD age was 12.0 ± 7.6 months, 38.5% (no difference between case and controls). The mean ± SD WHZ of cases and controls was −3.24 ± 1.01 versus −0.74 ± 0.95 (P < 0.001), respectively. Logistic regression analysis revealed that children with acute malnutrition were more likely than controls to be older (age > 1 year) (adjusted OR (AOR): 3.1, P = 0.004); have an undernourished mother (body mass index < 18.5), (AOR: 2.8, P = 0.017); have a father with no or a low-paying job (AOR: 5.8, P < 0.001); come from a family having a monthly income of <10,000 taka, (1 US\$ = 80 taka) (AOR: 2.9, P = 0.008); and often have stopped predominant breastfeeding before 4 months of age (AOR: 2.7, P = 0.013). Improved understanding of these characteristics enables the design and targeting of preventive-intervention programs of childhood acute malnutrition.

1. Introduction

One of every five children aged less than 5 years in low-income, developing countries is malnourished. Globally, undernutrition is associated with more than one-third of all deaths in this age group [1]. Acute malnutrition defined by weight-for-height z-score (WHZ) < −2 (i.e., wasting) in young children continues to be a major health problem in low-income countries, particularly Bangladesh. Despite recent advances in prevention and management of childhood malnutrition in Bangladesh, 16% of children under 5 years of age are acutely malnourished (WHZ < −2) [2]. UNICEF describes malnutrition in Bangladesh as a "silent emergency" [3]. Childhood malnutrition places a heavy burden on many families in Bangladesh and other developing countries. It not only directly increases mortality but also imposes significant national health and development costs due to associated morbidities, including impaired cognitive ability and indirect deaths.

It is well documented that poverty and malnutrition, regardless of location, are highly intertwined. Although risk factors for malnutrition have been identified, individual factors potentially change in specific areas over time and a current characterisation of risk factors provides the basis for preventative intervention programmes.

2. Methods

The study was conducted in the Dhaka Hospital of the International Centre for Diarrhoeal Disease Research (icddr,b) situated in Dhaka, Bangladesh, a metropolitan area (1,500 sq km) with a total population of ~15 million. Each year, the Dhaka Hospital provides care and treatment for over 120,000 patients with diarrhoea, with or without other associated health problems. The hospital also conducts research on enteric and other common infectious diseases as well as undernutrition and provides training on case management of diarrheal diseases, management of malnutrition, and research methodology. Under-five children constitute about 60% of the total patient population and most (~60%) are from poor socioeconomic communities in urban and periurban areas of Dhaka.

A nonmatched case-control study design was used to assess and identify potential risk factors associated with acute malnutrition/wasting among 6–59-month-old children. Children in this age group without any congenital anomaly or other chronic conditions causally associated with malnutrition (e.g., heart disease), who were admitted to the Dhaka Hospital of icddr,b from June to September 2012, were enrolled. Using the contemporary growth standards of the World Health Organization (2006) and ANTHRO software [4], weight-for-height z-score (WHZ), weight-for-age z-score (WAZ), height-for-age z-score (HAZ), and body mass index-for-age z-score (BMI-AZ) of all studied children were calculated. Children with moderate or severe wasting (WHZ < −2) but without bilateral pedal edema were considered cases. Children with a WHZ ≥ −2 and without bilateral pedal edema were enrolled as control children. Verbal consent from the attending guardian, usually the mother of the child, was obtained.

2.1. Data Collection. One of the investigators and/or a research assistant interviewed the mother/caregiver using a pretested, structured questionnaire. Data recorded from the interviews included age and sex of child, birth order, number of total and under-five siblings, feeding and immunisation history, type of house hold latrine, marital status of mother, monthly family income, and parental age, education, and occupation. Children's nude weight using a frequently standardised digital scale with 10 g precision (Seca, model 345, Hamburg, Germany) and recumbent length to the nearest mm using a calibrated, locally constructed length board were obtained. Mother's (if present) weight and height were measured using standard procedures [5]. The investigator(s) supervised the interview process and anthropometry and reviewed the data forms daily.

2.2. Data Analyses. Data were entered using SPSS software for Windows (version 11.5) (SPSS Inc., Chicago, IL, USA). For normally distributed continuous variables, means were compared using unpaired t-tests. For continuous variables not normally distributed, the Mann-Whitney U test was performed. Differences in proportions were compared by the chi-square test or Fisher's exact test if the expected number in any cell was ≤5. A probability of less than 0.05 was considered statistically significant. The strength of association of selected associated/risk factors for acute malnutrition was determined by estimating odds ratios (ORs) and their 95% confidence intervals (CIs). All independent variables, for example, birth order, number of siblings, socioeconomic status, parental characteristics, child feeding, and immunisation history, were analysed initially in univariate models and the attributes that were significantly associated with wasting (dependent variable) and biologically plausible were included in logistic regression models.

3. Results

A total of 449 children were enrolled, of whom 178 were cases (wasted children) and 271 were controls. Their overall mean ± SD age was 12.0 ± 7.6 months (cases were on an average 2 months older), and 38.5% were female without any group difference between case and control children. The mean ± SD WHZ and BMIAZ of case and control children were −3.24 ± 1.01 versus −0.74 ± 0.95 and −3.21 ± 1.04 versus −0.77 ± 0.96, respectively ($P < 0.001$). As dictated by the study design, the cases had significantly lower anthropometric values than the control children (Table 1). Cases had a shorter period than controls of exclusive or predominant breastfeeding. Maternal nutritional status, family income, and the fathers' educational levels were worse in the malnourished children (cases). Cases had worse immunization status (Bacillus Calmette-Guérin (BCG) and measles vaccine), breastfeeding duration, and parental and other socioeconomic characteristics than control children (Table 2). Logistic regression analysis revealed that children with acute malnutrition were more likely than control to be older (age > 1 year) (adjusted OR (AOR): 3.1, $P = 0.004$), have an undernourished mother (body mass index (BMI) < 18.5), (AOR: 2.8, $P = 0.017$), have a father with no or a low-paying job (AOR: 5.8, $P < 0.001$), come from a family having a monthly income of less than 10,000 taka, (1 US\$ = 80 taka) (AOR: 2.9, $P = 0.008$), and have shorter period of predominant breastfeeding (AOR: 2.7, $P = 0.013$) (Table 3).

4. Discussion

The aim of this study was to identify risk factors associated with acute malnutrition (WHZ < −2, which includes both moderate and severe wasting) in our population of 6–59-month-old children. Our study shows that the major associated/risk factors for acute malnutrition among these children were older age of the child, undernourished mother, jobless father or father with a low-paying job, low total family income, and poorer breastfeeding practices. Some of these factors may operate in synergy to increase the risk of acute malnutrition.

Older age as a risk/associated factor for acute malnutrition of children in our study might reflect a selection bias. However, Jeyaseelan and Lakshman from Tamil Nadu, India [6], and Kikafunda et al. from Uganda [7] also observed older age of a child to be significantly associated with malnutrition. Proper nutrition and child care are essential to begin in early childhood to prevent malnutrition and ensure maximum potential for normal psychomotor development as children grow older.

Similar to other studies from Bangladesh [8–11] and Africa [12], the current study observed maternal malnutrition (BMI less than 18.5) as an independent risk factor for children's wasting/acute malnutrition. Undernourished mothers often deliver low-birth-weight (LBW) infants [13], which is an attributable risk factor for increased childhood malnutrition, morbidity, and mortality. The last nationwide LBW survey in Bangladesh showed a high prevalence of 36%. The capacity to adequately breastfeed may also be compromised [14–16]

TABLE 1: Characteristics (continuous variables) of the cases (wasted) and controls (nonwasted) children.

Variable	Case $N = 178$	Control $N = 271$	P value
Child's age (months)	13.4 ± 4.0	11.2 ± 6.6	0.004
Weight-for-length z-score[a]	-3.24 ± 1.01	-0.74 ± 0.95	<0.001
Weight-for-age z-score[a]	-3.46 ± 1.34	-1.08 ± 1.19	<0.001
Length-for-age z-score[a]	-2.16 ± 1.84	-0.88 ± 1.45	<0.001
BMI-for-age z-score[a]	-3.21 ± 1.04	-0.77 ± 0.96	<0.001
Total number of children in the family	1.8 ± 1.0	1.7 ± 0.9	0.270
Exclusive/predominant breastfeeding (month)	4.0 ± 2.6	4.4 ± 2.4	0.042
Birth order	1.8 ± 1.0	1.7 ± 0.8	0.365
Mother's age (years)	23.7 ± 5.2	23.9 ± 4.7	0.737
Mother's weight (kg)	45.0 ± 7.8	50.4 ± 10.2	<0.001
Mother's height (meter)	1.49 ± 0.05	1.50 ± 0.06	<0.001
Mother's body mass index (kg/M^2)	20.4 ± 3.4	22.3 ± 4.0	<0.001
Mother's education (years)	5.0 ± 4.2	7.5 ± 3.9	<0.001
Father's age (years)	30.8 ± 6.8	31.5 ± 5.7	0.249
Father's education (years)	5.8 ± 4.6	8.3 ± 4.3	<0.001
Total family income per month (taka[b])	10128 ± 6647	16095 ± 16489	<0.001

All data are expressed as mean ± SD. [a]In relation to the WHO 2006 standard [4]; [b]taka (Bangladeshi currency: 1 UD$ = 80 taka, average rate during the study period).

TABLE 2: Characteristics (attributes) of the cases (wasted) and controls (nonwasted) children.

Variable	Case $N = 178$	Control $N = 271$	P value
Child's age > 1 year: n (%)	67 (37.6)	62 (22.9)	0.001
Girls: n (%)	74 (41.6)	99 (36.5)	0.283
Did not receive BCG: n (%)	5 (2.8)	1 (0.4)	0.038
Did not receive pentavalent/polio vaccine (or received less than age appropriate doses): n (%)	16 (9.0)	23 (8.5)	0.984
Did not receive measles vaccine (among >9 months old; $n = 109$ cases and 142 controls): n (%)	31 (28.4)	26 (18.3)	0.041
Predominant breastfeeding stopped before 4 months: n (%)	76 (42.7)	85 (31.4)	0.010
Teenaged mother (<20 years): n (%)	23 (13.4)	21 (7.9)	0.045
Shorter mother (height < 1.5 meters): n (%)	86 (54.4)	110 (44.5)	0.033
Undernourished mother (BMI < 18.5): n (%)	52 (32.5)	37 (14.9)	<0.001
Illiterate or less educated (<5 years' schooling) mother: n (%)	101 (56.7)	88 (32.5)	<0.001
Mother working outside of the home: n (%)	15 (8.4)	12 (4.4)	0.063
Divorced/widowed mother: n (%)	16 (9.0)	3 (1.1)	<0.001
Younger father (age < 25 years): n (%)	44 (25.4)	37 (14.3)	0.003
Illiterate or less educated (<5 years' schooling) father: n (%)	92 (52.6)	72 (27.0)	<0.001
Father with low-paid job: n (%) (e.g., rickshaw puller or day labourer): n (%)	149 (83.7)	139 (51.3)	<0.001
Monthly income < 10000 taka[a]: n (%)	121 (70.3)	136 (51.5)	<0.001
Using unsanitary latrine: n (%)	10 (5.6)	3 (1.1)	0.006
Child worn any thread or amulet: n (%)	94 (53.1)	157 (57.9)	0.331
Child worn kajal[b] at the side of fore head: n (%)	139 (78.1)	219 (80.8)	0.549

All data are expressed as number (%). [a]Taka (Bangladeshi currency: 1 UD$ = 80 taka, average rate during the study period); [b]a black mark/line used over eyelash by females and side of forehead in some children in Indo-Pak subcontinent.

TABLE 3: Factors associated with acute malnutrition (wasting): results of logistic regression model.

Attribute	Adjusted odds ratio	95% CI of adjusted OR		P value
		Lower	Upper	
Child's age > 1 year	3.144	1.431	6.904	0.004
Did not receive measles vaccine (among >9 months old; $n = 109$ cases and 142 controls)	2.492	0.973	6.378	0.057
Predominant breastfeeding stopped before 4 months	2.669	1.229	5.796	0.013
Teenaged mother (<20 years)	1.758	0.451	6.847	0.416
Shorter mother (height < 1.5 meters)	1.399	0.686	2.851	0.355
Undernourished mother (BMI < 18.5)	2.803	1.203	6.532	0.017
Illiterate or less educated (<5 years' schooling) mother	1.676	0.754	3.728	0.205
Younger father (age < 25 years)	1.614	0.682	3.815	0.276
Illiterate or less educated (<5 years' schooling) father	1.186	0.525	2.682	0.681
Father with low-paid job	5.778	2.537	13.157	<0.001
Monthly income < 10000 taka [a]	2.871	1.310	6.291	0.008
Using unsanitary latrine	1.505	0.078	29.173	0.787
Constant	0.016	—	—	0.001

[a] Taka (Bangladeshi currency: 1 UD$ = 80 taka, average rate during the study period).

in maternal malnutrition and such mothers might have less energy to appropriately nurture their children.

The fathers of most (84%) of the wasted children in our study were rickshaw pullers or day laborers. Likewise, a study from South India [17] also found that children of fathers who were day laborers were ~3 times more likely to be severely underweight. These occupations are among the lowest paid employment categories in Bangladesh. Moreover, they often result in erratic or insecure incomes, at times yielding little or no earnings on a particular day. Income insecurity leads to food insecurity forcing family members to consume poor food quality and/or amount. Low family income as a possible risk factor of acute malnutrition, as found in this study, was also reported by Ahmed et al. [8] in wasted children under 2 years old, by Nahar et al. [18] in severely underweight under-5 children in Bangladesh, and by Jeyaseelan and Lakshman [6] in undernourished children in Tamil Nadu, India.

Our finding of improper/inadequate breastfeeding as an associated factor with acute malnutrition is in accordance with the findings of several other studies [10, 19, 20] from Bangladesh and elsewhere, in which early supplementation with infant formula or cow's milk, early introduction of semisolid complementary foods, and inadequate breastfeeding were important risk factors for malnutrition in children. During the critical period of early infancy, proper breastfeeding and complementary feeding practices play critical roles. The hygienic and nutritional risks associated with bottle-feeding and artificial milk are well known [21–23], and previous studies also found that breastfeeding had a significant and substantial impact on overall survival of undernourished children [24, 25]. It is also possible that the association with a shorter duration of predominant breastfeeding could be an example of reverse causality, whereby children who were ill and undernourished stopped breastfeeding or were provided with other foods.

One of the possible limitations of the present study is that the same personnel who obtained the anthropometric measurements of the children and mothers also conducted the interviews, so interviewer biases could be there. However, most of the variables identified as risk/associated factors for acute malnutrition in our study were objective in type. The other limitation was the cross-sectional nature of the present study, which did not allow us to state the identified associated factors as definite causally related risk factors.

The children suffering from acute malnutrition often need supplementary food. In this regard it is worthwhile to mention that icddr,b has developed ready-to-use foods using locally available food ingredients. These foods can be used to prevent and to treat moderate wasting in children living in food-insecure communities. Moreover, the associated factors identified for acute malnutrition in this study can be incorporated into the design and targeting of preventive interventions. Factors such as breastfeeding practices are potentially modifiable. Interventions that motivate behaviours more consistent with recommended infant and young child feeding practices would be expected to have a positive impact. Certain factors and possible causes of acute malnutrition are complex and involve societal and broad-based preventive programs.

Conflict of Interests

None of the authors/investigators has any financial interests that might affect the results of this study.

Authors' Contribution

Each author has taken part in conception and design, analysis and interpretation of data, and drafting and/or revising the paper.

Acknowledgments

This study was supported by icddr,b. This research/study was funded by core donors which provide unrestricted support to icddr,b for its operations and research. Current donors providing unrestricted support include Australian Agency for International Development (AusAID), Government of the People's Republic of Bangladesh, Canadian International Development Agency (CIDA), Swedish International Development Cooperation Agency (Sida), and the Department for International Development, UK (DFID). The authors gratefully acknowledge these donors for their support and commitment to icddr,b's research efforts. They sincerely appreciate Professor G. J. Fuchs, Department of Pediatric Gastroenterology and Nutrition, Arkansas Children's Hospital, USA, for his excellent review and input in this study. The study and its reporting are approved by the institutional review board of icddr,b without any ethical concern.

References

[1] R. E. Black, L. H. Allen, Z. A. Bhutta et al., "Maternal and child undernutrition: global and regional exposures and health consequences," *The Lancet*, vol. 371, no. 9608, pp. 243–260, 2008.

[2] National Institute of Population Research and Training (NIPORT), Maitra and Associates, and Macro International, "Bangladesh Demographic and Health Survey 2011," National Institute of Population Research and Training, Maitra and Associates, and Macro International, Dhaka, Bangladesh and Calverton, Md, USA, 2012.

[3] S. Crowe, "'A silent emergency' as Bangladesh's poor suffer from economic downturn," Newsline, Unicef information by country, 2009, http://www.unicef.org/infobycountry/bangladesh_49247.html.

[4] WHO Multicentre Growth Reference Study Group, "WHO Child Growth Standards: Length/height-for-age, weight-for-age, weight-for-length, weight-for-height and body mass index-for-age: Methods and development," Geneva, Switzerland, World Health Organization, 2006, http://www.who.int/childgrowth/standards/technical_report/en/index.html.

[5] WHO, "Physical status. The use and interpretation of anthropometry," Report of a WHO Expert Committee WHO Technical Report Series 854, World Health Organization, Geneva, Switzerland, 1995.

[6] L. Jeyaseelan and M. Lakshman, "Risk factors for malnutrition in south Indian children," *Journal of Biosocial Science*, vol. 29, no. 1, pp. 93–100, 1997.

[7] J. K. Kikafunda, A. F. Walker, D. Collett, and J. K. Tumwine, "Risk factors for early childhood malnutrition in Uganda," *Pediatrics*, vol. 102, no. 4, article E45, 1998.

[8] A. S. Ahmed, T. Ahmed, S. K. Roy, N. Alam, and M. I. Hossain, "Determinants of under nutrition in children under 2 years of age from rural Bangladesh," *Indian Pediatrics*, vol. 49, pp. 821–824, 2012.

[9] M. I. Rayhan and M. S. H. Khan, "Factors causing malnutrition among under five children in Bangladesh," *Pakistan Journal of Nutrition*, vol. 5, no. 6, pp. 558–562, 2006.

[10] A. Rahman and S. Chowdhury, "Determinants of chronic malnutrition among preschool children in Bangladesh," *Journal of Biosocial Science*, vol. 39, no. 2, pp. 161–173, 2007.

[11] M. Aminul Islam, M. Mujibur Rahman, and D. Mahalanabis, "Maternal and socioeconomic factors and the risk of severe malnutrition in a child: a case-control study," *European Journal of Clinical Nutrition*, vol. 48, no. 6, pp. 416–424, 1994.

[12] F. Delpeuch, P. Traissac, Y. Martin-Prével, J. P. Massamba, and B. Maire, "Economic crisis and malnutrition: socioeconomic determinants of anthropometric status of preschool children and their mothers in an African urban area," *Public Health Nutrition*, vol. 3, no. 1, pp. 39–47, 2000.

[13] M. S. Kramer, "The epidemiology of adverse pregnancy outcomes: an overview," *Journal of Nutrition*, vol. 133, no. 5, pp. 1592S–1596S, 2003.

[14] T. S. Osteria, "Maternal nutrition, infant health, and subsequent fertility," *Philippine Journal of Nutrition*, vol. 35, no. 3, pp. 106–111, 1982.

[15] K. H. Brown, N. A. Akhtar, A. D. Robertson, and M. G. Ahmed, "Lactational capacity of marginally nourished mothers: relationships between maternal nutritional status and quantity and proximate composition of milk," *Pediatrics*, vol. 78, no. 5, pp. 909–919, 1986.

[16] K. H. Brown, A. D. Robertson, and N. A. Akhtar, "Lactational capacity of marginally nourished mothers: infants' milk nutrient comsumption and patterns of growth," *Pediatrics*, vol. 78, no. 5, pp. 920–927, 1986.

[17] K. Saito, J. R. Korzenik, J. F. Jekel, and S. Bhattacharji, "A case-control study of maternal knowledge of malnutrition and health- care-seeking attitudes in rural South India," *Yale Journal of Biology and Medicine*, vol. 70, no. 2, pp. 149–160, 1997.

[18] B. Nahar, T. Ahmed, K. H. Brown, and M. I. Hossain, "Risk factors associated with severe underweight among young children reporting to a diarrhoea treatment facility in Bangladesh," *Journal of Health, Population and Nutrition*, vol. 28, no. 5, pp. 476–483, 2010.

[19] F. J. Henry, A. Briend, V. Fauveau, S. A. Huttly, M. Yunus, and J. Chakraborty, "Gender and age differentials in risk factors for childhood malnutrition in Bangladesh," *Annals of Epidemiology*, vol. 3, no. 4, pp. 382–386, 1993.

[20] F. J. Henry, A. Briend, V. Fauveau, S. R. A. Huttly, M. Yunus, and J. Chakraborty, "Risk factors for clinical marasmus: a case-control study of Bangladeshi children," *International Journal of Epidemiology*, vol. 22, no. 2, pp. 278–283, 1993.

[21] J. M. Jason, P. Nieburg, and J. S. Marks, "Mortality and infectious disease associated with infant-feeding practices in developing countries," *Pediatrics*, vol. 74, no. 4, pp. 702–727, 1984.

[22] K. H. Brown, R. E. Black, G. Lopez de Romana, and H. Creed de Kanashiro, "Infant-feeding practices and their relationship with diarrheal and other diseases in Huascar (Lima), Peru," *Pediatrics*, vol. 83, no. 1, pp. 31–40, 1989.

[23] B. M. Popkin, L. Adair, J. S. Akin, R. Black, J. Briscoe, and W. Flieger, "Breast-feeding and diarrheal morbidity," *Pediatrics*, vol. 86, no. 6, pp. 874–882, 1990.

[24] A. Briend, B. Wojtyniak, and M. G. M. Rowland, "Breast feeding, nutritional state, and child survival in rural Bangladesh," *British Medical Journal*, vol. 296, no. 6626, pp. 879–882, 1988.

[25] A. Briend and A. Bari, "Breastfeeding improves survival, but not nutritional status, of 12–35 months old children in rural Bangladesh," *European Journal of Clinical Nutrition*, vol. 43, no. 9, pp. 603–608, 1989.

8

Free Radicals and Antioxidant Status in Protein Energy Malnutrition

M. Khare,[1] C. Mohanty,[1] B. K. Das,[2] A. Jyoti,[3] B. Mukhopadhyay,[3] and S. P. Mishra[3]

[1] Department of Anatomy, Institute of Medical Sciences, Banaras Hindu University, Varanasi, Uttar Pradesh, India
[2] Department of Pediatrics, Institute of Medical Sciences, Banaras Hindu University, Varanasi, Uttar Pradesh, India
[3] Department of Biochemistry, Institute of Medical Sciences, Banaras Hindu University, Varanasi, Uttar Pradesh, India

Correspondence should be addressed to S. P. Mishra; drsurendram2@gmail.com

Academic Editor: Namık Yaşar Özbek

Background/Objectives. The aim of this study was to evaluate oxidant and antioxidant status in children with different grades of Protein Energy Malnutrition (PEM). *Subjects/Methods.* A total of two hundred fifty (250) children (age range: 6 months to 5 years) living in eastern UP, India, were recruited. One hundred and ninety-three (193) of these children had different grades of PEM (sixty-five (65) children belong to mild, sixty (60) to moderate, and sixty-eight (68) to severe group). Grading in group was done after standardization in weight and height measurements. Fifty-seven (57) children who are age and and sex matched, healthy, and well-nourished were recruited from the local community and used as controls after checking their protein status (clinical nutritional status) with height and weight standardization. Redox homeostasis was assessed using spectrophotometric/colorimetric methods. *Results.* In our study, erythrocyte glutathione (GSH), plasma Cu, Zn-superoxide dismutase (Cu,Zn-SOD,EC 1.15.1.1), ceruloplasmin (Cp), and ascorbic acid were significantly ($P < 0.001$) more decreased in children with malnutrition than controls. Plasma malondialdehyde (MDA), and protein carbonyl (PC) were significantly ($P < 0.001$) raised in cases as compared to controls. *Conclusion.* Stress is created as a result of PEM which is responsible for the overproduction of reactive oxygen species (ROSs). These ROSs will lead to membrane oxidation and thus an increase in lipid peroxidation byproducts such as MDA and protein oxidation byproducts such as PC mainly. Decrease in level of antioxidants suggests an increased defense against oxidant damage. Changes in oxidant and antioxidant levels may be responsible for grading in PEM.

1. Introduction

Malnutrition is one of the major public health challenges in developing countries. Usually is referred to as a silent emergency as it has devastating effects on children, society, and future mankind. The net loss of body protein particularly skeletal muscle protein is likely to be a major factor responsible for PEM [1, 2]. Plasma albumin [3, 4], erythrocyte glutathione, and other endogenous antioxidant molecules such as bilirubin and uric acid [5] directly scavenge ROSs. Dietary deficiency of protein not only impairs the synthesis of plasma albumin and antioxidant enzymes but also reduces tissue concentrations of antioxidants, thereby resulting in a compromised antioxidant status [6, 7]. Copper-zinc and manganese are indispensable metals for the activities of Cu-Zn-SOD and Mn-SOD, respectively. Free radicals are very short lived and unstable, so they are difficult to measure. But their detrimental effects can be measured by estimating their byproducts. Markers of oxidative stress are MDA, a byproduct of lipid peroxidation and PC, a byproduct of protein oxidation. Defense capacity against ROS can be measured blood levels of GSH, glutathione peroxidase (GPx), Cu,Zn-SOD, Cp, and ascorbic acid. The pathogenesis of extreme muscle wasting (emaciation) and anemia commonly found in children with PEM has been suggested to be caused by an imbalance between the production of these toxic free radicals and antioxidant potential [8]. Very few studies of oxidant and antioxidant status in PEM children have been done so far. Therefore the aim of present study is to explore the status of oxidants and antioxidants in grades of PEM.

TABLE 1: Anthropometric measurements in cases of malnutrition and control.

Parameters	Mean ± SD				Intergroup comparison one way ANOVA	Post Hoc test significant pairs
	Control $n = 57$	Grade 1 $n = 65$	Grade 2 $n = 60$	Grades 3 and 4 $n = 68$		
Wt (kg)	12.09 ± 3.09	9.94 ± 2.28	8.11 ± 1.77	6.76 ± 2.04	$F = 75.392$ $P < 0.01$	All significant
Age (month)	29.52 ± 15.95	30.88 ± 15.33	27.77 ± 13.95	26.27 ± 17.64	$F = 1.221$ $P > 0.05$	
Ht (cm)	87.80 ± 12.03	88.76 ± 10.95	83.97 ± 10.69	80.91 ± 13.52	$F = 7.001$ $P < 0.001$	Control Grades 3 and 4 Grade 1 and Grades 3 and 4
HC (cm)	47.4 ± 2.18	47.7 ± 1.78	46.9 ± 2.10	46.8 ± 2.48	$F = 2.507$ $P > 0.05$	No group significant
MAC (cm)	14.9 ± 0.89	13.9 ± 0.86	12.04 ± 1.14	10.9 ± 0.97	$F = 263.723$ $P < 0.001$	All significant
CC (cm)	48.52 ± 3.59	49.02 ± 3.16	48.1 ± 3.10	47.7 ± 4.35	$F = 1.803$ $P > 0.05$	No group significant

2. Subjects and Methods

The study was conducted in the Department of Biochemistry and the Department of Pediatrics, SSLH, Institute of medical sciences, Banaras Hindu University, Varanasi. 250 children aged between 6 months to 5 years were selected. These children were examined for malnutrition, diagnosed, and classified according to nutrition subcommittee of IAP in 4 grades with various percentages of expected body weight for age [9].

All the chemicals and reagents required for the analysis were of analytical grade, and proper aseptic measures had been taken while study. Estimation was done by Spectrophotometer. The children were classified using the standard value, that is, 100% as 50th percentile of the standard NCHS growth standard, Normal > 80% of standard weight for age. Grade-I = 71–80%, Grade-II = 61–70%, Grade-III = 51–60%, and Grade IV = < 50%. According to this classification, 193 children were of strictly defined malnutrition cases; of these children, 65 belong to grade-I, 60 to grade-II, and 68 to grade-III, and none of the cases was of grade IV. 57 normal and healthy children presenting no clinical and anthropometric signs or symptoms suggestive of any form of malnutrition with age and sex matched were used as control group. The gradation was done on the basis of clinical examination and plasma protein level was not assayed. Male and female ratio was 5 : 4 in both case and control groups. The hemoglobin level of the control group was about 11.9 gm/dL (conventional unit, estimated by Drabkin's method) and hemoglobin levels in grade 1, grade 2, and grades (3 + 4) were about 11.5 gm/dL, 10.2 gm/dL, 8.41 gm/dL, respectively. Ethical clearance to conduct the present study was obtained from the ethical committee Institute of medical sciences, BHU. Informed consent was taken from the attendants of the patients. Blood samples were collected from strictly defined malnutrition cases and from normal subjects under aseptic condition. Random blood samples were taken from the patients attending the paediatric OPD of the Hospital (between 8AM and 2PM). Children suffering from severe infections, edema, taking micronutrient, and antioxidants supplement were excluded from the study. All patients and controls were asked about the history concerning their diet, and clinical examination was done for their anthropometric measurements. Five mL of venous blood was sampled from each subject. Three mL of blood was allowed for 30–60 minutes for spontaneous blood clotting. The serum was separated from the blood cells by centrifugation at 3000 rpm for 10 minutes at room temperature. The serum was decanted and centrifuged twice for 5 minutes at 3000 rpm to remove any blood cell remnants, decanted again, and then stored at −20°C in deionized eppendorf tube vials until assay. Two mL of whole blood in EDTA was stored separately for glutathione estimation and was stored at −20°C without any preservative. The red blood cells were lysed before estimating glutathione estimation. Oxidants such as MDA and PC were assayed by the thiobarbituric acid test [10] and Reznik and Packer [11], while antioxidants such as ascorbic acid, Cu,Zn-SOD, Cp, and glutathione levels by Roe [12]; S. Marklund and G. Marklund [13]; Ravin [14] and Beutler et al. [15], respectively. Statistical analysis was performed by one way analysis of variance (ANOVA), Post hoc analysis (Bonferroni test) and Pearson correlation coefficients using SPSS 11.5 software. Subjects with malnutrition were compared with nonmalnourished controls. The level of significance was considered at $P < 0.05$.

3. Results

Mean age, head circumference (HC), and chest circumference (CC) between malnourished and control groups were compared. Weight, height, and Mid arm circumference (MAC) were significantly reduced in malnourished children (Table 1; Figure 1). The mean oxidant damage products (MDA and PC) levels were significantly increased in malnourished group ($P < 0.001$) (Table 2; Figure 2) while the antioxidants (Cu,Zn-SOD, Cp, GSH, and ascorbic acid) were significantly reduced (Table 3; Figure 3). Significant negative correlations were observed between MDA and antioxidants (Cu,Zn-SOD,

TABLE 2: Oxidants in different grades of PEM.

Parameters	Mean ± SD				Intergroup comparison of one way ANOVA	Post HOC Test significant pairs
	Control	Grade 1	Grade 2	Grades 3 and 4		
MDA (μmoL/L)	0.46 ± 0.05	0.80 ± 0.07	1.80 ± 0.07	2.54 ± 0.52	$F = 605.395$ $P < 0.001$	All significant
PC (nmoL/mg)	13.99 ± 1.53	14.91 ± 1.48	31.27 ± 7.72	38.81 ± 10.24	$F = 241.998$ $P < 0.001$	All significant

TABLE 3: Serum antioxidants in cases of malnutrition and control.

Parameters	Mean ± SD				Intergroup comparison one way ANOVA	Post Hoc test significant pairs
	Control $n = 57$	Grade 1 $n = 65$	Grade 2 $n = 60$	Grades 3 and 4 $n = 68$		
Glutathione (mg/mL)	51.41 ± 4.52	40.90 ± 5.51	23.36 ± 5.0 0.59	11.75 ± 3.23	$F = 1173.572$ $P < 0.001$	All significant
SOD (μmoL/mL)	6.52 ± 0.72	4.78 ± 0.68	1.31 ± 0.89	0.35 ± 0.41	$F = 1351.690$ $P < 0.001$	All significant
Ceruloplasmin (mg/dL)	87.60 ± 8.21	76.31 ± 5.70	51.70 ± 9.69	30.30 ± 11.56	$F = 593.930$ $P < 0.001$	All pairs
Ascorbic acid (mg/L)	54.22 ± 8.46	31.41 ± 6.70	13.34 ± 2.94	10.69 ± 1.91	$F = 1001.035$ $P < 0.001$	All pairs

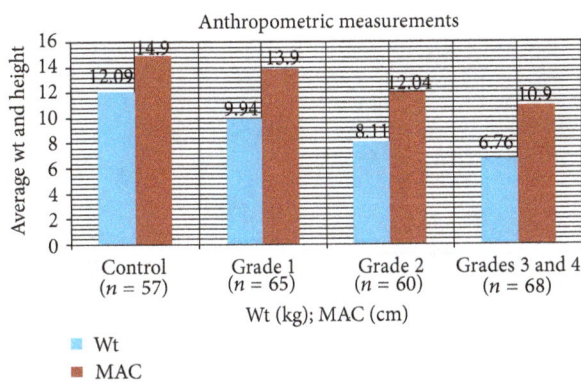

FIGURE 1: Anthropometric measurements in cases of PEM and Control. Results are expressed as mean ± S.D. $P < 0.01$ for Wt. and $P < 0.001$ for MAC while comparing Wt. and MAC of PEM (cases) with control by ANOVA test.

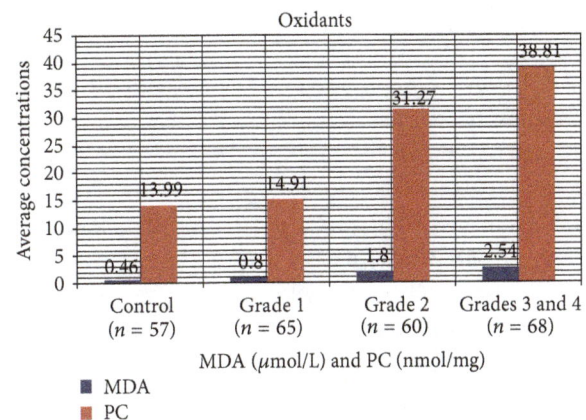

FIGURE 2: Serum MDA and PC conc. in PEM (cases of different grades, i.e., 1, 2, and 3) and control measured by thiobarbituric acid test [10] and Reznick and Packer [11] method, respectively. Results are expressed as mean ± S.D. $P < 0.001$ by ANOVA test.

glutathione, ceruloplasmin, and ascorbic acid) and PC and antioxidants (Table 4). Correlation between GPX and serum MDA in protein energy malnutrition ($P < 0.001$) in Figure 4, correlation between GPX and serum protein carbonyl in protein energy malnutrition ($P < 0.001$) in Figure 5, correlation between SOD and serum protein carbonyl in protein energy malnutrition ($P < 0.001$) in Figure 6, correlation between SOD and serum MDA in protein energy malnutrition ($P < 0.001$) in Figure 7.

4. Discussion

In the present work, we examined the status of both antioxidant and oxidant activities. Malnourished children were found to have more oxidant damage products and less antioxidant levels. Alternatively, the control group consisting of healthy children had comparatively less oxidant damage product and more antioxidant level. ROSs degrades polyunsaturated lipids, forming MDA. Raised levels of lipid peroxidation products in the serum are used as a marker for tissue damage, and MDA is regarded as one of the most stable products of lipid peroxidation. In present study, there is a significant increase in serum MDA in malnourished children as compared to control ($P < 0.001$) (Table 2; Figure 2). Increased plasma MDA levels have been demonstrated previously by other workers also. Boşnak et al. [16] in 2010 conducted a study on the oxidative stress in marasmus

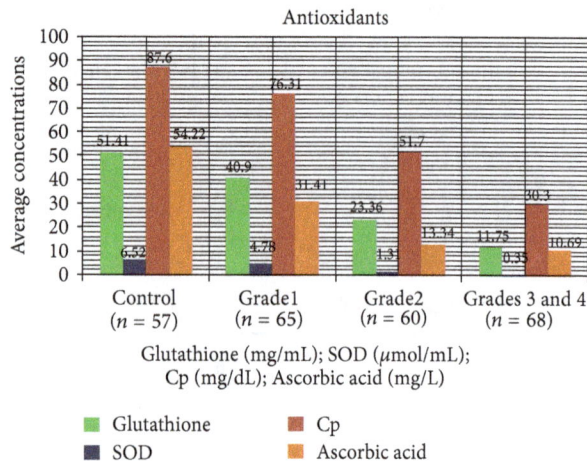

FIGURE 3: Glutathione; CU,ZN-SOD; Cp; ascorbic acid conc. in PEM (cases of different grades i.e, 1, 2, and 3) and control measured by Beutler et al. 1963 [15]; S. Marklund and G. Marklund [13]; Ravin [14]; Roe [12]; method, respectively. Results are expressed as mean ± S.D. $P < 0.001$ while comparing PEM (cases) with control by ANOVA test.

TABLE 4

Correlation between antioxidants and oxidants	Coefficient of correlation and its statistical significance between normal and malnourished
MDA and ceruloplasmin	$r = -0.904$, $P < 0.001$
MDA and Glutathione	$r = -0.901$, $P < 0.001$
MDA and CU, ZN-SOD	$r = -0.869$, $P < 0.01$
MDA and ascorbic acid	$r = -0.821$, $P < 0.001$
Protein carbonyl and glutathione	$r = -0.808$, $P < 0.01$
Protein carbonyl and CU, ZN-SOD	$r = -0.789$, $P < 0.01$
Protein carbonyl and ascorbic acid	$r = -0.727$, $P < 0.01$
Protein carbonyl and ceruloplasmin	$r = -0.851$, $P < 0.01$

children and concluded that MDA was significantly higher in marasmus children. In our present study, there was a significant increase in serum PC in malnourished children as compared to control ($P < 0.001$) (Table 2; Figure 2). PC is a byproduct of protein oxidation, and no related studies has been done earlier on PC in PEM children.

The plasma Cu,Zn-SOD level was found to be significantly decreased in cases. This supports its role as an antioxidant in cases of malnutrition where its level decreases to counteract the oxidative stress. In our present study however Cu,Zn-SOD level is more significant in grades III and IV. These results are in agreement with findings by Golden and Ramdath, 1987 [17]. However, Ashour et al. 1999 [18] had reported an increase of the antioxidant enzymatic activities in 40% of the marasmic children, whereas Sive et al. 1993 [19] found no changes in Cu,Zn-SOD level in marasmic children. In our present study, mean whole blood GPx activity is significantly decreased in malnourished children compared with control ($P < 0.001$) (Table 3; Figure 3). These results are

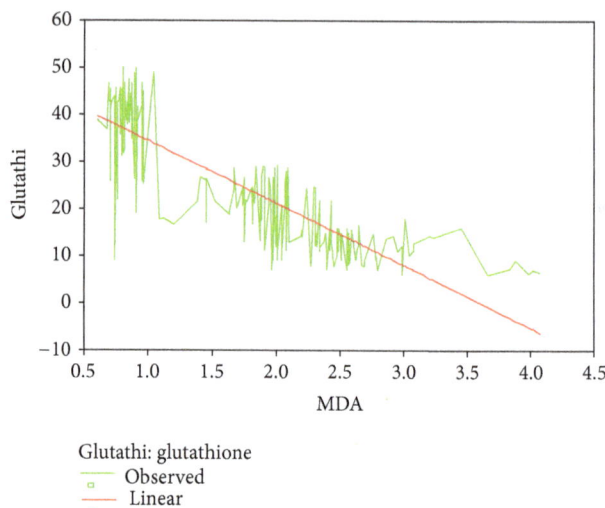

Glutathi: glutathione
— Observed
— Linear

FIGURE 4: Correlation between GPX and Serum MDA in protein energy malnutrition ($P < 0.001$).

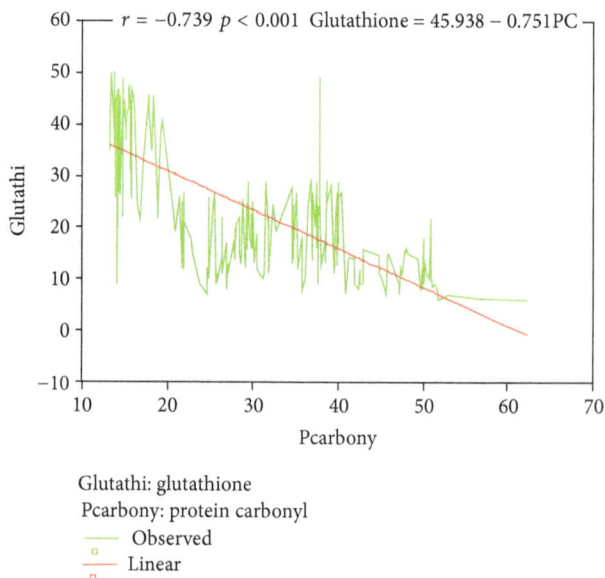

Glutathi: glutathione
Pcarbony: protein carbonyl
— Observed
— Linear

FIGURE 5: Correlation between GPX and Serum Protein Carbonyl in protein energy malnutrition ($P < 0.001$).

in agreement with those reported by Ashour et al. in 1999 [18], Golden and Ramdath in 1987 [17], and Sive et al. in 1993 [19]. In our present study, there is significantly depressed plasma ceruloplasmin level ($P < 0.01$) (Table 3; Figure 3) which is in agreement with the study done by Ashour et al. in 1999 [18] who also showed lower plasma concentration of ceruloplasmin in children with malnutrition. This reduction of the ceruloplasmin may be due to its excessive loss or destruction or its inability to synthesis ceruloplasmin. The concentration of ascorbic acid was markedly depressed in the malnourished group ($P < 0.001$) (Table 3; Figure 3). These results are in agreement with the results reported by Ashour et al. in 1999 [18]. Therefore it appears that these biochemical alterations are indicative of oxidative damage in

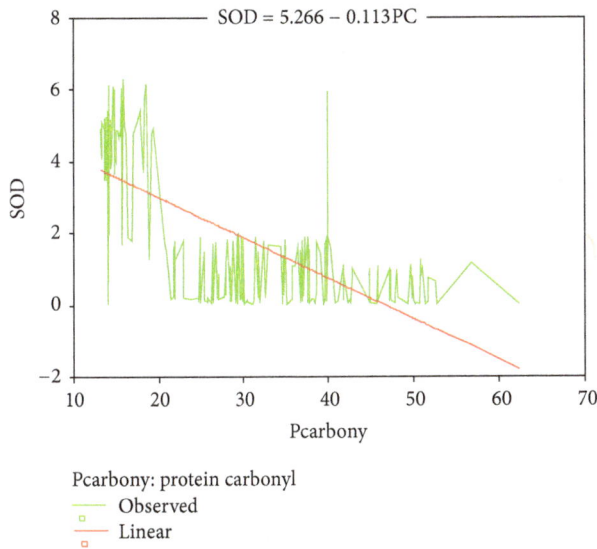

FIGURE 6: Correlation between SOD and Serum Protein Carbonyl in protein energy malnutrition ($P < 0.001$).

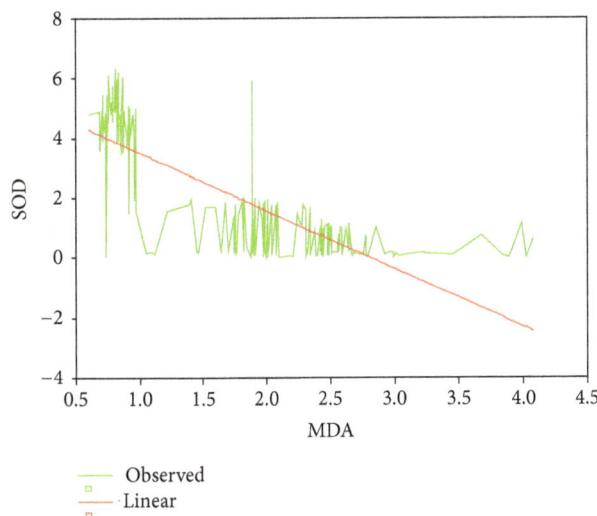

FIGURE 7: Correlation between SOD and Serum MDA in protein energy malnutrition ($P < 0.001$).

malnutrition. Negative correlations between oxidant (PC and MDA) and antioxidants (Cu,Zn-SOD, GPx, Cp, and ascorbic acid) (Table 4) indicate that the magnitude of initial oxidative stress was too high beyond the compensatory capacity of antioxidants. Aldehydes formed endogenously during lipid peroxidation such as MDA which reacts on cellular proteins to form adducts (ALEs) that induce protein dysfunctions and alter cellular responses [20]. Increased MDA levels in children with different grades of PEM may cause accelerated PC formation in plasma proteins especially in albumin. Increased oxidative stress may result from some deleterious effects of deficient caloric and micronutrient intake. In view of the reduced antioxidant defense capacity and the presence of increased oxidant stress, strategies should be developed to strengthen the antioxidant system of children

with protein energy malnutrition, so as to prevent further damage. Further studies are required to determine the cause-and-effect relationship and its prognostic value in patients with malnutrition.

The PC and MDA were measured as an estimate of free radical damage. So they do not give directly the values of the free radicals present in the serum. For more accurate estimation of free radicals, Electron Spin Resonance (ESR) should be used.

Conflict of Interests

The authors declare that there is no conflict of interests regarding the publication of this paper.

Acknowledgments

The authors are very much thankful to Director and Dean of IMS BHU for providing facilities for the above research work and for the kind support of the patients and attendants.

References

[1] H. W. Lane and L. O. Schulz, "Nutritional questions relevant to space flight," *Annual Review of Nutrition*, vol. 12, pp. 257–278, 1992.

[2] T. P. Stein, "Nutrition in the space station era," *Nutrition Research Reviews*, vol. 14, no. 1, pp. 87–117, 2001.

[3] Sitar, S. Aydin, and U. Cakatay, "Human serum albumin and its relation with oxidative stress," *Clinical Laboratory*, vol. 59, no. 9-10, pp. 945–952, 2013.

[4] P. Atukeren, S. Aydin, E. Uslu, M. K. Gumustas, and U. Cakatay, "Redox homeostasis of albumin in relation to alpha-lipoic acid and dihydrolipoic acid," *Oxidative Medicine and Cellular Longevity*, vol. 3, no. 3, pp. 206–213, 2010.

[5] A. M. Rizzo, P. Berselli, S. Zava et al., "Endogenous antioxidants and radical scavengers," *Advances in Experimental Medicine and Biology*, vol. 698, pp. 52–67, 2010.

[6] H. Sies, "Glutathione and its role in cellular functions," *Free Radical Biology and Medicine*, vol. 27, no. 9-10, pp. 916–921, 1999.

[7] L. J. Machlin and A. Bendich, "Free radical tissue damage: protective role of antioxidant nutrients," *The FASEB Journal*, vol. 1, no. 6, pp. 441–445, 1987.

[8] F. O. Jimoh, A. A. Odutuga, and A. T. Oladiji, "Status of lipid peroxidation and antioxidant enzymes in the tissues of rats fed low-protein diet," *Pakistan Journal of Nutritionm*, vol. 4, no. 6, pp. 431–434, 2005.

[9] Nutritional Sub-Committee of Indian Academy of Pediatrics, "Reports of the convener," *Indian Pediatrics*, vol. 9, p. 360, 1972.

[10] K. Satoh, "Serum lipid peroxide in cerebrovascular disorders determined by a new colorimetric method," *Clinica Chimica Acta*, vol. 90, no. 1, pp. 37–43, 1978.

[11] A. Z. Reznick and L. Packer, "Oxidative damage to proteins: spectrophotometric method for carbonyl assay," *Methods in Enzymology*, vol. 233, pp. 357–363, 1994.

[12] J. H. Roe, "Chemical determination of ascorbic, dehydroascorbic, and diketogulonic acids," *Methods of biochemical analysis*, vol. 1, pp. 137–140, 1954.

[13] S. Marklund and G. Marklund, "Involvement of the superoxide anion radical in the autoxidation of pyrogallol and a convenient

assay for superoxide dismutase," *European Journal of Biochemistry*, vol. 47, pp. 469–474, 1974.

[14] H. A. Ravin, "An improved colorimetric enzymatic assay of ceruloplasmin," *The Journal of Laboratory and Clinical Medicine*, vol. 58, pp. 161–168, 1961.

[15] E. Beutler, O. Duron, and B. M. Kelly, "Improved method for the determination of blood glutathione," *The Journal of laboratory and clinical medicine*, vol. 61, pp. 882–888, 1963.

[16] M. Boşnak, S. Kelekçi, S. Yel, Y. Koçyiğit, V. Şen, and A. Ece, "Oxidative stress in marasmic children: relationships with leptin," *European Journal of General Medicine*, vol. 7, no. 1, pp. 1–8, 2010.

[17] M. H. Golden and D. Ramdath, "Free radicals in the pathogenesis of kwashiorkor," *Proceedings of the Nutrition Society*, vol. 46, no. 1, pp. 53–68, 1987.

[18] M. N. Ashour, S. I. Salem, H. M. El-Gadban, N. M. Elwan, and T. K. Basu, "Antioxidant status in children with protein-energy malnutrition (PEM) living in Cairo, Egypt," *European Journal of Clinical Nutrition*, vol. 53, no. 8, pp. 669–673, 1999.

[19] A. A. Sive, B. F. Subotzky, H. Malan, and W. S. Dempster, "Red blood cell antioxidant enzyme concentration in PEM," *Annals of Tropical Pediatrics*, vol. 13, pp. 33–38, 1993.

[20] A. Negre-Salvayre, C. Coatrieux, C. Ingueneau, and R. Salvayre, "Advanced lipid peroxidation end products in oxidative damage to proteins. Potential role in diseases and therapeutic prospects for the inhibitors," *British Journal of Pharmacology*, vol. 153, no. 1, pp. 6–20, 2008.

9

Lipid Profile and Correlation to Cardiac Risk Factors and Cardiovascular Function in Type 1 Adolescent Diabetics from a Developing Country

Aashima Dabas,[1] Sangeeta Yadav,[1] and V. K. Gupta[2]

[1] Department of Paediatrics, Maulana Azad Medical College and Associated Lok Nayak Hospital,
 Bahadur Shah Zafar Marg, New Delhi 110002, India
[2] Department of Biochemistry, G. B. Pant Hospital, Jawahar Lal Nehru Marg, New Delhi 110002, India

Correspondence should be addressed to Aashima Dabas; dr.aashimagupta@gmail.com

Academic Editor: F. J. Kaskel

Objective. The adverse role of dyslipidemia in predicting cardiovascular outcomes has not been elucidated extensively among type 1 diabetics in the literature. *Methods.* We assessed dyslipidemia and its correlation to other cardiac risk factors in adolescents with type 1 diabetes. Total thirty type 1 adolescent diabetics were evaluated for their metabolic profile, including serum lipids and echocardiography was performed. *Results.* The average age of the cohort was 14.3 ± 3.09 yr with disease duration of 5.35 ± 2.94 yr. The mean HbA1C was 8.01%. The mean serum cholesterol, LDL, HDL, and triglyceride were normal. Serum cholesterol was high in patients with longer disease duration ($P = 0.011$, $r = 0.41$), high systolic blood pressure ($P = 0.04$, $r = 0.32$), and elevated HbA1C > 8% ($P = 0.038$, $r = 0.33$). Higher lipid values were associated with poorer carotid artery distensibility ($P > 0.05$) and higher carotid artery intimomedial thickness (cIMT) ($P < 0.05$ for cholesterol and LDL). Hyperglycemia adversely affected ejection fractions, though serum lipids did not show any significant effect on left ventricular parameters. Conclusions. Dyslipidemia and hyperglycemia can serve as biomarkers for cardiovascular dysfunction in at-risk adolescents with type 1 diabetes. Carotid artery parameters are adjunctive tools which may be affected early in the course of macrovascular disease.

1. Introduction

Early atherosclerotic lesions presenting as fatty streaks in blood vessels in childhood can progress in adolescence in the presence of risk factors like hyperlipidemia, hypertension, and diabetes mellitus (DM) [1]. There is enough evidence to support hyperglycemia as a risk factor for cardiovascular disease (CVD) in type 1 diabetes mellitus (T1DM). Hyperglycemia causes nonenzymatic glycation of proteins leading to formation of advanced glycation end products (AGEs) which are thought to be implicated in both microvascular and macrovascular complications of diabetes. They promote cross linking of proteins which can manifest as decreased cardiac compliance [2]. However, the role of lipids in causation of CVD has not been established in young adolescent diabetics.

The prevalence of hyperlipidemia in T1DM is approximately 20–40% [3]. There is enhanced foam cell formation and an increase in the formation of low density lipoprotein cholesterol (LDL-C) dienes, which increase the susceptibility of LDL for oxidation and predispose for atherosclerosis [1, 4]. Chronic hyperglycemia induces a state of oxidative stress which in turn promotes low density lipoprotein (LDL) oxidation and a decrease in nitric oxide availability. Diabetes also promotes the expression of E-selectin and vascular cell adhesion molecule (VCAM) by the endothelial cells. These promote leucocyte adhesion to the vessels which accumulate lipids and release proinflammatory cytokines, thus promoting plaque formation [3, 5].

Hypertension acts as an independent cardiac risk factor and is postulated to promote smooth muscle proliferation that can increase intimomedial thickness (IMT) and left ventricle mass. It also adversely affects diastolic heart functions [3, 6].

Early changes of atherosclerosis include increased arterial stiffness and increased arterial IMT. These are followed by cardiac dysfunction and left ventricular hypertrophy. The arterial distensibility is postulated to be a more sensitive marker of atherosclerosis than cIMT as it measures endothelial dysfunction [5, 6]. There is limited data on noninvasive evaluation of cardiovascular functions in diabetic children. The incidence of early cardiovascular complications in T1DM has not been elucidated in the setting of a developing country.

We thus undertook a study to assess the metabolic control in young adolescent diabetics. The cardiovascular status of these patients was assessed using echocardiography and risk factors for the same were evaluated, with emphasis on lipid profile.

2. Methods

The study was conducted at the pediatric endocrinology clinic of a referral tertiary care hospital.

2.1. Sample Characteristics. All adolescent (10–18 years) type 1 diabetic patients who had regular follow-up at the endocrine clinic were assessed for enrolment in the study. They were diagnosed based on clinical and laboratory criteria; facilities for diagnosing islet cell antibodies were not available. All patients were screened for celiac disease by serum tissue transglutaminase levels and none had elevated titres. The thyroid function tests and anti-thyroid peroxidase antibodies measured at their initial diagnosis were also normal in all patients. The subjects were on premeal insulin bolus regimen (short and long acting insulin). Out of forty five such subjects, thirty consented and were evaluated. Patients were excluded if there was:

(i) any history of hypertension or intake of antihypertensive or lipid lowering medication,

(ii) any history of substance abuse,

(iii) any co morbid coexistent chronic disease,

(iv) history of recent hospitalization/illness in the last month; such patients were evaluated after an interval of three months of apparent wellness.

The study design was prospective cross sectional. The study was approved by the institutional ethical committee. Informed consent was taken from the parents/guardians.

2.2. Clinical Evaluation. A general physical examination was performed and weight and height recorded. Body mass index (BMI) was calculated as weight (kg)/height^2 (m)^2. The BMI readings were interpreted using World Health Organization (WHO) charts and recorded to nearest percentile [7]. Baseline blood pressure (BP) was recorded using a standard sphygmomanometer in the supine position after a ten-minute rest period. An average of two readings was noted during any given measurement. The BP readings were interpreted against

height and age adjusted BP centiles and a value ≥ 95th centile was considered abnormal if measured at ≥3 separate occasions [8]. Mean Bp was calculated as [(2 × DBP) + SBP]/3 [8].

2.3. Laboratory Evaluation. Both fasting and postprandial blood samples were collected by venipuncture in appropriate BD vacutainers using sterile technique. Fasting and postprandial blood glucose values were measured by the glucose oxidase method. Glycated hemoglobin (HbA1C) and lipid profile were measured on fasting blood samples. HbA1C was assessed using immunoturbidimetric method which measured the absorbance of the glycosylated hemoglobin fraction and total hemoglobin fraction at 415 nm. The lipid profile (total cholesterol, serum triglyceride, and serum high density lipoprotein-cholesterol (HDL-C)) was measured using standard methods on an autoanalyzer. Total cholesterol and triglycerides were measured using enzymatic colorimetric method. HDL-C was estimated by an automated direct assay method. LDL-C was calculated by Friedewald's formula [9].

2.4. Cardiovascular Function Evaluation. This was assessed using high resolution ultrasound scanner (AGILENT SONOS 4500 ULTRASOUND MACHINE) which was connected to computer software and obtained images were stored for future reference. The prerequisites for echocardiography measurements included fasting for 8–12 hours (to avoid changes in flow mediated arterial dilatation by substances like caffeine, high fat) and rest for 15 minutes [10]. All parameters were evaluated by a single experienced vascular sonographer who was blinded to the metabolic profile of the patients.

2.4.1. Arterial Functions. The patients were placed supine with neck in slight hyperextension. The common carotid artery (below the carotid bulb and 1 cm proximal to bifurcation) was scanned on B mode (realtime) and Doppler imaging using a 7–12 MHz linear array transducer [1, 11]. Both right and left common carotid artery were evaluated and mean of three different recordings of both sides was taken as common final value.

(1) Physiological Changes. Flow mediated dilatation of the carotid artery (endothelium independent) was done to assess its distensibility. Distensibility is a measure of luminal diameter change in vessel with change in blood pressure [12]. Exogenous nitric oxide donor, for example, high dose nitroglycerine (NTG) tablet (0.4 mg sublingual) was given to obtain a vasodilator response. Peak vasodilatation occurs 3-4 minutes after drug administration during which blood pressure was monitored. Further evaluation was terminated on a patient if he developed hypotension or bradycardia. Images of the vessel before and after the drug administration were recorded and difference in diameter (distensibility) was noted.

A2. Anatomical Changes. Carotid intimal-medial thickness (cIMT) was assessed by measuring the near and far wall of the artery at two separate angles—anterior oblique and lateral. cIMT was measured as the difference between two echogenic lines of the vessel wall. The first line is the luminal-intimal interface while the second is collagen containing upper layer of adventitia [13, 14]. The normal limit for cIMT is arbitrary and is influenced by age, gender, and population. It is thus interpreted in terms of increased risk rather than statistical distribution; however a value of >1 mm is definitely abnormal [15].

2.4.2. Cardiac Functions. The cardiac parameters (*M*-mode measurements) were recorded using the standard parasternal long axis view just below the tip of the mitral leaflet using 5 MHz phased array scanner [16]. The following parameters were recorded: left ventricular systolic and end diastolic internal dimensions (LVIDs, LVIDd), thickness of interventricular septum (IVS), fractional shortening at systole and diastole (FSs, FSd), and ejection fraction (EF) [17]. The apical four-chamber view was obtained for diastolic function analysis which included measurement of peak mitral inflow velocity at early diastole and at late diastole. Left ventricular inflow signals were obtained in the pulse mode by placing the sample volume between the mitral leaflets and adjusting the position until the highest peaks of diastolic velocity were obtained. The peak early diastolic velocity (*E*) and peak late diastolic velocity (*A*) were measured and ratio (*E/A*) was determined [18–20].

2.5. Statistical Analysis. The results were analyzed using appropriate statistical tests on SPSS software. Quantitative data was expressed as mean ± 2 SD. Statistical significance of quantitative variables between different categories was analyzed using *t*-test. Pearson's correlation coefficient/Spearman's rank coefficient (*r*) was used to indicate significant linear relationship among quantitative variables and regression analysis was done. A *P* value <0.05 was considered as significant. Any *P* value <0.001 was taken as highly significant.

3. Results

A total of thirty diabetic patients were included in the study and all tolerated the study procedure well. There was an equal gender distribution with 15 boys and 15 girls. The mean age of patients was 14.3 ± 3.09 years. The body mass index (BMI) was in the range of 13.3–24 kg/m^2 (mean 17.1 ± 2.9 kg/m^2, at 25th centile of WHO chart). The average duration of the disease was 5.35±2.94 years; two patients had diabetes for >10 years. The mean insulin dose was 1.1 U/kg/day. The average BP was 111.4 ± 12.52 mmHg systolic/70.48 ± 9.16 mmHg diastolic. Two patients were hypertensive when interpreted as per age and height chart [8]. The measured laboratory and echocardiography data have been summarized in Table 1. The observed HbA1C range was 4–13.1% (mean = 8.01 ± 2.19; normal range = 6–8%). The normal range of the lipid parameters was cholesterol, 150–200 mg/dL; triglyceride, 60–150 mg/dL; LDL, <100 mg/dL, as per kit inserts. The mean HDL was less than the reference of 40–60 mg/dL.

3.1. Lipids and Traditional Cardiac Risk Factors. None of the lipid parameters had any significant correlation to age

TABLE 1: Mean laboratory and echocardiographic parameters of study population.

Parameter	Mean ± S. D.
Fasting blood glucose	223.8 ± 108.8 mg/dL
Postmeal glucose (2 hours later)	267.9 ± 114.79 mg/dL
HbA1C	8.01%
S. Cholesterol	152.70 ± 33.5 mg/dL
S. Triglyceride	111.8 ± 49.61 mg/dL
S.HDL	38.31 ± 11.38 mg/dL
S.LDL	92.39 ± 29.73 mg/dL
Carotid distensibility	0.097 ± 0.064 mm.
cIMT	0.698 ± 0.23 mm
LVID [s]/LVID [d]	3.65 ± 1.05 cm/4.69 ± 1.32 cm
Interventricular septal thickness	8.49 ± 1.20 mm
EF [s]/EF [d]	70.6 ± 7.3%/66.11 ± 6.6%
FS [s]/FS [d]	35.84 ± 3.6 cm/32.9 ± 3.42 cm
E/A ratio	1.25 ± 0.97

(*P* > 0.05). Among lipids, serum cholesterol had a significant positive correlation with SBP (*P* = 0.04, *r* = 0.32; Figure 1(a)) and weaker with DBP (*P* > 0.05; *r* = 0.26; Figure 1(b)); the rest of lipid parameters had weaker correlation with BP. A significant correlation was established between serum cholesterol and LDL with duration of disease (*P* = 0.011, *r* = 0.41, *P* = 0.049, *r* = 0.30, Figure 1(c)) unlike the rest of lipid parameters.

3.2. Cardiovascular Parameters. There was no difference in arterial distensibility or cIMT when compared with age or gender (*P* > 0.05). Table 2 depicts the relation of different cardiovascular variables evaluated on echocardiography with metabolic parameters. On multivariate analysis, the arterial distensibility remained unaffected by changes in blood pressure, duration of disease, fasting sugar, HbA1C, and lipid profile (*P* > 0.05). However, there was a significant inverse relation between postprandial sugar and arterial distensibility (*P* = 0.05; *r* = −0.43). Both serum cholesterol and LDL had a significant correlation with cIMT, (*P* = 0.002; *r* = 0.48 and *P* = 0.017; *r* = 0.44, resp. (Figure 1(d)). Serum triglycerides and HDL did not show any correlation to arterial parameters. There was no observed significance between cIMT and duration of disease or fasting/postprandial sugar (>0.05). Both SBP and DBP were significantly related to cIMT (*P* = 0.02; *r* = 0.37 and *P* = 0.005; *r* = 0.46, resp.). Serum lipid parameters did not affect left ventricular functions in our cohort (*P* > 0.05).

3.3. Glycemic Control and Analysis. Patients with a poorer sugar profile (HbA1C ≥ 8%) had longer disease duration (*P* = 0.009; *r* = 0.44), higher DBP (*P* = 0.047, *r* = 0.37), higher serum cholesterol (*P* = 0.011; *r* = 0.41), and higher serum LDL (*P* = 0.55; *r* = 0.29). The arterial distensibility was better with good glycemic (HbA1C < 8%) values unlike those with higher HbA1C, though the result was not significant (*P* = 0.75). The mean cIMT was significantly higher in

TABLE 2: Cardiovascular variables compared with metabolic parameters—showing significance values (P).

Echo parameter/metabolic parameter	HbA1C	Serum cholesterol	Serum triglyceride	Serum HDL	Serum LDL
Carotid distensibility	0.75	0.63	0.87	0.30	0.92
cIMT	0.02*	0.002*	0.06	0.10	0.017*
Ejection fraction (systole)	0.02*	0.197	0.142	0.463	0.501
Ejection fraction (diastole)	0.03*	0.204	0.090	0.590	0.513

*Significant value.

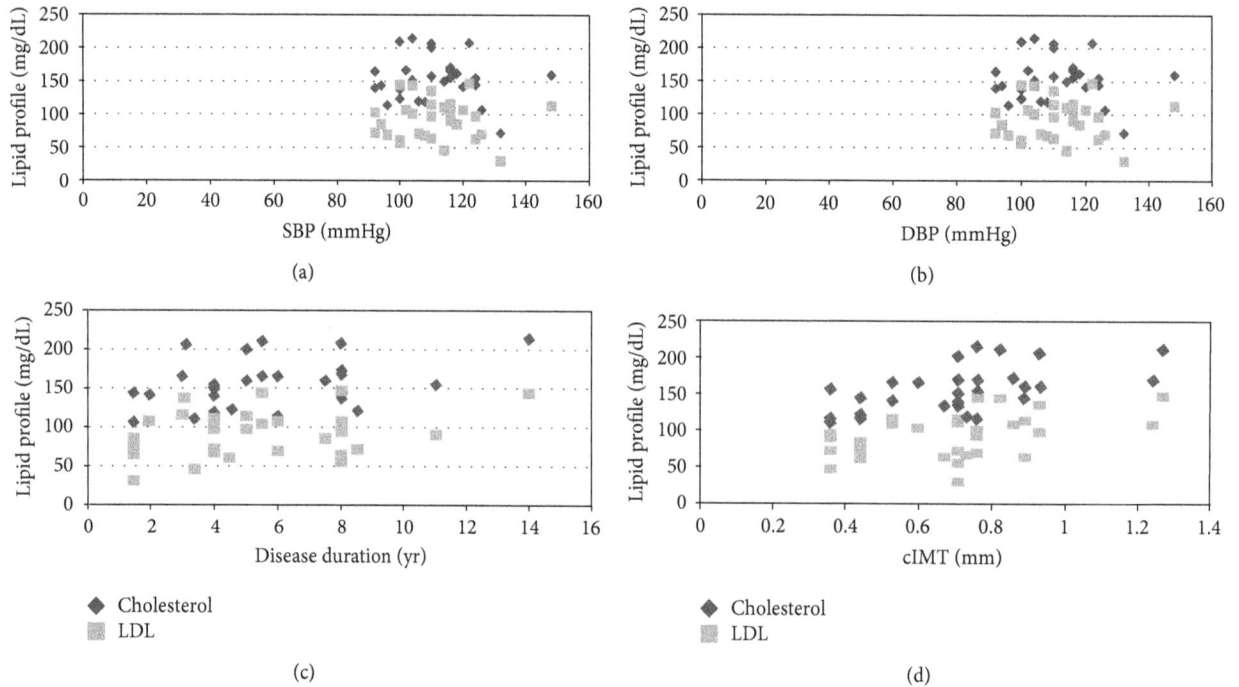

FIGURE 1: (a) Correlation of systolic BP with serum cholesterol and LDL. (b) Correlation of diastolic BP (DBP) with serum cholesterol and serum LDL. (c) Correlation of disease duration with serum cholesterol and serum LDL. (d) Correlation of cIMT with serum cholesterol and serum LDL. *(Each pair of points represents single subject).

patients with higher HbA1C; $P = 0.019$; $r = 0.43$. There was a significant difference with ejection fractions measured during systole (74.4 ± 7.2% in good control and 68.18 ± 6.3% in poor control); $P = 0.02$. The ejection fraction at diastole was also significantly higher in those with good control (69.1 ± 7.1%) as compared to those with poor control (64.07 ± 5.52); $P = 0.03$. Rest of the LV parameters did not establish a significant relation with HbA1C ($P > 0.05$).

LV internal diameters were directly influenced with cIMT values ($P = 0.048$ in systole and $P = 0.042$ in diastole). Five patients in our cohort had increased interventricular septal thickness; two of them also had high cIMT (>0.8 mm); ($P = 0.013$). The mitral inflow velocity in late diastole (A) was significantly associated with carotid artery distensibility ($P < 0.01$) and with cIMT ($P = 0.002$).

4. Discussion

The present cohort of adolescent diabetics had a near normal metabolic control with mean lipid profile being normal. Patients with high serum lipids (especially cholesterol and LDL)

were at high risk of CVD as they recorded higher blood pressure and had longer disease duration, poorer glycemic control (HbA1C > 8%), and deranged arterial parameters as measured on echocardiography.

Diabetic patients are prone to develop dyslipidemia (quantitative and qualitative) with reported prevalence of 24–40% [21–24]. Diabetics with suboptimal HbA1C may have deranged lipid values versus those with optimal HbA1C [25]. Serum HDL levels are generally optimum in T1DM and do not play a causative role in CVD [26, 27]. The mean lipids were higher in our patients with poorer glycemic control. Though our patients with longer disease duration had poorer glycemic control and higher serum cholesterol, they did not manifest any significant changes in the carotid artery parameters, similar to data reported by Gunczler et al. [28]. Conversely few other authors have identified early cardiac changes in the presence of longer diabetes duration [29, 30].

The coexistence of diabetes and hypertension has been considered as a major factor in the expression of the abnormalities in human diabetic myocardium [13, 15, 31]. Both serum cholesterol and glycemic control predicted higher systolic BP in our study. Abdelghaffar et al. and Carugo et al. have reported a similar difference in blood pressures of diabetics versus controls in their studies [32, 33]. However, Aepfelbacher et al. did not document any difference in BP of T1DM even after a documented improvement in HbA1C [34]. Hypertension emerged as a risk factor for increased cIMT in our cohort similar to prior conducted studies [35–38]. The American Diabetes Association (ADA) thus recommends blood pressure evaluation in all diabetics on follow-up visits for cardiovascular screening [39]. They have also defined optimal serum lipid levels in children with T1DM but the threshold to decide intervention is still under research [40].

BMI is a nonlipid cardiac risk factor for atherogenesis [41, 42] and is raised in T1DM [12, 32]. The BMI recorded in our cohort was low as poverty and lower socioeconomic status determined BMI in our setting.

There was no significant correlation between carotid artery distensibility and any of the lipid values, though serum cholesterol and LDL had significant relation to cIMT. Various study trials have reported hyperlipidemia to be associated with carotid atherosclerosis in T1DM [4, 32, 38, 43]; Järvisalo et al. concluded the role of both serum cholesterol and LDL levels in predicting arterial structural integrity in T1DM, even if they were present within the normal range in blood [1, 38]. However few like Peppa-Patrikiou et al. have reported inconclusive results [35]. These outcomes are variable probably because of various confounding factors like age, blood pressure, family history of dyslipidemia, disease duration, and HbA1C status.

Hyperglycemia was established as a cardiac risk factor in our study similar to earlier studies. Correlation of HbA1C was seen with arterial distensibility [12], cIMT [12, 32, 35, 38, 44], and few ventricular parameters [33, 34, 45–47] as described in past. In a recent publication by DCCT, cIMT has been established as a marker for atherosclerosis when associated with hyperglycemia [48]. However, there are few authors who have obtained normal cIMT [12, 28, 49] and normal LV functions in patients with T1DM [50].

Left ventricular changes are frequently reported in diabetes in existence of glucose intolerance [42]. There are limited available human studies where lipid values are correlated to cardiac functions in T1DM. There was no correlation between lipids and LV parameters in our study which was probably due to a short disease duration; as postulated earlier by Chen et al [51].

The study was one of the first pilot studies which assessed left ventricular functions in adolescent diabetics in relation to lipid profile. However the major limitation of our study was a small sample size and absence of healthy control population for comparison. The disease duration was also small to influence significant changes in LV functions. Future studies comparing diabetic population with healthy controls will be needed on a larger scale to reinforce the results of this first pilot study.

5. Conclusion

To summarize, both serum cholesterol and LDL were established as cardiac risk factors, in addition to HbA1C and blood pressure. Dyslipidemia can serve as early biomarker for cardiovascular dysfunction in adolescents with Type 1 Diabetes.

What is already known about this topic is as follows.

(1) Type 1 diabetes is associated with cardiovascular morbidity.

(2) Patients with type 1 diabetes need to be screened for dyslipidemia around puberty.

What this paper adds is as follows.

(1) Dyslipidemia may not be overt early in course of type 1 diabetes.

(2) Raised serum cholesterol and serum LDL can serve as biomarkers for cardiovascular morbidity in adolescents with type 1 diabetes.

(3) Echocardiography may be used as an adjunct to monitor cardiac status in diabetics with poor metabolic control to prevent complications.

Disclosure

The authors disclose that the paper represents valid work and that neither this paper nor one with substantially similar content under their authorship has been published or is being considered for publication elsewhere. The research was a self-funded project without any external financial aid.

Conflict of Interests

The authors declare that there is no conflict of interests regarding the publication of this paper.

Acknowledgment

Sangeeta Yadav conceptualized the study and played a critical role in drafting the paper. V. K. Gupta played an integral role in conduct of the research and provided expert inputs in revision of the paper. AD had full access to all the data in the study and is responsible for the integrity of the data and the accuracy of the data analysis. The authors will like to express sincere thanks to Dr. Rani Gera, Pediatric Cardiologist, for performing and supervising the conduct of echocardiography during the research.

References

[1] M. J. Järvisalo, A. Putto-Laurila, L. Jartti et al., "Carotid artery intima-media thickness in children with type 1 diabetes," *Diabetes*, vol. 51, no. 2, pp. 493–498, 2002.

[2] Z. Milicevic, I. Raz, S. D. Beattie et al., "Natural history of cardiovascular disease in patients with diabetes: role of hyperglycemia," *Diabetes Care*, vol. 31, supplement 2, pp. S155–S160, 2008.

[3] The DCCT Research Group, "Lipid and lipoprotein levels in patients with IDDM," *Diabetes Care*, vol. 15, no. 7, pp. 886–894, 1991.

[4] R. Kawamori, Y. Yamasaki, H. Matsushima et al., "Prevalence of carotid atherosclerosis in diabetic patients: ultrasound high-resolution B-mode imaging on carotid arteries," *Diabetes Care*, vol. 15, no. 10, pp. 1290–1294, 1992.

[5] N. Mitsuhashi, T. Onuma, S. Kubo, N. Takayanagi, M. Honda, and R. Kawamori, "Coronary artery disease and carotid artery intima-media thickness in Japanese type 2 diabetic patients," *Diabetes Care*, vol. 25, no. 8, pp. 1308–1312, 2002.

[6] P. Lacolley, P. Challande, S. Boumaza et al., "Mechanical properties and structure of carotid arteries in mice lacking desmin," *Cardiovascular Research*, vol. 51, no. 1, pp. 178–187, 2001.

[7] World Health Organization, "WHO Child Growth Standards. Methods and development. Department of Nutrition for Health and Development," WHO, Geneva, Switzerland, S41–S55, 2007, http://www.who.int/childgrowth/standards/en/.

[8] National High Blood Pressure Education Program Working Group on High Blood Pressure in Children and Adolescents, "The fourth report on the diagnosis, evaluation, and treatment of high blood pressure in children and adolescents," *Pediatrics*, vol. 114, no. 2, supplement, pp. 555–576, 2004.

[9] G. R. Warnick, R. H. Knopp, V. Fitzpatrick, and L. Branson, "Estimating low-density lipoprotein cholesterol by the Friedewald equation is adequate for classifying patients on the basis of nationally recommended cutpoints," *Clinical Chemistry*, vol. 36, no. 1, pp. 15–19, 1990.

[10] M. C. Corretti, T. J. Anderson, E. J. Benjamin et al., "Guidelines for the ultrasound assessment of endothelial-dependent flow-mediated vasodilation of the brachial artery: a report of the international brachial artery reactivity task force," *Journal of the American College of Cardiology*, vol. 39, no. 2, pp. 257–265, 2002.

[11] P. Pauciullo, A. Iannuzzi, R. Sartorio et al., "Increased intima-media thickness of the common carotid artery in hypercholesterolemic children," *Arteriosclerosis and Thrombosis*, vol. 14, no. 7, pp. 1075–1079, 1994.

[12] A. Parikh, E. B. Sochett, B. W. McCrindle, A. Dipchand, A. Daneman, and D. Daneman, "Carotid artery distensibility and cardiac function in adolescents with type 1 diabetes," *Journal of Pediatrics*, vol. 137, no. 4, pp. 465–469, 2000.

[13] S. Cosson and J. P. Kevorkian, "Left ventricular diastolic dysfunction: an early sign of diabetic cardiomyopathy?" *Diabetes and Metabolism*, vol. 29, no. 5, pp. 455–466, 2003.

[14] J. Larsen, M. Brekke, L. Sandvik, H. Arnesen, K. F. Haussen, and K. Dahl-Jorgensen, "Silent coronary atheromatosis in type 1 diabetic patients and its relation to long-term glycemic control," *Diabetes*, vol. 51, no. 8, pp. 2637–2641, 2002.

[15] A. Simon, J. Gariepy, G. Chironi, J.-L. Megnien, and J. Levenson, "Intima-media thickness: a new tool for diagnosis and treatment of cardiovascular risk," *Journal of Hypertension*, vol. 20, no. 2, pp. 159–169, 2002.

[16] D. J. Sahn, A. DeMaria, J. Kisslo, and A. Weyman, "Recommendations regarding quantitation in M-mode echocardiography: results of a survey of echocardiographic measurements," *Circulation*, vol. 58, no. 6, pp. 1072–1083, 1978.

[17] N. B. Schiller, P. M. Shah, M. Crawford et al., "Recommendations for quantitation of the left ventricle by two-dimensional echocardiography. American Society of Echocardiography Committee on Standards, Subcommittee on Quantitation of Two-Dimensional Echocardiograms," *Journal of the American Society of Echocardiography*, vol. 2, no. 5, pp. 358–367, 1989.

[18] M. Romanens, S. Fankhauser, B. Saner, L. Michaud, and H. Saner, "No evidence for systolic or diastolic left ventricular dysfunction at rest in selected patients with long-term type I diabetes mellitus," *European Journal of Heart Failure*, vol. 1, no. 2, pp. 169–175, 1999.

[19] T. K. Mishra, P. K. Rath, N. K. Mohanty, and S. K. Mishra, "Left ventricular systolic and diastolic dysfunction and their relationship with microvascular complications in normotensive, asymptomatic patients with type 2 diabetes mellitus," *Indian Heart Journal*, vol. 60, no. 6, pp. 548–553, 2008.

[20] A. Sato, L. Tarnow, and H.-H. Parving, "Increased left ventricular mass in normotensive type 1 diabetic patients with diabetic nephropathy," *Diabetes Care*, vol. 21, no. 9, pp. 1534–1539, 1998.

[21] D. M. Maahs, L. G. Ogden, D. Dabelea et al., "Association of glycaemia with lipids in adults with type 1 diabetes: modification by dyslipidaemia medication," *Diabetologia*, vol. 53, no. 12, pp. 2518–2525, 2010.

[22] D. B. Petitti, G. Imperatore, S. L. Palla et al., "Serum lipids and glucose control: the SEARCH for diabetes in youth study," *Archives of Pediatrics and Adolescent Medicine*, vol. 161, no. 2, pp. 159–165, 2007.

[23] K. C. Loh, A. C. Thai, K. F. Lui, and W. Y. Ng, "High prevalence of dyslipidaemia despite adequate glycaemic control in patients with diabetes," *Annals of the Academy of Medicine Singapore*, vol. 25, no. 2, pp. 228–232, 1996.

[24] A. K. Kershnar, S. R. Daniels, G. Imperatore et al., "Lipid abnormalities are prevalent in youth with type 1 and type 2 diabetes: the search for diabetes in youth study," *Journal of Pediatrics*, vol. 149, no. 3, pp. 314–319, 2006.

[25] J. Guy, L. Ogden, R. P. Wadwa et al., "Lipid and lipoprotein profiles in youth with and without type 1 diabetes: the SEARCH for diabetes in youth case-control study," *Diabetes Care*, vol. 32, no. 3, pp. 416–420, 2009.

[26] P. K. Merrin, S. Renton, C. Fisher et al., "Serum lipids and apolipoproteins and their relationship with macrovascular disease in type 1 diabetes," *Diabetic Medicine*, vol. 11, no. 4, pp. 402–406, 1994.

[27] N. Chaturvedi, J. H. Fuller, and M.-R. Taskinen, "Differing associations of lipid and lipoprotein disturbances with the macrovascular and microvascular complications of type 1 diabetes," *Diabetes Care*, vol. 24, no. 12, pp. 2071–2077, 2001.

[28] P. Gunczler, R. Lanes, E. Lopez, S. Esaa, O. Villarroel, and R. Revel-Chion, "Cardiac mass and function, carotid artery intima-media thickness and lipoprotein (a) levels in children and adolescents with type 1 diabetes mellitus of short duration," *Journal of Pediatric Endocrinology and Metabolism*, vol. 15, no. 2, pp. 181–186, 2002.

[29] E. Adal, G. Koyuncu, A. Aydin, A. Çelebi, G. Kavunoğlu, and H. Cm, "Asymptomatic cardiomyopathy in children and adolescents with type 1 diabetes mellitus: association of echocardiographic indicators with duration of diabetes mellitus and metabolic parameters," *Journal of Pediatric Endocrinology and Metabolism*, vol. 19, no. 5, pp. 713–726, 2006.

[30] B. Shivalkar, D. Dhondt, I. Goovaerts et al., "Flow mediated dilatation and cardiac function in type 1 diabetes mellitus," *American Journal of Cardiology*, vol. 97, no. 1, pp. 77–82, 2006.

[31] M. Barbagallo, R. K. Gupta, and L. M. Resnick, "Cellular ions in NIDDM: Relation of calcium to hyperglycemia and cardiac mass," *Diabetes Care*, vol. 19, no. 12, pp. 1393–1398, 1996.

[32] S. Abdelghaffar, M. El Amir, A. El Hadidi, and F. El Mougi, "Carotid intima-media thickness: an index for subclinical atherosclerosis in type 1 diabetes," *Journal of Tropical Pediatrics*, vol. 52, no. 1, pp. 39–45, 2006.

[33] S. Carugo, C. Giannattasio, I. Calchera et al., "Progression of functional and structural cardiac alterations in young normotensive uncomplicated patients with type 1 diabetes mellitus," *Journal of Hypertension*, vol. 19, no. 9, pp. 1675–1680, 2001.

[34] F. C. Aepfelbacher, S. B. Yeon, L. A. Weinrauch, J. D'Elia, and A. J. Burger, "Improved glycemic control induces regression of left ventricular mass in patients with type 1 diabetes mellitus," *International Journal of Cardiology*, vol. 94, no. 1, pp. 47–51, 2004.

[35] M. Peppa-Patrikiou, M. Scordili, A. Antoniou, M. Giannaki, M. Dracopoulou, and C. Dacou-Voutetakis, "Carotid atherosclerosis in adolescents and young adults with IDDM: relation to urinary endothelin, albumin, free cortisol, and other factors," *Diabetes Care*, vol. 21, no. 6, pp. 1004–1007, 1998.

[36] J. M. Sorof, A. V. Alexandrov, G. Cardwell, and R. J. Portman, "Carotid artery intimal-medial thickness and left ventricular hypertrophy in children with elevated blood pressure," *Pediatrics*, vol. 111, no. 1, pp. 61–66, 2003.

[37] X.-Z. Yang, Y. Liu, J. Mi, C.-S. Tang, and J.-B. Du, "Pre-clinical atherosclerosis evaluated by carotid artery intima-media thickness and the risk factors in children," *Chinese Medical Journal*, vol. 120, no. 5, pp. 359–362, 2007.

[38] M. J. Järvisalo, L. Jartti, K. Näntö-Salonen et al., "Increased aortic intima-media thickness: a marker of preclinical atherosclerosis in high-risk children," *Circulation*, vol. 104, no. 24, pp. 2943–2947, 2001.

[39] D. Power, "Standards of medical care in diabetes: response to position statement of the American Diabetes Association," *Diabetes Care*, vol. 29, no. 2, pp. 476–477, 2006.

[40] S. Krishnan and K. R. Short, "Prevalence and significance of cardiometabolic risk factors in children with type 1 diabetes," *Journal of the CardioMetabolic Syndrome*, vol. 4, no. 1, pp. 50–56, 2009.

[41] K. O. Schwab, J. Doerfer, W. Hecker et al., "Spectrum and prevalence of atherogenic risk factors in 27,358 children, adolescents, and young adults with type 1 diabetes: cross-sectional data from the German diabetes documentation and quality management system (DPV)," *Diabetes Care*, vol. 29, no. 2, pp. 218–225, 2006.

[42] M. K. Rutter, H. Parise, E. J. Benjamin et al., "Impact of glucose intolerance and insulin resistance on cardiac structure and function: sex-related differences in the Framingham Heart Study," *Circulation*, vol. 107, no. 3, pp. 448–454, 2003.

[43] S. D. J. M. Kanters, A. Algra, and J.-D. Banga, "Carotid intima-media thickness in hyperlipidemic type I and type II diabetic patients," *Diabetes Care*, vol. 20, no. 3, pp. 276–280, 1997.

[44] R. R. Rodriguez, R. A. Gómez-Díaz, J. T. Haj et al., "Carotid intima-media thickness in pediatric type 1 diabetic patients," *Diabetes Care*, vol. 30, no. 10, pp. 2599–2602, 2007.

[45] T. J. Berg, O. Snorgaard, J. Faber et al., "Serum levels of advanced glycation end products are associated with left ventricular diastolic function in patients with type 1 diabetes," *Diabetes Care*, vol. 22, no. 7, pp. 1186–1190, 1999.

[46] E. H. Kim and Y. H. Kim, "Left ventricular function in children and adolescents with type 1 diabetes mellitus," *Korean Circulation Journal*, vol. 40, no. 3, pp. 125–130, 2010.

[47] M. Salem, S. El Behery, A. Adly, D. Khalil, and E. El Hadidi, "Early predictors of myocardial disease in children and adolescents with type 1 diabetes mellitus," *Pediatric Diabetes*, vol. 10, no. 8, pp. 513–521, 2009.

[48] D. M. Nathan, J. Lachin, P. Cleary et al., "Intensive diabetes therapy and carotid intima-media thickness in type 1 diabetes mellitus," *The New England Journal of Medicine*, vol. 348, no. 23, pp. 2294–2303, 2003.

[49] T. Yavuz, A. Akçay, R. E. Ömeroğlu, R. Bundak, and M. Şükür, "Ultrasonic evaluation of early atherosclerosis in children and adolescents with type 1 diabetes mellitus," *Journal of Pediatric Endocrinology and Metabolism*, vol. 15, no. 8, pp. 1131–1136, 2002.

[50] J. Salazar, A. Rivas, M. Rodriguez, J. Felipe, M. D. Garcia, and J. Bone, "Left ventricular function determined by Doppler echocardiography in adolescents with type I (insulin-dependent) diabetes mellitus," *Acta Cardiologica*, vol. 49, no. 5, pp. 435–439, 1994.

[51] M.-R. Chen, Y.-J. Lee, C.-H. Hsu, H.-A. Kao, and F.-Y. Huang, "Cardiovascular function in young patients with type 1 diabetes mellitus," *Acta Paediatrica Taiwanica*, vol. 40, no. 4, pp. 250–254, 1999.

10

Off-Label Medicine Use in Pediatric Inpatients: A Prospective Observational Study at a Tertiary Care Hospital in India

Mohd Masnoon Saiyed,[1] Tarachand Lalwani,[1] and Devang Rana[2]

[1] Department of Pharmacology and Clinical Pharmacy, K.B. Institute of Pharmaceutical Education and Research,
GH 6, Sector 23, Gandhinagar, Gujarat 382024, India
[2] Department of Pharmacology, Smt. N.H.L. Municipal Medical College, Sheth V.S. General Hospital, Ellisbridge,
Ahmedabad, Gujarat 380006, India

Correspondence should be addressed to Mohd Masnoon Saiyed; saiyed78@gmail.com

Academic Editor: Julie Blatt

Background. In the absence of standard pediatric prescribing information, clinicians often use medicines in an off-label way. Many studies have been published across the globe reporting different rates of off-label use. There is currently no study based on Indian drug formulary. *Methods.* The prospective observational study included pediatric patients in ages between 0 and 12 years admitted in a tertiary care hospital. Off-label use was assessed using the National Formulary of India (NFI). Predictors of off-label use were determined by logistic regression. *Results.* Of the 1645 medications prescribed, 1152 (70%) were off-label based on 14 possible off-label categories. Off-label medicines were mainly due to dose difference and use in restricted age limits as indicated in NFI. Respiratory medicines (82%), anti-infectives (73%), and nervous system medicines (53%) had higher off-label use. Important predictors of off-label prescribing were pediatric patients in age of 0 to 2 years (OR 1.68, 95% CI; $P < 0.001$) and hospital stay of six to 10 days (OR 1.91, 95% CI; $P < 0.001$). *Conclusion.* Off-label prescribing is common among pediatric patients. There is need to generate more quality data on the safety and efficacy of off-label medicines to rationalize pediatric pharmacotherapy.

1. Introduction

The goal to achieve ideal pediatric drug therapy is a worldwide challenge for regulatory bodies and clinicians. Children are treated with medicines not tested for safety and efficacy and are frequently supported by the low quality of evidence [1]. In the absence of standard prescribing information, clinicians prescribe drugs in an off-label manner. Off-label use means use of medicine which is outside the terms of product license with respect to dose, route of administration, indication, or age [2]. Off-label medicine use among children represents an important health issue as the effects and health risks may be unexpected. Various national and international studies have been published about the amount of and problems associated with off-label medicines in children. The magnitude of off-label prescribing is accounted to be between 18% and 60% in infants but it may be up to 90% in neonates [3–9].

Most of these studies have been conducted outside India and may not be applicable as hospitalization and prescribing patterns differ based on culture, healthcare infrastructure, and health policies. There is a distinct lack of research on off-label prescribing in India. Only one previous study has been conducted in India which reported 50.62% of off-label prescribing based on British National Formulary [5]. Currently there is no study conducted in India based on National Formulary of India (NFI). Hence, the objective of the research study was to quantify off-label use based on NFI, various predictors and discusses some strategies to monitor it.

2. Methods

2.1. Data Collection. The prospective observational study was carried out at a tertiary care hospital in Ahmedabad (India) for the period of six months. All the pediatric patients in ages

TABLE 1: Off-label medicine use categories.

Sr. number	Category	Reason for off-label use	Examples based on NFI
1	Dose	Dose higher than recommended	Once daily dosing of gentamicin in children
2	Age	Drug not recommended in the patient below a certain age	Losartan used in children under 6 years
3	Indication	Drug prescribed for indications outside of those listed in the NFI	Diclofenac for abdominal pain
4	Route of administration	Drug administered by a route not described in the NFI	Adrenaline through inhalation route
5	Absence of pediatric information (PI)	No mention at all in the NFI regarding pediatric use	Nifedipine for hypertension

*NFI: National Formulary of India, 2011 [10].

between 0 and 12 years receiving at least one medication and admitted in pediatric ward were included in the study. The pediatric ward was of 60 bed size and attended by 10 academic pediatricians and 28 postgraduate students. Patients were not considered if they were in age of more than 12 years, not taking any prescription medication and undergoing surgery. Demographics, clinical characteristics, and medication usage were obtained from the medical records using predefined paper case record forms. The data collection was carried out by one of the researchers (MMS) who discussed each of the medicines with attending pediatrician and clinical pharmacologist (DR). Drugs were entered into the database using the World Health Organization Anatomical Therapeutic Chemical (WHO-ATC) classification system [11]. We utilized National Formulary of India (NFI, 4th edition, 2011) which is an official publication of Indian Pharmacopoeia Commission, Ministry of Health and Family Welfare, Government of India [10]. There were five off-label categories (Table 1). Categories for off-label use were allocated for each medicine according to the reason(s) why their use was deemed off-label when compared to the terms of the product labeling for that medicine in NFI. We followed a published algorithm and used these dimensions to determine whether there is strong scientific evidence for frequently prescribed off-label medicines [12] (Table 4).

2.2. Statistical Analysis. Variables such as age, number of medications, number of diagnoses, and length of hospital stay were regarded as continuous and expressed as mean with standard deviation (SD). Categorical variables are presented as numbers with percentages (%). Risk factors for off-label prescribing were analyzed with multivariate binary logistic regression. The odds ratio (OR) with 95% confidence interval (CI) was used to determine the predictors for off-label prescribing. A probability value of less than 0.05 was considered statistically significant for all analyses. The data were analyzed using Statistical Package for the Social Sciences (SPSS Inc., IBM).

2.3. Research Reporting. This study was reported according to the Strengthening the Reporting of Observational Studies in Epidemiology (STROBE) guidelines [13].

3. Results

3.1. Demographic and Clinical Characteristics. The study included a total of 320 patients admitted in pediatric general ward of the public teaching hospital over a period of six months. There were 206 (64%) male and 114 (36%) female patients. The mean age was 2.73 years (range = 0.1 to 12 years and standard deviation: 3.09). The most common age group was 0 to 1 years representing 43% of total sample size.

On average each patient had 1.2 number of diagnosis and 48 patients (mean = 2.5) had more than one diagnosis during hospitalization. The majority of patients suffered from respiratory diseases (33%), central nervous system diseases (16.5%), and gastrointestinal disease (11%). A total of 1645 medications were prescribed to the study cohort during hospitalization, with a total hospital stay of 1743 days. This constituted the mean number of five (SD = 2) medications prescribed per patient and 5.48 (SD = 3.62) days of hospital stay. The number of medications and hospital stay ranged from one to 13 and one to 33 days, respectively. The majority of patients received antibiotics, cough, and cold preparations, antipyretics, inhaled corticosteroids, bronchodilators, and antiepileptic drugs. Medications were mostly administered by oral route (40%) and intravenous route (35%) followed by inhalation route (25%).

3.2. Nature of Off-Label Prescribing. Of the 320 patients included in the study, 310 (97%) patients received at least one off-label medication. A total of 1645 medications were administered during the hospitalization; 1152 (70%) medicines were prescribed in off-label manner when its usage was validated with National Formulary of India, 2011, for five different off-label categories. Patients received on average (SD) 3.66 (2.13) off-label medicines within a range of one to 10. The most common cause of off-label prescribing 893 (63%) was due to higher dose use (category 1) than stated for particular pediatric patients. Mostly ceftriaxone, amikacin, paracetamol, and chlorpheniramine were prescribed in this category.

Off-label medicines use for age (category 2) and indication (category 3) was found to be 282 (19.8%) and 145 (10.2%), respectively. Those medicines which had no pediatric

TABLE 2: Proportion off-label medicine use in different age groups.

Age group	Total medicine	Off-label medicine	Off-label category				
			Dose	Age	Indication	Route	Absence of pediatric information
All age groups (n = 320)	1645	1152 (70)	893 (63)	282 (19.8)	145 (10.2)	24 (1.7)	76 (5.3)
1–12 months (n = 138)	683	472 (69)	391 (64)	147 (24)	44 (7.2)	8 (1.4)	21 (3.4)
>1-2 years (n = 63)	363	276 (76)	218 (63)	70 (20.3)	35 (10.3)	6 (1.8)	16 (4.6)
>2 years–6 years (n = 74)	393	269 (68)	204 (65.4)	46 (14.7)	37 (11.8)	5 (1.6)	20 (6.5)
>6–12 years (n = 45)	206	135 (65)	80 (52.6)	19 (12.5)	29 (19.1)	5 (3.3)	19 (12.5)

*Note: the total number of off-label uses exceeds that of off-label drugs because a drug may be off-label for more than one category. Figures in parentheses indicate percentage.

TABLE 3: Off-label medicine use according to ATC and drugs.

WHO-ATC system	Total medicine	Off-label medicine	Off-label category				
			Dose	Age	Indication	Route	Absence of pediatric information
Anti-infectives for systemic use	531	389 (73)	408 (87.8)	21 (4.5)	5 (1.1)	9 (1.9)	22 (4.7)
Respiratory system	463	378 (82)	244 (56.8)	170 (39.5)	6 (1.4)	7 (1.6)	3 (0.7)
Nervous system	411	220 (53)	168 (55.8)	49 (16.3)	68 (22.6)	0 (0)	16 (5.3)
Alimentary tract and metabolism	99	85 (86)	34 (27.7)	18 (14.6)	48 (39)	0 (0)	23 (18.7)
Hormonal preparation	40	32 (80)	30 (66.7)	15 (33.3)	0 (0)	0 (0)	0 (0)
Cardiovascular system	34	24 (71)	9 (28.1)	9 (28.1)	2 (6.3)	0 (0)	12 (37.5)
Blood and blood forming agents	18	16 (89)	0 (0)	0 (0)	16 (100)	0 (0)	0 (0)
Ant parasitic products	49	8 (16)	0 (0)	0 (0)	0 (0)	8 (100)	0 (0)

*Note: the total number of off-label uses may exceed that of off-label drugs because a drug may be off-label for more than one category. Figures in parentheses indicate percentage.

information (category 5) were 76 (5.3%). Use of ipratropium, salbutamol, and dextromethorphan was common for different dose and age limits. Lorazepam (seizures) and ondansetron (nausea and vomiting) were frequently used for off-label indication.

3.3. Off-Label Prescribing in Different Age Groups.
The study also attempted to distribute the receipt of off-label medicines in different age groups as shown in Table 2. The extent off-label prescribing was highest (76%) in age group of more than 1 to 2 years, followed by age group of more than 1 to 12 months which accounted for 69% of off-label use. Off-label use in dose (category 1) was consistent among the patients in age of 0 to 6 years. The use of medicines in patients for restricted age limits (category 2) was highest in 1–12-month age group.

Indication (category 3) and absence of pediatric information (category 5) were most prominent in 6–12-year patients.

3.4. Off-Label Prescribing by ATC Class and Drugs.
Highest proportion of off-label medicines were prescribed in anti-infectives for systemic use 389 (73%) and respiratory system 378 (82%) as shown in Table 3. The amount of off-label prescribing in nervous system and alimentary tract and metabolism system was 220 (53%) and 85 (86%), respectively. Majority of off-label medicines prescribed were ceftriaxone, amikacin, amoxicillin, and vancomycin in antibiotics class and inhaled corticosteroids, ipratropium, salbutamol, chlorpheniramine, phenylephrine corresponding to respiratory system. Blood and blood forming agents 16 (89%), hormonal preparation 32 (80%), and cardiovascular medicines 24 (71%) had substantial high amount of off-label use. Adrenaline,

TABLE 4: Most frequently prescribed off-label medicines.

Sr. number	System	Off-label medicine use (%)	Off-label category	Quality of evidence	Strength of recommendation
1	Alimentary tract and metabolism	Ondansetron (100%)	Indication	Strong	High
2	Respiratory system	Phenylephrine (91%)	Age, dose	Moderate	Medium
3	Respiratory system	Dextromethorphan (90%)	Age, dose	Moderate	Medium
4	Respiratory system	Chlorpheniramine (88%)	Dose	Moderate	Medium
5	Anti-infectives for systemic use	Ceftriaxone (81%)	Dose	Strong	High
6	Nervous system	Lorazepam (80%)	Indication	Strong	High
7	Respiratory system	Ipratropium (79%)	Age, Dose	Strong	High
8	Anti-infectives for systemic use	Amikacin (75%)	Dose	Strong	High
9	Respiratory system	Salbutamol (75%)	Age, dose	Strong	High
10	Nervous system	Paracetamol (56%)	Age, dose	Moderate	High

TABLE 5: Predictors of off-label medicine use (multivariate binary logistic regression model).

Sr. number	Parameter	Total number of patients	OR (95% CI)	P value
1	Age group			
	0–2 years	201	1.68 (1.26–2.24)	<0.001
	>2–6 years	74	1.40 (0.99–1.96)	0.052
	>6–12 years	45	1 (reference)	—
2	Gender			
	Female	114	1.41 (1.13–1.77)	0.002
	Male	206	1 (reference)	—
3	Number of diagnosis			
	Double or more	48	0.91 (0.73–1.12)	0.389
	Single	272	1 (reference)	—
4	Hospital stay			
	1–5	224	1.32 (0.97–1.81)	0.074
	6–10	66	1.91 (1.33–2.75)	<0.001
	More than 10	30	1 (reference)	—

*$P < 0.05$ indicates significant difference and $P >$ or $= 0.05$ indicates nonsignificant difference; OR: odd ratio and CI: confidence interval.

nifedipine, prednisolone, and dexamethasone were also used in off-label manner. Antiparasitic products 8 (16%) had minimum off-label use.

Antibiotics (75%) and inhaled corticosteroids (79%) were mostly prescribed in higher doses (category 1) than recommended. In respiratory system, many medicines (39.5%) were prescribed below age limits (category 2) as indicated in the formulary. Medicines used for unapproved indication (category 3) largely confined to alimentary tract and metabolism system and blood and blood forming agents. Medicines which had no pediatric information were predominantly in antihypertensive drug class.

3.5. Predictors of Off-Label Medicine Use. On multivariate regression analysis as shown in Table 5, we found that pediatric patients in age of 0 to 2 years (OR 1.68, 95% CI, 1.26–2.24,) were more likely to receive off-label medicines than any other age group. Female patients (OR 1.41, 95% CI, 1.13–1.77) received substantially high amount of off-label medicines compared to male. Hospital stay of six to 10 days

(OR 1.91, 95% CI, 1.33–2.75) also carried higher risk of off-label prescription.

4. Discussion

Using the data of the pediatric ward of a tertiary care hospital, we found that 70% of medicines were prescribed in off-label manner. The magnitude off-label prescribing is substantial higher than reported in the recent studies [14–16]. Cuzzolin et al. performed a literature review of published studies on off-label and unlicensed drug use in children [3]. A total of 30 studies from 1990 to 2006 were included. Seven studies involved neonatal intensive care units (NICUs), fifteen studies included pediatric wards, and twelve studies were conducted in community setting. Cuzzolin et al. found off-label prescribing in pediatric ward ranging between 18 and 60%. Various reasons for different rates of off-label use are off-label classification methods, sample sizes, pediatrician's prescribing habits, in-house treatment protocols, and diseases characteristics most importantly pediatric drug regulation.

Patients in ages between 0 and 2 years are most likely to receive off-label medicines and had highest representation in study sample. Previous studies also established that age group of 0 to 2 years is the highest recipient of off-label prescriptions [16, 17]. This is mainly due to absence of specific dosing guidelines and route administration in 0-to-2-year age group in NFI. Of the medicines prescribed during the period, it was observed that antibiotics, respiratory medicines, and nervous system medicines were frequently prescribed in off-label manner. Several studies had shown high rate of off-label prescribing in respiratory [18], antibiotics [19], analgesics [20], and antiepileptics [21]. About 82% of medicines in respiratory system were off-label which is more than what is reported in studies in US (n = 312 million, 70%) [22] and Portugal (n = 500, 77%) [23]. If asthma therapies are considered, inhaled corticosteroids are frequently prescribed (30.7% of all prescriptions). The mainstay therapy for asthma is inhaled corticosteroids (ICS), but guidelines often do not give specific recommendations for upper doses limits specially in children [24].

Various combinations of antihistaminics, decongestants, and/or analgesics were prescribed to patients in off-label doses for common cold. But the effectiveness in young children is still questionable [25]. During the study paracetamol was commonly used drug to treat fever and pain in children. Still, the off-label use of paracetamol is substantial, mainly due to off-label classification for dose or age. Although paracetamol is normally considered safe in pediatrics care, a previous Cochrane review pointed out that there is limited evidence regarding the efficacy and safety for paracetamol in the treatment of fever in children [26]. Lorazepam and ondansetron were widely prescribed for off-label indication but are supported by well conducted clinical studies [27, 28].

World Health Organization (WHO) adopted in 2007 the WHA60.20 Resolution "Better Medicines for Children" to improve monitoring medicine safety in the pediatrics and highlighted its concern on off-label medicines [29]. The strict drug approval procedure is the way to ensure quality data on quality, safety, and efficacy for different pediatric age groups. Despite many regulatory amendments and policies, we still have apathetic outlook to pediatric clinical trials [30].

The pharmaceutical companies should be convinced to have appropriate pediatric information in the label and they are not being permitted to market drugs likely to be used in children without suitable pediatric labeling. Indian drug regulatory authorities should also develop pediatric specific drug development regulation so that the tendency to market medicines without pediatric specific data is discouraged. This might ensure pediatric labeling for new medicines yet to be introduced in the market; but it is unlikely that drug companies will carry out trials to confirm pediatric use for drugs already marketed and used in children, although in an off-label manner.

Alternatively, the situation can be improved when prescribers report their pediatric experiences with different off-label medicines in form research articles or discussion at scientific platforms. When medicines are used as off-label, each patient is unique and risk-benefit pertaining to him should be assessed by high quality evidence. The doctor needs to be updated with latest evidence which could be accomplished by using several useful drug compendia like DRUGDEX, Clinical Pharmacology, and so forth. Only such focused and coordinated actions would make sure that children's right to safe, cost-effective, and quality medicines would be realized.

5. Conclusion

Based on National Formulary of India, our data suggest that magnitude of off-label prescribing in pediatric inpatients is considerable higher than reported in some of the countries. Dose discrepancy and use in restricted age limits were identified as main contributor to off-label prescribing. There is need for strict drug regulation for pediatric population to ensure safety and effectiveness of pharmacotherapy. Further studies are needed to examine why there are inadequate dosing guidelines and generation of more clinical data especially in respiratory medicines. Understanding various risk factors and spectrum of off-label medicine use can assist developing prevention strategies. Off-label prescribing is a reality and will not go soon. Implementing evidence based approach can significantly improve rationality of pediatric pharmacotherapy.

Ethical Approval

The study received ethical approval from Ethics Committee (Protocol no. 39), K.B. Institute of Pharmaceutical Education and Research, India.

Conflict of Interests

The authors report no conflict of interests that might bias the outcome of the paper.

References

[1] J. Dunne, "The European Regulation on medicines for paediatric use," *Paediatric Respiratory Reviews*, vol. 8, no. 2, pp. 177–183, 2007.

[2] E. Kimland and V. Odlind, "Off-label drug use in pediatric patients," *Clinical Pharmacology & Therapeutics*, vol. 91, no. 5, pp. 796–801, 2012.

[3] L. Cuzzolin, A. Atzei, and V. Fanos, "Off-label and unlicensed prescribing for newborns and children in different settings: a review of the literature and a consideration about drug safety," *Expert Opinion on Drug Safety*, vol. 5, no. 5, pp. 703–718, 2006.

[4] S. Turner, A. Longworth, A. J. Nunn, and I. Choonara, "Unlicensed and off label drug use in paediatric wards: prospective study," *British Medical Journal*, vol. 316, no. 7128, pp. 343–345, 1998.

[5] S. S. Jain, S. B. Bavdekar, N. J. Gogtay, and P. A. Sadawarte, "Off-label drug use in children," *Indian Journal of Pediatrics*, vol. 75, no. 11, pp. 1133–1136, 2008.

[6] S. B. Bavdekar, P. A. Sadawarte, N. J. Gogtay, S. S. Jain, and S. Jadhav, "Off-label drug use in a Pediatric Intensive Care Unit," *Indian Journal of Pediatrics*, vol. 76, no. 11, pp. 1113–1118, 2009.

[7] C. Pandolfini, P. Impicciatore, D. Provasi et al., "Off-label use of drugs in Italy: a prospective, observational and multicentre study," *Acta Paediatrica*, vol. 91, no. 3, pp. 339–347, 2002.

[8] H. Knopf, I.-K. Wolf, G. Sarganas, W. Zhuang, W. Rascher, and A. Neubert, "Off-label medicine use in children and adolescents: results of a population-based study in Germany," *BMC Public Health*, vol. 13, no. 1, article 631, 2013.

[9] S. Conroy, M. P. Raffaelli, F. Rocchi et al., "Survey of unlicensed and off label drug use in paediatric wards in European countries," *British Medical Journal*, vol. 320, no. 7227, pp. 79–82, 2000.

[10] *National Formulary of India*, 4th edition, 2011, http://cdsco.nic.in/writereaddata/NFI_2011.pdf.

[11] WHO Collaborating Centre for Drug Statistics Methodology, *Guidelines for ATC Classification and DDD Assignment*, Norwegian Institute of Public Health, Oslo, Norway, 14th edition, 2011.

[12] R. Harbour and J. Miller, "A new system for grading recommendations in evidence based guidelines," *British Medical Journal*, vol. 323, no. 7308, pp. 334–336, 2001.

[13] E. von Elm, D. G. Altman, M. Egger, S. J. Pocock, P. C. Gøtzsche, and J. P. Vandenbroucke, "The Strengthening the Reporting of Observational Studies in Epidemiology (STROBE) statement: guidelines for reporting observational studies," *Journal of Clinical Epidemiology*, vol. 61, no. 4, pp. 344–349, 2008.

[14] P. Langerová, J. Vrtal, and K. Urbánek, "Incidence of unlicensed and off-label prescription in children," *Italian Journal of Pediatrics*, vol. 40, no. 1, article 12, 2014.

[15] L. Dos Santos and I. Heineck, "Drug utilization study in pediatric prescriptions of a university hospital in southern Brazil: off-label, unlicensed and high-alert medications," *Farmacia Hospitalaria*, vol. 36, no. 4, pp. 180–186, 2012.

[16] C. Carnovale, V. Conti, V. Perrone et al., "Paediatric drug use with focus on off-label prescriptions in Lombardy and implications for therapeutic approaches," *European Journal of Pediatrics*, vol. 172, no. 12, pp. 1679–1685, 2013.

[17] E. Schirm, H. Tobi, and L. T. W. de Jong-van den Berg, "Risk factors for unlicensed and off-label drug use in children outside the hospital," *Pediatrics*, vol. 111, no. 2, pp. 291–295, 2003.

[18] G. W. Jong, I. A. Eland, M. C. J. M. Sturkenboom, J. N. van den Anker, and B. H. C. Stricker, "Unlicensed and off-label prescription of respiratory drugs to children," *European Respiratory Journal*, vol. 23, no. 2, pp. 310–313, 2004.

[19] S. Ekins-Daukes, J. S. McLay, M. W. Taylor, C. R. Simpson, and P. J. Helms, "Antibiotic prescribing for children. Too much and too little? Retrospective observational study in primary care," *British Journal of Clinical Pharmacology*, vol. 56, no. 1, pp. 92–95, 2003.

[20] S. Conroy and V. Peden, "Unlicensed and off label analgesic use in paediatric pain management," *Paediatric Anaesthesia*, vol. 11, no. 4, pp. 431–436, 2001.

[21] P. H. Novak, S. Ekins-Daukes, C. R. Simpson, R. M. Milne, P. Helms, and J. S. McLay, "Acute drug prescribing to children on chronic antiepilepsy therapy and the potential for adverse drug interactions in primary care," *British Journal of Clinical Pharmacology*, vol. 59, no. 6, pp. 712–717, 2005.

[22] A. T. F. Bazzano, R. Mangione-Smith, M. Schonlau, M. J. Suttorp, and R. H. Brook, "Off-label prescribing to children in the United States outpatient setting," *Academic Pediatrics*, vol. 9, no. 2, pp. 81–88, 2009.

[23] M. Morais-Almeida and A. J. Cabral, "Off-label prescribing for allergic diseases in pre-school children," *Allergologia et Immunopathologia*, vol. 42, no. 4, pp. 342–347, 2014.

[24] National Asthma Education and Prevention Program and Third Expert Panel on the Diagnosis and Management of Asthma, *Expert Panel Report 3: Guidelines for the Diagnosis and Management of Asthma*, 2014, http://www.ncbi.nlm.nih.gov/books/NBK7232/.

[25] A. I. De Sutter, M. L. van Driel, A. A. Kumar, O. Lesslar, and A. Skrt, "Oral antihistamine-decongestant-analgesic combinations for the common cold," *Cochrane Database of Systematic Reviews*, vol. 2, 2012.

[26] M. Meremikwu and A. Oyo-Ita, "Paracetamol for treating fever in children," *Cochrane Database of Systematic Reviews*, no. 2, Article ID CD003676, 2002.

[27] B. Carter and Z. Fedorowicz, "Antiemetic treatment for acute gastroenteritis in children: an updated Cochrane systematic review with meta-analysis and mixed treatment comparison in a Bayesian framework," *BMJ Open*, vol. 2, no. 4, Article ID e000622, 2012.

[28] K. Prasad, P. R. Krishnan, K. Al-Roomi, and R. Sequeira, "Anticonvulsant therapy for status epilepticus," *British Journal of Clinical Pharmacology*, vol. 63, no. 6, pp. 640–647, 2007.

[29] K. Hoppu, G. Anabwani, F. Garcia-Bournissen et al., "The status of paediatric medicines initiatives around the world—what has happened and what has not?" *European Journal of Clinical Pharmacology*, vol. 68, no. 1, pp. 1–10, 2012.

[30] S. Selvarajan, M. George, S. S. Kumar, and S. A. Dkhar, "Clinical trials in India: where do we stand globally?" *Perspectives in Clinical Research*, vol. 4, no. 3, pp. 160–164, 2013.

11

Associated Factors of Acute Chest Syndrome in Children with Sickle Cell Disease in French Guiana

Narcisse Elenga,[1] Emma Cuadro,[1] Élise Martin,[1] Nicole Cohen-Addad,[2] and Thierry Basset[1]

[1] *Pediatric Unit, Cayenne Medical Center, Andrée Rosemon Hospital, Rue des Flamboyants, BP 6006, 97306 Cayenne Cedex, French Guiana*
[2] *Pediatric Unit, Kourou Medical Center, Avenue des îles, BP 703, 97310 Kourou, French Guiana*

Correspondence should be addressed to Narcisse Elenga; elengafr@yahoo.fr

Academic Editor: Julie Blatt

A matched case-control study was performed in order to identify some associated factors for ACS or to confirm the published data. Controls were children hospitalized during the same period for pain crisis who did not develop an ACS during hospitalization. Between January 2006 and October 2010, there were 24 episodes of ACS distributed among 19 patients (8 girls and 11 boys). The median age was 7.5 years (range: 3 to 17 years) for the cases and 7 years (range: 3–18 years) for the controls. Four cases and 11 controls were treated with hydroxyurea (HU). In 75% of the cases, the ACS had arisen 24–72 hours following admission. The independent factors associated with ACS were average Hb rate <8 g/dL (OR = 4.96, 95% CI = 1.29–27.34, and P = 0.04), annual number of hospitalizations >3 (OR = 5.44, 95% CI = 3.59–8.21, and P = 0.003), average length of hospitalization >7 days (OR = 3.69, 95% CI = 3.59–8.21, and P = 0.003), and a pathological transthoracic echocardiography (TTE) (OR = 13.77, 95% CI = 2.07–91.46, and P = 0.003). Although the retrospective design and small sample size are weaknesses of the present study, these results are consistent with those of previous studies and allowed identifying associated factors such as a pathological TTE.

Sickle cell disease (SCD) is a major public health concern in French Guiana, a French region with 230,000 inhabitants located in South America [1]. The incidence of major SCD from birth screening is 1/227, and the overall frequency of AS carriers is 10% [2]. The major SCD groups include the three main genetic forms: hemoglobin (Hb) SS (68%), Hb SC (25%), and Sβ thalassemia (7%). The acute chest syndrome (ACS) is a complication of SCD characterized by pleuritic chest pain, fever, rales on lung auscultation, and pulmonary infiltrates on chest X-ray [3]. It is the most frequent cause of mortality in children with SCD [3–8]. In 1979, Charache et al. first suggested using the term acute chest disease (ACD) for this complication, acknowledging the difficulties in determining its pathogenesis [9].

We report here the results of a case-control study of risk factors for ACS in children with SCD in French Guiana, in order to find some associated factors for ACS or to confirm the published data. We hypothesized that HbSS, age, high Hb level, and high steady-state leukocyte count could be risk factors for ACS. This matched case-control study

concerned all cases of ACS hospitalized in the pediatric unit in French Guiana from 2006 to 2010. The cases were children hospitalized between January 2006 and October 2010 for pain crisis and who developed an ACS. The controls were children hospitalized during the same period for pain crisis and who did not develop an ACS during hospitalization. Each episode of ACS was matched on age, gender, and year of diagnosis.

The transthoracic echocardiography (TTE) was performed by a single pediatrician cardiologist, at baseline when the child was in a healthy state, during the annual evaluation. Patients with a pathological TTE were followed every six months by the same pediatrician cardiologist. All the TTE were obtained at true baseline and not during admissions. These TTE showed the following anatomical pathologies: an enlargement of the left heart chambers associated with an elevation in blood volume in seven cases and two controls and elevation in left ventricular myocardial indices in two cases and two controls. The Commission Nationale Informatique et Libertés approved our data collection. The factors associated with ACS were analyzed by logistic regression based on odds

TABLE 1: Case and control description and bivariate and multivariate analysis*.

Variables	Cases (%)	Controls (%)	Bivariate analysis		Multivariate analysis	
			Crude OR (95% CI)	P	Adjusted OR (95% CI)	P
Age (years)						
0–4	2 (8)	25 (33)	1			
5–9	14 (59)	21 (27)	0.12 (0.02, 0.59)	0.009		
10–14	6 (25)	15 (20)	0.2 (0.04, 1.12)	0.07		
15–19	2 (8)	15 (20)	0.6 (0.08, 4.72)	0.63		
Sex						
M	13 (54)	43 (57)	1			
F	11 (46)	33 (43)	1.1 (0.44, 2.77)	0.84		
Type of haemoglobin						
SS	20 (83)	45 (59)	1			
Sβ thal or SC	4 (17)	31 (41)	0.29 (0.09, 0.93)	0.038		
History of treatment by hydroxyurea						
Yes	4 (17)	11 (14)	1			
No	20 (83)	65 (86)	0.85 (0.24, 2.95)	0.79		
Duration of hospitalization (days)						
>7	14 (58)	12 (16)	4.23 (2.64, 6.3)	<0.01	**3.69 (2.30–5.56)**	*<0.01*
0–7	10 (42)	64 (84)	1			
Age during the first symptoms						
1 year	5 (21)	34 (45)	1			
Before 1 year	19 (79)	42 (55)	3.08 (1.04, 9.09)	0.04		
History of >3 annual hospitalisations						
Yes	19 (79)	26 (34)	7.31 (2.45, 21.8)	<0.01	**5.44 (3.59–8.21)**	*0.003*
No	5 (21)	50 (66)	1			
Basic haemoglobin level						
>8 g/dL	3 (12)	31 (41)	1			
0–8 g/dL	21 (88)	45 (59)	4.82 (1.32, 17.58)	0.15	**4.96 (1.29–27.34)**	*0.04*
Basic S haemoglobin level						
≥80%	20 (83)	39 (51)	1			
<80%	4 (17)	37 (49)	0.21 (0.07, 0.68)	0.009		
Transthoracic echocardiography						
Normal	15 (63)	70 (95)	1			
Abnormal	9 (37)	4 (5)	10.5 (2.85, 38.65)	<0.001	**13.77 (2.07–91.46)**	*0.003*
Transcranial echo-Doppler						
Normal	19 (79)	72 (97)	1			
Abnormal	5 (21)	2 (3)	9.47 (1.7, 52.69)	0.01		

*Obtained using conditional logistic regression with indicator variables for nonbinary variables.
Bold fonts: OR (95% CI) of multivariate analysis.
Italic fonts: P-value of multivariate analysis.

ratios (OR). For all tests performed, a *P* value of 0.05 or less was considered as statistically significant. The data were entered into Microsoft Excel 2007 and analyzed using R.2.10.0 (R project, CRAN R 2.10.0 version 2010) statistical software. All the factors numbered in Table 1 were included in this analysis. We included in our final model the covariates that were associated with the outcome in the univariate analysis and other factors associated with ACS, according to the literature.

Between January 2006 and October 2010, there were 24 episodes of ACS distributed among 19 patients (8 girls and 11 boys). One patient developed 3 events of ACS; 3 presented 2 events; and 15 patients presented 1 event of ACS. The median age was 7.5 years (range: 3 to 17 years) for the cases and 7 years (range: 3–18 years) for the controls (Mann-Whitney test). These two groups did not differ in age.

Four cases and 11 controls were treated with hydroxyurea (HU). The results are shown in Table 1. Among the cases, there were 20 HbSS, 3 HbSβ° thalassemia, and 1 HbSC. Among the controls, there were 45 HbSS, 12 HbSβ° thalassemia, 10 HbSβ+ thalassemia, and 9 HbSC. The more frequent hospitalization, longer hospital stays, lower Hb, higher % HbS, and earlier presentation in the cases may be explained, at least in part, by the difference in genotype and the severity of sickle cell anaemia.

In 75% of the cases, the ACS had arisen 24–72 hours following admission. All patients received rehydration, oxygen therapy, and pulmonary physiotherapy using stress spirometry and triple antibiotic therapy (cefotaxime, aminoglycoside, and a macrolide). In 16 cases, patients received a single red blood cell transfusion and in six other cases, the red blood cell transfusion was followed by a partial exchange transfusion (removing the patient's own blood and replacing it with 0.9% NaCl volume for volume, which was followed by a red blood cell transfusion). The target haemoglobin S value was under 30% and haemoglobin level 80–90 g/L, and in any of the cases, we obtained them. The more frequent hospitalization, longer hospital stays, lower Hb, higher % HbS, and earlier presentation in the cases may be explained, at least in part, by the difference in genotype and the severity of sickle cell anaemia. Two cases died. The cases who died did not receive a transfusion. The first was a 6-year-old girl in severe vasoocclusive crisis with fever and severe anemia (Hb of 4 g/dL), who presented 8 hours later with a frank ACS and whom endotracheal intubation was unsuccessful. The second was a 4-year-old girl also with frank ACS and bilateral pleural effusion, who died despite successful endotracheal intubation. The two cases who died had received a single dose of ceftriaxone. The proportion of death was high and due in part to low access to care in foreign patients. Although health is free of charge in French Guiana, the prevention is complicated by the fact that a number of persons are illiterate or do not understand the language. However, the health priorities of immigrants are often overridden by daily struggles to obtain food, shelter, and papers. Due to the low power of our study, certain factors such as lower Hb, higher % HbS, and earlier presentation in the cases as well as the transcranial Doppler, that were significant in bivariate analysis, were not statistically significant in multivariate analysis. However, the effect of including several episodes in single individuals was not analysed because of the small sample of our study.

Annual number of hospitalizations >3 (OR = 5.44, 95% CI = 3.59–8.21, and *P* = 0.003), average length of hospitalization >7 days (OR = 3.69, 95% CI = 3.59–8.21, and *P* = 0.003), average Hb rate <8 g/dL (OR = 4.96, 95% CI = 1.29–27.34, and *P* = 0.04), and a pathological TTE (OR = 13.77, 95% CI = 2.07–91.46, and *P* = 0.003) were independent associated factors for ACS. The TTE was performed to detect any abnormalities such as left heart chambers abnormalities and intracardiac shunts, including foramen ovale. According to a few studies [10], intracardiac shunting could be a risk factor for stroke in children with SCD because it predisposes to thrombosis and elevations of right heart pressure, which could promote paradoxical embolization across an intracardiac shunt. In our study, a pathological TTE was a strong factor associated with ACS. However, the role of cardiac abnormalities as associated factors for children with ACS was unknown. Defining the role of intracardiac shunting in pediatric ACS will require controlled studies with unified detection methods in stratified populations. HU is efficacious in children and adults with SCD, with an increase in Hb F%, reduction in hospitalizations and pain crises, and prevention of new episodes of ACS. However, in our study, because of its low power, this variable did not appear as a protective factor. Although the retrospective design and small sample size are weaknesses of the present study, our results are consistent with those of previous studies [3, 4, 9]. This study also allowed us to identify associated factors such as pathological TTE. Possible preventative measures consist of earlier use of red blood cell transfusion and/or early use of HU. The role of cardiac abnormalities in ACS deserves to be clarified by other studies.

Conflict of Interests

The authors declare that they have no conflict of interests.

References

[1] J. Zonzon and G. Prost, *Géographie De La Guyane*, Servedit, Paris, France, 1997.

[2] M. Etienne-Julan, G. Elana, G. Loko, N. Elenga, T. Vaz, and M. Muszlak :, "La drépanocytose dans les départements français d'outre-mer (Antilles, Guyane, la Réunion, Mayotte): données descriptives et organisation de la prise en charge," *BEH*, pp. 27–28, 2012.

[3] E. P. Vichinsky, L. D. Neumayr, A. N. Earles et al., "Causes and outcomes of the acute chest syndrome in sickle cell disease," *The New England Journal of Medicine*, vol. 342, no. 25, pp. 1855–1865, 2000.

[4] E. P. Vichinsky, L. A. Styles, L. H. Colangelo, E. C. Wright, O. Castro, and B. Nickerson, "Acute chest syndrome in sickle cell disease: clinical presentation and course," *Blood*, vol. 89, no. 5, pp. 1787–1792, 1997.

[5] S. K. Ballas, S. Lieff, L. J. Benjamin et al., "Definitions of the phenotypic manifestations of sickle cell disease," *American Journal of Hematology*, vol. 85, no. 1, pp. 6–13, 2010.

[6] C. T. Quinn, E. P. Shull, N. Ahmad, N. J. Lee, Z. R. Rogers, and G. R. Buchanan, "Prognostic significance of early vaso-occlusive complications in children with sickle cell anemia," *Blood*, vol. 109, no. 1, pp. 40–45, 2007.

[7] J. M. Knight-Madden, T. S. Forrester, N. A. Lewis, and A. Greenough, "Asthma in children with sickle cell disease and its association with acute chest syndrome," *Thorax*, vol. 60, no. 3, pp. 206–210, 2005.

[8] M. E. Nordness, J. Lynn, M. C. Zacharisen, P. J. Scott, and K. J. Kelly, "Asthma is a risk factor for acute chest syndrome and cerebral vascular accidents in children with sickle cell disease," *Clinical and Molecular Allergy*, vol. 3, article no. 2, 2005.

[9] S. Charache, J. C. Scott, and P. Charache, "'Acute chest syndrome' in adults with sickle cell anemia. Microbiology, treatment, and prevention," *Archives of Internal Medicine*, vol. 139, no. 1, pp. 67–69, 1979.

[10] M. M. Dowling, N. Lee, C. T. Quinn et al., "Prevalence of intracardiac shunting in children with sickle cell disease and stroke," *Journal of Pediatrics*, vol. 156, no. 4, pp. 645–650, 2010.

12

Critical Analysis of PIM2 Score Applicability in a Tertiary Care PICU in Western India

Vivek V. Shukla,[1] Somashekhar M. Nimbalkar,[1,2] Ajay G. Phatak,[2] and Jaishree D. Ganjiwale[2]

[1] Department of Pediatrics, Pramukhswami Medical College, Karamsad, Anand, Gujarat 388325, India
[2] Central Research Services, Charutar Arogya Mandal, Karamsad, Anand, Gujarat 388325, India

Correspondence should be addressed to Somashekhar M. Nimbalkar; somu_somu@yahoo.com

Academic Editor: Hans Juergen Laws

Objective. Children have limited physiological reserve that deteriorates rapidly. Present study profiled patients admitted to PICU and determined PIM2 score applicability in Indian setting. *Patients and Methods.* Prospective observational study. *Results.* In 742 consecutive admissions, male : female ratio was 1.5 : 1, 35.6% patients were ventilated, observed mortality was 7%, and 26.4% were <1 year. The profile included septicemia and septic shock (29.6%), anemia (27.1%), pneumonia (19.6%), and meningitis and encephalitis (17.2%). For the first year, sensitivity of PIM2 was 65.8% and specificity was 71% for cutoff value at 1.9 by ROC curve analysis. The area under the curve was 0.724 (95% CI: 0.69, 0.76). This cutoff was validated for second year data yielding similar sensitivity (70.6%) and specificity (65%). Logistic regression analysis (LRA) over entire data revealed various variables independently associated with mortality along with PIM2 score. Another logistic model with same input variables except PIM2 yielded the same significant variables with Nagelkerke R square of 0.388 and correct classification of 78.5 revealing contribution of PIM2 in predicting mortality is meager. *Conclusion.* Infectious diseases were the commonest cause of PICU admission and mortality. PIM2 scoring did not explain the outcome adequately, suggesting need for recalibration. Following PALS/GEM guidelines was associated with better outcome.

1. Introduction

Infant and childhood mortality is very high in resource-limited countries. According to the 2010 United Nations reports, infant mortality rate (IMR) ranges from 1.92 (Singapore) to 135 (Afghanistan) with IMR of India at 52.9 deaths per 1000 live births [1]. About 60% of these deaths are neonatal yet many of the remaining deaths are preventable by appropriate and timely interventions. Mortality rates have declined in the last decade due to economic growth and better health care facilities, yet the rates still remain very high especially in rural areas [1]. The diseases accounting for the mortality also vary geographically.

Children have poor physiological reserve that deteriorates rapidly during life-threatening emergencies. Following evidence based guidelines for management of pediatric emergencies by implementing the Pediatric Advanced Life Support [2] guidelines (American Academy of Pediatrics) and the Golden Hour Emergency Management [3] of pediatric illnesses laid down by the Indian Academy of Pediatrics offers the possibility of a better outcome. Mortality and morbidity of pediatric illness depend on the rapidity of response and target oriented therapy [4].

For planning of future healthcare and emergency policies in pediatric population, it is imperative to understand the comprehensive profile of pediatric emergencies. Most of the studies depicting profile of patients presenting in emergency departments and those treated in PICU are either from the developed countries [5–12] or from the metropolitan cities of India [13–15]. Even continent-wide directories of profiles and outcomes of patients attending emergency care and admitted to pediatric intensive care have been prepared [16, 17].

There is paucity of data from rural and western part of India. Such data would be helpful in identification of the prevalent serious diseases likely to present at emergency department and also to form an early intervention strategy as well as prioritize and plan appropriate resource allocation. The present study is undertaken to assess the clinical profile of patients presenting to the emergency room of a rural, tertiary care center in western India, which will allow us to devise specific responses [9, 18, 19].

Illness severity and mortality risk scoring systems are used for predicting the outcome of children admitted to PICU [20]. These scoring systems cannot give individual risk very accurately but aid in comparing severity in patients with similar disease and presentation [21] for comparing the efficiency of different PICU [22, 23]. Many studies have validated the use of prognostic scores like PIM2, PRISM3, and so forth and their association with outcome of patients receiving intensive care in the west. Few such studies have been conducted in rural settings in the developing world. These areas account for large number of critical cases and global mortality burden. The most validated and widely studied score is pediatric index of mortality 2 score [24–27].

Shann et al. introduced pediatric index of mortality (PIM) in 1997 for prediction of outcome of patients admitted in PICUs of Australia, United Kingdom, and New Zealand [28, 29]. This system was updated in 2003 (PIM2) and is better than the previous version in outcome predictability [29]. A valid score should predict mortality with reasonable sensitivity and the variables used in calculating the score should be appropriate and in accordance with course of clinical management [30–32]. The main objective of our study was to assess the clinical profile of patients requiring pediatric intensive care and determine applicability of PIM2 score in a rural, tertiary care center in western India.

2. Methods

2.1. Study Setting. We conducted a prospective observational study covering patients admitted to pediatric (1 month to 18 years) intensive care units from January 2010 to December 2011. The study was approved and the human research ethics committee of the institute granted a waiver of informed consent.

2.2. Data Collection. The clinical and general profile variables were noted at the time of admission in PICU. All the profile data variables and observations were noted at the time of admission to PICU latest by the first 24 h after admission. Scoring was done with the laboratory investigations, which were clinically indicated in management of the patients. The interventions done at emergency care department and pediatric intensive care unit within the first 24 h of admission were recorded. The admission source, time taken to enter PICU from the point of admission, and interventions carried by emergency team and pediatric emergency team were noted. The interventions of both the emergency team at emergency department and pediatric emergency team at emergency department and at pediatric intensive care department for the first 24 h after admission were studied, and adherence to management of patients according to the PALS and GEM guidelines and protocol was assessed. Deviation from protocol was noted in every patient included in the study.

All the intensive and life support interventions were noted. At each step the interventions were classified as appropriate or inappropriate according to the PALS and GEM guidelines. The outcome of the patients was recorded at the time of discharge. According to the diagnosis at the time of discharge the patients were classified according to the systems involved and major disease groups. Most of the patients who took discharge against medical advice (DAMA) did it for financial reasons in spite of the hospital policy to manage patients till alternative means are ensured. Further, most of them were in very critical condition and less likely to survive. Hence the DAMA patients were classified as Death for statistical analysis. The variable, namely, protein energy malnutrition, was removed from the analysis due to technical difficulties faced in weighing of critically ill patients with ongoing life support modalities.

2.3. Statistical Methods. The baseline data of the patients was expressed using descriptive statistics like mean, standard deviation, frequencies, proportions, and so forth. Various associations at the univariate level were expressed as cross tabulations and chi square statistics for qualitative variables. Independent sample t-test was used to express the associations for the continuous independent variables. The optimal cutoff value of PIM2 scores in this population was determined by ROC analysis. The independent contribution of various factors to mortality was determined using the multivariable stepwise logistic regression model with backward likelihood ratio (LR) method. The data was analyzed using SPSS 14.

3. Results

A total of 742 patients were admitted to PICU during the study period (Figure 1). Three patients were excluded because of transfer to another hospital and incomplete follow-up. There was seasonal fluctuation in PICU admissions. The median age of patients was 36 months (range 1–216 months). Out of 742 patients included in study, 445 (60.2%) were males and 294 (39.8%) were females. Two hundred and sixty-one patients (35.3%) were mechanically ventilated during their PICU stay. Observed mortality was $N = 52/739$ (7%). After DAMA patients were considered dead, the mortality was $N = 243/739$ (32.8%). The most frequent diagnoses were clinically septicemia and septicemic shock 219 (29.6%), significant anemia $N = 200$ (27.1%), pneumonia $N = 145$ (19.6%), meningitis and encephalitis $N = 127$ (17.2%), multiple organ dysfunction $N = 66$ (8.9%), and congenital heart disease $N = 42$ (5.7%). The major causes of death were septicemic shock ($N = 34$, 65%), multiple organ dysfunction syndrome ($N = 25$, 48%), and meningitis/encephalitis ($N = 11$, 21.2%).

The numbers of patients with Death/DAMA were significantly more than those discharged in diagnoses subcategories of septicemic shock, multiple organ dysfunction, and meningitis/encephalitis.

The sensitivity of the PIM2 was found for the first year data as 65.8%, and the specificity was 71% for a cutoff value at 1.9 by the receiver operating characteristic curve (ROC) analysis. The area under the curve was 0.724 (95% CI: 0.69,

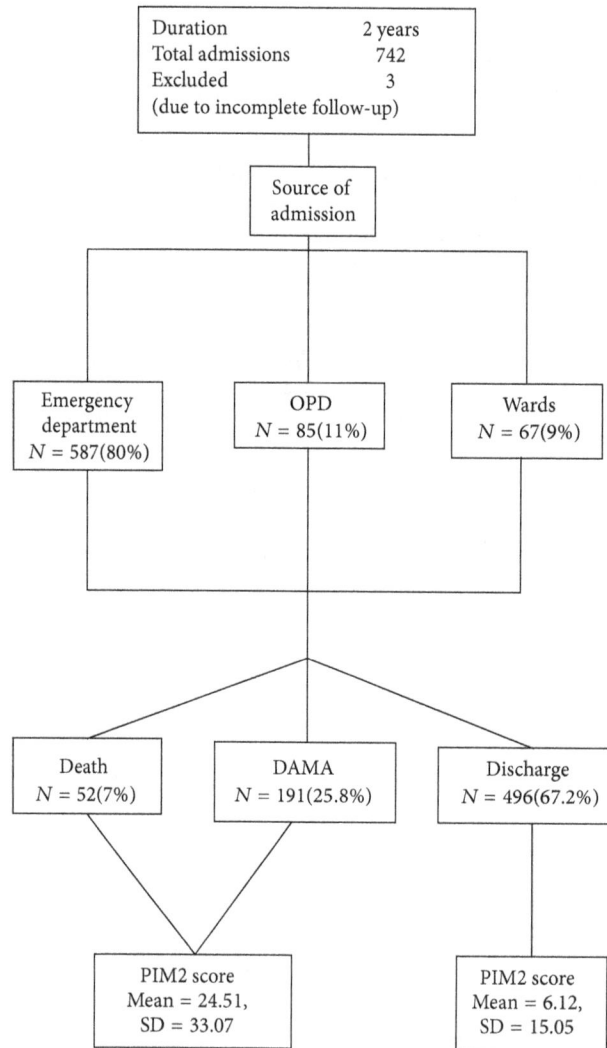

FIGURE 1: Flowchart of study participants. OPD: outpatient department, DAMA: discharge against medical advice, PIM2: pediatric index of mortality 2, and SD: standard.

0.76). This cutoff was validated for the second year data, which yielded the similar sensitivity (70.6%) and specificity (65%). In univariate analysis, PIM2 score was observed to be significantly higher ($P < 0.001$) in patients who died (243) (mean = 24.51, SD = 33.07) as compared to those who survived (496) (mean = 6.12, SD = 15.05).

The logistic regression analysis (LRA) with backward likelihood ratio method was used to obtain independent relationship between the predictor variables and the mortality. The variables included in the model were age (completed years), gender, time to reach PICU (minutes), presence or absence of anemia, pneumonia, multiple organ dysfunction syndrome, meningitis, congenital heart disease, emergency team following guidelines, pediatric team following guidelines, volume administration, airway stabilization, oxygen administration, shock, ventilator therapy given, and PIM2. Results of LRA showed that the overall correct classification rate was good (79.7%). The Nagelkerke R square = 0.409

implies that 40.9% of the variation in the outcome variable is explained by the variables in the model.

Age, PIM2, meningitis/meningoencephalitis, multiple organ dysfunction syndrome, congenital heart disease, following PALS/GEM guidelines, and shock are significantly associated with mortality (Table 1).

Another logistic model with the same input variables except PIM2 in the model yielded the same significant variables at the end with Nagelkerke R square of 0.388 and correct classification of 78.5 implying that the contribution of PIM2 in predicting mortality is meager (data not shown).

4. Discussion

Eighty percent of total PICU admissions were through the emergency department, 11% were admitted from OPD, and 9% were admitted from the hospital wards. Majority were unplanned admissions. Similar trends are seen in Indian

TABLE 1: Findings of logistic regression analysis with PIM2 as a predictor in the model.

Variable	Categories	OR	P value	95% CI for OR
PIM2	Continuous	1.017	0.0001	1.007, 1.026
Age (completed years)	Continuous	0.955	0.028	0.917, 0.995
MODS	Yes (ref)			
	No	0.161	0.001	0.062, 0.417
Meningitis	Yes (ref)			
	No	0.239	0.001	0.145, 0.395
CHD	Yes (ref)			
	No	0.396	0.035	0.167, 0.936
PALS/GEM guidelines followed	Yes (ref)			
	No	6.351	0.0001	3.008, 13.412
Shock	Yes (ref)			
	No	0.325	0.001	0.205, 0.513

PIM2: pediatric index of mortality 2, OR: odds ratio, CI: confidence interval, MODS: multiple organ dysfunction syndrome, and CHD: congenital heart disease.

studies [14] but western studies and registries show that significant proportions (approx. 85%) of the total admissions in PICU are planned and postsurgical [17]. Thus emergency care services in India should be more prepared for handling critically ill children. This will require training the teams in implementing protocol-based management of patients rapidly.

$N = 261$ patients (35.3%) were mechanically ventilated during their PICU stay. $N = 496/739$ patients were discharged after completion of their treatment. Observed mortality was $N = 52/739$ (7%); the major causes of death were septicemic shock, multiple organ dysfunction syndrome, and meningitis/encephalitis. If DAMA patients were considered dead, the mortality was $N = 243/739$ (32.8%). In analysis of outcomes DAMA patients were considered dead as most of them were very critical at the time of DAMA. Most of DAMA cases were due to financial constraints which are particularly a very important factor in Indian settings due to lack of state run insurance coverage. During the course of the study insurance was not available, but subsequently there has been a move towards insurance for below poverty line families. This insurance, referred to as Rashtriya Swasthya Bima Yojna (RSBY), covers emergency care too. However many eligible patients do not carry RSBY cards as the process of getting enrolled is not known to many eligible families, and getting a card often involves corruption at the local self-government level. The mortality percentage is similar to other PICUs [1, 9, 14, 16, 17, 24]. Infectious diseases were the most common cause of PICU admission and mortality which is also seen in some recent studies [13–15, 18], in contrast to very low contribution of the same in western countries [16, 17, 24].

Higher numbers of males were admitted with a male: female ratio of 1.5 : 1 (445 versus 294). Even if we discount liberally for the skewed sex distribution in the study population, this difference in admission is stark. This difference is common in countries such as India which have a preference for male gender. However the possibility of males requiring more intensive care cannot be ruled out as similar results are also seen in studies performed in developed countries [16, 17, 25, 26].

Infants less than 1 year comprised 40% of total admissions. More than 50% of patients admitted were below 2 years of age. The median age of patients was 36 months (range 1–216 months). A higher vulnerability of infants and young children is present and a need for special consideration of these groups in healthcare planning is required. Similar results were also seen in other studies [9, 16–18].

Age group of age less than 2 years is associated with significantly higher disease frequency as well as higher chances of mortality and higher need for invasive life support. The association of pneumonia with age was significant ($P < 0.0001$). It was significantly higher in younger age groups and the disease frequency declined as the age increased. Significant associations with lower age group were noted in ventilatory requirements, meningitis/encephalitis, and septicemia/septic shock subgroups. Distribution of anemia and MODS was not correlating with age. Similar findings are also seen in other studies [17].

Analysis of monthwise frequency of different diseases showed a definite trend in disease frequency. Infectious diseases such as septicemia and septic shock, meningitis/encephalitis, and pneumonia had significant variation seasonally. Rainy season of June to August had significant increase in frequency of meningitis/encephalitis. Pneumonia frequency was seen more in winter months from August to December. Similar seasonal trends were also reported in other studies [16–18].

Only 1% of total patients were fully insured. The analysis showed that the outcome in insured patients was significantly better with no patients taking DAMA or dying as compared to uninsured groups. Patients (3%) having even a partial insurance (KAS) had a significantly better outcome. Category wise outcome analysis showed significantly better outcomes with patients having insurance (P value = 0.02).

The sensitivity (65.4%) and specificity (70.8%) of PIM2 were significantly lower in our study as compared to those in western studies [24–27]. These results show that PIM2 score is not well calibrated and not useful to predict mortality with low specificity and sensitivity, and recalibration of PIM2 score is needed according to Indian settings.

The stepwise logistic regression analysis (LRA) was used to obtain a risk adjusted relationship between the predictor variables and the probability of death. The LRA showed significant predictability of variables such as septicemic shock, meningitis/encephalitis, acute renal failure, and dialysis and ventilation during PICU stay with respect to the outcome which shows the need of incorporating these variables in prognostic mortality score in Indian setting.

Improvement of outcome on adherence to PALS and GEM guidelines indicates the need for proper implementation of guidelines for improving outcome in pediatric emergency care. The providers of emergency care to a child should have appropriate and proper training in managing critical children according to PALS/GEM guidelines. Similar results were also seen in another study [4].

4.1. PIM2 Applicability in Indian Settings. The PIM2 score was calibrated to predict mortality with a level of healthcare facilities available in Australia, New Zealand, and United Kingdom at the time of study, that is, 1997 around 16 years back so it cannot be generalized without proper recalibration. The study population is 1 month to 18 years as compared to original study of PIM2 including the patients <16 years of age by Lemeshow and Gall [30]. The score validity would differ with changes in treatment and management approaches, level of healthcare, referral practices, and admission criteria [29]. The high risk and low risk diagnosis in PIM2 were analyzed according to those of Australia, New Zealand, and United Kingdom [29], none of which are suitable for southeast Asian countries including India.

The laboratory parameters and ventilation during the first hour of admission which are significant variables in calculating PIM2 are subjective to availability of laboratory tests, treatment approaches, and intervention thresholds which changes the mortality score calculation even with same disease severity [29]. Many patients admitted in tertiary level Indian PICU are referred from local hospitals. These patients are stabilized before referrals which alters the parameters included in calculation of score. PIM2 does not take into account the referred status and the treatment received; this hampers the assessment of actual risk of mortality.

It can only compare groups but cannot predict risk in individual patients [29]. Normal systolic blood pressure is taken as 120 mmHg whereas most of pediatric patients have much less than 120 mmHg.

Age is not taken into account while calculating risk in PIM2 score when it is well evident that young children have higher vulnerability. The low risk diagnoses such as croup, bronchiolitis, asthma, and diabetic ketoacidosis have significant mortality in a resource-limited country like India.

The high risk diagnoses which are included in PIM2 such as severe combined immunodeficiency, leukemia, neurodegenerative disorders, spontaneous cerebral hemorrhage, and hypoplastic left heart are infrequent causes of mortality in India, whereas infectious diseases, septicemia, septicemic shock, meningitis and encephalitis, multiple organ dysfunction syndrome, acute renal failure, and disseminated intravascular coagulation which account for majority of deaths in developing countries are not considered in calculation of PIM2 scoring [30]. These lacunae make PIM2 score inappropriate for use in Indian setting without proper recalibration.

5. Conclusion

PIM2 score is not applicable without proper recalibration in Indian settings where the disease patterns and frequency are markedly different and the standard of care provided is not as good as that provided in developed countries where PIM2 was devised and validated.

In our setup there is delay in seeking health and most patients end up in ICU because of late care received. This contributes to severe physiologic derangements and increased chances of mortality which is in contrast to western and developed countries due to availability of good referral and immediate healthcare assistance. There is need for proper intervention and management at the primary centers and well-structured referral system.

6. Implications

6.1. Generalizability. This study done in Indian settings may also be applicable to other developing and underdeveloped countries of the world.

6.2. Strengths and Limitations. The study has been carried out over a fairly large period and can avoid the changes in results due to differences in seasons and patterns of admissions. Though it is a single center study, being a referral center it receives most of the sick patients in the region due to a large referral. This study is the only study till date from India to validate PIM2 score, which is validated across many developed countries and a few developing countries.

Due to financial constraints many patients took DAMA and this might result in variations in outcome when reproduced in a more affluent setting. We did not collect data related to prematurity in the study population as often this data is not available and may be unreliable as patients may have been delivered at home or delivered by trained birth attendants who cannot assess prematurity. Our patient population extended until 18 years and collecting this data over the entire population would have been challenging.

6.3. Further Research. Further research is needed to confirm the findings of present study in a multicentric study from areas of developing countries. There is a need to have risk scoring calibrated to local disease prevalence, treatment expertise, malnutrition status, and other factors contributing to mortality.

There cannot be a compact risk scoring system because the smaller the variable size the lesser the sensitivity and specificity. So there is a need of mortality predictor score with sufficient variables which takes into account wider range of medical problems and possible contributors to mortality, without having much emphasis on laboratory parameters, and which does not get biased by different thresholds of interventions.

Many diseases occurring in tropical countries, which account for significant mortality, evolve over a period of time and the prediction of outcome at the admission time is flawed largely in such patients. This denotes a need for a score, which continuously estimates the risk over a period.

What Is Known on This Subject

PIM2 score is a validated and widely used mortality prediction score in pediatric critical care. It has been proved to be most accurate in mortality prediction in developed country setting.

What This Study Adds

PIM2 is a poor mortality prediction model for developing country settings due to resource-poor conditions and difference in disease prevalence. This study highlights factors associated with mortality in these settings that can be considered for mortality prediction models.

Abbreviations

DAMA: Discharge against medical advice
LRA: Logistic regression analysis
MODS: Multiple organ dysfunction syndrome
PIM2: Pediatric index of mortality 2
PICU: Pediatric intensive care unit
ROC: Receiver operating characteristic curve.

Conflict of Interests

None of the authors have any conflict of interests to disclose.

Authors' Contribution

Vivek V. Shukla contributed to concept and design, data acquisition, data analysis, drafting, and revision of the paper for important intellectual content and final approval of this paper. Somashekhar M. Nimbalkar contributed to the design of the study, analysis, drafting the paper, and final approval of this paper. Jaishree D. Ganjiwale contributed to concept and design, analysis of data, writing of the paper, and final approval of this paper. Ajay G. Phatak contributed to concept and design, data analysis, revision of the paper, and final approval of this paper.

Acknowledgments

The authors would like to thank Dr. Ashish Dongara, MD, for reviewing the paper and Ms. Amee Amin for proofreading of English (US).

References

[1] "2011 revision of United Nations world population prospects reports by 5 years average," http://esa.un.org/wpp/Other-Information/faq.htm.

[2] American Heart Association, "PALS Course Guide," http://www.heart.org/HEARTORG/CPRAndECC/Healthcare-Training/Pediatrics/Pediatric-Advanced-Life-Support-PALS_UCM_303705_Article.jsp.

[3] "Pediatric golden hour of emergency management," Indian Academy of Pediatrics. Course guide.

[4] J. A. Carcillo, B. A. Kuch, Y. Y. Han et al., "Mortality and functional morbidity after use of PALS/APLS by community physicians," Pediatrics, vol. 124, no. 2, pp. 500–508, 2009.

[5] P. Fulbrook and D. Foxcroft, "Measuring the outcome of paediatric intensive care," Intensive and Critical Care Nursing, vol. 15, no. 1, pp. 44–51, 1999.

[6] G. Pearson, P. Barry, C. Timmins, J. Stickley, and M. Hocking, "Changes in the profile of paediatric intensive care associated with centralisation," Intensive Care Medicine, vol. 27, no. 10, pp. 1670–1673, 2001.

[7] D. A. Harrison, A. R. Brady, and K. Rowan, "Case mix, outcome and length of stay for admissions to adult, general critical care units in England, Wales and Northern Ireland: the Intensive Care National Audit & Research Centre Case Mix Programme Database," Critical Care, vol. 8, no. 2, pp. R99–R111, 2004.

[8] C. Pileggi, G. Raffaele, and I. F. Angelillo, "Paediatric utilization of an emergency department in Italy," European Journal of Public Health, vol. 16, no. 5, pp. 565–569, 2006.

[9] S. Kinney, J. Tibballs, L. Johnston, and T. Duke, "Clinical profile of hospitalized children provided with urgent assistance from a medical emergency team," Pediatrics, vol. 121, no. 6, pp. e1577–e1584, 2008.

[10] E. Ben-Isaac, S. M. Schrager, M. Keefer, and A. Y. Chen, "National profile of nonemergent pediatric emergency department visits," Pediatrics, vol. 125, no. 3, pp. 454–459, 2010.

[11] A. Downing and G. Rudge, "A study of childhood attendance at emergency departments in the West Midlands region," Emergency Medicine Journal, vol. 23, no. 5, pp. 391–393, 2006.

[12] K. M. S. Choi, D. K. K. Ng, S. F. Wong et al., "Assessment of the Pediatric Index of Mortality (PIM) and the Pediatric Risk of Mortality (PRISM) III score for prediction of mortality in a paediatric intensive care unit in Hong Kong," Hong Kong Medical Journal, vol. 11, no. 2, pp. 97–103, 2005.

[13] S. Singhi, G. Gupta, and V. Jain, "Comparison of pediatric emergency patients in a tertiary care hospital vs. a community hospital," Indian Pediatrics, vol. 41, no. 1, pp. 67–72, 2004.

[14] P. Khilnani, D. Sarma, R. Singh et al., "Demographic profile and outcome analysis of a tertiary level pediatric intensive care unit," Indian Journal of Pediatrics, vol. 71, no. 7, pp. 587–591, 2004.

[15] P. Garg, "Pediatric hospitalizations at two different setting community hospitals in north India: implications for regionalization of care," Indian Journal of Pediatrics, vol. 76, no. 7, pp. 711–716, 2009.

[16] PICANeT Paediatric Intensive Care Audit Network, "University of Leeds and University of Leicester Annual Report of the Paediatric Intensive Care Audit Network," 2008, http://www.picanet.org.uk.

[17] Report of the Australian and New Zealand Paediatric Intensive Care Registry, Australian and New Zealand Intensive Care Society (ANZICS), 2010, http://www.anzics.com.au/core/reports.

[18] S. Singhi, V. Jain, and G. Gupta, "Pediatric emergencies at a tertiary care hospital in India," Journal of Tropical Pediatrics, vol. 49, no. 4, pp. 207–211, 2003.

[19] I. Santhanam, M. Pai, K. R. Kasturi, and M. P. Radhamani, "Mortality after admission in the pediatric emergency department: a prospective study from a referral children's hospital in

Southern India," *Pediatric Critical Care Medicine*, vol. 3, no. 4, pp. 358–363, 2002.

[20] P. E. Marik and J. Varon, "Severity scoring and outcome assessment: computerized predictive models and scoring systems," *Critical Care Clinics*, vol. 15, no. 3, pp. 633–646, 1999.

[21] J. Rogers and H. D. Fuller, "Use of daily Acute Physiology and Chronic Health Evaluation (APACHE) II scores to predict individual patient survival rate," *Critical Care Medicine*, vol. 22, no. 9, pp. 1402–1405, 1994.

[22] J. E. Zimmerman, "Measuring intensive care unit performance: a way to move forward," *Critical Care Medicine*, vol. 30, no. 9, pp. 2149–2150, 2002.

[23] R. B. Becker and J. E. Zimmerman, "ICU scoring systems allow prediction of patient outcomes and comparison of ICU performance," *Critical Care Clinics*, vol. 12, no. 3, pp. 503–514, 1996.

[24] J. Mestrovic, G. Kardum, B. Polic, A. Omazic, L. Stricevic, and A. Sustic, "Applicability of the Australian and New Zealand Paediatric Intensive Care Registry diagnostic codes and Paediatric Index of Mortality 2 scoring system in a Croatian paediatric intensive care unit," *European Journal of Pediatrics*, vol. 164, no. 12, pp. 783–784, 2005.

[25] D. K. Ng, T.-Y. Miu, W.-K. Chiu, N.-T. Hui, and C.-H. Chan, "Validation of Pediatric Index of Mortality 2 in three pediatric intensive care units in Hong Kong," *Indian Journal of Pediatrics*, vol. 78, no. 12, pp. 1491–1494, 2011.

[26] S. Hariharan, K. Krishnamurthy, and D. Grannum, "Validation of Pediatric Index of Mortality-2 scoring system in a pediatric intensive care unit, Barbados," *Journal of Tropical Pediatrics*, vol. 57, no. 1, pp. 9–13, 2011.

[27] A. Wolfler, P. Silvani, M. Musicco et al., "Pediatric Index of Mortality 2 score in Italy: a multicenter, prospective, observational study," *Intensive Care Medicine*, vol. 33, no. 8, pp. 1407–1413, 2007.

[28] F. Shann, G. Pearson, A. Slater, and K. Wilkinson, "Paediatric Index of Mortality (PIM): a mortality prediction model for children in intensive care," *Intensive Care Medicine*, vol. 23, no. 2, pp. 201–207, 1997.

[29] A. Slater, F. Shann, and G. Pearson, "PIM2: a revised version of the Paediatric Index of Mortality," *Intensive Care Medicine*, vol. 29, no. 2, pp. 278–285, 2003.

[30] S. Lemeshow and J.-R. le Gall, "Modeling the severity of illness of ICU patients: a systems update," *The Journal of the American Medical Association*, vol. 272, no. 13, pp. 1049–1055, 1994.

[31] S. Lemeshow, J. Klar, and D. Teres, "Outcome prediction for individual intensive care patients: useful, misused, or abused?" *Intensive Care Medicine*, vol. 21, no. 9, pp. 770–776, 1995.

[32] A. Laupacis, N. Sekar, and I. G. Stiell, "Clinical prediction rules: a review and suggested modifications of methodological standards," *The Journal of the American Medical Association*, vol. 277, no. 6, pp. 488–494, 1997.

13

Decision Making in the PICU: An Examination of Factors Influencing Participation Decisions in Phase III Randomized Clinical Trials

Laura E. Slosky,[1] Marilyn Stern,[2] Natasha L. Burke,[3] and Laura A. Siminoff[4]

[1] Division of Developmental and Behavioral Sciences, Children's Mercy Hospital, 2401 Gillham Road, Kansas City, MO 64108, USA
[2] Department of Rehabilitation and Mental Health Counseling, University of South Florida, 13301 Bruce B. Downs Boulevard, MHC 1632, P.O. Box 12, Tampa, FL 33612, USA
[3] Department of Psychology, University of South Florida, 4202 East Fowler Avenue, PCD4118G, Tampa, FL 33620, USA
[4] Department of Social and Behavioral Health, Virginia Commonwealth University, P.O. Box 980149, Richmond, VA 23298, USA

Correspondence should be addressed to Laura E. Slosky; lslosky@cmh.edu

Academic Editor: Julie Blatt

Background. In stressful situations, decision making processes related to informed consent may be compromised. Given the profound levels of distress that surrogates of children in pediatric intensive care units (PICU) experience, it is important to understand what factors may be influencing the decision making process beyond the informed consent. The purpose of this study was to evaluate the role of clinician influence and other factors on decision making regarding participation in a randomized clinical trial (RCT). *Method.* Participants were 76 children under sedation in a PICU and their surrogate decision makers. Measures included the Post Decision Clinician Survey, observer checklist, and post-decision interview. *Results.* Age of the pediatric patient was related to participation decisions in the RCT such that older children were more likely to be enrolled. Mentioning the sponsoring institution was associated with declining to participate in the RCT. Type of health care provider and overt recommendations to participate were not related to enrollment. *Conclusion.* Decisions to participate in research by surrogates of children in the PICU appear to relate to child demographics and subtleties in communication; however, no modifiable characteristics were related to increased participation, indicating that the informed consent process may not be compromised in this population.

1. Introduction

Obtaining informed consent prior to subject participation in an experimental protocol is vital to maintain ethical standards and ensure respect for persons. Even with a number of national and international guidelines to ensure true informed consent [1–5], some in the field believe the concept is an elusive ideal [6]. Patients who participated in clinical trials were unaware of the particulars of the research (e.g., randomization, treatment arms, etc.) or that the treatment was experimental in nature [7–9], and information presented in the consent form was not always taken into account when making medical decisions [10]. Moreover, for nearly two-thirds of those approached for study participation, the consent form played no part in their participation decision [10].

Problems with comprehension and readability [11], a misconception of direct therapeutic benefit [9, 12], and not recognizing the ability to discontinue [9] or opt out of treatment [13] also impede the function of the informed consent process. Importantly, the decision making process involving informed consent may be flawed, especially in high pressure environments [14]. Given the profound and sometimes clinical levels of distress that surrogates (i.e., parents or legal guardians) of children in pediatric intensive care units (PICU) experience [15], it is important to understand what factors may be influencing the decision making process beyond the informed consent process. Properly addressing such factors would help protect the integrity of the informed consent process.

Although the informed consent process precludes coercion and denial of services, it may nevertheless be challenging for physicians (i.e., medical doctors) to fully disengage from the role of health care provider during the informed consent process. Physicians have significant influence on medical decisions that are made by their patients [16–18], and communication with the physician during clinical encounters is an important factor in the final decision to participate in clinical trials [19–21]. In a study involving oncology patients, 68% of the time physicians recommended that their patients participate in a clinical trial, which was related to the resultant decision to participate [22]. Surrogates often rely on their child's physicians for their knowledge and expertise in the medical care of their child [16, 17]. Therefore, it is hypothesized that treating physicians play a significant role in the decisions that surrogates make regarding research trial participation. Based on previous findings [23], it is expected that physicians recommending these research opportunities have a significant influence on their patients' decisions to participate in clinical trials.

The PICU is a multidisciplinary environment, and although the patient's physician may present trial information to eligible study participants, other health care providers (e.g., nurses and respiratory therapists) may also serve in this role. Clinician understanding and actual or perceived endorsement of the trial being presented [24, 25] and potential benefits to the patient are associated with participation decisions [24]. A personal physician may be more apt to handle these types of questions depending on the type of study and clinician training [24], and it is possible that a physician's explanation may have a stronger impact on decision to participate than another health care provider (HCP). Lastly, distrust of sponsoring institutions has been noted as a reason for declining participation in research studies [3, 26]. Therefore, mention of the sponsoring institution to potential participants will also be examined as a potential factor in the surrogate decision-making process.

This study provides insight into how influential physician recommendations are in this unique population of surrogate decision makers for critically ill children in potentially life threatening situations. It also provides insight into the role of different HCPs and additional putative factors in the decision-making process. There are three primary hypotheses. First, it is expected that a HCP's overt recommendation to participate in the RCT will be related to participation decisions such that surrogates will be more likely to enroll their child into the RCT. Second, it is expected that surrogates receiving RCT information from a physician will be more likely to enroll their child in the RCT than those receiving the information from another HCP. Third, it is expected that surrogates who are given information about the institution supporting the RCT will be more likely to enroll their child in the protocol than those not receiving this information.

2. Method

2.1. Participants. Participants were recruited from Rainbow Babies and Children's Hospital Pediatric Intensive Care Unit. Data were collected from a total of 76 surrogate decision makers of hospitalized children in the PICU, with each surrogate

TABLE 1: Demographics.

Variable	n	%
Female surrogate	70	92.0
Male pediatric Patient	44	57.1
Surrogate race		
Caucasian	28	36.8
African American	44	57.9
Other	4	5.3
Single parent Household	35	48.7
12 or fewer years Surrogate education	31	41.9
Income above 25 K Annually	40	49.3

Variable	Mean	SD	Range
Age of pediatric Patient (years)	5.76	4.84	0–17
Age of surrogate (years)	32.13	8.02	17–59

representing one pediatric case (see Table 1). Hospitalized children had suffered a wide range of illnesses and accidents and were all in need of mechanical ventilation for at least a 24-hour period.

2.2. Procedure. This study was part of a larger study on informed consent. On call research nurses were contacted once a child became eligible to participate in a greater than minimal risk phase III clinical trial. This individual first provided an explanation of the present study on informed consent and obtained written informed consent. Surrogates then participated in an informed consent conference regarding participation in a drug RCT with their child's HCP. In this conference, the HCP presented an opportunity to participate in a clinical trial to test the efficacy of an experimental pharmaceutical treatment. Randomization procedures were explained, safety concerns addressed, and voluntary participation stressed. If the surrogates expressed an interest in enrolling their child, they were given a consent form to read and provided written informed consent for the drug RCT. Some HCPs presenting trial information were study investigators and others were not. HCP involvement in the RCT presented was controlled for in study analyses. Conferences with surrogates were observed and audio-recorded by research assistants. Following this conference, surrogates participated in a private structured interview about this HCP interaction. Both the drug RCT and the current informed consent study were approved by University Internal Review Boards.

2.3. Measures

2.3.1. Semistructured Post-Decision Interview. A brief interview was conducted with the surrogates after they finished the informed consent conference. The interview was conducted in private, without the child's HCP present. The purpose of this interview was to obtain participant specific characteristics and to assess understanding of the clinical trial and treatment options. Participant specific characteristics included

TABLE 2: Demographic factors associated with decision to participate in the RCT.

Variable	χ^2	df	P	t	df	P
Surrogate gender	.03	1	>.05			
Surrogate race	.001	1	>.05			
Marital status	2.27	2	>.05			
Surrogate Education level	3.04	2	>.05			
Income level	2.23	4	>.05			
Surrogate age				.80	20.09	>.05
Pediatric patient age				3.00	22.30	<.005*

Note: df = degrees of freedom, * significant.

decision making preferences, risk taking inclinations, quality of relationship with their HCP, subject assessment of treatment risks and benefits, comprehension of trial participation requirements, their final decision regarding participation in the clinical trial, and the rationale behind their decision.

2.3.2. Post-Decision Clinician Survey. The HCP that participated in the informed consent conference completed a survey after the informed consent conference. This measure was used to gather information about the HCP and his or her level of involvement in the randomized clinical trial. Demographic data for the HCP was recorded and included type of HCP, specialty, board certification, membership in clinical trials groups, exposure to trials during training, whether or not the HCP was an investigator in the drug trial, age, gender, and race. The HCP also provided their perception of the strength of their recommendation regarding participation in the RCT and the likelihood of the patient to benefit from the clinical trial.

2.3.3. The Observer Checklist. This instrument was developed for the current study and was used to document and assess the interactions between surrogates and their child's HCP. The checklist was completed by research assistants who observed the informed consent process; the audiotape was used for coding purposes. The measure lists specific information categories related to informed consent that were dichotomously coded as occurring or not occurring. Examples of information coded included whether the informed consent process included an explanation of risks, benefits, funding, and alternatives. Content initiators were also coded in relation to each topic area raised. Past studies achieved between 88 and 93% agreement on this measure among independent raters [14, 21], and the current study achieved an interrater reliability within this range at approximately 90% agreement. The measure was developed and chosen to capture unique aspects and interactions of the consent process not addressed by previously validated measures.

2.4. Statistical Analyses. A series of Chi-square analyses and *t*-tests were conducted to identify demographic factors significantly associated with the decision to participate in the RCT. Hierarchical logistic regression analyses were performed to test the primary hypotheses. Demographic factors associated with the decision to participate in the RCT were entered as control variables in the first step of the regression analyses followed by the specific research question (i.e., HCP's verbal recommendation to participate (coded as yes or no), HCP presenting trial information (coded as physician or other), or HCP mention of the sponsoring institution (coded as yes or no)). Each regression was then compared to a constant-only model to determine whether the proposed hypothesis was statistically significant. Effect sizes were analyzed with Cox and Snell R-square and Nagelkerke R-square. All analyses were performed using the statistical package for the social sciences (SPSS) version 16.0.

3. Results

Participation in the RCT was not associated with any surrogate level data (see Table 2). However, participation was associated with patient age such that surrogates of older children (M_{AGE} = 6.212) were more likely to consent to participate than surrogates of younger children (M_{AGE} = 3.055). Patient age was controlled for in study analyses.

For the first hypothesis, it was hypothesized that if a HCP gave a verbal statement to the surrogate decision maker advocating enrollment in the RCT, the surrogate would be more likely to enroll their child in the RCT. The model with age and HCP recommendation was not statistically different from the constant-only model, and the effect size of HCP recommendation was small (see Table 3). Since the results were contrary to previous findings, the model was evaluated without controlling for the age of the pediatric patient. This model was compared to a constant only model, and the results were still not significant, $X^2(1) = .14, P > .05$. The effect size of physician recommendation was even smaller, with Cox and Snell R-square = .002 and Nagelkerke R-square = .003. However, a post hoc correlation was used to examine the relationship between strength of HCP recommendation and the decision to enroll in the RCT, and the results were significant. The stronger the recommendation, the less likely the surrogate was to enroll their child; $r = -.33, P < .05$.

For the second hypothesis, it was hypothesized that the type of HCP presenting the trial to the surrogate decision maker would predict trial participation such that those receiving the information from a physician would be more likely to participate than those being informed by another type of HCP (e.g., nurse or respiratory therapist). The model with age and the HCP presenting the trial was not statistically

TABLE 3: β Weights and Chi-Square Results for Logistic Regression Analysis.

Hypothesis	β	χ^2	P	Cox & Snell R^2	Nagelkerke R^2
(1) Age of Pediatric Patient	−0.19				
HCP Recommendation	−0.001	4.90	>.05	.06	.11
(2) Age of Pediatric Patient	−0.20				
Type of HCP Presenting	−0.40	5.08	>.05	.07	.12
(3) Age of Pediatric Patient	−0.09				
Mention Sponsoring Institution	−2.30	11.05	<.005*	.14	.14

Note: HCP = Health Care Provider, *significant.

different from the constant-only model, and the effect size of the HCP presenting the trial was small (see Table 3).

Lastly, it was hypothesized that if a clinician referenced the name of the institution supporting the trial and indicated that the study was approved by the institution's Internal Review Board, the surrogate would be more likely to enroll their child in the experimental protocol. The model with age and mention of the sponsoring institution was significantly different from the constant-only model, and the effect size of mentioning the sponsoring institution was moderate (see Table 3). The change in odds associated with a one-unit change in reference to the supporting institution was −2.30, indicating that if the supporting institution was mentioned, the surrogate was 2.30 times less likely to enroll their child in the experimental protocol.

4. Discussion

The purpose of the current study was to elucidate factors that influence surrogate decision makers in the PICU to participate in RCTs. This is particularly important given the informed consent process has previously been found to be flawed, particularly in stressful environments [14]. It is therefore important to understand what may be influencing such decisions in this vulnerable population. Demographic variables were analyzed as potential covariates and putative factors predicting trial participation were analyzed including explicit verbal recommendation by the HCP to participate, the type of HCP presenting the trial, and HCP mention of the institution supporting the trial. Results from the majority of demographic variables were not significant; those who chose to participate in the RCT were not significantly different from those who elected standard treatment on most demographic domains. However, age of the pediatric patient was related to surrogates' decisions to enroll their child in the RCT. Surrogates who had an older child in the PICU were more likely to enroll them in the RCT than those with a younger child. A younger child in the PICU may be perceived as more vulnerable and unable to handle treatment when little is known about its safety and side effects. Younger children generally are seen as more vulnerable and less able to handle both adverse and normative events; however, this view may or may not be well founded [27, 28]. Nevertheless, patient age was controlled for in study analyses.

The relationship between an explicit HCP recommendation to participate in the RCT and the decision to participate was not significant, which indicates that a HCP recommending participation in the RCT did not predict whether a surrogate enrolled their child in the RCT. This was contrary to previous research findings, so the analysis was repeated without controlling for the age of the pediatric patient. The model still did not achieve statistical significance after age was excluded indicating that age of the pediatric patient was not accounting for the nonsignificant relationship. A larger sample size may be needed to detect a significant effect of physician recommendation on participation. However, it is possible that the levels of extreme stress that are unique to this time pressured situation may affect decision making in a manner differently than previously hypothesized, particularly in this population of surrogates that has children with acute complications of chronic conditions. Stress affects brain regions that are responsible for complex cognitive processes [29]. This potential change in cognitive functioning may cause surrogate decision makers to make decisions regarding clinical trial participation before the information is presented to them. In fact, previous research has found that this decision prior to information presentation is one of the strongest predictors of participation [30]. This type of informed consent study has also never been conducted in such a high stress environment or with such a fragile population. These changes in environmental stress and potential harm to the patient may be more salient when making decisions related to decision making regarding research participation. Further, participants had already agreed to participate in a study of informed consent which likely impacted their thought processes surrounding drug trial participation which is also likely to play a contributory role in current findings. Overall, however, the HCP's endorsement not affecting participant enrollment is a positive outcome and consistent with the ultimate goals of the informed consent process.

No relationship was found between the type of HCP presenting trial information and a surrogate's decision to participate. This indicates that a physician presenting the RCT to the surrogate did not reliably predict trial participation over another type of HCP presenting the same information. This implies that one type of clinician does not have more persuasive power than another, regardless of rank and role in the child's care. This has important implications for the informed consent process and supports the ultimate goal of this construct, protecting the patient. If a given individual had

Decision Making in the PICU: An Examination of Factors Influencing Participation Decisions...

77

more persuasive power in these acutely stressful situations, they could more easily manipulate the outcome [31, 32]. This would present a significant conflict of interest within clinical practice, which could become especially problematic if the presenting clinician was a primary investigator for the trial desiring to recruit participants. The possible conflict of interest would have the potential to compromise patient care and the best interests of the child. However, as this study has revealed, the type of HCP presenting does not impact the resultant decision to participate. It therefore appears that this aspect of protection of human subjects is not compromised.

The third hypothesis examined the relationship between clinician mention of the institution sponsoring the RCT and participation. The results indicated that the mention of the institution supporting the trial reliably distinguished between surrogates enrolling their child in the experimental protocol from those surrogates who did not enroll their child. While this predictive relationship was significant, the direction of the relationship was unexpected. Specifically, analyses revealed that when the institution was mentioned, surrogates were less likely to enroll their child in the experimental protocol. This finding suggests that mention of the supporting institution may remind the surrogate of the experimental nature of the protocol, leading to a lower participation rate. Previous research has clearly shown a deficit in patient knowledge regarding RCTs during enrollment [14, 33]. However, giving particular information about the sponsoring institution may lead surrogates to feel the research is in the best interests of the institution versus the best interests of current or future patients. This approach may seem less personal to the surrogates and perhaps leads to the lower likelihood of participation.

A few limitations of this study are noted. First, a small yet clinically significant sample was used to test hypotheses. Second, the applicability of results to other surrogates may be limited given parents in the PICU are significantly more stressed and more prone to symptoms of posttraumatic stress than parents with children on other hospital services [32]. Nevertheless, this is an important population to study, particularly because of the unique and stressful circumstances of the PICU. Third, there may be other relevant factors that may affect the decision-making process which were not addressed in the study; however, the goal was to address particular factors that would be relevant across sites and populations. Finally, the education level and SES measures were likely not sufficiently sensitive as categories were notably broad. Additional control of these variables may be informative in future studies. The study also showcases strengths as multiple informants were used whenever possible, nonmodifiable participant characteristics were considered as relevant covariates, and findings represent a contribution to a clinically significant body of literature surrounding decision making in a unique environment.

5. Conclusion

The critical role that physicians play in medical decision making is well known [16, 17]. Physicians undoubtedly play a role in treatment decisions made by their patients' families in the pediatric intensive care unit. However, this influence is reduced in the context of recruitment in clinical trials in the PICU, which is consistent with ethical standards related to the consenting process. In addition, type of HCP is not related to the decision making process, which also highlights the equity in the decision-making process and adherence to ethical standards. Nevertheless, there are subtle communication factors that play a role in this process. For instance, participants may possibly feel deceived or pressured when the sponsoring institution is mentioned or strong recommendations to participate are given. As any kind of pressure to participate is counter to the informed consent process, such techniques should be strongly discouraged and avoided. The current study indicates that subtleties of HCP communication merit further investigation regarding their influence on participation in a pediatric RCT. It also suggests that the age of the child is likely a significant factor in this decision making process. The influence of these subtle factors on decision making as well as the impact of direct recommendations should be evaluated in more depth and with additional participants in future studies. Further, the significant HCP influences may not only play a role in the high stress environment of the PICU, but also play a role in other areas of pediatrics. Expansion of the current study to other pediatric populations (e.g., those with chronic illnesses) would represent a significant contribution to the literature related to decision making in RCTs beyond the informed consent process to ensure protection for these vulnerable populations.

Conflict of Interests

The authors declare that there is no conflict of interests regarding the publication of this paper.

Acknowledgments

This study was supported by Grant no. R01- CA78210 from the National Cancer Institute awarded to Laura A. Siminoff. Work was performed at Case Western Reserve University and Virginia Commonwealth University.

References

[1] Nuremburg Code, U.S. National Institutes of Health, Office of Human Subjects Research, 2008.

[2] World Medical Association, The Declaration of Helsinki, 1964, http://www.wma.net/en/30publications/10policies/b3/.

[3] J. Jones, Bad Blood: The Tuskegee Syphilis Experiment, Free Press, New York, NY, USA, 1993.

[4] R. Nelson, "Research involving children," in Institutional Review Board Management and Function, E. Bankert and R. Amdur, Eds., pp. 366–372, Jones & Bartlett Publishers, Boston, Mass, USA, 2006.

[5] R. E. Shaddy and S. C. Denne, "Guidelines for the ethical conduct of studies to evaluate drugs in pediatric populations," Pediatrics, vol. 125, no. 4, pp. 850–860, 2010.

[6] L. A. Siminoff, C. Burant, and S. J. Youngner, "Death and organ procurement: public beliefs and attitudes," *Social Science & Medicine*, vol. 59, no. 11, pp. 2325–2334, 2004.

[7] G. F. Bahna, J. C. Holland, D. T. Penman et al., "Informed consent for investigational chemotherapy: patients'and physicians'perceptions," *Journal of Clinical Oncology*, vol. 2, no. 7, pp. 849–855, 1984.

[8] B. R. Cassileth, D. Volckmar, and R. L. Goodman, "The effect of experience on radiation therapy patients' desire for information," *International Journal of Radiation Oncology Biology Physics*, vol. 6, no. 4, pp. 493–496, 1980.

[9] D. Das, P. Y. Cheah, F. Akter et al., "Participants' perceptions and understanding of a malaria clinical trial in Bangladesh," *Malaria Journal*, vol. 13, article 217, 2014.

[10] C. Gallo, F. Perrone, S. de Placido, and C. Giusti, "Informed versus randomised consent to clinical trials," *The Lancet*, vol. 346, no. 8982, pp. 1060–1064, 1995.

[11] D. B. Friedman, S. H. Kim, A. Tanner, C. D. Bergeron, C. Foster, and K. General, "How are we communicating about clinical trials? An assessment of the content and readability of recruitment resources," *Contemporary Clinical Trials*, vol. 38, no. 2, pp. 275–283, 2014.

[12] R. Dal-Ré, F. Morell, J. C. Tejedor, and D. Gracia, "Therapeutic misconception in clinical trials: fighting against it and living with it," *Revista Clínica Española*, 2014.

[13] T. T. Raymond, T. G. Carroll, G. Sales, and M. C. Morris, "Effectiveness of the informed consent process for a pediatric resuscitation trial," *Pediatrics*, vol. 125, no. 4, pp. e866–e875, 2010.

[14] L. A. Siminoff, "Improving communication with cancer patients," *Oncology*, vol. 6, no. 10, pp. 83–87, 1992.

[15] E. Iverson, A. Celious, C. R. Kennedy et al., "Factors affecting stress experienced by surrogate decision makers for critically ill patients: implications for nursing practice," *Intensive and Critical Care Nursing*, vol. 30, no. 2, pp. 77–85, 2014.

[16] J. L. Brody, D. G. Scherer, R. D. Annett, C. Turner, and J. Dalen, "Family and physician influence on asthma research participation decisions for adolescents: the effects of adolescent gender and research risk," *Pediatrics*, vol. 118, no. 2, pp. e356–e362, 2006.

[17] W. C. McCormick, T. S. Inui, and D. Roter, "Interventions in physician-elderly patient interactions," *Research on Aging*, vol. 18, no. 1, pp. 103–136, 1996.

[18] L. E. Marsillio and M. C. Morris, "Informed consent for bedside procedures in the pediatric intensive care unit: a preliminary report," *Pediatric Critical Care Medicine*, vol. 12, no. 6, pp. e266–e270, 2011.

[19] C. Tournoux, S. Katsahian, S. Chevret, and V. Levy, "Factors influencing inclusion of patients with malignancies in clinical trials: a review," *Cancer*, vol. 106, no. 2, pp. 258–270, 2006.

[20] T. L. Albrecht, C. Blanchard, J. C. Ruckdeschel, M. Coovert, and R. Strongbow, "Strategic physician communication and oncology clinical trials," *Journal of Clinical Oncology*, vol. 17, no. 10, pp. 3324–3332, 1999.

[21] L. A. Siminoff, A. Zhang, N. Colabianchi, C. M. Saunders Sturm, and Q. Shen, "Factors that predict the referral of breast cancer patients onto clinical trials by their surgeons and medical oncologists," *Journal of Clinical Oncology*, vol. 18, no. 6, pp. 1203–1211, 2000.

[22] S. Eggly, T. Albrecht, F. Harper, T. Foster, M. Franks, and J. Ruckdeschel, "Oncologists recommendations of clinical trial participation to patients," *Journal of Pediatrics*, vol. 151, no. 1, pp. 50–55, 2007.

[23] C. L. Lewis, L. C. Hanson, C. Golin et al., "Surrogates' perceptions about feeding tube placement decisions," *Patient Education and Counseling*, vol. 61, no. 2, pp. 246–252, 2006.

[24] F. W. S. M. Verheggen and F. C. B. van Wijmen, "Informed consent in clinical trials," *Health Policy*, vol. 36, no. 2, pp. 131–153, 1996.

[25] K. Menon, R. E. Ward, I. Gaboury et al., "Factors affecting consent in pediatric critical care research," *Intensive Care Medicine*, vol. 38, no. 1, pp. 153–159, 2012.

[26] M. Glover, A. Kira, V. Johnston, N. Walker, D. Thomas, and A. Change, "A systematic review of barriers and facilitators to participation in randomized controlled trials by indigenous people from New Zealand, Australia, Canada and the United States," *Global Health Promotion*, 2014.

[27] M. Green and A. J. Solnit, "Reactions to the threatened loss of a child: a vulnerable child syndrome," *Pediatrics*, vol. 34, pp. 58–66, 1964.

[28] A. J. Sameroff and M. J. Chandler, "Reproductive risk and the continuum of caretaking casualty," in *Review of Child Development Research*, F. D. Horowitz, Ed., vol. 4, pp. 187–244, University of Chicago Press, Chicago, Ill, USA, 1975.

[29] B. S. McEwen, "Stressed or stressed out: what is the difference?" *Journal of Psychiatry & Neuroscience*, vol. 30, no. 5, pp. 315–318, 2005.

[30] *Advisory Committee on Human Radiation Experiments: Final report*, US Government Printing Office, Washington, DC, USA, 1995.

[31] S. Orbell and M. Hagger, "Temporal framing and the decision to take part in type 2 diabetes screening: effects of individual differences in consideration of future consequences on persuasion," *Health Psychology*, vol. 25, no. 4, pp. 537–548, 2006.

[32] J. Berenbaum and J. Hatcher, "Emotional distress of mothers of hospitalized children," *Journal of Pediatric Psychology*, vol. 17, no. 3, pp. 359–372, 1992.

[33] J. Katz, *The Silent World of Doctor and Patient*, Free Press, New York, NY, USA, 1984.

14

Effects of Whole Body Therapeutic Hypothermia on Gastrointestinal Morbidity and Feeding Tolerance in Infants with Hypoxic Ischemic Encephalopathy

Kimberly M. Thornton,[1,2] **Hongying Dai,**[3] **Seth Septer,**[2,4] **and Joshua E. Petrikin**[1,2]

[1] *Department of Neonatology, Children's Mercy Hospital, 2401 Gillham Road, Kansas City, MO 64108, USA*
[2] *School of Medicine, University of Missouri-Kansas City, 2401 Gillham Road, Kansas City, MO 64108, USA*
[3] *Research Development and Clinical Investigation, Children's Mercy Hospital, 2401 Gillham Road, Kansas City, MO 64108, USA*
[4] *Department of Gastroenterology, Children's Mercy Hospital, 2401 Gillham Road, Kansas City, MO 64108, USA*

Correspondence should be addressed to Kimberly M. Thornton; kimmcdonaldthornton@gmail.com

Academic Editor: Tonse N. K. Raju

Objective. This retrospective cohort study evaluated the effects of whole body therapeutic hypothermia (WBTH) on gastrointestinal (GI) morbidity and feeding tolerance in infants with moderate-to-severe hypoxic ischemic encephalopathy (HIE). *Study Design.* Infants ≥ 35 weeks gestational age and ≥1800 grams birth weight with moderate-to-severe HIE treated from 2000 to 2012 were compared. 68 patients had documented strictly defined criteria for WBTH: 32 historical control patients did not receive WBTH (non-WBTH) and 36 cohort patients received WBTH. *Result.* More of the non-WBTH group infants never initiated enteral feeds (28% versus 6%; $P = 0.02$), never reached full enteral feeds (38% versus 6%, $P = 0.002$), and never reached full oral feeds (56% versus 19%, $P = 0.002$). Survival analyses demonstrated that the WBTH group reached full enteral feeds (median time: 11 versus 9 days; $P = 0.02$) and full oral feeds (median time: 19 versus 10 days; $P = 0.01$) sooner. The non-WBTH group had higher combined outcomes of death and gastric tube placement (47% versus 11%; $P = 0.001$) and death and gavage feeds at discharge (44% versus 11%; $P = 0.005$). *Conclusion.* WBTH may have beneficial effects on GI morbidity and feeding tolerance for infants with moderate-to-severe HIE.

1. Introduction

Perinatal HIE is associated with high morbidity and mortality in the neonatal period as well as long-term neurocognitive deficits. Although slightly different inclusion criteria were used among studies, multiple randomized controlled trials demonstrate that WBTH has a statistically significant improvement in neurodevelopmental disability at 18 to 24 months of [1–3] followup and 6 to 7 years of followup [4] for infants with moderate-to-severe HIE at birth. However, the effects of a perinatal hypoxic ischemic event extend beyond the brain and neurodevelopment. Decreased perfusion to the GI tract [5] and decreased motility leading to feeding intolerance [6] may follow perinatal asphyxia. Patients can present with symptoms of GI bleeding, vomiting, diarrhea,

and even necrotizing enterocolitis (NEC) following HIE [7, 8]. Since WBTH acts to prevent secondary damage to the brain from ischemia and reperfusion injury that occurs following periods of perinatal anoxia, it is plausible to believe that WBTH could have similar preventative effects on the ischemic damage to the GI system.

Previous studies demonstrate conflicting results. There were some indications of hepatic dysfunction and feeding disturbances seen in subjects involved in a few of the major studies for therapeutic hypothermia, but none of those studies focused specifically on the effects to the GI system as a primary outcome. For example, the *Cool Cap* study, using selective head cooling, reported elevated liver enzymes (aspartate transaminase > 200 IU/L and alanine transaminase > 100 IU/L) in 38% of the cooled subjects versus 53% of controls ($P = 0.02$) [9]. Another selective head cooling trial, performed by Zhou et al., reported raised liver enzymes (not defined) in 35% of the cooled subjects versus 28% of the controls ($P > 0.05$) [10]. The *ICE* study reported 35% of subjects who received WBTH with hepatic dysfunction (alanine aminotransferase level > 100 U/L) versus 45% of controls ($P > 0.05$). This study also found a higher incidence of GI impairment (sloughing of the bowel, rectal bleeding, or NEC) in 4% of cooled subjects versus 2% of controls ($P > 0.05$) [2]. Another WBTH study, sponsored by the National Institute of Child Health and Human Development (NICHD), reported hepatic dysfunction (aspartate aminotransferase level > 200 IU and alanine aminotransferase level > 100 IU) in 20% of cooled subjects versus 15% of controls (significance not reported but calculated $P > 0.05$). In the cooled group, 11% of patients were discharged on gavage feeds versus 7% of controls (significance not reported but calculated $P > 0.05$) and 7% of patients were discharged with a gastric tube (GT) versus 17% of controls (significance not reported but calculated $P > 0.05$) [3]. Finally, the *TOBY* trial for WBTH reported only one case of NEC in a cooled patient and no cases of NEC in the control group (<1% versus 0%, no significance) [1].

To our knowledge, there are no published clinical trials evaluating the effects of therapeutic hypothermia for GI ischemia and reperfusion injury following HIE in humans, but several animal studies suggest a benefit. Pierro and Eaton [11] developed a rat model of intestinal ischemia-reperfusion by surgically isolating and temporarily occluding the superior mesenteric artery for 30-minute duration and then assessing signs of metabolic and histologic damage incurred to the GI tract after 60 minutes of reperfusion. They demonstrated evidence of liver energy failure, intestinal damage, and 100% mortality in the animals within 4 hours of reperfusion at normothermia. However, when the rats were kept hypothermic (32-33°C) by controlling the environmental temperature, there was a significant decrease in metabolic and histologic damage as well as 100% survival [11]. Hassoun et al. used a similar rat model with 45 minutes of induced ischemia and 6 hours of reperfusion to demonstrate decreased levels of inflammatory markers (nuclear factor kappa-B and inducible nitric oxide synthase); an increased level of a protective marker (heme oxygenase-1) and decreased histologic intestinal damage after direct hypothermia was applied to the GI tract during the ischemic period [12]. Finally, Stefanutti and colleagues [13] used the same rat model with "rescue" hypothermia applied by controlling the environmental temperature only during the reperfusion period. After 60 minutes of ischemia and 2 to 5 hours of reperfusion, hypothermia led to 100% survival and reduced inflammation, metabolic injury, and histologic damage to the GI tract [13].

We wanted to apply this evidence for WBTH use in animal models with ischemia-reperfusion injury to clinical practice. The purpose of our study was to evaluate the effects of WBTH on GI function and feeding tolerance in infants diagnosed with moderate-to-severe HIE. The primary objective was to determine the number of days to reach full enteral feeds and to reach full oral feeds in a group of infants with HIE treated with WBTH compared to a historical

control group of infants with HIE prior to the routine use of WBTH. Our hypothesis was that WBTH would have a protective effect on GI function and feeding tolerance status post-moderate-to-severe HIE.

2. Methods

2.1. Study Population: Total. Study approval was obtained from the Institutional Review Board of Children's Mercy Hospitals (Kansas City, MO). There were 435 total patients identified for retrospective analysis: 347 in the non-WBTH group and 88 in the WBTH group. 287 total patients were excluded from the study because they did not meet criteria for moderate-to-severe HIE, because they had a significant congenital defect at birth, because they were enrolled in another research study involving WBTH, or because there was insufficient data available in the medical record. There were 78 patients in the non-WBTH general criteria (defined below) group and 70 patients in the WBTH general criteria group. There were 32 patients in the non-WBTH strict criteria (defined below) group and 36 patients in the WBTH strict criteria group (Figure 1).

2.2. Study Population: Non-WBTH Group. Medical charts were reviewed for all infants ≥ 35 weeks of gestational age and ≥ 1800 grams of birth weight admitted to our institution from January 2000 to December 2008 with at least one of the following diagnoses on admission: hypoxic ischemic encephalopathy, birth asphyxia, meconium aspiration, nuchal cord, placental abruption, seizure, depression at birth, acidosis at birth, and/or shoulder dystocia. Strict criteria for the use of WBTH at our institution are based on previously published data [1–3, 9, 10, 14] and defined as a history of birth asphyxia, severe metabolic acidosis on cord blood gases or blood gas obtained within 1 hour of life (pH ≤ 7 or base deficit ≥ 16 or pH 7.01–7.15 or base deficit 10–16 and 10-minute APGAR score ≤ 5 or assisted ventilation at birth continued ≥ 10 minutes), and seizures or other evidence of moderate-to-severe encephalopathy (decreased consciousness, decreased-to-no activity, distal flexion or decerebrate posturing, hypotonia, decreased or absent reflexes, abnormal pupillary response, and abnormal breathing pattern) as documented in the medical record. Patients with adequate documentation were included in the study as historical controls and defined as the non-WBTH strict criteria group. When data for these criteria was missing, the record was reviewed further to identify other evidence of significant HIE. If patients had indirect evidence of moderate-to-severe HIE (abnormal lab values, abnormal neuroimaging, death, etc.), they were included as historical controls in the larger non-WBTH general criteria group. If the degree of HIE was considered to be mild or insufficient evidence was ultimately found to determine HIE status, the patient was excluded from the analysis. Patients with significant congenital anomalies at birth (congenital heart disease, gastroschisis, omphalocele, intestinal atresia, chromosomal trisomy, hydrocephalus, etc.) or patients involved in another study protocol using WBTH were also excluded.

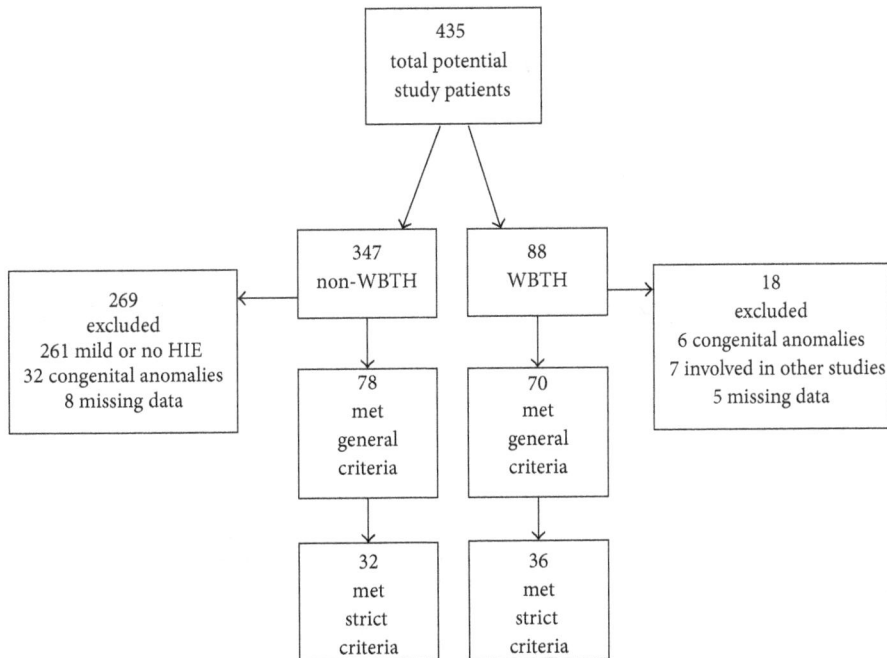

FIGURE 1: Study population.

2.3. Study Population: WBTH Group. A data set had been previously collected for quality purposes on all patients receiving WBTH from the start of standard practice use at our institution in December 2008 up to December 2012. These patients had been diagnosed with moderate-to-severe HIE based on the aforementioned criteria and completed 72 hours of WBTH at 33-34°C. In some instances, inadequate documentation existed so that all of the criteria were not found for each patient. The WBTH strict criteria group included only those patients with all criteria clearly documented, while the WBTH general criteria group included all patients who received WBTH. Again, patients with significant congenital anomalies at birth (congenital heart disease, gastroschisis, omphalocele, intestinal atresia, hydrocephalus, etc.) or patients involved in another study protocol using WBTH were excluded. Of note, patients with moribund conditions or congenital/chromosomal anomalies with poor likelihood of survival in the neonatal period were not treatment candidates as per the standard protocol for WBTH at our institution.

2.4. Study Design. We performed a twofold analysis of the data by comparing infants in the strict criteria group who received WBTH to those who did not and comparing infants in the general criteria group who received WBTH to those who did not. If information was missing in the medical record for the individual research parameters, the patient was excluded only from the statistical analysis of that specific parameter. Primary outcomes were day of life (DOL) enteral feeds started, DOL full enteral feeds reached, and DOL full oral feeds reached. Secondary outcomes included never started enteral feeds, never reached full enteral feeds, never reached full oral feeds, death, GT, combined death and GT, discharge with gavage feeds, combined death and discharge with gavage feeds, NEC, use of extracorporeal membrane

oxygenation (ECMO), elevated liver enzymes, elevated coagulation parameters, and days to hospital discharge or death. These outcomes were chosen as objective measures of GI morbidity and feeding tolerance that could be easily determined from the electronic medical documentation. Other variables such as gastric residuals and withholding of feeds were considered for outcome measures but were not well documented in the electronic medical record and could not be used for this study.

2.5. Statistical Methods. Data are expressed as mean ± standard deviation (SD) for continuous outcome variables and percentage for categorical outcome variables. Characteristics of WBTH and non-WBTH patients were compared using Chi-square test, Fisher's exact test, and t-test. Patients who did not start or reach full enteral feeds due to death were treated as censored data. Patients who did not reach full oral feeds due to death, GT placement, or discharge with gavage feeds were also treated as censored data. Kaplan-Meier survival curves were generated for WBTH and non-WBTH patients. We then performed the log-rank test to compare survival curves between the two groups. All analyses were performed using SAS 9.2 (Cary, NC) and SPSS 20. Statistical significance was claimed at 95% confidence level ($P < 0.05$).

3. Results

3.1. Comparison of Demographic Data. Overall, there were more males (59% of total study population) than females and more Caesarean sections performed (66% of total study population) than vaginal deliveries for infants with moderate-to-severe HIE. There were slight differences in birth weight, gestational age, and maternal age between the groups, but we do not feel that these differences affected our results. The

TABLE 1: Demographics for all subjects.

Variable	WBTH	Non-WBTH	P value
General criteria group	(n = 70)	(n = 78)	
Gender (% male)	44 (63%)	44 (56%)	0.50
Birth weight (grams)	3447.1 ± 524.2	3262.0 ± 570.3	0.04*
Gestational age (weeks)	39.0 ± 1.5	38.4 ± 1.9	0.02*
Maternal age (years)	25.4 ± 6.3	29.8 ± 15.6	0.03*
Cesarean delivery	45 (64%)	52 (67%)	0.86
5-minute APGAR score	3.0 ± 2.1	3.3 ± 2.0	0.29
Strict criteria group	(n = 36)	(n = 32)	
Gender (% male)	18 (50%)	18 (56%)	0.63
Birth weight (grams)	3510 ± 523.7	3120.1 ± 568.6	<0.01*
Gestational age (weeks)	39.2 ± 1.5	38.3 ± 1.7	0.02*
Maternal age (years)	25.4 ± 6.9	27.9 ± 7.6	0.17
Cesarean delivery	21 (58%)	23 (72%)	0.31
5-minute APGAR score	4.1 ± 1.8	2.2 ± 1.8	<0.001*

*Significance defined by $P < 0.05$.

degree of HIE, defined by the 5-minute APGAR score, was similar for the general criteria group, but the strict WBTH group had lower APGAR scores at 5 minutes when compared with the non-WBTH group (2.2±8 versus 4.1±1.8, $P < 0.001$). However, the mean score was below 5 at 5 minutes for both groups, suggesting that the groups had comparable degrees of depression at birth (Table 1).

3.2. Comparison between WBTH (n = 36) and Non-WBTH (n = 32) Using Strict Criteria. The non-WBTH group had more infants who never started on enteral feeds due to death (28% versus 6%, $P = 0.02$), more infants who never reached full enteral feeds due to death (38% versus 6%, $P = 0.002$), and more infants who never reached full oral feeds due to death, GT placement, or discharge with gavage feeds (56% versus 19%, $P = 0.002$) as compared to the WBTH group. The non-WBTH group has a higher mortality rate than the WBTH group (32% versus 6%, OR (95% CI): 7.9 (1.6–39.5), $P = 0.009$). The non-WBTH group had a higher rate of combined death and GT placement (46.9% versus 11.1%, $P = 0.001$) and combined death and gavage feeds at discharge (43.8 versus 11.1, $P = 0.005$). Survival analysis was performed to take the censoring into account. The Kaplan Meier curves demonstrated that infants in the WBTH group reached full enteral feeds (median time: 11 versus 9 days, $P = 0.02$) and full oral feeds (median time: 19 versus 10 days, $P = 0.01$) sooner than those in the non-WBTH group (Figure 2). There were only 3 cases of NEC, but they were all in the non-WBTH group (9% versus 0%, $P = 0.1$) There was no difference in elevation of liver enzymes (63% versus 63.9%, $P = 0.94$) or abnormal coagulation factors (91.3% versus 100%, $P = 0.15$) between groups (Table 2).

3.3. Comparison between WBTH (n = 70) and Non-WBTH (n = 78) Using General Criteria. There was no statistical significance between groups for primary outcomes, mortality, or GI morbidity measures. There were few cases of NEC, and there was no statistical significance of occurrence of NEC

between groups (5% versus 3%, $P = 0.68$). However, there were an increased number of infants who never reached full oral feeds due to death, GT placement, or discharge with gavage feeds in the non-WBTH group versus the WBTH group (42% versus 26%, $P = 0.03$). Also, infants who received WBTH had elevated coagulation parameters (prothrombin time > 15.6 seconds and partial thromboplastin time > 41.5 seconds) (80% versus 100%, $P = 0.0001$) more often than those not treated with WBTH, but there was no difference in the number of infants with elevated liver enzymes between groups (54.6% versus 62.9%, $P = 0.33$) (Table 3).

4. Discussion

Our analysis suggests that infants treated with WBTH for moderate-to-severe HIE may have improved feeding tolerance, GI morbidity, and overall mortality compared with those not treated with WBTH. Infants treated with WBTH strict criteria group reached full enteral feeds and full oral feeds sooner than those not treated. The WBTH strict criteria group had a lower overall mortality as well as combined GI morbidity (defined as GT placement or gavage feeds at discharge) and mortality.

Our results show that the majority of subjects had elevated liver enzymes and elevated coagulation parameters, expected sequelae of HIE [15, 16]. Other studies have reported that these effects were only temporary with improvement in liver enzymes and coagulation parameters over time, and our results were consistent (data not shown). There was, however, no significant difference in the number of infants with elevated liver enzymes between the WBTH and non-WBTH groups in our study.

Interestingly, there was no difference in the DOL feeds initiated between groups in either analysis. This retrospective study covered a wide time frame during which many changes occurred in medical practice, including the standard use of WBTH for moderate-to-severe HIE and the use of standardized feeding protocols. The feeding protocols are

TABLE 2: Primary and secondary outcome variables for strict criteria group.

Variable	WBTH ($n = 36$)	Non-WBTH ($n = 32$)	P value
Primary outcomes (mean ± SD)			
DOL enteral feeds started	5.6 ± 2	6 ± 3	0.12
DOL full enteral feeds reached	10.1 ± 3.7	11.3 ± 5.6	0.02[*]
DOL full oral feeds reached	11.5 ± 5.6	12.7 ± 6.7	0.01[*]
Secondary outcomes (%)			
Never started enteral feeds	5.6	28.1	0.02[*]
Never reached full enteral feeds	5.6	37.5	0.002[*]
Never reached full oral feeds	19.4	56.3	0.002[*]
Death	5.7	32.3	0.009[*]
GT	5.6	15.6	0.24
Combined death and GT	11.1	46.9	0.001[*]
Discharged with gavage feeds	5.6	9.4	0.66
Combined death and discharged with gavage feeds	11.1	43.8	0.005[*]
NEC[+]	0	9.4	0.1
ECMO	8.3	0	0.24
Elevated liver enzymes[†]	63.9	63	0.94
Elevated coagulation parameters[∞]	100	91.3	0.15
Days to hospital discharge or death	16.9 ± 11.1	16.9 ± 12	1

[*] Significance defined by $P < 0.05$.
[+] Grossly bloody stool (Bell's stage IIA or greater).
[†] Aspartate aminotransferase level >200 IU and alanine aminotransferase level >100 IU.
[∞] Prothrombin time >15.6 seconds and partial thromboplastin time >41.5 seconds.

TABLE 3: Primary and secondary outcome variables for general criteria group.

Variable	WBTH ($n = 70$)	Non-WBTH ($n = 78$)	P value
Primary outcomes (mean ± SD)			
DOL enteral feeds started	5.4 ± 2.2	5.8 ± 2.6	0.39
DOL full enteral feeds reached	9.9 ± 4.3	10.4 ± 6.1	0.12
DOL full oral feeds reached	11.4 ± 6.2	11.4 ± 6.9	0.13
Secondary outcomes (%)			
Never started enteral feeds	12.9	21.8	0.15
Never reached full enteral feeds	12.9	25.6	0.05
Never reached full oral feeds	25.7	42.3	0.03[*]
Death	15.9	23.4	0.26
GT	10	12.8	0.29
Combined death and GT	26	36.4	0.21
Discharged with gavage feeds	2.9	7.7	0.28
Combined death and discharged with gavage feeds	17.4	31.2	0.06
NEC[+]	2.9	5.1	0.68
ECMO	5.7	1.3	0.19
Elevated liver enzymes[†]	62.9	54.6	0.33
Elevated coagulation parameters[∞]	100	80.4	0.0001[*]
Days to hospital discharge or death	15.8 ± 10.2	16.2 ± 10.9	0.83

[*] Significance defined by $P < 0.05$.
[+] Grossly bloody stool (Bell's stage IIA or greater).
[†] Aspartate aminotransferase level >200 IU and alanine aminotransferase level >100 IU.
[∞] Prothrombin time >15.6 seconds and partial thromboplastin time >41.5 seconds.

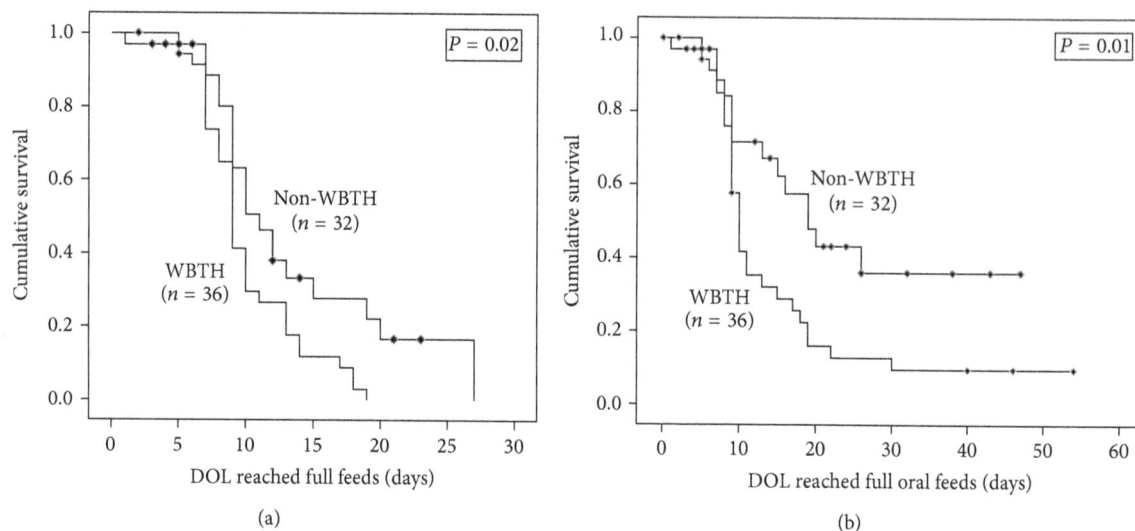

FIGURE 2: Survival curves for subjects with strict criteria*. *Censored subjects are labeled.

primarily used for the initiation and advancement of feeds in preterm infants. There is no current standardized practice for initiating feeds in late-preterm and term infants with HIE at our institution. However, we expected to see a difference in practice for initiation of feeds over the twelve-year timeframe of our study, believing that many providers would feel more comfortable starting feeds sooner in the group of infants treated with WBTH. Since this was not the case, our results are actually strengthened by the fact that both groups were fed similarly.

Limitations of the study include the small sample size and retrospective analysis of data. A historical cohort study was performed because therapeutic hypothermia has been accepted as the standard of care for infants with moderate-to-severe HIE; a prospective analysis or randomized controlled trial is not an ethical option to evaluate the effects of WBTH on GI morbidity and feeding following a perinatal hypoxic event. We estimate that fewer infants with HIE were referred to our tertiary care institution prior to use of WBTH due to the lack of therapeutic options, further limiting the number of patients available for analysis. The study was also limited by the quality of documentation in the medical record. This was the reason for dividing the groups into strict and general criteria based on the level of documentation available. When there was a lack of adequate information, the research team either determined an infant that met criteria for moderate-to-severe HIE based on other findings in the medical record (such as multiple abnormal lab values or even death) or decided to exclude the infant from the study if insufficient evidence was found. Although the 5 minute APGAR score was lower in the non-WBTH strict group versus the WBTH strict group, both groups had a mean score <5 at 5 minutes of life to suggest a considerable level of depression after birth in each one. The lower mortality seen specifically in the WBTH strict criteria group may arguably be explained by the fact that these infants were already a subgroup of infants with more

significant illness. However, the lower mortality combined with more significant results seen in the groups of infants with clear evidence of moderate-to-severe HIE by a more strict definition validates the strict use of cooling criteria used by our institution.

It should be noted that a requirement for GT placement or gavage feeds at discharge or the number of days to reach full oral feeds could all be reflections of oral skills. Those differences seen in our study could arguably be similar to the known improvements in neurologic function seen with WBTH. However, advancement of enteral feeds is a more specific measure of GI motility and the decreased number of days to reach full enteral feeds alone suggests a nonneural benefit to WBTH.

Future implications for study may include use of therapeutic hypothermia for other causes of gastrointestinal ischemia-reperfusion injury such as NEC. NEC is a unique form of gastrointestinal ischemia that occurs most often in preterm infants. Its exact etiology is not fully elucidated and felt to be multifactorial. In 2010, Hall et al. [17] published a small randomized prospective pilot study establishing the safety of using WBTH in preterm infants with advanced stage surgical NEC. The authors of the study plan to complete a larger multicenter randomized controlled trial evaluating the use of therapeutic hypothermia to decrease the amount of GI ischemic injury and surgical intervention required for NEC. Although our study was not powered for the incidence of NEC, we see interesting trends in the small numbers of patients with NEC and moderate-to-severe HIE. Our study strongly supports the need for further research in this area. Next steps could include a larger, multicentered cohort study evaluating the incidence of NEC in infants with HIE before and after the use of WBTH.

In conclusion, WBTH use for moderate-to-severe HIE may have beneficial effects to the newborn that extend beyond neurocognitive and neurodevelopmental outcomes.

Our findings suggest that WBTH improves GI morbidity and feeding tolerance for infants with moderate-to-severe HIE when strict criteria for cooling are applied.

Conflict of Interests

The authors declare no conflict of interests.

References

[1] D. V. Azzopardi, B. Strohm, A. D. Edwards et al., "Moderate hypothermia to treat perinatal asphyxial encephalopathy," *The New England Journal of Medicine*, vol. 361, no. 14, pp. 1349–1358, 2009.

[2] S. E. Jacobs, C. J. Morley, T. E. Inder et al., "Whole-body hypothermia for term and near-term newborns with hypoxic-ischemic encephalopathy: a randomized controlled trial," *Archives of Pediatrics and Adolescent Medicine*, vol. 165, no. 8, pp. 692–700, 2011.

[3] S. Shankaran, A. R. Laptook, R. A. Ehrenkranz et al., "Whole-body hypothermia for neonates with hypoxic-ischemic encephalopathy," *The New England Journal of Medicine*, vol. 353, no. 15, pp. 1574–1584, 2005.

[4] S. Shankaran, A. Pappas, S. A. McDonald et al., "Childhood outcomes after hypothermia for neonatal encephalopathy," *The New England Journal of Medicine*, vol. 366, no. 22, pp. 2085–2092, 2012.

[5] H. Akinbi, S. Abbasi, P. L. Hilpert, and V. K. Bhutani, "Gastrointestinal and renal blood flow velocity profile in neonates with birth asphyxia," *Journal of Pediatrics*, vol. 125, no. 4, pp. 625–627, 1994.

[6] C. L. Berseth and H. H. McCoy, "Birth asphyxia alters neonatal intestinal motility in term neonates," *Pediatrics*, vol. 90, no. 5, pp. 669–673, 1992.

[7] A. Martin-Ancel, A. Garcia-Alix, F. Gaya, F. Cabanas, M. Burgueros, and J. Quero, "Multiple organ involvement in perinatal asphyxia," *Journal of Pediatrics*, vol. 127, no. 5, pp. 786–793, 1995.

[8] R. N. Goldberg, D. W. Thomas, and F. R. Sinatra, "Necrotizing enterocolitis in the asphyxiated full-term infant," *The American Journal of Perinatology*, vol. 1, no. 1, pp. 40–42, 1983.

[9] P. D. Gluckman, J. S. Wyatt, D. Azzopardi et al., "Selective head cooling with mild systemic hypothermia after neonatal encephalopathy: multicentre randomised trial," *The Lancet*, vol. 365, no. 9460, pp. 663–670, 2005.

[10] W. Zhou, G. Cheng, X. Shao et al., "Selective head cooling with mild systemic hypothermia after neonatal hypoxic-ischemic encephalopathy: a multicenter randomized controlled trial in China," *Journal of Pediatrics*, vol. 157, no. 3, pp. 367–372, 2010.

[11] A. Pierro and S. Eaton, "Intestinal ischemia reperfusion injury and multisystem organ failure," *Seminars in Pediatric Surgery*, vol. 13, no. 1, pp. 11–17, 2004.

[12] H. T. Hassoun, R. A. Kozar, B. C. Kone, H. J. Safi, and F. A. Moore, "Intraischemic hypothermia differentially modulates oxidative stress proteins during mesenteric ischemia/reperfusion," *Surgery*, vol. 132, no. 2, pp. 369–376, 2002.

[13] G. Stefanutti, A. Pierro, E. J. Parkinson, V. V. Smith, and S. Eaton, "Moderate hypothermia as a rescue therapy against intestinal ischemia and reperfusion injury in the rat," *Critical Care Medicine*, vol. 36, no. 5, pp. 1564–1572, 2008.

[14] H. B. Sarnat and M. S. Sarnat, "Neonatal encephalopathy following fetal distress: a clinical and electroencephalographic study," *Archives of Neurology*, vol. 33, no. 10, pp. 696–705, 1976.

[15] P. Shah, S. Riphagen, J. Beyene, and M. Perlman, "Multiorgan dysfunction in infants with post-asphyxial hypoxic-ischaemic encephalopathy," *Archives of Disease in Childhood: Fetal and Neonatal Edition*, vol. 89, no. 2, pp. F152–F155, 2004.

[16] S. Shankaran, E. Woldt, T. Koepke, M. P. Bedard, and R. Nandyal, "Acute neonatal morbidity and long-term central nervous system sequelae of perinatal asphyxia in term infants," *Early Human Development*, vol. 25, no. 2, pp. 135–148, 1991.

[17] N. J. Hall, S. Eaton, M. J. Peters et al., "Mild controlled hypothermia in preterm neonates with advanced necrotizing enterocolitis," *Pediatrics*, vol. 125, no. 2, pp. e300–e308, 2010.

15

Current Neonatal Resuscitation Practices among Paediatricians in Gujarat, India

Satvik C. Bansal,[1] Archana S. Nimbalkar,[2] Dipen V. Patel,[1] Ankur R. Sethi,[1] Ajay G. Phatak,[3] and Somashekhar M. Nimbalkar[1]

[1] *Department of Paediatrics, Pramukhswami Medical College, Karamsad, Anand, Gujarat 388325, India*
[2] *Department of Physiology, Pramukhswami Medical College, Karamsad, Anand, Gujarat 388325, India*
[3] *Central Research Services, Charutar Arogya Mandal, Karamsad, Anand, Gujarat 388325, India*

Correspondence should be addressed to Satvik C. Bansal; satvikcb@charutarhealth.org

Academic Editor: Dharmapuri Vidyasagar

Aim. We assessed neonatal resuscitation practices among paediatricians in Gujarat. *Methods.* Cross-sectional survey of 23 questions based on guidelines of Neonatal Resuscitation Program (NRP) and Navjaat Shishu Suraksha Karyakram (NSSK) was conducted using web-based tool. Questionnaire was developed and consensually validated by three neonatologists. *Results.* Total of 142 (21.2%) of 669 paediatricians of Gujarat, India, whose e-mail addresses were available, attempted the survey and, from them, 126 were eligible. Of these, 74 (58.7%) were trained in neonatal resuscitation. Neonatal Intensive Care Unit with mechanical ventilation facilities was available for 54% of respondents. Eighty-eight (69.8%) reported correct knowledge and practice regarding effective bag and mask ventilation (BMV) and chest compressions. Knowledge and practice about continuous positive airway pressure use in delivery room were reported in 18.3% and 30.2% reported use of room air for BMV during resuscitation. Suctioning oral cavity before delivery in meconium stained liquor was reported by 27.8% and 38.1% cut the cord after a minute of birth. Paediatricians with NRP training used appropriate method of tracheal suction in cases of nonvigorous newborns than those who were not trained. *Conclusions.* Contemporary knowledge about neonatal resuscitative practices in paediatricians is lacking and requires improvement. Web-based tools provided low response in this survey.

1. Introduction

The life of a foetus in utero and the independent existence of a newborn are two vastly varied conditions requiring complex transitions. Birth asphyxia contributes to 19% of the 4 million neonatal deaths worldwide every year. In addition to its contribution to mortality, birth asphyxia can result in cognitive impairment, epilepsy, cerebral palsy, and chronic diseases in later life [1]. These numbers assume significance in Indian settings where neonatal mortality rate of 33 contributes to about 75% of the infant mortality rate of 47 as figures from 2010 reveal. This contribution of neonatal mortality to infant mortality has been increasing over the past decade as measures to reduce infant mortality are becoming effective [2].

Approximately 10% of newborns (4–7 million per year) require some form of assistance at birth. This makes neonatal resuscitation a frequently performed medical intervention [3–5]. As per the updated (October 2010) recommendations of International Liaison Committee on Resuscitation (ILCOR), Neonatal Resuscitation Program (NRP) of American Heart Association (AHA) and American Academy of Paediatrics (AAP), at least one trained person is required to be present during delivery [4]. This requires that the healthcare personnel involved need to be abreast with the latest recommendations and should follow them in their clinical practice. The Indian Academy of Pediatrics (IAP) and National Neonatology Forum (NNF) of India currently follow NRP guidelines. IAP in collaboration with National Rural Health Mission of Government of India developed Basic

Newborn Care and Resuscitation Programme (BNCRP) of Navjaat Shishu Suraksha Karyakram (NSSK) adopted from NRP guidelines for grass root workers as well as paediatricians [6].

A questionnaire based survey from Haryana, India, showed poor knowledge and practices of neonatal resuscitation among the healthcare personnel attending deliveries [7].

There is lack of information regarding neonatal resuscitation practices prevalent among paediatricians of Gujarat. This study assesses this issue with the help of web-based tool.

2. Materials and Methods

2.1. Setting. This survey was conducted amongst paediatricians within the state of Gujarat over a period of 4 months from April to July 2012. The study was approved by the Human Research Ethics Committee of HM Patel Centre for Medical Care and Education, Karamsad.

2.2. Data Collection. The questionnaire was based on revised 2010 NRP guidelines as well as NSSK guidelines and was developed, pilot-tested, and consensually validated by SMN, DVP, and ASN. It consisted of 23 multiple-choice clinical knowledge based questions, and responses were based on common interventions performed during neonatal resuscitation (the Appendix). The questionnaire was placed on an online survey website, https://www.surveymonkey.com/. The recruitment process is summarized in Figure 1. The access to the data collected over the server was password-protected. Due care was taken to prevent data loss or data entry error. The paediatricians who did not provide delivery room resuscitation in their setup were excluded.

Data were downloaded as MS Excel 2010 spreadsheets and analysed using SPSS (version 14). Univariate analysis was done to compare the practices between trained and untrained care givers. A P value less than 0.05 was considered significant.

3. Results

Out of 1,169 registered paediatricians in the state of Gujarat, e-mail addresses of 669 paediatricians were available. Over the span of 4 months, 142 (24.9%) paediatricians responded from 569 working email addresses and from them 126 were eligible for the survey (Figure 1).

Out of 126 paediatricians, 68 (54%) were associated with Neonatal Intensive Care Unit (NICU) with mechanical ventilation facility, 84 (66.7%) performed more than 20 resuscitation, and 67 (53.2%) attended more than 100 deliveries in the last one year. Only 73 (57.9%) reported to conduct resuscitation of high risk/unstable infants in the new-born corner in the delivery room under radiant warmer. Most of the participants 93 (73.8%) reported having saturation monitor in the delivery room, but only 34 (27%) reported availability of oxygen blender. Although recommended, only 23 (18.3%) reported using continuous positive airway pressure (CPAP) in the delivery room. Forty-six (36.5%) of the paediatricians had NSSK training, while 55 (43.7%) were trained in NRP in

the last three years. Practice of positive pressure ventilation in delivery room was performed by self-inflating bag flow inflating bag and Neopuff (T piece resuscitator) in 103 (81.7%), 2 (1.5%), and 18 (14.2%) respondents, respectively.

Of 126 paediatricians, 88 (69.8%) reported correct knowledge and practice regarding effective bag and mask ventilation and chest compressions. Only 46 (36.5%) of the paediatricians applied plastic/thermal wraps for extremely low birth weight newborns, which is a recommended practice. Similarly, only 48 (38.1%) participants followed the recommended practice of cutting the umbilical cord after a delay of one minute. Many participants 78 (61.9%), adopted the current recommendations of endotracheal suctioning of nonvigorous newborn in cases of meconium stained liquor. Thirty-five (27.8%) followed oral cavity suctioning before delivery of shoulder.

The participants who underwent NRP training were following correct practices as compared to those without the training with respect to meconium stained liquor (80% versus 53.1%, $P = 0.002$), but no significant difference was found with respect to application of plastic/thermal wraps for extremely low birth weight babies (43.6% versus 34.9%, $P = 0.33$) and timing of cutting of the umbilical cord (45.5% versus 36.1%, $P = 0.30$). The use of bag and mask with room air was not significantly different (84.4% versus 82.4%, $P = 0.49$) between those who underwent NSSK/BNCRP training and those who did not.

4. Discussion

This survey on resuscitation practices in Gujarat represents the difference between practices of the individual providers and the latest 2010 NRP guidelines. The results obtained are mostly reflective of the practices followed in advanced neonatal units as the majority (54%) of participants were from NICU with ventilation facility.

There was marked variation amongst the respondents regarding the time of clamping and cutting of umbilical cord; 61.9% of the respondents immediately cut the cord, whereas the rest waited for one minute. Consensus on Science with Treatment Recommendations (CoSTR) recommend delayed clamping of cord in both term and preterm uncomplicated deliveries [3, 8]. This practice is associated with decreased incidence of IVH and higher blood pressures during stabilization and thus improved neonatal outcome.

The practice of the intrapartum suctioning of oropharynx and nasopharynx before the delivery of the shoulder is no longer recommended [9], but 27.8% of respondents in this survey still did it. Majority of the respondents agreed on endotracheal suctioning of nonvigorous babies only, which is recommended. Earlier endotracheal suction of all infants, whether vigorous or nonvigorous, was performed in an effort to decrease the incidence of meconium aspiration syndrome; then, two large randomized controlled trials, questioned this practice [10, 11]. As a result, endotracheal suctioning of vigorous infants with meconium stained amniotic fluid (MSAF) is no longer recommended [8].

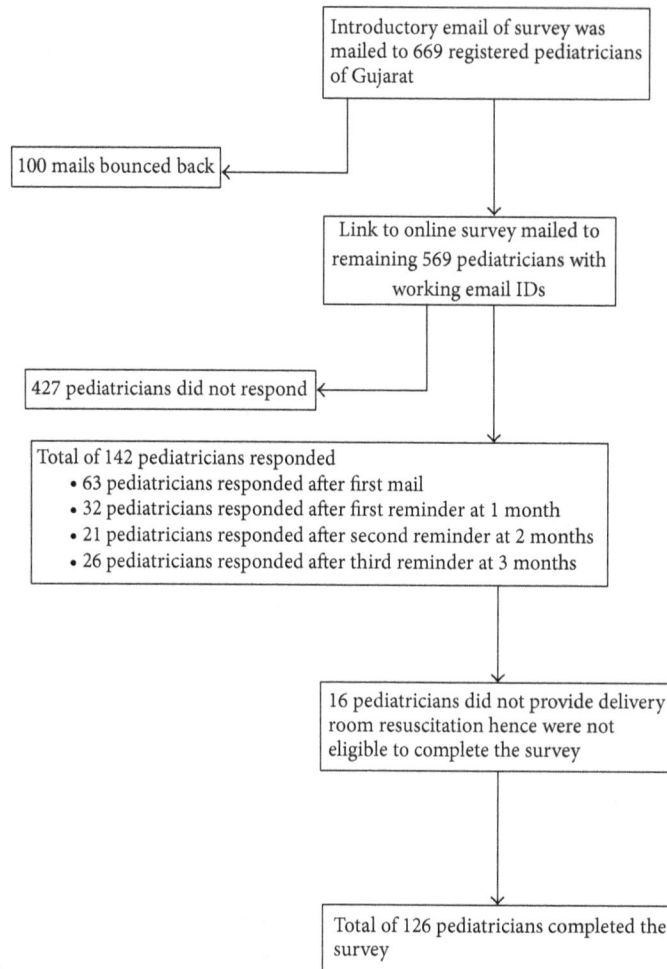

FIGURE 1: Recruitment process.

The latest NRP guidelines based on few studies [12, 13] recommend the monitoring of saturation of newborns in the delivery room. Pulse oximeter gives a continuous audible heart rate signal in addition to providing oxygen saturations, thereby allowing the resuscitators to concentrate on other tasks. In the delivery room, ideally a pulse oximeter should be used—one with highest sensitivity and lowest average signal detection time. In our survey, 73.8% of the paediatricians had saturation monitors in the delivery room. This information is encouraging for a resource-limited country like India, especially, as a recent survey in UK showed that only 58% of tertiary units and 29% of nontertiary units regularly used pulse oximeters [14].

The latest NRP and ILCOR guidelines recommend the use of room air for initial resuscitation of term infants [3, 4]. This survey shows that 63.5% of the respondents still initiate resuscitation with oxygen. This finding may reflect a gap in knowledge or lack of universal acceptance of NRP guidelines or both. A similar survey conducted in 2012 in UK [14] showed that 84.5% of individuals were using room air whereas 90% of the participants from level-three units in Canada [15] were following the same. This shows an

earlier adaptation of the newer guidelines, although room air has been incorporated in the guidelines since 2005 in Canada. In an earlier survey in 2004 from Australia and New Zealand, most healthcare personnel utilized oxygen as per the guidelines prevalent during those times [5]. Thus, there is a better adherence to guidelines in the developed world. In our survey, only 27% of paediatricians had oxygen blenders in the delivery room. In contrast, 97% of neonatologists working in tertiary care settings in Canada [15] and 71.7% participants in UK [16] were using oxygen blenders. This shortcoming though unacceptable, is a reality in a resource-limited nation like India. Appropriate emphasis must be endowed to ensure availability of basic infrastructural requirements for high quality resuscitation.

The temperature of all newborns should be maintained at $37.0 \pm 0.5°C$ [17]. In very low birth weight infants there is greater incidence of heat loss and about 25% have temperature $<35°C$ at the time of admission [18]. This hypothermia gravely affects the prognosis of the newborns [19]. To prevent insensible heat loss, wrapping of high-risk infants is recommended [3, 8, 20]. The EPICure study showed that hypothermia (temperature $< 35°C$) was associated with increased mortality rates in extremely low birth weight (ELBW) newborns [19]. These led to two prospective randomized trials that reported the benefit of polythene wraps for preventing heat loss amongst ELBW infants [21, 22]. The infant's head was dried and the polythene wrap was covered over the body without drying. This direct application reduces evaporative and convective heat losses [23]. In this survey, 36.5% of the respondents used plastic/thermal wraps. Lack of awareness, financial constraints, and unavailability of proper sterilization facilities appear to hinder its global acceptance.

The latest NRP algorithm and ILCOR recommend the use of CPAP in delivery room. Many animal studies have demonstrated the utility of peak end expiratory pressure (PEEP) in maintaining functional residual capacity and surfactant function and reducing lung injury [24–26]. In this survey, we found only 18.3% of paediatricians using delivery room CPAP. However, there was no significant difference noted in the practice by those who have attended any neonatal resuscitation training program in the past three years and those who have not, probably reflecting infrastructural and financial constraints. But, it has also been shown previously that the knowledge gained by participating in such training courses is high but is only partially retained [27]. Hence, this noncompliance can be attributed to both of these factors.

There is a need to follow up the process of knowledge and skills gained by the trainees into clinical practice, by periodical refresher courses and evaluations. This would lead to baseline improvement in competence by adherence to recommended resuscitation guidelines and thereby improve quality of care provided to newborns immediately after birth [28, 29]. The respondents were accustomed to basic resuscitative practices, but there were undeniably certain grey areas, where awareness needs to be increased. There were a total of 5 NRP trainings conducted in the years 2011 to July 2012 involving 40 participants in each training programme. From these 200 trained participants, only 28 were paediatricians and the rest were resident doctors, in paediatrics, MBBS doctors and nurses. From 559 persons trained in NSSK during the same period, only 73 were paediatricians. As there is no legal requirement by the regulatory authorities to complete NRP/NSSK before attending deliveries, it is expected that this gap in knowledge will continue. Innovative methodologies in training and flexible courses need to be devised so that new knowledge reaches those who can use it the most. Varied adoption of practises followed by trained paediatricians in this study can be explained by theory of Diffusion of Innovations of Everett Rogers [30]. However, we did not evaluate the causes of failure of adoption of the current practices of neonatal resuscitation.

There was no difference in the practice like cutting the umbilical cord, applying plastic/thermal wraps or utilizing BMV between trained and nontrained paediatricians. Studies on neonatal resuscitation practices have been conducted in various countries. In Canada, a clear gap in recommendations and practices was observed. It was also found that certification in NRP did not ensure competency and compliance with established standards of care [31]. Similar gaps have been reported in studies done in Muscat, Poland, Spain, Nepal, and United Kingdom [16, 32–35].

We observed a low response rate for the survey and this may be a threat to the generalizability of surveys conducted by e-mail or through internet-based modalities. The low response rate in this study is in contrast with the higher response rates reported in Canada (55%) and Australia (64%) which utilized the similar methodology [15, 36].

This web-linked survey method merged the process of data collection and data entry allowing the investigators to proceed with analysing the data. It has a greater reach and an option of real time monitoring. There are also less chances of data loss. More experience with such web-linked surveys is needed to establish their overall effectiveness. In this survey, we did not differentiate between paediatrician and neonatologist. There is an issue of compliance in web-linked method of surveys and it is more complex than traditional methods. In this survey, we did not include the question pertaining to total duration of practice in paediatrics.

5. Conclusions

This survey has identified areas of nonuniformity and lack of awareness amongst paediatricians for practices followed for neonatal resuscitation. There are evident gaps in the knowledge and compliance for the latest NRP and NSSK norms amongst the paediatricians of Gujarat. Research into effective dissemination of these guidelines is imperative. The web-based survey though reported low response rate had greater reach.

What Is Already Known on This Topic. Resuscitation at birth has a major role in improving morbidity and mortality of neonates. The guidelines are repeatedly revised; last revision in NRP based on ILCOR is done during 2010. Updating the practice needs to be done to improve birth outcomes.

What This Paper Adds. The contemporary knowledge of current neonatal resuscitation guidelines is low even in trained paediatricians in Gujarat. Research into effective dissemination of guidelines is imperative.

Appendix

Web-Based Questionnaire

Name:

Institution:

If you do not provide delivery room resuscitation in your setup, please go to last question and return the form

(1) Please indicate the level of NICU in your center

  (a) Stabilization of newborn babies and referral

  (b) Admission of LBW babies for sepsis, jaundice, exchange transfusion, feeding problems, and so forth

  (c) Facilities available for ventilation

(2) Number of neonates resuscitated by you in the last year

    (a) 1-2
    (b) 3–7
    (c) 8–16
    (d) More than 20

(3) Number of deliveries (vaginal or LSCS) attended in the last year

    (a) Less than 10
    (b) 10–50
    (c) 50–100
    (d) More than 100

(4) Where do you resuscitate high-risk/unstable infants after delivery?

    (a) In the dedicated newborn corner in the delivery room
    (b) In a separate room near the delivery room
    (c) In the NICU or separate adjacent room
    (d) Anywhere

(5) Device of your choice when providing positive pressure ventilation with a mask in the delivery room

    (a) Self-inflating resuscitation bag
    (b) Anaesthesia bag
    (c) Neopuff T-piece resuscitator
    (d) Other

(6) How do you begin ventilation of the term neonate with bag and mask during resuscitation?

    (a) Oxygen attached to bag and mask but without reservoir
    (b) Oxygen attached to bag and mask with reservoir
    (c) Only bag and mask without any reservoir or oxygen
    (e) Neopuff

(7) At what rate do you give breaths by bag and mask while resuscitating term neonates?

    (a) 20–30/min
    (b) 20–30 in 90 sec
    (c) 20–30 in 30 sec
    (d) 20–30 in 15 sec

(8) Do you have a saturation monitor in the resuscitation area of delivery room?

    (a) Yes
    (b) No

(9) Do you have an oxygen blender in the resuscitation area of delivery room?

    (a) Yes
    (b) No

(10) Do you use CPAP or PEEP in the delivery room?

    (a) Yes
    (b) No

(11) If you use CPAP/PEEP in the delivery room, what level of pressure do you use?

    (a) 4
    (b) 5
    (c) 6
    (d) 7

(12) Which of the following is true about chest compressions?

    (a) Area is below the xiphoid process of sternum
    (b) Area is above the nipple line
    (c) Done at compression: ventilation ratio of 1 : 2
    (d) Using palm for compression
    (e) Using thumbs for compression

(13) Free flow oxygen can be given reliably by a mask attached to self-inflating bag

    (a) True
    (b) False

(14) For persistent apnea, just after birth, what would you do?

    (a) Continue tactile stimulation a little bit more vigorously
    (b) Give positive pressure ventilation promptly
    (c) Give free flow oxygen

(15) The best indicator of effective bag and mask ventilation is

    (a) Rising heart rate and audible breath sounds
    (b) Rise in oxygen saturation
    (c) Chest movements
    (d) None of the above

(16) During chest compression how much pressure do you use?

    (a) Depress the sternum to 1/3rd of AP diameter of chest
    (b) Depress the sternum to 1/2 of AP diameter of chest
    (c) There is no strict guideline; it varies depending upon the weight of the baby
    (d) Go on increasing pressure till there is no response

(17) Have you undergone the NSSK/BNCNRP program of the IAP in the last three years?

   (a) Yes

   (b) No

(18) Have you undergone the NRP program of the NNF in the last three years?

   (a) Yes

   (b) No

(19) How long do you resuscitate a neonate who has asystole and not improving with all measure?

   (a) 5 minutes

   (b) 10 minutes

   (c) 15 minutes

   (d) 20 minutes

(20) For term babies born through meconium stained liquor, one of the following is to be done

   (a) Suction of oral cavity before delivery of shoulder

   (b) Endotracheal suction of active baby (vigorous)

   (c) Endotracheal suction of nonvigorous baby

   (d) Endotracheal suction of all babies born through meconium stained liquor

(21) Do you routinely apply plastic/thermal wraps for extremely low birth weight (ELBW) babies immediately after birth?

   (a) Yes

   (b) No

(22) What is the routine practice in your delivery room regarding cutting of the umbilical cord?

   (a) Cord is cut immediately after the delivery of the baby

   (b) Cord is cut after a delay of a minute of the delivery of the baby

   (c) Cord is cut after pulsations stop

   (d) Cord is cut after 5 minutes

(23) After vaginal delivery, the baby is placed at the following place in your primary area of practice

   (a) Under the radiant warmer in newborn care corner

   (b) On the side of the mother

   (c) On the chest/abdomen of the mother.

Abbreviations

AAP:	American Academy of Paediatrics
AHA:	American Heart Association
BMV:	Bag-mask ventilation
BNCRP:	Basic Neonatal Care Resuscitation Program
CPAP:	Continuous positive airway pressure
HREC:	Human Research and Ethics Committee
ILCOR:	International Liaison Committee on Resuscitation
LBW:	Low birth weight
LSCS:	Lower segment caesarean section
NICU:	Neonatal Intensive Care Unit
NNF:	National Neonatology Forum
NRP:	Neonatal Resuscitation Program
NSSK:	Navjaat Shishu Suraksha Karyakram
PEEP:	Peak end expiratory pressure
USA:	United States of America.

Disclosure

This paper is self-funded.

Conflict of Interests

None of the authors have any conflict of interests to disclose.

References

[1] J. E. Lawn, S. Cousens, and J. Zupan, "4 Million neonatal deaths: when? Where? Why?" *The Lancet*, vol. 365, no. 9462, pp. 891–900, 2005.

[2] *Infant and Child Mortality in India: Levels, Trends and Determinants*, UNICEF, 2010.

[3] J. M. Perlman, J. Wyllie, J. Kattwinkel et al., "Neonatal resuscitation: 2010 International consensus on cardiopulmonary resuscitation and emergency cardiovascular care science with treatment recommendations," *Pediatrics*, vol. 126, no. 5, pp. e1319–e1344, 2010.

[4] J. Kattwinkel, J. M. Perlman, K. Aziz et al., "Neonatal resuscitation: 2010 American Heart Association Guidelines for Cardiopulmonary Resuscitation and Emergency Cardiovascular Care," *Pediatrics*, vol. 126, no. 5, pp. e1400–e1413, 2010.

[5] C. P. F. O'Donnell, P. G. Davis, and C. J. Morley, "Neonatal resuscitation: review of ventilation equipment and survey of practice in Australia and New Zealand," *Journal of Paediatrics and Child Health*, vol. 40, no. 4, pp. 208–212, 2004.

[6] B. Dhingra and A. K. Dutta, "National rural health mission," *Indian Journal of Pediatrics*, vol. 78, no. 12, pp. 1520–1526, 2011.

[7] D. Louis, P. Kumar, and A. Gupta, "Knowledge and practices of healthcare providers about essential newborn care and resuscitation in a district of Haryana," *The Journal of the Indian Medical Association*, vol. 111, no. 2, pp. 114–117, 2013.

[8] J. M. Perlman, J. Wyllie, J. Kattwinkel et al., "Part 11: Neonatal resuscitation: 2010 International Consensus on Cardiopulmonary Resuscitation and Emergency Cardiovascular Care Science with Treatment Recommendations," *Circulation*, vol. 122, no. 16, pp. S516–S538, 2010.

[9] "ACOG Committee Opinion No. 379: Management of delivery of a new-born with meconium-stained amniotic fluid," *Obstetrics & Gynecology*, vol. 110, no. 3, p. 739, 2007.

[10] N. Linder, J. V. Aranda, M. Tsur et al., "Need for endotracheal intubation and suction in meconium-stained neonates," *Journal of Pediatrics*, vol. 112, no. 4, pp. 613–615, 1988.

[11] T. E. Wiswell, C. M. Gannon, J. Jacob et al., "Delivery room management of the apparently vigorous meconium-stained neonate: results of the multicenter, international collaborative trial," *Pediatrics*, vol. 105, no. 1 I, pp. 1–7, 2000.

[12] M. J. Sendak, A. P. Harris, and R. T. Donham, "Use of pulse oximetry to assess arterial oxygen saturation during newborn resuscitation," *Critical Care Medicine*, vol. 14, no. 8, pp. 739–740, 1986.

[13] L. G. Maxwell, A. P. Harris, M. J. Sendak, and R. T. Donham, "Monitoring the resuscitation of preterm infants in the delivery room using pulse oximetry," *Clinical Pediatrics*, vol. 26, no. 1, pp. 18–20, 1987.

[14] C. Mann, C. Ward, M. Grubb et al., "Marked variation in newborn resuscitation practice: a national survey in the UK," *Resuscitation*, vol. 83, no. 5, pp. 607–611, 2012.

[15] W. El-Naggar and P. J. McNamara, "Delivery room resuscitation of preterm infants in Canada: current practice and views of neonatologists at level III centers," *Journal of Perinatology*, 2011.

[16] V. Murthy, N. Rao, G. F. Fox, A. D. Milner, M. Campbell, and A. Greenough, "Survey of UK newborn resuscitation practices," *Archives of Disease in Childhood: Fetal and Neonatal Edition*, vol. 97, no. 2, pp. F154–F155, 2012.

[17] J. Perlman, J. Kattwinkel, J. Wyllie et al., "Neonatal resuscitation: in pursuit of evidence gaps in knowledge," *Resuscitation*, vol. 83, no. 5, pp. 545–550, 2012.

[18] A. R. Laptook, W. Salhab, and B. Bhaskar, "Admission temperature of low birth weight infants: predictors and associated morbidities," *Pediatrics*, vol. 119, no. 3, pp. e643–e649, 2007.

[19] K. Costeloe, E. Hennessy, A. T. Gibson, N. Marlow, and A. R. Wilkinson, "The EPICure study: outcomes to discharge from hospital for infants born at the threshold of viability," *Pediatrics*, vol. 106, no. 4 I, pp. 659–671, 2000.

[20] A. Singh, J. Duckett, T. Newton, and M. Watkinson, "Improving neonatal unit admission temperatures in preterm babies: exothermic mattresses, polythene bags or a traditional approach?" *Journal of Perinatology*, vol. 30, no. 1, pp. 45–49, 2010.

[21] S. Vohra, G. Frent, V. Campbell, M. Abbott, and R. Whyte, "Effect of polyethylene occlusive skin wrapping on heat loss in very low birth weight infants at delivery: a randomized trial," *Journal of Pediatrics*, vol. 134, no. 5, pp. 547–551, 1999.

[22] S. Vohra, R. S. Roberts, B. Zhang, M. Janes, and B. Schmidt, "Heat Loss Prevention (HeLP) in the delivery room: a randomized controlled trial of polyethylene occlusive skin wrapping in very preterm infants," *Journal of Pediatrics*, vol. 145, no. 6, pp. 750–753, 2004.

[23] G. Sedin, "To avoid heat loss in very preterm infants," *Journal of Pediatrics*, vol. 145, no. 6, pp. 720–722, 2004.

[24] A. Hartog, D. Gommers, J. J. Haitsma, and B. Lachmann, "Improvement of lung mechanics by exogenous surfactant: effect of prior application of high positive end-expiratory pressure," *British Journal of Anaesthesia*, vol. 85, no. 5, pp. 752–756, 2000.

[25] N. Mulrooney, Z. Champion, T. J. M. Moss, I. Nitsos, M. Ikegami, and A. H. Jobe, "Surfactant and physiologic responses of preterm lambs to continuous positive airway pressure," *American Journal of Respiratory and Critical Care Medicine*, vol. 171, no. 5, pp. 488–493, 2005.

[26] A. H. Jobe, B. W. Kramer, T. J. Moss, J. P. Newnham, and M. Ikegami, "Decreased indicators of lung injury with continuous positive expiratory pressure in preterm lambs," *Pediatric Research*, vol. 52, no. 3, pp. 387–392, 2002.

[27] D. Trevisanuto, P. Ferrarese, P. Cavicchioli, A. Fasson, V. Zanardo, and F. Zacchello, "Knowledge gained by pediatric residents after neonatal resuscitation program courses," *Paediatric Anaesthesia*, vol. 15, no. 11, pp. 944–947, 2005.

[28] J. Singh, S. Santosh, J. P. Wyllie, and A. Mellon, "Effects of a course in neonatal resuscitation—evaluation of an educational intervention on the standard of neonatal resuscitation," *Resuscitation*, vol. 68, no. 3, pp. 385–389, 2006.

[29] T. Xu, H.-S. Wang, H.-M. Ye et al., "Impact of a nationwide training program for neonatal resuscitation in China," *Chinese Medical Journal*, vol. 125, no. 8, pp. 1448–1456, 2012.

[30] R. Hornik, "Some reflections on diffusion theory and the role of Everett Rogers," *Journal of Health Communication*, vol. 9, no. 1, pp. 143–148, 2004.

[31] A. Mitchell, P. Niday, J. Boulton, G. Chance, and C. Dulberg, "A prospective clinical audit of neonatal resuscitation practices in Canada," *Adv Neonatal Care*, vol. 2, no. 6, pp. 316–326, 2002.

[32] S. Manzar, A. K. Nair, M. G. Pai, and S. M. Al-Khusaiby, "Use of structured question format in neonatal resuscitation assessment," *Journal of the Pakistan Medical Association*, vol. 54, no. 11, p. 583, 2004.

[33] R. Lauterbach, E. Musialik-Swietlińska, J. Swietliński et al., "Current neonatal resuscitation practices in Polish neonatal units—national survey," *Medycyna Wieku Rozwojowego*, vol. 12, no. 4, part 1, pp. 837–845, 2008.

[34] M. Iriondo, M. Thió, E. Burón, E. Salguero, J. Aguayo, and M. Vento, "A survey of neonatal resuscitation in Spain: gaps between guidelines and practice," *Acta Paediatrica, International Journal of Paediatrics*, vol. 98, no. 5, pp. 786–791, 2009.

[35] C. A. Nelson and J. M. Spector, "Neonatal resuscitation capacity in Nepal," *Journal of Paediatrics and Child Health*, vol. 47, no. 3, pp. 83–86, 2011.

[36] K. Bhola, K. Lui, and J. L. Oei, "Use of oxygen for delivery room neonatal resuscitation in non-tertiary Australian and New Zealand hospitals: a survey of current practices, opinions and equipment," *Journal of Paediatrics and Child Health*, vol. 48, no. 9, pp. 828–832, 2012.

16

Bacterial Pathogens and Antimicrobial Resistance Patterns in Pediatric Urinary Tract Infections: A Four-Year Surveillance Study (2009–2012)

Seyed Reza Mirsoleymani,[1] **Morteza Salimi,**[2] **Masoud Shareghi Brojeni,**[3] **Masoud Ranjbar,**[3] **and Mojtaba Mehtarpoor**[4]

[1] *Department of Nursing, Faculty of Nursing and Midwifery, Shahid Beheshti University of Medical Sciences, Tehran 1985717443, Iran*
[2] *Department of Physiology, Faculty of Medicine, Shahid Beheshti University of Medical Sciences, Tehran 1985717443, Iran*
[3] *Student Research Committee, Hormozgan University of Medical Sciences, Bandar Abbas 7914964153, Iran*
[4] *Department of Health Management and Economics, School of Public Health, Tehran University of Medical Sciences, Tehran 1417614411, Iran*

Correspondence should be addressed to Masoud Ranjbar; masoudranjbar857@gmail.com

Academic Editor: Hans Juergen Laws

The aims of this study were to assess the common bacterial microorganisms causing UTI and their antimicrobial resistance patterns in Bandar Abbas (Southern Iran) during a four-year period. In this retrospective study, samples with a colony count of $\geq 10^5$ CFU/mL bacteria were considered positive; for these samples, the bacteria were identified, and the profile of antibiotic susceptibility was characterized. From the 19223 samples analyzed, 1513 (7.87%) were positive for bacterial infection. UTI was more frequent in male (54.9%). *E. coli* was reported the most common etiological agent of UTI (65.2%), followed by *Klebsiella* spp. (26%), *Pseudomonas aeruginosa* (3.6%), and *Staphylococcus* coagulase positive (3.7%). Results of antimicrobial susceptibility analysis for *E. coli* to commonly used antibiotics are as follows: Amikacin (79.7%), Ofloxacin (78.3%), Gentamicin (71.6%), Ceftriaxone (41.8), Cefotaxime (41.4%), and Cefixime (27.8%). Empirical antibiotic selection should be based on awareness of the local prevalence of bacterial organisms and antibiotic sensitivities rather than on universal or even national guidelines. In this study, Amikacin and Gentamicin were shown to be the most appropriate antibiotics for empiric therapy of pyelonephritis, but empirical therapy should only be done by specialist physicians in cases where it is necessary while considering sex and age of children.

1. Introduction

Urinary tract infection (UTI) is a common health problem during the childhood period and it is an important cause of morbidity and mortality in the first 2 years of life [1–4]. The reported incidence of UTI is 7% among girls and 2% among boys during the first 6 years of life [5]. The main objects in childhood urinary tract infections are rapid recovery from complaints and prevention of related complications, such as urosepsis, urolithiasis, and renal abscess, as well as the prevention of permanent renal parenchymal damage [6]. To achieve these aims, empirical antibiotic prescription is often endorsed even before the culture results are available [7]. On the other hand, antibiotic resistance of urinary tract pathogens has been known to increase worldwide, especially to commonly used antimicrobials [8, 9]. The increasing antibiotic resistance trends are likely to have important clinical implications for the empirical use of antibiotics [10]. For this reason, knowledge of the etiology pathogens of UTIs and their antimicrobial resistance patterns in specific geographical locations may aid clinicians in choosing the appropriate antimicrobial empirical treatment [11]. Prior to this study, the frequency of bacterial species causing UTI and their susceptibility patterns to most commonly used antibiotics has not been previously determined in the southern provinces of Iran; so the aim of this study was to characterize these factors in this region of Iran.

2. Methods

This retrospective study analyzed the bacteria isolated from patients with UTI at the Children's Hospital, the main center for newborns and children located in Bandar Abbas, capital of Hormozgan Province, South of Iran. Urine samples were obtained from outpatients and inpatients with suspected UTI and those who were admitted in pediatric wards with signs and symptoms of UTI to document the common bacterial species causing UTI and their antibacterial susceptibility profile. The period of study was from 2009 to 2012. Patients were children aged from 1 week to 16 years without history of genitourinary abnormalities, recent hospitalization, or antibiotic usage. Patients were hospitalized for evaluation and treatment with signs and symptoms of acute pyelonephritis, including: temperature $\geq 38°C$, chills, frequency, dysuria, urgency, suprapubic and/or flank tenderness, pyuria (defined as ≥ 5 WBC/Hpf), and fever with unknown source in children and in neonates (7–30 days of age) with clinical evidences of sepsis.

Data on age, sex, result of urine culture, the etiological agent, and susceptibility pattern were obtained from the medical records of patients. Urine samples were collected using midstream method in toilet-trained children and using clean-catch methods or sterile bladder catheter in younger children and infants.

Samples were inoculated on blood agar and eosin methylene blue agar plates and then were read after overnight incubation at 37°C. After incubation, the urine culture samples were classified as negative, positive, and contaminated. When polymorphic bacterial growth (two or more bacterial species growth in one plate) was observed, the samples were classified as contaminated (exclusion criteria). The urine cultures were considered as negative when bacterial growth was lower than 10^3 CFU/mL (exclusion criteria). Growth of two or more bacterial species (polymorphic bacterial growth) was considered as an exclusion criterion. When monomorphic bacterial growth was higher than 10^5 CFU/mL, the culture was classified as positive (inclusion criteria) and, for these cases, the antimicrobial susceptibility test (AST) was performed. The AST was also performed when the result of urine culture was between 10^4 and 10^5 CFU/mL. Identification of bacterial microorganisms was made on the basis of gram reaction, morphology and biochemical features. The AST was performed by Kirby-Bauer disk diffusion method. A bacterial suspension in physiological saline solution was prepared by picking up 1-2 colonies from pure cultures. The suspension was spread on Mueller-Hinton Agar plate by a swab. Antibiotic disks were placed onto the cultures medium surface. The culture plates were incubated at 37°C for 24 hours; then inhibition zones were measured and hereby the antimicrobial efficacy was determined [12]. The commercial antibiotics used for isolates included Ciprofloxacin,

Trimethoprim-sulfamethoxazole (Cotrimoxazole), Gentamicin, Tobramycin, Ampicillin, Nitrofurantoin, Nalidixic acid, Ceftriaxone, Cefotaxime, Cefalexin, Cefazolin, Amoxicillin, Oxacillin, Cefixime, Ceftazidime, Erythromycin, Tetracycline, Clindamycin, Ofloxacin, and Amikacin; in addition to these antibiotics, Penicillin and Erythromycin were used for gram positive bacteria. The data were analyzed using the Statistical Package for the Social Sciences (SPSS) 16.0 for Windows. The normality of data and homogeneity of variance were checked before analysis. As most of the variables failed, these statistical method assumptions and the nonparametric Kruskal-Wallis test, as well as chi square test, were used.

3. Results

From January 2009 to 2012, a total of 19223 urine samples were submitted for analysis and culture. These samples showed 1513 (7.87%; 95% CI 7.49–8.2%) bacterial growth higher than 10^5 CFU/mL. The prevalence of UTI among male and female children suspected to have UTI was 5.1% (845/16282; 95% CI 4.78–5.43%) and 22.4% (659/2941; 95% CI 20.9–23.9%), respectively. Only the first urine sample of one patient and monomorphic bacterial growth samples was considered in this study. 176 of these samples were *Staphylococcus* coagulase negative (rather a contamination microorganism) and were excluded from the study. So, finally, 1209 samples were included. 664 (54.9%) of these patients were males and 545 (45.1%) were females. Of these patients, 437 (36.1%), 377 (31.2%), and 395 (32.7%) were neonates (<28 days), infants (28 days to 1 years), and children (1 years to 14 year), respectively. The predominant agents of UTI were successively *E. coli* (65.2%; 95% CI 62.5–67.8%), *Klebsiella* spp. (26%; 95% CI 23.6–28.4%), *Pseudomonas aeruginosa* (3.6%; 95% CI 2.6–4.6%), *Staphylococcus* coagulase positive (3.7%; 95% CI 2.7–4.7%), *Citrobacter* (0.9%; 95% CI 0.4–1.3%), *Enterobacter* spp. (0.4%; 95% CI 0.1–0.7%), and *Proteus mirabilis* (0.2%; 95% CI 0.0–0.4%) (Table 1).

Analysis of the results according to patient gender represented that, although *E. coli* is the predominant isolated pathogen from both sexes, it occurred more frequently in females (70.8% in females compared to 60.5% in males: significant at $\rho = 0.001$ (chi square = 11.359)), whereas the prevalence of UTI due to *Klebsiella* spp. was higher in males than in females (28.3% in males compared to 23.1% in females, respectively. Significant at $\rho = 0.001$ (chi square = 11.359)). And the prevalence of UTI caused by *Pseudomonas aeruginosa* was significantly higher in males at $\rho = 0.035$ (chi square = 4.45).

Table 1 illustrates incidence of the main bacterial pathogens implicated in urinary tract infection, according sex and age during the study period. Significant (Kruskal-Wallis test, $\rho < 0.05$) changes in the main bacterial pathogens responsible for UTI were observed during the study period. In general, the incidence of *Staphylococcus* coagulase positive increased and the incidence of *Klebsiella* spp. decreased during the period of the study (Figure 1).

In vitro sensitivity testing showed that the mean susceptibility *E. coli* had a sensitivity rate of 79.7% to Amikacin and

TABLE 1: The main bacterial pathogens implicated in urinary tract infection by sex and age throughout the study period.

| Bacteria | Neonates | | | Infants | | | Children | | |
	Total[a] (N = 437)	Male[b] (n = 260)	Female[b] (n = 177)	Total[a] (N = 377)	Male[b] (n = 217)	Female[b] (n = 160)	Total[a] (N = 395)	Male[b] (n = 187)	Female[b] (n = 208)
E. coli	57.7	54.2	62.7	70.8	66.8	76.3	68.1	62.0	73.6
Klebsiella	36.2	38.1	33.3	19.4	21.2	16.8	21	23.0	19.2
P. aeruginosa	2.3	3.1	1.1	5.0	6.0	3.8	3.8	5.3	2.4
S. coagulase positive	1.6	2.3	0.6	3.2	4.1	1.8	6.6	9.2	4.3
Citrobacter	1.6	1.5	1.7	0.8	0.5	1.3	0.3	0.0	0.5
Enterobacter	0.6	0.8	0.6	0.5	0.9	0.0	0.0	0.0	0.0
Proteus	0.0	0.0	0.0	0.3	0.5	0.0	0.3	0.5	0.0

[a]Percentage determined in relation to N; [b]percentage determined in relation to n.

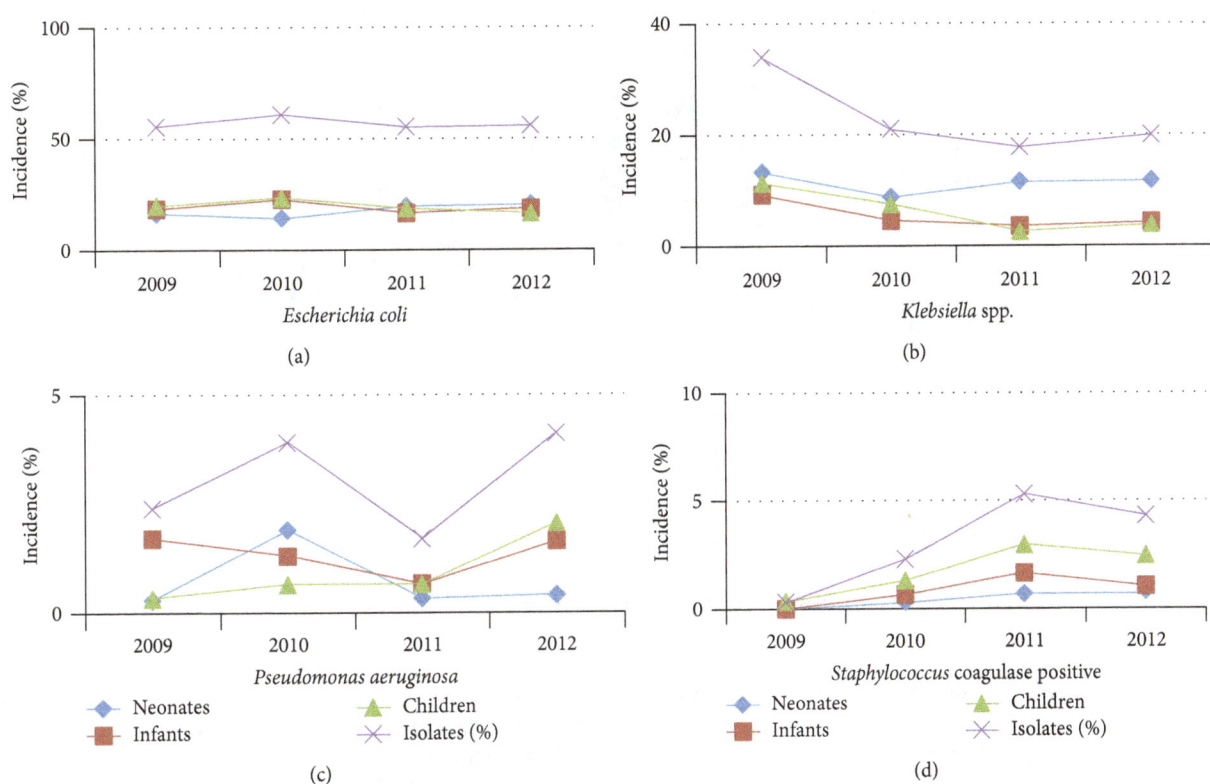

FIGURE 1: Incidence of the main bacteria implicated in UTI by age during the study period.

77.1% to Ciprofloxacin. In this study, the highest resistance rate of this germ was to Ampicillin (83.5%) followed by Trimethoprim-sulfamethoxazole (75.4%). The E. coli resistance to Trimethoprim-sulfamethoxazole (one of the most important UTI empirical therapy options) changed significantly over the study period (chi square test, $\rho < 0.001$). In general, the resistance rate has been increased in females but has been reduced in males (Table 2). Klebsiella spp., the second common germ producing UTI, showed the highest sensitivity to Ciprofloxacin (81.3%) and Amikacin (73.1%) and the highest resistance to Ampicillin (86.3%) and Cephalothin (62.4%). Pseudomonas was 100% resistant to

Trimethoprim-sulfamethoxazole in this study. It showed the highest sensitivity to Tobramycin (100%), Amikacin (86.4%), and Gentamycin (84%). The antibiotic resistance patterns of E. coli (the most common germ) and Pseudomonas aeruginosa (the most antibiotic resistant germ) agents of UTI are presented in Figures 2 and 3.

4. Discussion

Urinary tract infection (UTI) is of major clinical importance owing to considerably high morbidity and mortality rates among children [3]. In this study, of 19223 patients who were

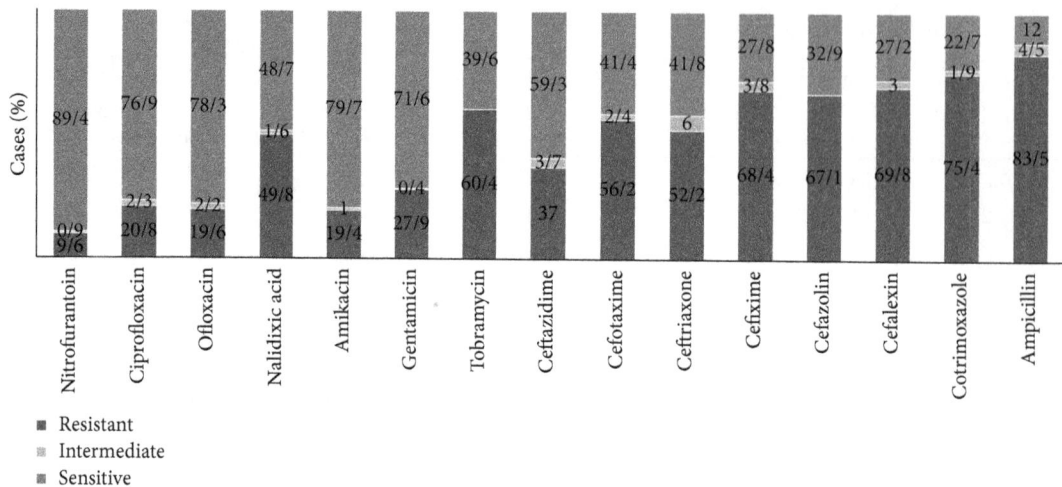

FIGURE 2: *E. coli* sensitivity and resistance pattern of bacteria causing UTI to antibiotics.

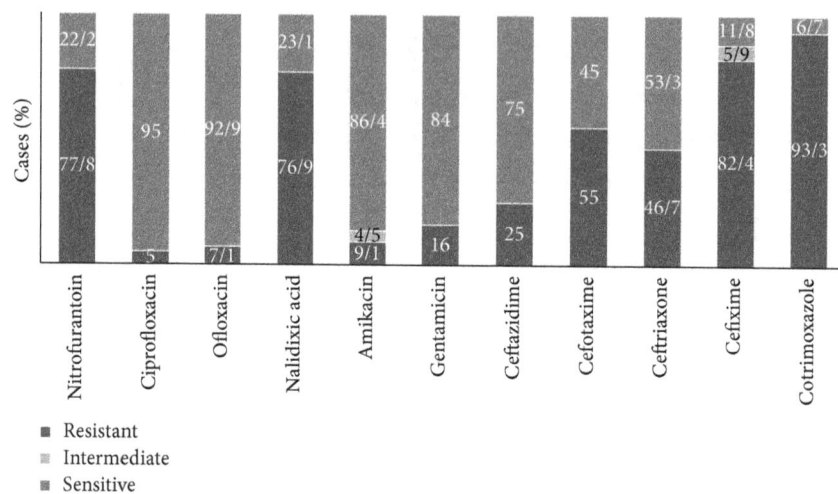

FIGURE 3: *Pseudomonas aeruginosa* sensitivity and resistance pattern of bacteria causing UTI to antibiotics.

TABLE 2: The *E. coli* resistance to Trimethoprim-sulfamethoxazole over the study period.

	Year				P value	chi square
	2009	2010	2011	2012		
Male	72.7%	81.7%	47.9%	64.0%	<0.001	33.961
Female	68.4%	72.3%	66.7%	86.9%	0.004	19.201
Total	70.6%	77.6%	56.6%	73.5%	<0.001	40.589

suspected to UTI and from whom urine samples were taken, only 7.87% had a urinary tract infection. Its relative ratio varies in different areas of Iran. In studies carried out in Tabriz and Qazvin, 13.2% and 7.2% of pediatric suspected of urinary tract infection had a positive urine culture [10, 13] that was similar to our results. This is possibly because UTI symptoms are not a dependable indicator of infection and in children younger than 2 years of age are nonspecific [10] therefore, urine culture of suspected children is necessary for a definitive diagnosis of UTI.

In this study, *E. coli*, as the most common pathogen, incidence among females was significantly higher than in males and incidence of *Klebsiella*, as the second most common pathogen, was significantly higher in males. On the other hand, in this study, 70.5% of UTI caused by *Pseudomonas aeruginosa* were in males and only 29.5% were in females. *Pseudomonas aeruginosa* is an opportunistic uropathogen for community-acquired UTI [12] and also totally resistant to first line empirical antibiotics (special importance of this pathogen) [14]. Be male, received recent antibiotic therapy, have a neurogenic bladder and have a history of urinary tract procedures such as catheterization are known as risk factors for UTI caused by *Pseudomonas aeruginosa* [15]. So similar to other literature, sex might influence the etiology of UTI and most be considered in empirical therapy [12].

In this study, among children who have a positive urine culture, 55.9% were males and 44.1% were females. Also, most of the participants were infants and neonates (65.2%) and 34.8% were children. Male children are infected more than girls during the first 3 months of their life but, incidence of

UTI among girls who have more than one year old is much more [16] possibly because the structural anomalies incidence in first 3 months among boys is more. Boys were more at risk of wrong diagnosis of UTI than female children too. In this study, the frequencies of positive cultures were 5.1% for males and 22.4% for females (ratio~1 : 4). Farajnia et al. reported this ratio 1 : 2 [10] and Farrell et al. reported this ratio 1 : 4.1 [17]. The cause of this needs more study.

Chi square test showed that pathogens differed significantly ($p < 0.001$) across the three age groups of study. *E. coli* prevalence was higher in infants (63.1%), incidence of *Klebsiella* was higher in neonate (32.9%), and *Pseudomonas aeruginosa* incidence was higher in infants, but the *Staphylococcus* coagulase positive prevalence was higher in children (5.4%). So age might influence the etiology of urinary tract infection as has been shown in the study of Afsharpaiman et al. [16]. Overall, these results indicate that urine culture is necessary for a definitive diagnosis of UTI and that empirical therapy should only be done by specialist physicians in case where it is necessary while considering sex and age of children.

E. coli is the leading uropathogen and was isolated from 56.6–84.6% of Iranian children with febrile UTI [16, 18]. The results of this study in this context are in agreement with previous literature findings. *E. coli* was the most causative organism responsible for 65.2% of urinary tract infections. But the resistance pattern of this germ to antibiotics was very different in comparison with other studies. For example Sharifian et al. reported the highest susceptibility percentage of *E. coli* to Ceftriaxone (97.8%) and Cefotaxime (95.2%) in 2006 in Tehran [19]. But, in this study, *E. coli* specimens were 52.2% and 56.2% resistant to Ceftriaxone and Cefotaxime, respectively, probably because the pattern of the sensitivity of microorganisms to antibiotics varies over time and between different geographical locations. There was no study before this study for physicians of this region to estimate the most common pathogen and its resistant pattern in pediatrics, but they empirically consider *E. coli* as the most causative agent and Ceftriaxone and Cefixime as the most appropriate choice for UTI treatment but the results of this study have shown that Ceftriaxone probably cannot be the best choice hereafter. On the other hand, according to the results of this study, *E. coli* specimens were 64.8% resistant to Cefixime and 75.4% resistant to Trimethoprim-sulfamethoxazole. Although Cefixime probably cannot be the best choice, it is better than Trimethoprim-sulfamethoxazole for outpatient treatment option.

In a study conducted in Khartoum, Ali and Osman reported that the mean susceptibility of all isolates was too high to Gentamicin (96%), Ciprofloxacin (94%), and Ceftriaxone (90%) whereas the lowest percentages of susceptibility were reported for Amoxicillin clavulanate (19%) and Ampicillin (14%) [20]. In a study conducted in the US hospitals, resistance among *E. coli* was highest for Trimethoprim-sulfamethoxazole (24%) but lower for Nitrofurantoin (<1%) and Cephalothin (15%) [5]. This study revealed a high *E. coli* resistance rate to antibiotics. Except for Nitrofurantoin and Ciprofloxacin that are not appropriate options for UTI treatment in children [19], the highest percentages of susceptibility

were seen for Amikacin (79.7%), Ofloxacin (78.3%), and Gentamicin (71.6%), whereas the highest percentages of resistance for this pathogen were found for Ampicillin (83.5%), Cotrimoxazol (75.4%), and Cefalexin (69.8%). Other studies in Iran have also indicated a high resistance rate to antibiotics. For example, Farajnia et al. reported resistance rate of 90.7% to Ampicillin, 51.8% to Cotrimoxazol, and 26.5% to Cefalexin, whereas the highest percentages of susceptibility were seen for Amikacin (96.6%) and Gentamicin (92.9%) in 2008 in Tabriz [10]. These significantly higher bacterial resistance rates to antibiotics in our country in comparison with other countries seem to be the result of two factors: first, a higher rate of antibiotic usage by families even in the absence of a prescription and, second, a population with a high percentage of young individuals since UTI is more common in the early years of life (UTI is most common in girls aged 3 to 5 years) [19]. The other factor that probably caused this study to show higher bacterial resistant rates of antibiotic is the empirical therapy itself because the results of this study showed that only 7.87%, of who were suspected to UTI, had a urinary tract infection in reality. Probably a high rate of antibiotics using resulted in various antibiotic resistance patterns in different parts of Iran.

In conclusion, we suggest that empirical antibiotic selection should be based on knowledge of the local prevalence of bacterial organisms and antibiotic sensitivities rather than on universal or even national guidelines. In this study, Amikacin and Gentamicin were shown to be the most appropriate antibiotics for empiric therapy of pyelonephritis, but, empirical therapy should only be done by specialist physicians in cases where it is necessary while considering sex and age of children.

Conflict of Interests

The authors declare that there is no conflict of interests regarding the publication of this paper.

Acknowledgments

The authors would like to hereby thank the Student Research Committee of Hormozgan University of Medical Sciences, Bandar Abbas, Iran, specially Ms. Soghra Fallahi and Mr. Mohammad Esmaeil Shahrzad for sharing their invaluable advice.

References

[1] L. P. Jadresić, "Diagnosis and management of urinary tract infections in children," *Paediatrics and Child Health*, vol. 20, no. 6, pp. 274–278, 2010.

[2] O. Adjei and C. Opoku, "Urinary tract infections in African infants," *International Journal of Antimicrobial Agents*, vol. 24, no. 1, pp. S32–S34, 2004.

[3] F. Mortazavi and N. Shahin, "Changing patterns in sensitivity of bacterial uropathogens to antibiotics in children," *Pakistan Journal of Medical Sciences*, vol. 25, no. 5, pp. 801–805, 2009.

[4] S. Habib, "Highlights for management of a child with a urinary tract infection," *International Journal of Pediatrics*, vol. 2012, Article ID 43653, 6 pages, 2012.

[5] R. S. Edlin, D. J. Shapiro, A. L. Hersh, and H. L. Copp, "Antibiotic resistance patterns in outpatient pediatric urinary tract infections," *The Journal of Urology*, vol. 190, no. 1, pp. 222–227, 2013.

[6] R. Beetz and M. Westenfelder, "Antimicrobial therapy of urinary tract infections in children," *International Journal of Antimicrobial Agents*, vol. 38, pp. 42–50, 2011.

[7] F. E. Abdullah, A. A. Memon, M. Y. Bandukda, and M. Jamil, "Increasing ciprofloxacin resistance of isolates from infected urines of a cross-section of patients in Karachi," *BMC Research Notes*, vol. 5, no. 1, pp. 696–701, 2012.

[8] A. Alemu, F. Moges, Y. Shiferaw, K. Tafess, A. Kassu, B. Anagaw et al., "Bacterial profile and drug susceptibility pattern of urinary tract infection in pregnant women at University of Gondar Teaching Hospital, Northwest Ethiopia," *BMC Research Notes*, vol. 5, no. 1, pp. 197–204, 2012.

[9] G. Schmiemann, I. Gagyor, E. Hummers-Pradier, and J. Bleidorn, "Resistance profiles of urinary tract infections in general practice-an observational study," *BMC Urology*, vol. 12, no. 1, pp. 33–38, 2012.

[10] S. Farajnia, M. Y. Alikhani, R. Ghotaslou, B. Naghili, and A. Nakhlband, "Causative agents and antimicrobial susceptibilities of urinary tract infections in the northwest of Iran," *International Journal of Infectious Diseases*, vol. 13, no. 2, pp. 140–144, 2009.

[11] N. Kashef, G. E. Djavid, and S. Shahbazi, "Antimicrobial susceptibility patterns of community-acquired uropathogens in Tehran, Iran," *Journal of Infection in Developing Countries*, vol. 4, no. 4, pp. 202–206, 2010.

[12] I. Linhares, T. Raposo, A. Rodrigues, and A. Almeida, "Frequency and antimicrobial resistance patterns of bacteria implicated in community urinary tract infections: a ten-year surveillance study (2000–2009)," *BMC Infectious Diseases*, vol. 13, no. 1, article 19, 2013.

[13] F. Vaezzadeh and M. Sharifi-Yazdi, "Laboratory evaluation of urine culture and drug resistance in children clinically suspected of urinary tract infection (UTI)," *Iranian Journal of Public Health*, vol. 30, pp. 123–127, 2001.

[14] M. Bitsori, S. Maraki, S. Koukouraki, and E. Galanakis, "Pseudomonas aeruginosa urinary tract infection in children: Risk factors and outcomes," *Journal of Urology*, vol. 187, no. 1, pp. 260–264, 2012.

[15] J. H. Tabibian, J. Gornbein, A. Heidari et al., "Uropathogens and host characteristics," *Journal of Clinical Microbiology*, vol. 46, no. 12, pp. 3980–3986, 2008.

[16] S. Afsharpaiman, F. Bairaghdar, M. Torkaman, Z. Kavehmanesh, S. Amirsalari, M. Moradi et al., "Bacterial pathogens and resistance patterns in children with community-acquired urinary tract infection: a cross sectional study," *Journal of Comprehensive Pediatrics*, vol. 3, no. 1, pp. 16–20, 2012.

[17] D. J. Farrell, I. Morrissey, D. de Rubeis, M. Robbins, and D. Felmingham, "A UK multicentre study of the antimicrobial susceptibility of bacterial pathogens causing urinary tract infection," *Journal of Infection*, vol. 46, no. 2, pp. 94–100, 2003.

[18] Y. Panahi, F. Beiraghdar, Y. Moharamzad, Z. K. Matinzadeh, and B. Einollahi, "The incidence of urinary tract infections in febrile children during a two-year period in Tehran, Iran," *Tropical Doctor*, vol. 38, no. 4, pp. 247–249, 2008.

[19] M. Sharifian, A. Karimi, S. R. Tabatabaei, and N. Anvaripour, "Microbial sensitivity pattern in urinary tract infections in children: a single center experience of 1,177 urine cultures," *Japanese Journal of Infectious Diseases*, vol. 59, no. 6, pp. 380–382, 2006.

[20] E. Ali and A. Osman, "Acute urinary tract infections in children in Khartoum State: pathogens, antimicrobial susceptibility and associated risk factors," *Arab Journal of Nephrology and Transplantation*, vol. 2, no. 2, pp. 11–16, 2009.

17

Magnitude and Reasons for Harmful Traditional Practices among Children Less Than 5 Years of Age in Axum Town, North Ethiopia, 2013

Kahsu Gebrekirstos, Atsede Fantahun, and Gerezgiher Buruh

Department of Nursing, College of Health Sciences, Mekelle University, Mekelle, 18713 Tigray, Ethiopia

Correspondence should be addressed to Kahsu Gebrekirstos; kahsu75@gmail.com

Academic Editor: Lavjay Butani

Background. In addition to beneficial traditional practices, there are around 140 harmful traditional practices affecting mothers and children in almost all ethnic groups of Ethiopia. Therefore this study might give a clue about their practice and associated factors. The objective of this study was to assess magnitude of harmful traditional practices among children less than 5 years of age in Axum Town, North Ethiopia. *Methods.* Community based cross-sectional study was conducted on 752 participants who were selected using multistage sampling. Simple random sampling method was used to select ketenas from all kebelles of Axum Town. After proportional allocation of sample size to eachketena, systematic random sampling method was used to get the study participants. Data was collected using interviewer administered questionnaire; it was entered and analyzed using SPSS version 16 and descriptive statistics was calculated. *Results.* Majority of the respondents (81.2%) were Orthodox, 78.2% of the mothers had no work, and majority of mothers had no formal education. Among the harmful traditional practices performed on children, uvula cutting alone was performed on 72.8% of children followed by milk teeth extraction and uvula cutting with eyebrow incision. *Conclusion.* The leading harmful traditional practice performed on children in this study was uvula cutting.

1. Introduction

WHO defined traditional medicine in 1978 as "the sum total of all the knowledge and practices, whether explicable or not, used in diagnosis, prevention and elimination of physical, mental or social imbalance and relying exclusively on practical experience and observation handed down from generation to generation whether verbally or in writing" [1, 2]. Even though the prevalence and degree may vary, harmful traditional practices (HTPs) which have numerous long term devastating effects are also performed in all continents of the world [3]. United Nations (UN) agencies and human right bodies started addressing HTP in the early 1990s but there was little progress [4]. There are now a number of important international instruments endorsed by most of the governments and could serve as a basis for a struggle against HTPs [5]. In addition to deep-rooted beliefs, customs, and rational

attitudes, lack of knowledge and being unaware of the effects of the practices help maintain these problems. HTPs such as uvulectomy, tonsillectomy, female circumcision, milk teeth extraction, and eyebrow incision are widely practiced with no or little attention to hygiene in Ethiopia [1]. Sometimes a harmful practice is so deeply rooted that it seems impossible to change. But in every country people have pushed forward positive social changes, and harmful practices have been ended [6]. Unlike in developing countries where traditional practices are performed by more than 80% of the population, populations in some countries in the Middle East as well as immigrants to Europe and USA have abandoned these practices [7].

Traditional medical and behavioral practices in sub-Saharan Africa have been evaluated infrequently in relation to risk of infectious disease transmission [8]. Kupeli et al. reported adverse effects and immediate, short-term, and long-term complications immediately after the procedure; the most common risks include excessive bleeding, infection, tetanus, meningitis, transmission of infectious diseases (HIV and hepatitis), and death [9].

It is said that there are around 140 HTPs affecting mothers and children in almost all ethnic groups of Ethiopia. HTPs that affect children are female genital mutilation (FGM), milk teeth extraction (MTE), food taboo, uvula cutting (UC), forbidding food and fluids during diarrhea, keeping babies from exposure to sun, and feeding new born babies with fresh butter [7].

In Ethiopia, two important national surveys have been conducted by EGLDAM (Ye Ethiopia Goji Lemadawi Dirgitoch Aswagaj Mahber) and the Former National Committee for Traditional Practices of Ethiopia (NCTPE). The survey identified five top priority HTPs including FGM, uvula cutting, MTE, early marriage, and marriage by abduction at national level [10]. Based on the baseline survey (BLS) on HTPs in Ethiopia conducted in 1997, the prevalence of uvula cutting in Tigray Region was 92.8% but 66.4% on the follow-up survey. The prevalence of FGM in Tigray Region was 48.1% in BLS with marked decrease to 21.2% in follow-up survey. The prevalence of MTE in Tigray Region decreased from 52.4% (baseline survey) to 26.6% (follow-up survey) [4].

The Objective of this study was to assess the magnitude and reasons associated with HTPs among Children less than 5 years of age in Axum Town, North Ethiopia. In this study we tried to assess the current status of HTPs in the study area. It might also have an implication in improving child health care practice and in reducing child morbidity and mortality.

2. Materials and Methods

Community based cross-sectional study was conducted in Axum Town, North Ethiopia, in 2013. The sample population was all mothers who have children less than 5 years old. The town is divided into 4 kebeles and kebeles also subdivided into ketenas (districts). A total of 9 ketenas, 3 ketenas from kebelle hawelti, and 2 ketenas from each of the rest of kebeles were selected. Afterwards, proportional allocation of samples systematic sampling method was used to select 752 mothers. Structured questionnaire adapted from the follow-up survey of HTPs in Ethiopia by EGLDAM in 2008 was used. Data was collected from mothers who have children less than 5 years old using interviewer administered questionnaire. Correction was done based on the feedback from the pretest. Data was checked and cleaned daily for completeness and consistency during data collection. Data was entered and analyzed using SPSS software (version 18.0) and descriptive statistics was calculated. It was coded and cleaned before analysis. The proposal was submitted to College of Health Sciences, Department of Nursing and Midwifery Institutional Review Board (IRB), Addis Ababa University for approval. Following approval, official letter of cooperation was written to Axum Town Administration Office from the Department of Nursing and Midwifery of Addis Ababa University. After getting permission from Axum Town Administration, data collectors were trained about the study. Study participants were informed OF the purpose, advantage, and disadvantage of the study, with the right to refuse at any stage of the interview. Confidentiality was assured for all the information provided and informed verbal consent was obtained prior to interview.

3. Results

3.1. Sociodemographic Characteristics. In this study a total of 752 mothers who had children less than five years old were interviewed with a response rate of 100%. The number of female children was 381 (50.7%) and mean age of children was 26.28 months (SD = +15.98; range: 1–59 months) while mean age of mothers was 30.55 years (SD = +6.22; range: 19–51 years). Majority of the respondents, 611 (81.2%), were Orthodox and 141 (18.8%) were Muslim. Regarding occupational status, about 588 (78.2%) of respondents had no work and 6 (0.8%) had other works like local clothes makers, Tella makers, and beauty salon workers. 379 (50.4%) attended primary school, 196 (26.1%) attended secondary school, and 100 (13.3%) were illiterate (Table 1).

3.2. Magnitude of Harmful Traditional Practices. Out of the 752 respondents 746 (99.2%) had information on at least one harmful traditional practice and 301 (40%) of them had information on all of the mainly recognized HTPs (uvula cutting, milk teeth extraction, FGM, and eyebrow incision), 588 (78.2%) knew about uvula cutting, and 493 (65.5%) knew about female genital mutilation. Three hundred seventy-two (49.5%) mothers mentioned family members as source of information and there was also another source mentioned by 4 (0.5%) respondents which was school. Most of mothers, 618 (82.2%), participating in this study had HTPs performed on themselves and of them 599 (79.6%) mothers reported that uvula cutting was performed on them. The mean age of children to perform HTPs was 4.61 weeks (SD = +10.5; range: 1–112). All of the HTPs, 660 (100%) cases, performed by traditional healers at their home. Minor complications like difficulty of swallowing, bleeding, swelling, and signs of infection happened in only in 80 (10.6%) cases after the procedure (Table 2).

From the total number of participants, 660 (87.8%) had performed at least one HTPs on their children. Among the HTPs performed on children, uvula cutting alone was practiced on 548 (72.8%) children and uvula cutting with milk teeth extraction as well as with eyebrow incision was performed on 89 (11.8%) and 17 (2.3%) children, respectively (Figure 1).

3.3. Reasons to Perform Harmful Traditional Practices. The main reasons to perform uvula cutting mentioned by mothers were to prevent swelling, pus, and rapture of the uvula which can lead the child to death as mentioned by 515 (68.5%) mothers. Having no better medical cure and its ability to prevent sore throat were mentioned by 96 (12.8%) and 97 (12.9%) respondents, respectively. Out of the respondents who practice milk teeth extraction, 62 (8.2%) reason out to prevent diarrhea and vomiting, prevention of teething

TABLE 1: Sociodemographic characteristics of children less than five years old in Axum Town, North Ethiopia, 2013.

Variable	Frequency ($n = 742$)	Percent
Sex		
Male	371	49.3
Female	381	50.7
Age of child in months		
0–4	47	6.2
5–9	92	12.2
10–14	107	14.2
15–19	51	6.8
20–24	87	11.6
25–29	40	5.3
30–34	62	8.2
35+	266	35.4
Age of mothers		
15–19	6	0.8
20–24	115	15.3
25–29	222	29.5
30–34	168	22.3
35–39	159	21.1
40–44	71	9.4
45+	11	1.5
Religion		
Orthodox	611	81.2
Muslim	141	18.8
Occupation		
Jobless	588	78.2%
Civil servant	56	7.4
Merchant	98	13.0
Farmer	4	0.5
Others*	6	0.8
Ethnic group		
Tigraway	748	99.5
Amhara	4	0.5
Educational status		
Illiterate	100	13.3
Religious	17	2.3
Primary school	379	50.4
Secondary school	196	26.1
Higher education	60	8.0

*Others = local clothes makers, beauty salon workers, and local drinks makers.

problem as well as cure or prevention diseases were other reasons. All mothers who practice eyebrow incision, 18 (2.4%) explain only one reason to perform eyebrow incision which was to treat eye diseases (Table 3).

TABLE 2: Harmful traditional practices among children less than five years old in Axum Town, North Ethiopia, 2013.

Variable	Frequency (n)	Percent (%)
Information about HTPs		
Yes	746	99.2
No	6	0.8
Information by type of HTPs*		
Uvula cutting	588	78.2
Female genital mutilation (FGM)	493	65.5
Milk teeth extraction (MTE)	380	50.5
Eyebrow incision	362	48.1
Bloodletting	308	40.9
Source of information*		
Mass media	314	41.7
Health personnel	410	54.5
Family members	372	49.5
Meeting	127	16.9
Others**	4	0.5
Any HTPs performed on mother		
Yes	618	82.2
No	134	17.8
Type of HTPs performed on mother*		
Uvula cutting	599	79.6
Female genital mutilation	5	0.7
Milk teeth extraction	43	5.7
Eyebrow incision	116	15.4
Bloodletting	16	2.13
HTPs performed on children		
Yes	660	87.8
No	92	12.2
In how many children		
All children	209	27.8
Only one child	158	21.0
Two children	175	23.3
Three and above	118	15.7
Minor problems happened after HTPs were performed		
Yes	80	10.6
No	580	77.1
Which problems happened after HTPs were performed		
Bleeding	16	2.1
Swelling	8	1.1
Difficulty of swallowing	45	6.0
Wound or infection	11	1.5

*More than one answer was given; **others = school.

4. Discussion

The purpose of this study was to assess the magnitude of harmful traditional practices among children less than 5 years old in Axum Town, North Ethiopia. Almost all (99.2%) study participants had information about HTPs. This was higher

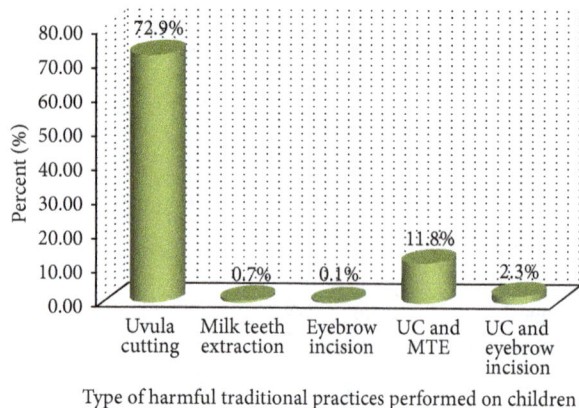

Type of harmful traditional practices performed on children

FIGURE 1: Types of harmful traditional practices among children less than 5 years in Axum Town, North Ethiopia, 2013.

TABLE 3: Reasons associated with harmful traditional practices among children less the 5 years old in Axum Town, North Ethiopia, 2013.

Variable	Frequency ($n = 742$)	Percent (%)
Reasons for performing uvula cutting*		
To prevent swelling, pus, and rupture of uvula	515	68.5
No better cure in modern medicine	96	12.8
To prevent sore throat	97	12.9
To prevent vomiting	2	0.3
Reasons for performing MTE*		
Prevents diarrhea and vomiting	62	8.2
Prevents problems of growth development	5	0.7
Root of teeth grows worms	21	2.8
MTE prevents or cures disease	9	1.2
Prevents teething problems	8	1.1
Reason for performing eyebrow incision		
Treatment of eye disease	18	2.4
Thinking if HTPs are harmful		
Yes	484	64.4
No	268	35.6
Which HTPs are harmful*		
FGM	472	62.7
Eye borrow incision	338	44.9
bloodletting	336	44.7
Milk teeth extraction	315	41.9
Uvula cutting	168	22.3

*More than one response was given.

than the study conducted in SNNPR which showed that a little higher number to half of the respondents (65.3%) had

information about HTPs [11]. About 78.2% of mothers had information about uvula cutting; this was higher than the follow-up survey conducted in 2008 by EGLDAM which was 73.5% nationally but almost inline in Tigray Region 79.8% [4]. This difference might be because of time gap; the study area as well as sample size was smaller than the survey.

This study showed that uvula cutting was practiced on 87% of children which was lower than a study conducted in Dembia district, Northwest Ethiopia, in which uvula cutting was practiced by 99.5% of respondents [1]. But this was higher than the follow-up survey conducted in 2008 by EGLDAM in Ethiopia in which the prevalence of uvula cutting was 66.4% in Tigray Region [4]. The variation might be because of time gap. The second common HTP in this study was milk teeth extraction which was performed on 12.5% of children but it was much lower than a study conducted in Dembia district, Northwest Ethiopia, in 2001 (95.6%) [1]. In addition to that it was also much lower than the follow-up survey conducted in 2008 by EGLDAM in Ethiopia that reported prevalence of milk teeth extraction as 26.6% [4]. This might be because awareness of families of milk teeth extraction has been improved but not for uvula cutting because of the easily accessible medical service. The third common HTP identified was eyebrow incision which was performed on 2.4% of children, but it was almost null as compared to the study conducted in Dembia district, Northwest Ethiopia (82%) [1]. It might be due to the fact that fear of HIV/AIDS transmission as well as awareness of mothers of modern medicine to treat eye infections or diseases has been improved. In this study there was no FGM practiced on children. This was in line with the study conducted in Dembia district, in which the practice of female circumcision was limited to only some areas and was supported by a small number of people. But, according to the study, in SNNPR prevalence of FGM was 33% [11]. In Tigray Region as well, the prevalence of FGM was 21.2% according to the follow-up survey conducted in 2008 by EGLDAM [4]. The difference might be because awareness of families of the complications of FGM was improved by health education by health personnel and mass media.

The reason for performing uvula cutting mentioned by most (68.5%) mothers was to prevent swelling, pus, and rupture of the uvula which can lead the child to death. This was much higher than the same reason (21.7%) reported in the follow-up survey conducted in Ethiopia by EGLDAM in 2008 [4]. But, contrary to this study, a study conducted in Nigeria in 2011 suggested that the majority of patients (65.5%) did not know the indication for uvula cutting being performed on them [12]. This variation might be due to difference of cultural diversity of the respondents. Out of the respondents who practice milk teeth extraction (12.5%) the reasons mentioned were to prevent diarrhea and vomiting (8.2%), to prevent teething problem (1.1%), and to cure or prevent diseases. This was in line with the reasons mentioned in the follow-up survey conducted in Ethiopia by EGLDAM in 2008 [4]. This study was also in line with study of HTPs in SNNPR, in 2005 [11]. In this study eyebrow incision was performed to treat eye disease as mentioned by all mothers who performed it. This was also similar to the reasons listed in the follow-up survey conducted in 2008 by EGLDAM [4].

5. Conclusion

In the study we tried to assess magnitude of harmful traditional practices among children less than five years old in Axum Town, North Ethiopia. Participants of this study were mothers who had children less than five years old. Based on this study the following was concluded.

(i) Almost all of the respondents had information about the commonly recognized HTPs which were uvula cutting, milk teeth extraction, FGM, and eyebrow incision; family members were the main source of information.

(ii) Majority of the mothers had uvula cutting, milk teeth extraction, and eyebrow incision performed on them.

(iii) The common HTPs performed on children in this study were uvula cutting, MTE, and eyebrow incision. Uvula cutting was practiced alone as well as together with MTE and eyebrow incision.

(iv) As mentioned by mothers the main reason of uvula cutting was to prevent swelling, pus, and rupture of the uvula which can lead the child to death.

(v) Prevention of diarrhea, vomiting, and teething problem was the reason described by mothers for performing milk teeth extraction.

Conflict of Interests

The authors declare that there is no conflict of interests regarding the publication of this paper.

Acknowledgments

The authors extend their appreciation to College of Health Sciences, Department of Nursing, Mekelle University, and Department of Nursing, Addis Ababa University. They want to thank also those who supported them from the beginning to the end of this paper.

References

[1] G. D. Alene and M. Edris, "Knowledge, attitudes and practices involved in harmful health behavior in Dembia district, Northwest Ethiopia," *Ethiopian Journal of Health Development*, vol. 16, no. 2, pp. 199–207, 2002.

[2] WHO Technical Report Series. Promotion and Development of Traditional Medicine. 622, 38:8: WHO, Geneva, Switzerland, 1978.

[3] Malawi Human Rights Commission. Cultural Practices and their Impact on the Enjoyment of Human Rights, Particularly the Rights of Women and Children in Malawi. Malawi, 2005.

[4] EGLDAM, Follow up National Survey on Harmful Traditional Practices in Ethiopia. Addis Ababa, Ethiopia, 2008.

[5] M. F. Zuberi, Assessment of violence against children in the eastern and southern Africa region, Results of initial desk review for the UN secretary general's study on violence against children, 2006.

[6] F. Worku and S. Gebresilassie, *Reproductive Health for Health Science Students*, Ethiopian Public Health Training Institute, University of Gondar, 2008.

[7] A. Dawit, W. Eshetu, G. Masresha, B. Misganaw, and M. Atsinaf, *Harmful Traditional Practices Module for Ethiopian Health Center Team*, Awassa College, Ethiopian Public Health Training Institute, 2004.

[8] J. M. Wojcicki, C. Kankasa, C. Mitchell, and C. Wood, "Traditional practices and exposure to bodily fluids in Lusaka, Zambia," *Tropical Medicine and International Health*, vol. 12, no. 1, pp. 150–155, 2007.

[9] E. Kupeli, I. Orhan, G. Toker, and E. Yesilada, "Anti-inflammatory and antinociceptive potential of Maclura pomifera (Rafin.) Schneider fruit extracts and its major isoflavonoids, scandenone and auriculasin," *Journal of Ethnopharmacology*, vol. 107, no. 2, pp. 169–174, 2006.

[10] ATEM Consultancy Service. Baseline Survey on the Most Prevalent HTP and Sanitation Practices among the Community of the Hamer, Dassenech, and Nyangatom Woredas of the South Omo Zone in the SNNPR. Addis Ababa, Ethiopia, 2011.

[11] Southern Nations, Nationalities and Peoples' Regional State, Bureau of Statistics and Population (BoSP). The Study of Harmful Traditional Practices (HTPs) on Demographic Structure and Socio-economic Development in the SNNPR, 2005.

[12] A. A. Adoga and T. L. Nimkur, The Traditionally Amputated Uvula amongst Nigerians: Still an Ongoing Practice. Clinical Study International Scholarly Research Network ISRN Otolaryngology, 2011.

18

Early Blood Gas Predictors of Bronchopulmonary Dysplasia in Extremely Low Gestational Age Newborns

Sudhir Sriram,[1] **Joy Condie,**[1] **Michael D. Schreiber,**[1] **Daniel G. Batton,**[2]
Bhavesh Shah,[3] **Carl Bose,**[4] **Matthew Laughon,**[4] **Linda J. Van Marter,**[5,6,7]
Elizabeth N. Allred,[8,9,10] **and Alan Leviton**[8,10]

[1] *Department of Pediatrics, University of Chicago, 5841 South Maryland Avenue MC 6060, Chicago, IL 60637, USA*
[2] *Department of Pediatrics, Southern Illinois School of Medicine, 301 North 8th Street, Springfield, IL 62794, USA*
[3] *Department of Pediatrics, Bay State Medical Center, 759 Chestnut Street, Springfield, MA 01199, USA*
[4] *Department of Pediatrics, University of North Carolina, 101 Manning Drive, Chapel Hill, NC 27599, USA*
[5] *Department of Pediatrics, Harvard Medical School, 220 Longwood Drive, Boston, MA 02115, USA*
[6] *Division of Newborn Medicine, Children's Hospital, 300 Longwood Avenue, Boston, MA 02115, USA*
[7] *Division of Newborn Medicine, Brigham and Women's Hospital, 75 Francis Street, Boston, MA 02115, USA*
[8] *Department of Neurology, Harvard Medical School, 220 Longwood Drive, Boston, MA 02115, USA*
[9] *Department of Biostatistics, Harvard School of Public Health, 655 Huntington Avenue, Boston, MA 02115, USA*
[10]*Department of Neurology, Children's Hospital, 300 Longwood Avenue, Boston, MA 02115, USA*

Correspondence should be addressed to Sudhir Sriram; ssriram@peds.bsd.uchicago.edu

Academic Editor: F. J. Kaskel

Aim. To determine among infants born before the 28th week of gestation to what extent blood gas abnormalities during the first three postnatal days provide information about the risk of bronchopulmonary dysplasia (BPD). *Methods.* We studied the association of extreme quartiles of blood gas measurements (hypoxemia, hyperoxemia, hypocapnea, and hypercapnea) in the first three postnatal days, with bronchopulmonary dysplasia, among 906 newborns, using multivariable models adjusting for potential confounders. We approximated NIH criteria by classifying severity of BPD on the basis of the receipt of any O_2 on postnatal day 28 and at 36 weeks PMA and assisted ventilation. *Results.* In models that did not adjust for ventilation, hypoxemia was associated with increased risk of severe BPD and very severe BPD, while infants who had hypercapnea were at increased risk of very severe BPD only. In contrast, infants who had hypocapnea were at reduced risk of severe BPD. Including ventilation for 14 or more days eliminated the associations with hypoxemia and with hypercapnea and made the decreased risk of very severe BPD statistically significant. *Conclusions.* Among ELGANs, recurrent/persistent blood gas abnormalities in the first three postnatal days convey information about the risk of severe and very severe BPD.

1. Introduction

Despite the improved survival of extremely low gestational age newborns (ELGANs) defined as infants born at <28 weeks' gestation, bronchopulmonary dysplasia (BPD) remains prevalent and an important healthcare burden to patients, their families, and society [1–4]. Identifying early, perhaps remediable, indicators of later pulmonary disorders has the potential to contribute to the reduction of the risk of these disorders.

Blood gas abnormalities and acid-base disturbances can occur as a result of lung immaturity that can be complicated by comorbidities, such as perinatal infection or pulmonary hypoplasia [5–10]. Likewise, medical management, including permissive hypercapnea, also can predispose, intentionally or unintentionally, to blood gas abnormalities [11–13].

In the presurfactant era, low PCO_2 levels were associated with increased risk, and high PCO_2 levels were associated with decreased risk of BPD [15–17]. In the postsurfactant era, BPD has been predicted by oxygen requirement, abnormal chest X-ray, and ventilator dependency at 4 days of age [18]. The relationship between early blood gas abnormalities and the development of BPD has not been well studied since the wide-spread acceptance of antenatal steroids, surfactant replacement therapy, and permissive hypercapnea.

The objective of the present study was to examine the relationship between blood gas abnormalities in the first three postnatal days and BPD risk.

2. Subjects and Methods

The ELGAN study was originally designed to detect structural and functional neurological abnormalities in infants born before 28 weeks of gestational age at 14 participating centers in the USA during the years 2002–2004 [19]. Approval was obtained from the institutional review board (IRB) at each participating institution. Consent was obtained from mothers, either antenatally or after delivery, based on the human research committee recommendations and/or individual clinical situation. Of 1506 infants enrolled, information on placental microbiology, blood gases, and BPD diagnosis was available for 906 infants.

The estimates of gestational age (GA) were based on availability of information to best determine the most accurate gestational age. The most accurate GA estimates were obtained from dates of embryo retrieval, intrauterine insemination, or by fetal ultrasound prior to 14 weeks (62%). The next reliable GA estimate was given to fetal ultrasound at greater than 14 weeks (29%), LMP (7%), and postnatal estimation of gestational age, as recorded in the neonatal intensive care unit log book (1%). The birth weight Z-score reflects the number of standard deviations the infant's birth weight is above or below the median weight of infants of the same gestational age in a standard data set [14].

We collected all the physiology, laboratory, and therapy data for the first 12 hours needed to calculate a score for neonatal acute physiology (SNAP-II) and a score for neonatal acute physiology perinatal extension (SNAPPE-II) [20].

We classified infants by the number of days they received mechanical ventilation (either high-frequency or conventional mechanical ventilation) from birth to 36 weeks' postmenstrual age (PMA). For the analyses presented here, we limited our analyses to the trichotomy of <7 days, 7–13 days, and 14 or more days of ventilation.

2.1. Blood Gas Collection and Classification. PO_2 and PCO_2 were measured almost routinely on the first three postnatal days and we collected the lowest, modal, and highest values on each day [21, 22]. The first postnatal day was defined as the first 24 hours after delivery plus the additional hours until midnight. Each successive day then began and ended at midnight [2]. The median number of blood gases obtained on each day declined rapidly from 8 on day 1 to 4 on day 3. With the exception of 7 ELGANs on day 1, 15 ELGANs on day 2, and 60 ELGANs on day 3 who had venous/capillary measurements, all other values were from arterial specimens.

ELGANs were classified by gestational age (23-24, 25-26, and 27 weeks) and blood specimens were classified by the

postnatal day they were obtained (1, 2, 3). Quartiles of PaO_2 and PCO_2 were calculated for each of 9 gestational age and postnatal day groups, separately for arterial and venous values (i.e., 18 groups), and blood gases of each infant were assigned to his/her quartile based on membership in one of these 18 groups. We considered an infant to be exposed to abnormal blood gas values, if she/he had a measurement in the lowest quartile and, separately, the highest quartile on at least two of three postnatal days. Values in the lowest or highest quartile on just one postnatal day were not considered an exposure.

Because we collected the minimum and maximum blood gas values each day, we cannot tell if the values of PCO_2 and/or PO_2 are from the same specimen. Since no protocol was established for sampling blood gases, all measurements were obtained at the discretion of the clinical team caring for each infant.

2.2. Modified Definitions of BPD. Because we did not collect information about percentage of oxygen delivered on postnatal day 28 or at 36 weeks PMA, we could not use NIH criteria for BPD [23, 24].

We approximated the NIH criteria as best as we could by replacing <30% and >30% with any oxygen. Thus, mild and moderate BPD are defined as a need for supplemental oxygen ≥28 days, but not at 36 weeks PMA, while severe BPD is defined as a need for supplemental oxygen at 36 weeks PMA, but not requiring ventilation assistance, and a classification of very severe BPD required a need for both supplemental oxygen and ventilation assistance at 36 weeks PMA.

2.3. Placenta. Delivered placentas were placed in a sterile exam basin and transported to a sampling room, where they were biopsied under sterile conditions. Eighty-two percent of the samples were obtained within 1 hour of delivery. The microbiologic and histologic procedures are described in detail elsewhere [25, 26]. Briefly, inflammation was defined as any of the following four lesions: (a) chorionic plate inflammation of grade 3 (neutrophils up to amnionic epithelium) and stage 3 (>20 neutrophils/20x), (b) external membrane inflammation of grade 3 (numerous large or confluent foci of neutrophils), (c) umbilical cord inflammation of grade 3 or higher (neutrophils in perivascular Wharton's jelly), and (d) neutrophilic infiltration into fetal stem vessels in the chorionic plate.

2.4. Statistical Analysis. We evaluated the hypothesis that ELGANs who have a blood gas value in an extreme quartile on at least 2 of the first 3 postnatal days are at increased risk for developing BPD. Four extremes in blood gases were considered: lowest and highest quartiles of PO_2 and PCO_2. Because only 80 of the 906 infants in our sample did not have any BPD by our minor modification of NIH criteria, having this group of infants serve as the referent group for multivariable analyses prominently limited statistical power. Consequently, we decided to group these infants who were not oxygen dependent on day 28 with those who were not dependent at 36 weeks PMA ($N = 314$) to form the referent group for all multivariable analyses of BPD risk.

TABLE 1: The values that define the lowest and highest quartiles of each blood gas on each day in each gestational age group.

Blood gas quartile →	Lowest PO_2 (mm Hg)			Highest PO_2 (mm Hg)		
Postnatal day →	1	2	3	1	2	3
Gestational age (wks) ↓						
23-24	39	43	44	152	98	104
25-26	42	45	45	145	100	95
27	40	44	46	142	92	96
Blood gas quartile →	Lowest PCO_2 (mm Hg)			Highest PCO_2 (mm Hg)		
Postnatal day →	1	2	3	1	2	3
Gestational age (wks) ↓						
23-24	27	33	34	65	68	63
25-26	29	35.5	35	60	64	60
27	29	35	36	58	57	56

We selected variables as confounders if in our data they were associated with both a blood gas extreme and with one of the pulmonary disorders with probabilities ≤0.25 [27]. After reviewing a broad range of potential confounders, we found that six variables were associated with both a blood gas extreme and severe or very severe BPD, including conception assistance, maternal fever during pregnancy, relative fetal growth restriction (defined as a birth weight more than one standard deviation below the expected median), recovery of *Mycoplasma* from the placenta, and illness severity indicators (SNAP-II and SNAPPE-II). The number of days ventilated was also associated with both blood gas disturbances and BPD, but we elected not to include this variable in the top part of Table 4 because it might have been an intervening variable between the blood gas abnormality and BPD. Rather, we added this potential confounder to the bottom part of Table 4. Comparison of the top to the bottom part of Table 4 allows an appreciation of how much the duration of ventilation variable might be an intervening variable between each blood gas disturbance and BPD.

All models included a hospital cluster term to account for the likelihood that infants born at one hospital are more alike and more likely to have received the same respiratory care than those born at another hospital [28]. The contributions of blood gas abnormalities to severity of BPD are given as odds ratios with 95% confidence intervals, controlling for potential confounders. In an effort to balance the risks of type 1 and type 2 errors, while evaluating only 4 highly related blood gas extremes, we chose to describe the precision of odds ratio estimates with 95% confidence intervals.

3. Results

Of the 1506 infants enrolled in the ELGAN Study, 1172 had blood gas assessments and 906 survived until 36 weeks PMA and had information about all variables in the multivariable models. Infants who did not have a blood gas measurement on all 3 of the first 3 postnatal days were less likely than others to have a high SNAPPE-II, lower mean arterial pressures, and to have had day-2 blood gas measurements that were in an extreme quartile. Fully 29% had a SNAPPE-II ≥45.

The values that define the lowest and highest quartiles of PO_2 and PCO_2 were fairly consistent for all gestational age groups on all 3 postnatal days (Table 1). By and large, gestational age groups differed minimally in the boundaries for what defines an extreme quartile of lowest and highest PO_2 and lowest and highest PCO_2 quartiles. Invariably, measurements that define an extreme quartile tended to be most extreme on day 1.

Infants who had an abnormal blood gas measurement on multiple days were more likely than others to have had a high SNAPPE-II (Table 2). Newborns who had recurrent/persistent hypoxemia were more likely than their peers to have required 14 or more days of ventilation assistance. Those who had hypercapnea were more likely than others to have developed very severe BPD and showed a predilection to be having a birth weight that was low for gestational age, to be born to a woman who had fever during the pregnancy, and to have required 14 or more days of ventilation assistance.

The univariable risk profiles of severe and very severe BPD are similar (Table 3). Both are characterized by a tendency to include an overrepresentation of newborns in the lowest gestational age category, those born to a woman who experienced fever during this pregnancy, those with a high SNAPPE-II, and very high rates of ventilation on 14 or more days.

In multivariable analyses, hypoxemia was associated with both severe and very severe BPD, while hypocapnea was associated with a reduced risk of BPD not accompanied by a need for assisted ventilation (Table 4, top set). Hypercapnea however was associated with ventilator-dependent BPD. Adding a variable for 14 or more days of ventilation prominently reduced or eliminated the associations with hypoxemia and hypercapnea (Table 4, bottom set). On the other hand, doing so did not influence the association between hypocapnea and severe BPD and allowed the association between hypocapnea and very severe BPD to become statistically significant.

4. Discussion

In the present study, the first of its kind in the surfactant era, recurring/persistent blood gas abnormalities during the

TABLE 2: The distribution of infants who had a blood gas extreme (defined as a P_aO_2 or PCO_2 in the highest or lowest quartile for gestational age on at least two of the first three postnatal days) listed at the top of each column within strata of potential confounders, listed on the left. These are column percents.

Potential confounder	Blood gas extreme								Row
	Lowest P_aO_2		Highest P_aO_2		Lowest PCO_2		Highest PCO_2		
	Yes	No	Yes	No	Yes	No	Yes	No	N
Gestational age (weeks)									
23-24	23	25	24	25	25	24	26	24	223
25-26	47	46	44	47	46	46	44	47	418
27	30	29	32	29	28	30	30	29	265
Birth weight Z-score <-1[§]									
Yes	25	20	25	20	23	20	30	18	59
Maternal fever[†]									
Yes	8	6	7	6	7	7	10	5	209
Placenta *Mycoplasma*									
Yes	9	10	10	10	14	9	7	11	109
SNAPPE-II ≥ 45									
Yes	33	28	37	28	34	28	47	24	263
Days ventilated									
<7	14	22	19	21	21	20	6	25	186
7–13	9	11	8	11	9	10	10	10	92
14+	77	67	74	68	69	69	84	65	628
BPD									
None	9	9	8	9	9	9	7	9	80
Mild/moderate	30	36	33	35	42	32	25	37	314
Severe	47	45	48	45	39	48	50	44	474
Very severe	14	10	11	11	9	11	17	9	98
Maximum column N	195	711	189	717	201	705	197	709	906

[§]Birth weight Z-scores based on Yudkin et al. [14] standard.

[†]Maternal temperature >100.4°F during pregnancy.

first three postnatal days convey information about the risk of severe and very severe BPD in ELGANs above and beyond the information conveyed by indicators of prematurity and risk of dying. The finding that some of the risk information is diminished when intervening ventilation is considered suggests that some of the blood gas disturbances are indicative of the need for ventilation, which in turn contributes to such late respiratory disorders as BPD.

In the ELGAN study sample, blood gas abnormalities on two of the first three postnatal days were associated with sustained or recurrent systemic inflammation in the week and a half that followed [22]. In addition, "prolonged" ventilation, defined as ventilation on 14 or more days between birth and 36 weeks PMA, was also associated with sustained or recurrent early systemic inflammation [29] and early sustained or recurrent systemic inflammation was associated with heightened BPD risk [30]. Consequently, we hypothesized that the blood gas derangements that predicted BPD probably contributed to BPD via an increased likelihood of "prolonged" ventilation, which, in turn, might promote inflammation [29]. The differences seen between the two sets of Table 4, which reflect addition of only the ventilation variable to multivariable models of BPD risks, indicate that

ventilation is likely to be an intermediary between the blood gas derangements and the BPD.

In a previous study, components of SNAP-II contributed to the prediction of the need for CPAP and/or ventilator assistance 72 hours after birth among newborns whose gestational age was ≥ 34 weeks [31]. Thus, we consider the SNAPPE-II worthy of inclusion among variables adjusting for endogenous risk of BPD in ELGANs.

A previous study found an association between early hypercapnea and BPD [32], while another found an association between hypercapnea and BPD but only among the premature infants whose clinical course complicated by PDA [4]. We, too, found that hypercapnea was associated with very severe BPD, but not with severe BPD. The association with very severe BPD was diminished and lost its statistical significance when we added a variable for duration of ventilation. These findings are compatible with the view that the association of hypercapnea with very severe BPD reflects phenomena associated with prolonged ventilation, perhaps more than early gas adjustments.

The apparent protective effect of hypocapnea against BPD in the present study is in contrast to a report from the early surfactant era that hypocapnea before surfactant therapy was

TABLE 3: The distribution of infants who had the form of bronchopulmonary dysplasia listed at the top of each column within strata of potential confounders, listed on the left. These are column percents.

Potential confounder	None	Bronchopulmonary dysplasia Mild/moderate O_2 at 28 weeks	Severe O_2 – no vent at 36 weeks	Very severe O_2 + vent at 36 weeks	Row N
Gestational age (weeks)					
23-24	0	17	33	34	223
25-26	30	50	45	52	418
27	70	33	22	14	265
Maternal fever[†]					
Yes	10	11	25	41	59
Birth weight Z-score <-1[§]					
Yes	6	6	6	7	209
Placenta *Mycoplasma*					
Yes	10	12	10	5	109
SNAPPE-II ≥ 45					
Yes	6	20	36	49	263
Days ventilated					
<7	66	32	8	0	186
7–13	20	16	6	2	92
14	14	52	86	98	628
P_aO_2 quartile on ≥ 2 days					
Lowest	23	18	22	29	195
Highest	19	20	22	21	189
PCO_2 quartile on ≥ 2 days					
Lowest	23	27	19	19	201
Highest	18	16	24	35	197
Maximum column N	80	314	414	98	906

[§]Birth weight Z-scores based on Yudkin et al. [14] standard.

[†]Maternal temperature >100.4°F during pregnancy.

associated with an increased risk of BPD [15]. It is unclear how hypocapnea might protect against BPD.

We are reluctant to infer that exposure to the observed blood gas extremes contributed to BPD. Rather, we consider it highly probable that the blood gas extremes are the first indicators of the severity of the respiratory dysfunction that will result in severe and very severe BPD. Nevertheless, we are not yet prepared to dismiss the possibility that improved care to minimize the occurrence of some of the blood gas abnormalities might reduce the occurrence of severe BPD.

We minimized confounding by indication. To avoid attributing to hypocarbia what might more appropriately be attributed to its antecedents, one group of investigators created a hypocarbia propensity score when evaluating the presumed consequences of hypocarbia [33].

Among the variables that comprised the propensity score were low gestational age <26 weeks, low birth-weight Z-score, and ventilation. We included these in multivariable models of BPD risk. Other propensity score components, including labor, membrane rupture, maternal leukocytosis, and antenatal antibiotic treatment, are closely related to other variables we adjusted for (e.g., maternal fever during pregnancy and recovery of *Mycoplasma* from the placenta). Similarly, such hypocarbia propensity score components such as systemic hypotension on day 1, neonatal leukopenia

on day 1, and administration of volume expanders and/or vasopressors on day 1, are closely related to high values of SNAPPE-II. Consequently, to a considerable extent we have approximated the hypocarbia-propensity score used previously. We acknowledge that our efforts might not have achieved the goal we set for our multivariable analyses.

Compared to infants exposed to pressure-limited ventilation equipment, those treated with volume-targeted ventilation have lower rates of hypocarbia, and the combined outcome of BPD/death [34, 35]. These types of findings appear to be contributing to a replacement of pressure-limited ventilation equipment with volume-targeted equipment. Such changes in ventilation might contribute to a reduced occurrence of BPD [36].

Our study is not without limitations. Our findings are based on *post hoc* analyses of data collected for a study of indicators of brain damage in ELGANs [19]. The boundaries for blood gas extremes were pooled values available for all ELGANs involved in this study who happened to have a wide range of respiratory illness severity. In addition, our definition of hypoxemia is not severe at all. Children, who died of their severe respiratory dysfunction before a BPD diagnosis could be made, are not included in the analyses. We did not have any specific index to evaluate the association between subsequent BPD and volutrauma/barotrauma. As

TABLE 4: Odds ratios (and 95% confidence intervals)§ of the association between blood gas abnormalities (defined as the extreme quartile for gestational age on at least two of the first three days) and BPD. The referent group consists of all infants who did not have severe or very severe BPD. The sets of tables differ in the inclusion/exclusion of one variable in the multivariable models. In the top set, days of ventilation during the NICU stay (<7, 7–13, ≥14) are not included in the model, while this variable is included in the bottom set.

(a) Without a variable for days of ventilation during the first 2 weeks (<7, 7–13, and ≥14)

BPD	Blood gas abnormalities			
	Low PO$_2$	High PO$_2$	Low PCO$_2$	High PCO$_2$
Severe	1.5 (1.02, 2.3)	0.9 (0.6, 1.4)	*0.6 (0.4, 0.96)*	1.3 (0.9, 2.0)
Very severe	2.5 (1.3, 5.0)	0.7 (0.3, 1.5)	0.5 (0.3, 1.03)	2.5 (1.2, 5.0)

(b) With a variable for days of ventilation during the first 2 weeks (<7, 7–13, ≥14)

BPD	Blood gas abnormalities			
	Low PO$_2$	High PO$_2$	Low PCO$_2$	High PCO$_2$
Severe	1.2 (0.8, 1.9)	0.9 (0.6, 1.5)	*0.6 (0.4, 0.96)*	0.9 (0.6, 1.5)
Very severe	1.7 (0.8, 3.5)	0.8 (0.3, 1.8)	*0.4 (0.2, 0.9)*	1.9 (0.9, 4.2)

§All models are adjusted for conception assistance, maternal fever during pregnancy, birth weight Z-score <−1, recovery of a *Mycoplasma* from the placenta, and SNAPPE ≥45. These models also include a hospital group/cluster term to account for the possibility that infants born at a particular hospital are more like each other than infants born at other hospitals.

with all observational studies, we are unable to distinguish between causation and association as explanations for what we found. Finally, even though we included SNAPPE-II scores in our multivariate regression models, we cannot completely rule out that the sickest infants were more likely to be treated aggressively than others who were not quite so sick, making our study prone to confounding by indication [37, 38].

Our study has several strengths. First, we included a large number of infants, making it unlikely that we missed important associations due to lack of statistical power, or claimed associations that might have reflected the instability of small numbers. Second, we selected infants based on gestational age, not birth weight, in order to minimize confounding due to factors related to fetal growth restriction [39]. This is especially important in light of the increased risk of BPD among infants in the ELGAN study who were born with severe growth restriction [30]. Third, we collected all of our data prospectively.

In conclusion, blood gas abnormalities in the first three postnatal days were associated with BPD, but adding a variable for duration of ventilation to the multivariable model left only hypocapnea associated with BPD. One reasonable implication of these findings is that hypoxemia and hypercapnea are probably not in the causal chain leading to BPD.

Rather, they are likely indicators of the need for ventilation, which is more likely to contribute to BPD risk.

Another implication of our findings is that hypocapnea is also probably not in the causal chain. Future studies are recommended to identify why hypocapnea conveys information about the reduced risk of BPD.

Conflict of Interests

All the authors stated that there is no conflict of interests regarding the publication of this paper.

Acknowledgments

This study was supported by The National Institute of Neurological Disorders and Stroke (NINDS; 5U01NS040069) and the National Institute of Child Health and Human Development (5P30HD018655-28).The authors wish to acknowledge their ELGAN study colleagues: Olaf Dammann, Tufts Medical Center, Boston, MA; Camilia Martin, Beth Israel Deaconess Medical Center, Boston, MA; Robert Insoft, Brigham & Women's Hospital, Boston, MA; Karl Kuban, Boston Medical Center, Boston, MA; Francis Bednarek (deceased), U Mass Memorial Health Center, Worcester, MA; John Fiascone, Tufts Medical Center, Boston, MA; Richard A. Ehrenkranz, Yale University School of Medicine, New Haven, CT; T. Michael O'Shea, Wake Forest University/Baptist Medical Center, Winston-Salem, NC; Stephen C. Engelke, University Health Systems of Eastern Carolina, Greenville, NC; Mariel Poortenga, Ed Beaumont, DeVos Children's Hospital, Grand Rapids, MI; Nigel Paneth, Sparrow Hospital, Lansing, MI; Greg Pavlov, Frontier Science and Technology Research Foundation, Amherst, NY, and our project officer, Deborah Hirtz.

References

[1] A. A. Fanaroff, M. Hack, and M. C. Walsh, "The NICHD neonatal research network: changes in practice and outcomes during the first 15 years," *Seminars in Perinatology*, vol. 27, no. 4, pp. 281–287, 2003.

[2] M. Laughon, E. N. Allred, C. Bose et al., "Patterns of respiratory disease during the first 2 postnatal weeks in extremely premature infants," *Pediatrics*, vol. 123, no. 4, pp. 1124–1131, 2009.

[3] M. C. Walsh, S. Szefler, J. Davis et al., "Summary proceedings from the bronchopulmonary dysplasia group," *Pediatrics*, vol. 117, no. 3, pp. S52–S56, 2006.

[4] D. D. Marshall, M. Kotelchuck, T. E. Young, C. L. Bose, P. A.-C. Lauree Kruyer, and T. M. O'Shea, "Risk factors for chronic lung disease in the surfactant era: a North Carolina population-based study of very low birth weight infants," *Pediatrics*, vol. 104, no. 6, pp. 1345–1350, 1999.

[5] R. Harding, M. L. Tester, T. J. Moss et al., "Effects of intra-uterine growth restriction on the control of breathing and lung development after birth," *Clinical and Experimental Pharmacology and Physiology*, vol. 27, no. 1-2, pp. 114–119, 2000.

[6] J. M. Abu-Shaweesh, "Maturation of respiratory reflex responses in the fetus and neonate," *Seminars in Neonatology*, vol. 9, no. 3, pp. 169–180, 2004.

[7] V. Polimeni, N. Claure, C. D'Ugard, and E. Bancalari, "Effects of volume-targeted synchronized intermittent mandatory ventilation on spontaneous episodes of hypoxemia in preterm infants," *Biology of the Neonate*, vol. 89, no. 1, pp. 50–55, 2006.

[8] C. Esquer, N. Claure, C. D'Ugard, Y. Wada, and E. Bancalari, "Mechanisms of hypoxemia episodes in spontaneously breathing preterm infants after mechanical ventilation," *Neonatology*, vol. 94, no. 2, pp. 100–104, 2008.

[9] S. Orgeig, T. A. Crittenden, C. Marchant, I. C. McMillen, and J. L. Morrison, "Intrauterine growth restriction delays surfactant protein maturation in the sheep fetus," *American Journal of Physiology: Lung Cellular and Molecular Physiology*, vol. 298, no. 4, pp. L575–L583, 2010.

[10] K. S. Sobotka, S. B. Hooper, B. J. Allison et al., "An initial sustained inflation improves the respiratory and cardiovascular transition at birth in preterm lambs," *Pediatric Research*, vol. 70, no. 1, pp. 56–60, 2011.

[11] W. A. Carlo, A. R. Stark, L. L. Wright et al., "Minimal ventilation to prevent bronchopulmonary dysplasia in extremely-low-birth-weight infants," *The Journal of Pediatrics*, vol. 141, no. 3, pp. 370–375, 2002.

[12] J. D. Miller and W. A. Carlo, "Safety and effectiveness of permissive hypercapnia in the preterm infant," *Current Opinion in Pediatrics*, vol. 19, no. 2, pp. 142–144, 2007.

[13] J. Kamper, N. Feilberg Jørgensen, F. Jonsbo et al., "The Danish national study in infants with extremely low gestational age and birthweight (the ETFOL study): respiratory morbidity and outcome," *Acta Paediatrica*, vol. 93, no. 2, pp. 225–232, 2004.

[14] P. L. Yudkin, M. Aboualfa, and J. A. Eyre, "New birthweight and head circumference centiles for gestational ages 24 to 42 weeks," *Early Human Development*, vol. 15, no. 1, pp. 45–52, 1987.

[15] J. S. Garland, R. K. Buck, E. N. Allred, and A. Leviton, "Hypocarbia before surfactant therapy appears to increase bronchopulmonary dysplasia risk in infants with respiratory distress syndrome," *Archives of Pediatrics & Adolescent Medicine*, vol. 149, no. 6, pp. 617–615, 1995.

[16] M. E. Avery, W. H. Tooley, and J. B. Keller, "Is chronic lung disease in low birth weight infants preventable? A survey of eight centers," *Pediatrics*, vol. 79, no. 1, pp. 26–30, 1987.

[17] E. N. Kraybill, D. K. Runyan, C. L. Bose, and J. H. Khan, "Risk factors for chronic lung disease in infants with birth weights of 751 to 1000 grams," *The Journal of Pediatrics*, vol. 115, no. 1, pp. 115–120, 1989.

[18] S. W. Ryan, J. Nycyk, and B. N. Shaw, "Prediction of chronic neonatal lung disease on day 4 of life," *European Journal of Pediatrics*, vol. 155, no. 8, pp. 668–671, 1996.

[19] T. M. O'Shea, E. N. Allred, O. Dammann et al., "The ELGAN study of the brain and related disorders in extremely low gestational age newborns," *Early Human Development*, vol. 85, no. 11, pp. 719–725, 2009.

[20] D. K. Richardson, J. D. Corcoran, G. J. Escobar, and S. K. Lee, "SNAP-II and SNAPPE-II: simplified newborn illness severity and mortality risk scores," *The Journal of Pediatrics*, vol. 138, no. 1, pp. 92–100, 2001.

[21] A. Leviton, E. Allred, K. C. K. Kuban et al., "Early blood gas abnormalities and the preterm brain," *American Journal of Epidemiology*, vol. 172, no. 8, pp. 907–916, 2010.

[22] A. Leviton, E. N. Allred, K. C. K. Kuban et al., "Blood protein concentrations in the first two postnatal weeks associated with early postnatal blood gas derangements among infants born before the 28th week of gestation. The ELGAN study," *Cytokine*, vol. 56, no. 2, pp. 392–398, 2011.

[23] A. H. Jobe and E. Bancalari, "Bronchopulmonary dysplasia," *American Journal of Respiratory and Critical Care Medicine*, vol. 163, no. 7, pp. 1723–1729, 2001.

[24] R. A. Ehrenkranz, M. C. Walsh, B. R. Vohr et al., "Validation of the National Institutes of Health consensus definition of bronchopulmonary dysplasia," *Pediatrics*, vol. 116, no. 6, pp. 1353–1360, 2005.

[25] A. B. Onderdonk, J. L. Hecht, T. F. McElrath, M. L. Delaney, E. N. Allred, and A. Leviton, "Colonization of second-trimester placenta parenchyma," *American Journal of Obstetrics and Gynecology*, vol. 199, no. 1, pp. 52.e1–52.e10, 2008.

[26] J. L. Hecht, A. Onderdonk, M. Delaney et al., "Characterization of chorioamnionitis in 2nd-trimester C-section placentas and correlation with microorganism recovery from subamniotic tissues," *Pediatric and Developmental Pathology*, vol. 11, no. 1, pp. 15–22, 2008.

[27] L. G. Dales and H. K. Ury, "An improper use of statistical significance testing in studying covariables," *International Journal of Epidemiology*, vol. 7, no. 4, pp. 373–375, 1978.

[28] M. D. Begg and M. K. Parides, "Separation of individual-level and cluster-level covariate effects in regression analysis of correlated data," *Statistics in Medicine*, vol. 22, no. 16, pp. 2591–2602, 2003.

[29] C. L. Bose, M. M. Laughon, E. N. Allred et al., "Systemic inflammation associated with mechanical ventilation among extremely preterm infants," *Cytokine*, vol. 61, pp. 315–322, 2013.

[30] C. Bose, M. Laughon, E. N. Allred et al., "Blood protein concentrations in the first two postnatal weeks that predict bronchopulmonary dysplasia among infants born before the 28th week of gestation," *Pediatric Research*, vol. 69, no. 4, pp. 347–353, 2011.

[31] G. J. Escobar, S. M. Shaheen, E. M. Breed et al., "Richardson score predicts short-term adverse respiratory outcomes in newborns ≥34 weeks gestation," *The Journal of Pediatrics*, vol. 145, no. 6, pp. 754–760, 2004.

[32] L. J. van Marter, E. N. Allred, M. Pagano et al., "Do clinical markers of barotrauma and oxygen toxicity explain interhospital variation in rates of chronic lung disease?" *Pediatrics*, vol. 105, no. 6, pp. 1194–1201, 2000.

[33] O. Dammann, E. N. Allred, K. C. K. Kuban et al., "Hypocarbia during the first 24 postnatal hours and white matter echolucencies in newborns or = 28 weeks gestation," *Pediatric Research*, vol. 49, no. 3, pp. 388–393, 2001.

[34] K. Wheeler, C. Klingenberg, N. McCallion, C. J. Morley, and P. G. Davis, "Volume-targeted versus pressure-limited ventilation in the neonate," *Cochrane Database of Systematic Reviews*, no. 11, Article ID CD003666, 2010.

[35] K. I. Wheeler, C. Klingenberg, C. J. Morley, and P. G. Davis, "Volume-targeted versus pressure-limited ventilation for preterm infants: a systematic review and meta-analysis," *Neonatology*, vol. 100, no. 3, pp. 219–227, 2011.

[36] W. Peng, H. Zhu, H. Shi, and E. Liu, "Volume-targeted ventilation is more suitable than pressure-limited ventilation for preterm infants: a systematic review and meta-analysis," *Archives of Disease in Childhood Fetal and Neonatal Edition*, vol. 99, pp. F158–F165, 2014.

[37] A. M. Walker, "Confounding by indication," *Epidemiology*, vol. 7, pp. 335–336, 1996.

[38] L. B. Signorello, J. K. McLaughlin, L. Lipworth, S. Friis, H. T. Sørensen, and W. J. Blot, "Confounding by indication in epidemiologic studies of commonly used analgesics," *American Journal of Therapeutics*, vol. 9, no. 3, pp. 199–205, 2002.

[39] C. C. Arnold, M. S. Kramer, C. A. Hobbs, F. H. McLean, and R. H. Usher, "Very low birth weight: a problematic cohort for epidemiologic studies of very small or immature neonates," *American Journal of Epidemiology*, vol. 134, no. 6, pp. 604–613, 1991.

19

Fall in Vitamin D Levels during Hospitalization in Children

Devi Dayal,[1] **Suresh Kumar,**[1] **Naresh Sachdeva,**[2] **Rakesh Kumar,**[1]
Meenu Singh,[1] **and Sunit Singhi**[1]

[1] *Department of Pediatrics, Postgraduate Institute of Medical Education and Research, Chandigarh 160012, India*
[2] *Department of Endocrinology, Postgraduate Institute of Medical Education and Research, Chandigarh 160012, India*

Correspondence should be addressed to Meenu Singh; meenusingh4@gmail.com

Academic Editor: F. J. Kaskel

Plasma levels of 25-hydroxyvitamin D [25(OH)D] were measured by competitive Electrochemiluminescence Immunoassay (ECLIA) in 92 children (67 boys, 25 girls) aged 3 months to 12 years at admission to hospital (timepoint 1, T1) and at discharge (timepoint 2, T2). There was a significant fall in the mean 25(OH)D from T1 (71.87 ± 27.25 nmol/L) to T2 (49.03 ± 22.25 nmol/L) (mean change = 22.84 nmol/L, P value = 0.0004). Proportion of patients having VDD (levels <50 nmol/L) at admission (25%, 23/92) increased significantly at the time of discharge (51.09%, 47/92) ($P = 0.0004$). There was a trend towards longer duration of hospital stay, requirement of ventilation and inotropes, development of healthcare-associated infection, and mortality in vitamin D deficient as compared to nondeficient patients though the difference was statistically insignificant. In conclusion, vitamin D levels fall significantly and should be monitored during hospital stay in children. Large clinical studies are needed to prospectively evaluate the effect of vitamin D supplementation in vitamin D deficient hospitalized children on various disease outcome parameters.

1. Introduction

Hospitalized children are prone to vitamin D deficiency (VDD) or exacerbate their existing deficiency due to multitude of reasons; many have VDD at the time of hospitalization due to widespread VDD, no additional vitamin D source due to poor oral intake and any sun exposure, and lack of practice of supplementation during hospitalization. Vitamin D has several skeletal as well as extraskeletal functions that include immunomodulation and cardioprotection as well as improvement of antimicrobial action, all of which may affect the outcomes in hospitalized patients [1, 2]. Several recent studies in adults suggest that VDD is associated with longer hospital stay and increases in morbidity and mortality [3–5]. A few intervention trials suggest some beneficial effect of vitamin D supplementation on outcomes in hospitalized vitamin D deficient patients although definite evidence is lacking [6, 7]. These studies have predominantly been conducted on patients admitted to intensive care units (ICUs). A few studies in pediatric population have shown similar results underlining the importance of estimating vitamin D levels in children with critical illness [8, 9]. All these

studies have correlated the initial vitamin D levels with disease parameters. There is little information available on the change in vitamin D levels during hospitalization in children although one previous study done on adults indicates a significant fall in levels [10]. We thus planned to study the prevalence of VDD in children at the time of admission and the change in levels after a variable period of stay in a general pediatrics unit of our hospital.

2. Material and Methods

2.1. Subjects and Protocols. Children aged 3 months–12 years admitted to a General Pediatrics unit of a tertiary care hospital in North India were prospectively enrolled over a period of 4 months (July–October, 2012). Children with renal and liver disorders and malabsorption syndromes, those receiving multivitamins or calcium supplements and antiepileptic drugs, and those hospitalized for <7 days were excluded. The Ethics Committee of the Institute approved the study. Informed written consent from the parents/caretakers was obtained and assent of the child was taken wherever possible before recruitment into the study.

Demographic data, medical history, anthropometric measurements, and detailed physical examination were recorded at admission. Clinical signs suggestive of VDD if present and risk factors for VDD were also noted. Blood samples were taken for analyses of 25-hydroxyvitamin D [25(OH)D], calcium, phosphorus, and alkaline phosphatase at admission (timepoint 1, T1) and at discharge from hospital (timepoint 2, T2). In patients who died, their most recent stored sample was used to assess 25(OH)D and other biochemical parameters. Patients were followed up till discharge from hospital or death.

2.2. Laboratory Methods. Blood samples for 25(OH)D measurement were collected in heparinized amber colored glass vials to prevent its photodegradation. Plasma was extracted after centrifugation and stored at −20°C until analyzed. Plasma total 25-OHD measurement was done by competitive Electrochemiluminescence Immunoassay (ECLIA) (E-2010, Roche Diagnostics, Germany) using kits, calibrators, and controls from the same manufacturer. The detection limit of the method used is 3.75 nmol/L (1.5 ng/mL).

2.3. Definition of Vitamin D Deficiency and Insufficiency. Depending on their 25(OH)D level, patients were classified into 3 categories [11, 12]:

(1) vitamin D deficiency: 25(OH)D level <50 nmol/L (<20 ng/mL);

(2) vitamin D insufficiency: 25(OH)D levels 50–75 nmol/L (20–30 ng/mL);

(3) vitamin D sufficiency: 25(OH)D levels >75 nmol/L (>30 ng/mL).

2.4. Outcomes. Primary outcome was the prevalence of VDD at timepoints 1 and 2 and secondary outcomes were relationship of 25(OH)D with clinically important outcomes including duration of stay in hospital, requirement of ventilation (invasive or noninvasive methods to assist or replace spontaneous breathing, e.g., continuous positive airway pressure, manual ventilation, and mechanical ventilation), requirement of inotropes (agents used to augment cardiac contractility, e.g., dopamine, dobutamine, adrenaline, nor-adrenaline, and milrinone), incidence of nosocomial infection (any infection that a patient acquired within the hospital setting that was not present at the time of admission), and death.

3. Data Analysis

Appropriate data entry and statistical analysis were performed on Microsoft Excel 2007 (Microsoft, Redmond, WA) and SPSS software version 15 (SPSS, Inc, Chicago, IL). Demographic variables were tested with chi-square test and reported as mean, SD, range, and percentages, as applicable. Dichotomous outcomes were compared by chi-square test or Fisher's exact test, as applicable. Continuous variables were compared by Student's *t*-test. Association of vitamin D level with patient characteristics and outcome variables

was measured by using chi-square test and Fisher's tests for categorical variables and *t*-tests, Wilcoxon rank sum, Mann-Whitney, or Kruskal-Wallis tests for continuous variables, where appropriate. The regression of T1 and T2 on hospital duration was also calculated. All tests were two-tailed and $P < 0.05$ was taken as significant.

4. Results

4.1. Clinical Characteristics of Study Population. Over the study period, 146 patients were admitted to the unit; out of these 92 patients were enrolled. Reasons for nonenrollment included refusal of consent ($n = 8$), age <3 months ($n = 9$), renal disorder ($n = 6$), liver disorder ($n = 4$), malabsorption syndrome ($n = 3$), on calcium and vitamin D supplements ($n = 4$), on antiepileptic drugs ($n = 3$), and duration of stay <7 days ($n = 17$). Their clinicodemographic characteristics and final outcomes are shown in Table 1.

4.2. Prevalence of Vitamin D Deficiency and Insufficiency. There were a significant increase from T1 to T2 in the percentage of 25(OH)D deficient patients (25% versus 51.09%, $P = 0.0004$) and a decrease in 25(OH)D sufficient patients (30.43% versus 15.22%, $P = 0.02$) (Table 2). Similarly the fall in the mean levels of 25(OH)D from T1 to T2 (71.87 ± 27.25 versus 49.03 ± 22.25 nmol/L, mean change = 22.84 nmol/L, P value = 0.0004) was statistically significant (Table 3).

4.3. Distribution of Serum 25(OH)D, Calcium, Phosphorus, and Alkaline Phosphatase. Total calcium and phosphorus levels were also significantly lower at T2, whereas alkaline phosphatase levels were similar at the 2 timepoints (Table 3).

The mean levels of 25(OH)D at timepoint 1 and timepoint 2 were lower in cases who required ventilation, received inotropes, developed nosocomial sepsis, and those who died though the difference was not statistically different (Table 4). Similarly when the comorbidities were pooled, the levels of 25(OH)D at the 2 timepoints were lower in patients with either of these comorbidities as compared to those without any comorbidity but the differences were statistically insignificant (66.37 ± 24.67 nmol/L versus 72.90 ± 28.95 nmol/L, $P = 0.71$ and 47.55 ± 22.95 nmol/L versus 49.52 ± 22.27 nmol/L, $P = 0.48$, resp.).

Vitamin D deficiency at timepoint 1 was more likely to be associated with failure to thrive ($P = 0.03$), short stature ($P = 0.025$), exclusive breastfeeding ($P = 0.03$), inadequate sun exposure ($P = 0.02$), calcium levels ($P = 0.009$), and alkaline phosphatase levels ($P = 0.008$) (Table 5). However, multivariate analysis did not show an independent association of any of these factors with VDD at timepoint 1. On linear regression, 25(OH)D levels at timepoints 1 and 2 were inversely correlated with duration of hospital stay (in days) though statistically insignificant ($r^2 = 0.011$, $P = 0.31$ and $r^2 = 0.012$, $P = 0.30$, resp.). Vitamin D deficient patients were supplemented with adequate doses of vitamin D and calcium at the time of discharge. Of the 6 patients who died during the study period, the underlying diagnoses were tubercular meningitis in 2, acute viral meningoencephalitis

TABLE 1: Clinicodemographic characteristics and final outcomes of patients.

Characteristics	Total patients, $n = 92$
Mean age (years) (range, ±SD)	5.27 (0.3–12, 4.32)
Sex (male : female)	67 : 25
Weight (kgs), mean (range, ±SD)	15.45 (3–48, 9.9)
Height (cms), mean, (range, ±SD)	99.55 (52–156, 30.57)
Failure to thrive, n (%)	12 (13.04)
Short stature, n (%)	9 (9.78)
Diagnosis	
CNS infections, n (%)	16 (17.39)
Sepsis, n (%)	15 (16.3)
Pneumonia, n (%)	14 (15.22)
Cardiac disease, n (%)	13 (14.13)
Diabetes mellitus/diabetic ketoacidosis	9 (9.78)
Malaria, n (%)	5 (5.43)
DSS, n (%)	3 (3.26)
Other, n (%)	17 (18.48)
Signs of rickets	8 (8.69)
Rachitic rosary, n (%)	6 (6.52)
Frontal bossing, n (%)	6 (6.52)
Harrison sulcus, n (%)	5 (5.43)
Wrist widening, n (%)	5 (5.43)
Wide anterior fontanelle, n (%)	4 (4.35)
Double malleolus, n (%)	3 (3.26)
Craniotabes, n (%)	2 (2.17)
Bowing of legs, n (%)	2 (2.17)
Risk factors for vitamin D deficiency	
Family size, mean (range, ±2SD)	4.4 (3–8, 1.1)
Birth order, mean (range, ±2SD)	2.02 (1–6, 1.0)
Exclusive breast feeding, n (%)	51 (55.43)
Sun exposure, n (%)	47 (51.1)
Dark skin color, n (%)	7 (7.61)
Final outcomes	
Duration of stay in hospital (in days), mean (range, ±SD)	13.87 (8–23, 3.52)
Required ventilation, n (%)	21 (22.83)
Required inotropes, n (%)	15 (16.30)
Nosocomial sepsis, n (%)	9 (9.78)
Died, n (%)	6 (6.52)

TABLE 2: Distribution of patients in four categories according to 25(OH)D levels at timepoint 1 and timepoint 2.

25(OH)D levels (nmol/L)	Timepoint 1	Timepoint 2	P value
<50, n (%)	23 (25)	47 (51.09)	0.0004
50–75, n (%)	41 (44.56)	31 (33.69)	0.173
<75, n (%)	64 (69.57)	78 (84.78)	0.02
>75, n (%)	28 (30.43)	14 (15.22)	0.02

in 1, diabetic ketoacidosis with disseminated fungal infection in 1, disseminated staphylococcal disease in 1 and pneumonia with nosocomial infection in 1.

5. Discussion

The data on prevalence of VDD obtained in this study is similar to the data in control subjects of a previously conducted study by us on vitamin D levels in type 1 diabetes patients [13]. The present study demonstrated a significant change in vitamin D status during hospitalization. The mean 25(OH)D levels fell by almost one-third and the proportion of vitamin D deficient patients doubled over a hospital duration of approximately 2 weeks. This fall in 25(OH)D levels may be related to factors that operate in a hospitalized child. Vitamin D deficiency is common in India as well as around the world and many children may be vitamin D deficient at the time of hospitalization [14, 15]. Poor oral intake and intestinal absorption due to illness and no sun exposure may exacerbate the existing deficiency. Additionally there is lack of practice of supplementation during hospitalization. The exact reasons for the significant fall in 25(OH)D concentrations (half-life approximately 3 weeks) within days of hospitalization are unclear. Recent studies have indicated that the catabolic pathways of vitamin D become predominant during critical illness and infection [9]. Also lower levels of vitamin D binding proteins due to interstitial extravasation resulting from increased vascular permeability during inflammatory responses and decreased synthesis may contribute to lower 25(OH)D levels [16]. In addition the dilutional effect of fluid supplementation during hospitalization may reflect in lower 25(OH)D concentrations. While the prevalence of VDD in hospitalized individuals is well documented [3–5, 8, 9, 17, 18], the clinical significance of this deficiency remains to be fully ascertained. Initial studies indicated that VDD affects most outcome parameters in adults as well as children admitted to ICUs and suggested supplementation to reduce morbidity and mortality [3–5, 8, 9, 17, 18]. Other studies, however, have failed to produce similar data on outcomes [19, 20]. We also could not demonstrate significant change attributable to vitamin D status on clinically relevant outcome parameters in our patients. Similarly the intervention trials with vitamin D have shown mixed results with most showing insignificant effects on various hospital outcomes [6, 7]. It is opined that this lack of significant effect on outcomes may be related to caveats in study design, vitamin D doses, and administration routes [6, 7, 21]. An alternative explanation may be related to efficiency of the vitamin D induced local as well as systemic immunity [22, 23]. A robust immune response is expected in those who are vitamin D replete at the time of acquiring infection and may help eliminate infection by augmenting the antibiotics' ability. The process of attaining this vitamin D sufficient state (with normal elicitation of vitamin D related immunity) after supplementation may take several days depending on vitamin D pharmacokinetics in body [24]. Thus, the initial supplementation in hospitalized persons may not have significant effect on the outcomes of presenting illness but may be beneficial in preventing the hospital-related morbidity if hospitalization becomes prolonged. In this context the fall in 25(OH)D levels shown in our study may be proposed as a ground for vitamin D supplementation in all hospitalized children to maintain an optimal 25(OH)D status. It will also be interesting to see the impact of routine

TABLE 3: Levels of 25(OH)D, calcium, phosphate, and alkaline phosphatase in study population at timepoint 1 and timepoint 2.

Characteristics	Timepoint 1	Timepoint 2	P value
25(OH)D level (nmol/L), mean (range, ±SD)	71.87 (20–167, 27.25)	49.03 (7.5–110, 22.25)	0.000
Calcium (mg/dL), mean (range, ±SD)	8.79 (5.9–12, 0.86)	8.53 (5–12, 0.93)	0.02
Phosphorus (mg/dL), mean (range, ±SD)	4.60 (2–6, 1.07)	4.29 (2–5, 1.17)	0.002
Alkaline phosphatase (IU/L), mean (range, ±SD)	229 (71–1004, 160)	236 (80–1135, 153)	0.32

TABLE 4: Mean (±SD) 25(OH)D levels at timepoints 1 and 2 among patients who required ventilation and inotropes, those who developed nosocomial sepsis, and those who died versus those who did not.

Characteristics	Yes	No	P value
Required ventilation, n (%)	21 (22.83)	71 (77.17)	
25(OH)D levels at timepoint 1	65.7 (21.1)	76.55 (28.95)	0.19
25(OH)D levels at timepoint 2	45.86 (20.15)	52.15 (23)	0.42
Required inotropes, n (%)	15 (16.30)	77 (83.70)	
25(OH)D levels at timepoint 1	66.88 (27.15)	75.91 (27.12)	0.16
25(OH)D levels at timepoint 2	44.62 (24.75)	53.78 (21.82)	0.32
Nosocomial sepsis, n (%)	9 (9.78)	83 (90.22)	
25(OH)D levels at timepoint 1	64.67 (27)	78.9 (29.4)	0.22
25(OH)D levels at timepoint 2	47 (27.8)	51 (28.3)	0.13
Died, n (%)	6 (6.52)	86 (93.48)	
25(OH)D levels at timepoint 1	65.8 (15.47)	75 (27.7)	0.16
25(OH)D levels at timepoint 2	42.85 (19.47)	56.15 (22.4)	0.17

TABLE 5: Comparison of various variables between vitamin D deficient and nondeficient children at timepoint 1.

Characteristics	Deficient, n = 23	Non-deficient, n = 69	P value
Mean age (±SD) (years)	5.1 (4.4)	5.36 (4.32)	0.73
Boys, n (%)	14 (60.87)	53 (76.81)	0.13
Girls, (%)	9 (39.13)	16 (23.19)	
Weight (in kgs), mean (±SD)	15.3 (10.91)	15.59 (9.64)	0.93
Height (in cms), mean (±SD)	97.43 (30.83)	100.2 (30.67)	0.70
Failure to thrive, n (%)	6 (26.09)	6 (8.69)	0.03
Short stature, n (%)	5 (21.74)	4 (5.80)	0.02
Risk factors for vitamin D deficiency			
Family size, mean (range, ±SD)	4.30 (1.03)	4.42 (1.15)	0.92
Birth order, mean (range, ±SD)	1.87 (0.96)	2.07 (1.02)	0.41
Exclusive breast feeding, n (%)	17 (73.91)	34 (49.27)	0.03
Adequate sun exposure, n (%)	7 (30.43)	40 (57.97)	0.02
Dark skin color, n (%)	4 (17.39)	3 (4.34)	0.25
Biochemical parameters			
Vitamin D levels (nmol/L), mean (±SD)	48.45 (22)	89.92 (24.1)	0.000
Calcium (mg/dL), mean (±SD)	8.39 (0.95)	8.93 (0.79)	0.009
Phosphorus (mg/dL), mean (±SD)	4.46 (1.0)	4.74 (0.92)	0.66
Alkaline phosphatase (units/L), mean (±SD)	309 (221)	149 (141)	0.008
Outcomes			
Hospital stay (in days), mean (±SD)	14.70 (3.21)	13.12 (3.59)	0.74
Required ventilation, n (%)	8 (34.78)	13 (18.84)	0.11
Required inotropes, n (%)	5 (21.74)	10 (14.49)	0.41
Nosocomial sepsis, n (%)	4 (17.39)	5 (7.24)	0.15
Died, n (%)	3 (13.04)	3 (4.35)	0.14

childhood vitamin D supplementation aimed at achieving an optimal vitamin D status on hospitalization rates and hospital outcomes in children in future.

The decrease in calcium and phosphorus levels in our study paralleled the decrease in 25(OH)D levels as expected [25]. A higher percentage of vitamin D deficient children had history of exclusive breast feeding and inadequate sun exposure, risk factors observed in previous studies as well [14]. The clinical signs of VDD were seen in far less number of cases than biochemical VDD as they develop only when the VDD persists for some duration [26]. So, relying only on clinical signs will miss a significant number of cases with VDD, which would otherwise be identified by measuring 25(OH)D levels. Our data collected during summer and monsoon seasons may have underestimated the actual prevalence of VDD in the studied subjects as 25(OH)D levels fluctuate throughout the year [27].

The data on change in vitamin D status during hospitalization is virtually nonexistent. Only one previous study conducted prospectively on adult patients demonstrated significant decrease in 25(OH)D levels in all patients after 3 days that remained significantly lower through 10 days in the ICU [10]. Our study appears to be the first one to have documented a fall in 25(OH)D levels in hospitalized children.

In conclusion, there are a significant fall in vitamin D levels over short duration hospitalization in children and a need to routinely screen all hospitalized children for VDD. Large multicentered trials are needed to prospectively evaluate the effect of vitamin D supplementation in vitamin D deficient hospitalized children on various disease outcome parameters.

Conflict of Interests

The authors declare that there is no conflict of interests regarding the publication of this paper.

References

[1] P. Pludowski, M. F. Holick, S. Pilz et al., "Vitamin D effects on musculoskeletal health, immunity, autoimmunity, cardiovascular disease, cancer, fertility, pregnancy, dementia and mortality—a review of recent evidence," *Autoimmunity Reviews*, vol. 12, no. 10, pp. 976–989, 2013.

[2] C. F. Gunville, P. M. Mourani, and A. A. Ginde, "The role of vitamin D in prevention and treatment of infection," *Inflammation & Allergy*, vol. 12, no. 4, pp. 239–245, 2013.

[3] S. Venkatram, S. Chilimuri, M. Adrish, A. Salako, M. Patel, and G. Diaz-Fuentes, "Vitamin D deficiency is associated with mortality in the medical intensive care unit," *Critical Care*, vol. 15, no. 6, article R292, 2011.

[4] Y. Arnson, I. Gringauz, D. Itzhaky, and H. Amital, "Vitamin D deficiency is associated with poor outcomes and increased mortality in severely ill patients," *Quarterly Journal of Medicine*, vol. 105, no. 7, pp. 633–639, 2012.

[5] A. B. Braun, F. K. Gibbons, A. A. Litonjua, E. Giovannucci, and K. B. Christopher, "Low serum 25-hydroxyvitamin D at critical care initiation is associated with increased mortality," *Critical Care Medicine*, vol. 40, no. 1, pp. 63–72, 2012.

[6] C. Schnedl, T. R. Pieber, and K. Amrein, "Vitamin D intervention trials in critical illness," *Inflammation & Allergy*, vol. 12, no. 4, pp. 282–287, 2013.

[7] M. Izadpanah and H. Khalili, "Potential benefits of vitamin D supplementation in critically ill patients," *Immunotherapy*, vol. 5, no. 8, pp. 843–853, 2013.

[8] K. Madden, H. A. Feldman, E. M. Smith et al., "Vitamin D deficiency in critically ill children," *Pediatrics*, vol. 130, no. 3, pp. 421–428, 2012.

[9] J. D. McNally, K. Menon, P. Chakraborty et al., "The association of vitamin D status with pediatric critical illness," *Pediatrics*, vol. 130, no. 3, pp. 429–436, 2012.

[10] D. M. Higgins, P. E. Wischmeyer, K. M. Queensland, S. H. Sillau, A. J. Sufit, and D. K. Heyland, "Relationship of vitamin D deficiency to clinical outcomes in critically ill patients," *Journal of Parenteral & Enteral Nutrition*, vol. 36, no. 6, pp. 713–720, 2012.

[11] B. Dawson-Hughes, R. P. Heaney, M. F. Holick, P. Lips, P. J. Meunier, and R. Vieth, "Estimates of optimal vitamin D status," *Osteoporosis International*, vol. 16, no. 7, pp. 713–716, 2005.

[12] B. W. Hollis, "Circulating 25-hydroxyvitamin D levels indicative of vitamin D sufficiency: implications for establishing a new effective dietary intake recommendation for vitamin D," *The Journal of Nutrition*, vol. 135, no. 2, pp. 317–322, 2005.

[13] V. V. Borkar, V. S. Devidayal, and A. K. Bhalla, "Low levels of vitamin D in North Indian children with newly diagnosed type 1 diabetes," *Pediatric Diabetes*, vol. 11, no. 5, pp. 345–350, 2010.

[14] S. Puri, R. K. Marwaha, N. Agarwal et al., "Vitamin D status of apparently healthy schoolgirls from two different socioeconomic strata in Delhi: relation to nutrition and lifestyle," *British Journal of Nutrition*, vol. 99, no. 4, pp. 876–882, 2008.

[15] M. F. Holick and T. C. Chen, "Vitamin D deficiency: a worldwide problem with health consequences," *The American Journal of Clinical Nutrition*, vol. 87, no. 4, pp. 1080S–1086S, 2008.

[16] S. A. Quraishi and C. A. Camargo Jr., "Vitamin D in acute stress and critical illness," *Current Opinion in Clinical Nutrition & Metabolic Care*, vol. 15, no. 6, pp. 625–634, 2012.

[17] P. Lee, J. A. Eisman, and J. R. Center, "Vitamin D deficiency in critically ill patients," *The New England Journal of Medicine*, vol. 360, no. 18, pp. 1912–1914, 2009.

[18] O. Lucidarme, E. Messai, T. Mazzoni, M. Arcade, and D. du Cheyron, "Incidence and risk factors of vitamin D deficiency in critically ill patients: results from a prospective observational study," *Intensive Care Medicine*, vol. 36, no. 9, pp. 1609–1611, 2010.

[19] A. Cecchi, M. Bonizzoli, S. Douar et al., "Vitamin D deficiency in septic patients at ICU admission is not a mortality predictor," *Minerva Anestesiologica*, vol. 77, no. 12, pp. 1184–1189, 2011.

[20] L. X. Su, Z. X. Jiang, L. C. Cao et al., "Significance of low serum vitamin D for infection risk, disease severity and mortality in critically ill patients," *Chinese Medical Journal*, vol. 126, no. 14, pp. 2725–2730, 2013.

[21] R. M. Perron and P. Lee, "Efficacy of high-dose vitamin D supplementation in the critically ill patients," *Inflammation & Allergy*, vol. 12, no. 4, pp. 273–281, 2013.

[22] S. Hansdottir, M. M. Monick, S. L. Hinde, N. Lovan, D. C. Look, and G. W. Hunninghake, "Respiratory epithelial cells convert inactive vitamin D to its active form: potential effects on host defense," *The Journal of Immunology*, vol. 181, no. 10, pp. 7090–7099, 2008.

[23] P. T. Liu, S. Stenger, H. Li et al., "Toll-like receptor triggering of a vitamin D-mediated human antimicrobial response," *Science*, vol. 311, no. 5768, pp. 1770–1773, 2006.

[24] J. I. Boullata, "Vitamin D supplementation: a pharmacologic perspective," *Current Opinion in Clinical Nutrition & Metabolic Care*, vol. 13, no. 6, pp. 677–684, 2010.

[25] R. P. Heaney, "Vitamin D and calcium interactions: functional outcomes," *The American Journal of Clinical Nutrition*, vol. 88, no. 2, pp. 541S–544S, 2008.

[26] C. L. Wagner and F. R. Greer, "Prevention of rickets and vitamin D deficiency in infants, children, and adolescents," *Pediatrics*, vol. 122, no. 5, pp. 1142–1152, 2008.

[27] V. Jain, N. Gupta, M. Kalaivani, A. Jain, A. Sinha, and R. Agarwal, "Vitamin D deficiency in healthy breastfed term infants at 3 months & their mothers in India: seasonal variation & determinants," *Indian Journal of Medical Research*, vol. 133, no. 3, pp. 267–273, 2011.

20

Utility of Gastric Lavage in Vigorous Neonates Delivered with Meconium Stained Liquor: A Randomized Controlled Trial

Jatin Garg, Rupesh Masand, and Balvir Singh Tomar

Department of Pediatrics, National Institute of Medical Sciences, 4 Govind Marg, NIMS City Center, Jaipur, Rajasthan 302004, India

Correspondence should be addressed to Jatin Garg; drjatingarg@yahoo.co.in and Rupesh Masand; masand.rupesh72@gmail.com

Academic Editor: Dharmapuri Vidyasagar

Objective. To determine the incidence of feed intolerance in vigorous babies with meconium stained liquor (MSL) who received prophylactic gastric lavage as compared to those who were not subjected to this procedure. *Design.* Randomized controlled trial. *Setting.* Tertiary care teaching hospital. *Participants/Intervention.* 330 vigorous babies delivered with MSL and satisfying the predefined inclusion criteria were randomized either to receive gastric lavage (group A, $n = 165$) or to not receive gastric lavage (group B, $n = 153$). Clinical monitoring was subsequently performed and recorded in prestructured proforma. *Results.* There was no significant statistical difference ($P > 0.05$) in incidence of feed intolerance in "lavage" and "no lavage" groups. *Secondary Outcome.* There was no evidence of secondary respiratory distress in either group. None of the patients in the lavage group exhibited adverse effects owing to the procedure. *Conclusions.* There is no role of prophylactic gastric lavage in neonates born with MSL.

1. Introduction

Meconium is a blackish-green sticky material composed of debris of intestinal cells, lanugo hair, vernix, liquor, and bile pigments [1, 2]. The incidence of meconium stained liquor (MSL) varies between 7% and 22% of life births [3–7]. Although unsubstantiated, it is thought that the presence of meconium in the stomach can act as a chemical irritant and can cause feeding problems [8]. These are 2.8 times more frequent in neonates born with MSL than those born without it, regardless of consistency of the amniotic fluid [9]. It has been hypothesized that some cases of meconium aspiration syndrome might be caused by postnatal aspiration of gastric contents into the airways [10]. Gastric lavage has been routinely employed with this belief to evacuate the gastric contents and avoid feeding problems but like other procedures it has been associated with complications [8, 11, 12].

Looking at the almost universal practice [11] of prophylactic gastric lavage in neonates delivered with MSL and its recommendation by pediatric textbooks [12–15], despite negligible scientific evidence and evidence-based recommendations, this study was designed with the objective of determining if gastric lavage in well babies with MSL led to the development of less feed intolerance as compared to those who were not subjected to this procedure.

2. Methodology

This randomized control trial was conducted in NICU of a tertiary care teaching hospital between August 2011 and July 2012, after approval from The Institutional Ethical Committee. For the purpose of the study, 330 vigorous neonates delivered with MSL and bearing a birth weight ≥1800 grams and gestational age ≥34 weeks were included. Neonates with hypoxic ischemic encephalopathy (HIE), major congenital malformation, Downes' score [16] for respiratory distress >3, and requiring CPR at the time of birth were excluded. An informed written consent was obtained by the attending resident doctor from the precounseled parents/guardians, immediately after birth of their neonate, who satisfied the required study criteria.

After initial care and stabilization, neonates were randomized either to receive gastric lavage (group A) or to not receive lavage (group B). Randomization was done using small square slips with computer generated numbers from 1 to 330. These prenumbered slips were folded and shuffled in

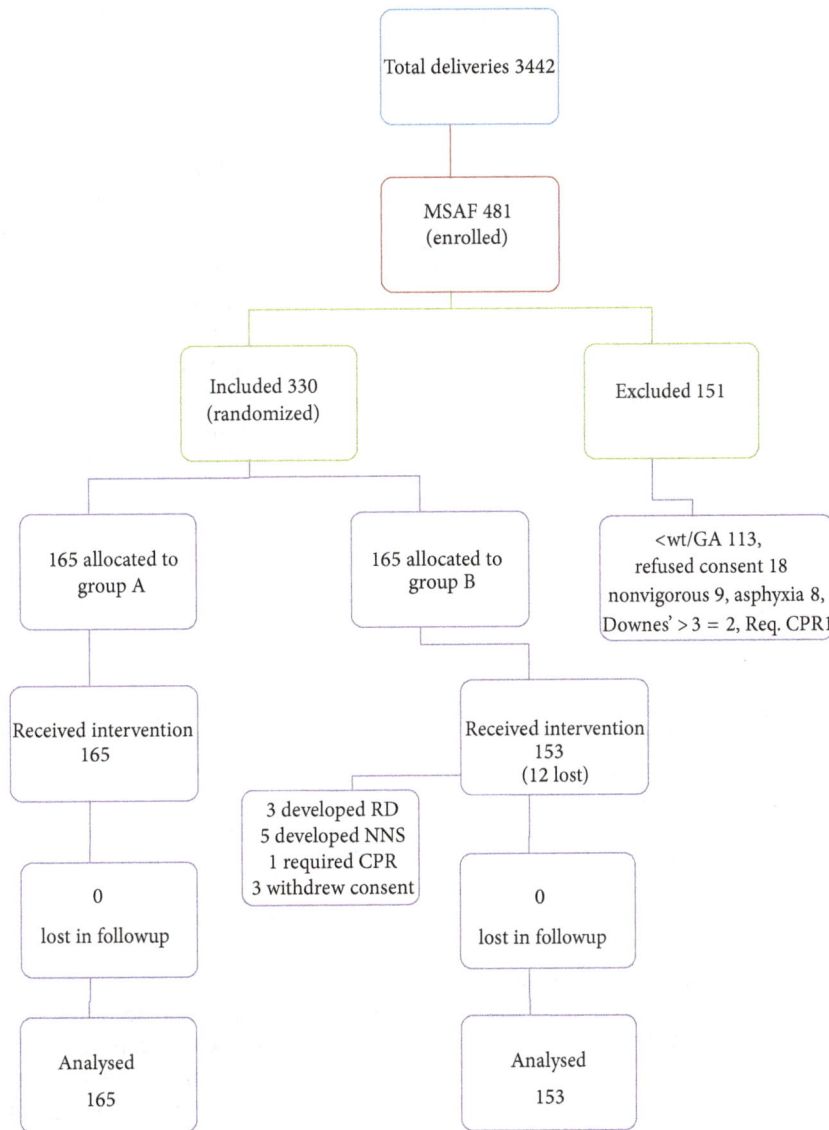

FIGURE 1: Study flow chart. MSL: meconium stained liquor; group A: the "gastric lavage" group; group B: the "no gastric lavage" group; GA: gestational age; <wt/GA: birth weight ≦1800 grams and gestational age ≦34 weeks; req. CPR: requiring cardiopulmonary resuscitation; RD: respiratory distress; NNS: neonatal sepsis.

a box and opened for each neonate to decide the intervention. Neonates with odd-numbered slips were allotted group A, while withdrawal of even-numbered slips rendered the study subjects in group B. A sample size of 165 in each group with an α error of 5% and 90% power in a two sided test was required. Blinding of intervention/outcome was not done; that is, the doctors and nursery staff were aware of the intervention (Figure 1).

Details of name, age, sex, weight, gestational age, mode of delivery, and vital parameters pre- and postgastric lavage were recorded in a prestructured proforma by resident duty doctors.

In group A, all neonates were subjected to lavage using a nasogastric tube of 6Fr/8Fr size and 10 mL/kg normal saline with aliquots of 5 mL each time, till the fluid aspirated was grossly clear. One of the authors (Jatin Garg) conducted

the procedure in the first 30 minutes after birth and it was recorded by the posted residents in the NICU on study proforma. Neonates in group B were not subjected to lavage. All babies were exclusively breast-fed on demand (group B) and after 1 hr of lavage under supervision of nursing staff who counseled the mothers and observed feed intolerance, if there was any. Feed intolerance was defined as (i) >2 vomiting episodes in 4 hr period or >3 in 24 hr and/or (ii) presence of abdominal distension defined as an increase in abdominal girth by 2 cm from baseline (checked only if repeated vomiting episodes were present) and/or (iii) if gastric residual volume is >2 mL of undigested milk or bile colored (checked only if abdominal distension noted) [17]. Neonates were monitored clinically for at least 15 minutes after the procedure and then subsequently at 1, 13, 24, and 48 hrs of life in the observation area of NICU. On

TABLE 1: Comparison of baseline variables in study groups and their association with feed intolerance.

	Total	Group A (165)	Group B (153)	P	Odd ratio	95% CI
	Over all feed intolerance	16	21	0.253	0.67	0.338–1.3475
GA*	34–36 wks 6 days	Group A (98)	Group B (69)	P	Odd ratio	95% CI
		9	12	0.1207	0.4803	0.1903–1.2126
	37–40 wks	Group A (67)	Group B (84)	P	Odd ratio	95% CI
		7	9	0.9578	0.9722	0.3421–2.7629
B.Wt	<2 kg	Group A (21)	Group B (19)	P	Odd ratio	95% CI
		7	5	0.6292	1.4000	0.3572–5.4874
	2-3 kg	Group A (140)	Group B (122)	P	Odd ratio	95% CI
		7	6	0.9878	1.0088	0.3296–3.0875
	>3 kg	Group A (4)	Group B (12)	P	Odd ratio	95% CI
		2	10	0.2032	0.200	0.0168–2.3864
Gender	M	Group A (86)	Group B (80)	P	Odd ratio	95% CI
		9	11	0.5171	0.7332	0.2867–1.8750
	F	Group A (79)	Group B (73)	P	Odd ratio	95% CI
		7	10	0.5574	0.7350	0.2628–2.0558
MOD#	Vaginal	Group A (92)	Group B (93)	P	Odd ratio	95% CI
		7	11	0.33	0.61	0.22–1.66
	C/S	Group A (73)	Group B (60)	P	Odd ratio	95% CI
		9	10	0.47	0.70	0.26–1.86
COM**	Thick	Group A (40)	Group B (42)	P	Odd ratio	95% CI
		7	8	0.85	0.90	0.29–2.76
	Thin	Group A (125)	Group B (111)	P	Odd ratio	95% CI
		9	13	0.23	0.58	0.23–1.42

Group A: the "gastric lavage" group; group B: the "no gastric lavage" group; CI: confidence interval; GA*: gestational age; B.Wt: birth weight; wks: weeks; kg: kilograms; M: male; F: female; MOD#: mode of delivery; C/S: cesarean section; COM**: consistency of meconium.

every occasion, heart rate, respiratory rate, abdominal girth, gastric residue, vomiting episodes, chest examination, and signs of respiratory distress were noted and Downes' scoring was performed, if required. Neonates in lavage group were monitored for complications secondary to nasogastric tube insertion, like apnea, bradycardia, and trauma to the nasal cavity. Appropriate statistical analysis was performed using SPSS 17 software. P value <0.05 was considered significant.

3. Results

There was no significant statistical difference (P > 0.05) in the incidence of feed intolerance in group A (9.70%) and group B (13.73%) (Table 1). None of the baseline characteristics like sex, birth weight, gestational age, mode of delivery, and consistency of meconium were significantly associated (P > 0.05) with occurrence of feed intolerance in our study subjects with meconium stained liquor. There was no evidence of secondary respiratory distress in either group A or group B. None of the patients in the lavage group exhibited adverse effects owing to the procedure, that is, apnea, bradycardia, or any trauma to nasal or oral cavity.

4. Discussion

The performance of gastric lavage in neonates remains a common practice in India and has been mentioned in

neonatal protocols of other regions of the world [18]. It is based on this belief that meconium acts as a chemical irritant in the stomach which can cause gastritis and secondary meconium aspiration syndrome upon regurgitation of gastric contents. Thus, gastric lavage was justified in order to prevent feed intolerance and to increase the success of breast-feeding during the first few hours of life. This randomized controlled trial, however, demonstrated that there was no significant difference in incidence of feed intolerance in the "gastric lavage" (group A) or the "no gastric lavage" (group B) group. The incidence of feed intolerance was 9.7% in the Group A as compared to 13.72% in the Group B (P > 0.05) which was comparable with other studies [17, 19]. This statistically insignificant difference in our study can be explained by the hypothesis proposed by Sharma et al. [19] that vigorous neonates have reduced exposure to meconium in-utero as compared to non-vigorous babies. Early feeding postnatally, further dilutes the meconium and its irritant properties. In our study, there was no association of feed intolerance to sex of the study subjects in either of the two groups as observed similarly by Cuello-García et al. [11]. Wiswell et al. [3] documented male neonates to be more prone to feed intolerance than female neonates (P = 0.022). There was no association of birth weight and gestational age with feed intolerance in either group which was similar to the observations by Ameta et al. [17].

Feed intolerance had no association with the consistency of the meconium, which was in consonance with other studies [11, 17].

None of the babies in the "no gastric lavage" (group B) developed secondary respiratory distress owing to pulmonary aspiration of meconium containing regurgitated gastric fluid which was similar to the observation by other studies [8, 17, 19]. This is contrary to the belief that neonates with MSL are prone to such complications if lavage is not carried out. Narchi and Kulaylat [8] concluded that neonates with MSL are not prone to develop secondary respiratory distress whether lavage is done or not done.

In the present study, gastric lavage was well tolerated in all subjects; that is, there were no procedural complications like apnea, bradycardia, or trauma to the nasal cavity. This finding was in consonance with other studies [8, 11, 17, 19]. However, Widstrom et al. [20] reported small elevation in mean arterial blood pressure, increased retching, and disrupted sequence of prefeeding behavior in neonates who had undergone gastric suction. The physiological side effects induced by gastric suction are minor, but it seemed to be unpleasant for the neonates [20], which could not be evaluated in this study. It has been demonstrated that the aspiration of the gastric contents through a catheter in newborns can be a noxious stimulus. All noxious stimuli especially if repeated can increase functional disorders in adulthood [21]. Inability to perform blinding and, on the part of the nursing staff, to differentiate between regurgitation and vomiting (in spite of prior training) constituted the shortcomings of this study.

5. Conclusion

This study is a randomized control trial which evaluated a common practice in neonatal care without availability of scientific evidence.

Gastric lavage has been mentioned as part of essential newborn care during management of babies with meconium aspiration [12–15]. However, this study demonstrated that feeding problems are not significant in neonates born with meconium stained liquor (MSL) and that there is no role of routine prophylactic gastric lavage in reducing their incidence. In resource poor settings, this may help in saving equipments, nursing time, clinical attention, and preventing procedure-related complications.

This study concludes that gastric lavage should be reserved for treating the rather rare occurrence of feed intolerance in neonates born with MSL instead of being performed on a routine prophylactic basis.

Conflict of Interests

The authors declare that there is no conflict of interests regarding the publication of this paper.

References

[1] J. Davy, "Composition of meconium," *Medico-Chirurgical Transactions*, vol. 27, pp. 189–197, 1844.

[2] H. H. Burris, "Meconium aspiration," in *Manual of Neonatal Care*, chapter 35, p. 429, A Lippincott Manual, 7th edition, 2012.

[3] T. E. Wiswell, J. M. Tuggle, and B. D. Turner, "Meconium aspiration syndrome. Have we made a difference?" *Pediatrics*, vol. 85, no. 5, pp. 715–721, 1990.

[4] E. M. Rossi, E. H. Philipson, T. G. Williams, and S. C. Kalhan, "Meconium aspiration syndrome: intrapartum and neonatal attributes," *American Journal of Obstetrics and Gynecology*, vol. 161, no. 5, pp. 1106–1110, 1989.

[5] C. Hernandez, B. B. Little, J. S. Dax, L. C. Gilstrap, and C. R. Rosenfeld, "Prediction of the severity of meconium aspiration syndrome," *American Journal of Obstetrics and Gynecology*, vol. 169, no. 1, pp. 61–70, 1993.

[6] P. J. Meis, M. Hall, J. R. Marshall, and C. J. Hobel, "Meconium passage: a new classification for risk assessment during labor," *American Journal of Obstetrics and Gynecology*, vol. 131, no. 5, pp. 509–513, 1978.

[7] A. Narang, P. M. C. Nair, O. N. Bhakoo, and K. Vashisht, "Management of meconium stained amniotic fluid: a team approach," *Indian Pediatrics*, vol. 30, no. 1, pp. 9–13, 1993.

[8] H. Narchi and N. Kulaylat, "Is gastric lavage needed in neonates with meconium-stained amniotic fluid?" *European Journal of Pediatrics*, vol. 158, no. 4, pp. 315–317, 1999.

[9] H. Narchi and N. Kulayat, "Feeding problems with the first feed in neonates with meconium—stained amniotic fluid," *Paediatr Child Health*, vol. 4, no. 5, pp. 327–330, 1999.

[10] M. G. Karlowicz, "More on meconium aspiration," *Pediatrics*, vol. 86, no. 6, pp. 1007–1008, 1990.

[11] C. Cuello-García, V. González-lópez, A. Soto-González, V. López-Guevara, S. J. Fernandez-Ortiz, and M. C. Cortez-Hernandez, "Gastric lavage in healthy term newborns: a randomized controlled trial," *Anales de Pediatría*, vol. 63, no. 6, pp. 509–513, 2005.

[12] M. Singh, "Care of the baby in the labour room," in *Care of Newborn*, p. 104, Sagar Publications, 7th edition, 2010.

[13] R. Ballard, T. Hansen, and A. Corbet, "Respiratory failure in the term infant," in *Avery's Diseases of the Newborn*, R. A. Ballard, Ed., pp. 705–722, Elsevier Saunders, Philadelphia, Pa, USA, 8th edition, 2005.

[14] M. Levene, D. Tudehope, and M. Thearle, "Neonatal depression at birth and resuscitation of the new born," in *Essential of Neonatal Medicine*, M. Levene, D. Tudehope, and M. Thearle, Eds., pp. 12–23, Blackwell Science, Oxford, UK, 3rd edition, 2000.

[15] D. R. Marlow and B. A. Redding, "The high risk neonate," in *Textbook of Pediatric Nursing*, D. R. Marlow and B. A. Redding, Eds., pp. 386–439, WB Saunders, Philadelphia, Pa, USA, 6th edition, 1988.

[16] M. Singh, "Care of the baby in the labour room," in *Care of Newborn*, p. 277, Sagar Publications, 7th edition, 2010.

[17] G. Ameta, A. Upadhyay, and S. Gothwal, "Role of gastric lavage in vigorous neonates born with meconium stained amniotic fluid," *Indian Journal of Pediatrics*, vol. 80, no. 3, pp. 195–198, 2013.

[18] R. Jimenez, "normal newborn care," in *Diagnostic and Therapeutic Protocols in Pediatrics Neonatology*, A. Delgado-Rubio, Ed., 2002, http://www.aeped.es/protocols/neonatology/care-rn-normal.pdf.

[19] P. Sharma, S. Nangia, S. Tiwari, A. Goel, B. Singla, and A. Saili, "Gastric lavage for preventionof feeding problems in neonates with meconium stained amniotic fluid: a randomized controlled trial," *PaediatrInt Child Health*. In press.

[20] A.-M. Widstrom, A. B. Ransjo-Arvidson, and K. Christensson, "Gastric suction in healthy newborn infants: effects on circulation and developing feeding behavior," *Acta Paediatrica Scandinavica*, vol. 76, no. 4, pp. 566–572, 1987.

[21] K. J. S. Anand, B. Runeson, and B. Jacobson, "Gastric suction at birth associated with long-term risk for functional intestinal disorders in later life," *Journal of Pediatrics*, vol. 144, no. 4, pp. 449–454, 2004.

21

Validation of the Breastfeeding Experience Scale in a Sample of Iranian Mothers

Forough Mortazavi,[1] **Seyed Abbas Mousavi,**[2] **Reza Chaman,**[3] **and Ahmad Khosravi**[4]

[1] Department of Midwifery, Faculty of Nursing and Midwifery, Sabzevar University of Medical Sciences, Sabzevar 9613873136, Iran
[2] Research Center of Psychiatry, Golestan University of Medical Sciences, Golestan 4918936316, Iran
[3] School of Medicine, Yasuj University of Medical Sciences, Yasuj 7591741418, Iran
[4] Center for Health Related Social and Behavioral Sciences Research, Shahroud University of Medical Sciences, Shahroud 3614773955, Iran

Correspondence should be addressed to Forough Mortazavi; frmortazavi@yahoo.com

Academic Editor: Namık Yaşar Özbek

Objectives. The aim of this study was to validate the breastfeeding experience scale (BES) in a sample of Iranian mothers. *Methods.* After translation and back translation of the BES, an expert panel evaluated the items by assessing the content validity ratio (CVR) and content validity index (CVI). 347 of mothers visiting health centers completed the Farsi version of the BES in the first month postpartum. Exploratory factor analysis (EFA) and confirmatory factor analysis (CFA) were performed to indicate the scale constructs. Reliability was assessed by Cronbach's alpha coefficient. *Results.* CVR and CVI scores for the BES were 0.96 and 0.87, respectively. Cronbach's alpha coefficient for the BES was 0.83. The results of the EFA revealed a new 5-factor model. The results of the CFA for the BES indicated a marginally acceptable fit for the proposed model and acceptable fit for the new model (RMSEA = 0.064, SRMR = 0.064, $\chi^2/df = 2.4$, and CFI = 0.95). Mothers who were exclusively breastfeeding at the first month postpartum had less breastfeeding difficulties score (30.3 ± 7.6) than mothers who were on partial breastfeeding (36.7 ± 11.3) ($P < 0.001$). *Conclusions.* The Farsi version of the BES is a reliable and valid instrument to assess postpartum breastfeeding difficulties in Iranian mothers.

1. Introduction

Breastfeeding brings benefits for both mother and baby [1]. The World Health Organization recommended exclusive breastfeeding (EBF) for all infants up to six months [2].

Iranian government has encouraged breastfeeding since the 1990s and significant success has been achieved, so that the rate of any breastfeeding at one year of age has reached 90% [3]. However, the rate of EBF is decreasing [4]. EBF rates at 4 and 6 months of age at national level averaged 56.8% and 27.7% [3]. Results of a study in Kerman, Iran, showed that partial breastfeeding rate at the end of the first month postpartum averaged 60% [5].

Breastfeeding difficulties are common. Previous studies in Iran, Sweden, and Canada revealed that 34%, 27%, and 87% of mothers in early postpartum period reported a breastfeeding difficulty, respectively [6, 7]. Sore nipple, engorgement, fatigue, feeling tired, difficult latching on, fussy baby, and insufficient supply of breast milk were the common breastfeeding problems [5].

Most breastfeeding difficulties are a relatively normal experience [8]; however, due to wide range of severity, they can be very stressful [9] and have been a risk factor for breastfeeding discontinuation in different studies [6, 10]. A study in the USA showed that mothers who had experienced breastfeeding difficulties in the first month postpartum had a higher risk for discontinuing full breastfeeding before 6 months and any breastfeeding before 12 months [11]. On the other hand, studies showed that support during early postpartum period was associated with increased EBF duration [12]. It is therefore necessary that breastfeeding difficulty be measured routinely during early postpartum period; however, due to the lack of a valid instrument for this purpose, for use in primary health care settings, most mothers with breastfeeding difficulty in the postpartum period remain undiagnosed. It is therefore important to validate an appropriate instrument for the task of measuring breastfeeding difficulty in the postpartum period. Since the breastfeeding experience includes multiple factors related to infant and mother, it is recommended to measure difficulties more multidimensionally and in the form of a continuous variable [9, 13, 14].

The instrument that was developed and validated to measure common breastfeeding difficulty in the form of a continuous variable in the postpartum period is the breastfeeding experience scale (BES) [15]. The first 18 items of the BES measure the severity of breastfeeding difficulties. The validity and reliability of this instrument have been examined and confirmed [13, 16, 17]. The aim of this study, therefore, was to translate and investigate the reliability and validity of the BES in a sample of Iranian mothers. To our best knowledge, no study has validated the BES in mothers in Iran.

2. Materials and Methods

This study was part of a larger study on the assessment of breastfeeding attrition prediction tools and was conducted on 358 pregnant women in late pregnancy of which 347 mothers visited 10 health clinics affiliated to Shahroud University of Medical Sciences in Shahroud, Iran, in 2011, for postpartum visit. The sampling method was convenient and the inclusion criteria were as follows: having a healthy baby and the ability to read and write. The subjects were informed that their participation was voluntary and all their information will be kept confidential. The Ethics Committee of the Shahroud University of Medical Sciences approved the study protocol (Approval no. 900.02). We obtained permission to use the BES from the author. The mothers completed the Farsi version of the BES and GHQ-28 at the end of the first and second month postpartum, respectively. Infant-feeding practice was evaluated at the end of the first month postpartum using the BES.

2.1. Instruments.
Participants completed a questionnaire consisting of sociodemographic and obstetrical information (age, level of education, employment status, family income, parity, mode of delivery, and infant birth weight) at the 2-week postpartum visit. In addition, intention to breastfeed was assessed by a question using a 5-point numerical rating scale in late pregnancy (1: definitely breastfeed, 6: definitely not breastfeed).

2.1.1. GHQ-28.
The General Health Questionnaire (GHQ-28) is one of the screening tools used in epidemiological studies of psychiatric disorders [18]. It contains 28 questions in four subscales: somatic symptoms, anxiety and insomnia, social dysfunction, and severe depression. Each item is scored on a 4-point Likert scale ranging from zero to 3. The total score ranges from 0 to 84, where a higher score indicates lower psychological well-being. The validity of the Farsi version of the instrument has been supported in previous study

[19]. The clinical cut-off point for screening general health in Iran has been estimated at 24, which represent probable psychological health problems requiring more evaluation.

2.1.2. Breastfeeding Experience Scale (BES).
Breastfeeding experiencescale (BES) [17] is a questionnaire that consists of 30 items. The first 18 items measure presence or absence and severity of common breastfeeding difficulties in the early postpartum period. Scores range from "not at all" (1) to "unbearable" (5). The total score ranges from 18 to 90, with a higher score representing increased problem severity. The scale includes five subscales as follows: breast concerns (three items: sore nipples, cracked nipples, and breast infection), process concerns (five items: leaking breasts, baby reluctant to nurse due to sleepiness, breast engorgement, baby nursing too frequently, and feeling very tired), mechanic concerns (five items: baby having sucking difficulty, baby having difficulty in latching on, baby reluctant to nurse due to fussiness, feeling tense and overwhelmed, and difficulty in positioning baby), milk insufficiency concerns (three items: worry about not having enough milk, worry about baby's weight gain, and worry that baby was not getting enough milk), and social concerns (two items: feeling embarrassed when nursing and difficulty in combining work and breastfeeding). Content validity and internal consistency of this scale (alpha = 0.76) were demonstrated during early development of the BES [17]. In another study, the internal consistency of the questionnaire at 3 and 6 weeks postpartum was 0.79 and 0.72, respectively [20]. Also, in a study on 31 mothers with mastitis, the α-coefficient for the 18 items was 0.81 [16]. The last 12 items of the BES assess whether breastfeeding was continued, formula was added or substituted breast milk, how often formula was introduced, and what breastfeeding difficulties were related to mother's weaning decision in case of early weaning.

2.2. Statistical Analysis.
Data analyses were conducted by SPSS version 18 (SPSS Inc., Chicago, IL, USA) and LISREL version 8.80 (Scientific Software International Inc., 2007). The reliability of the Farsi version of the BES was assessed by Cronbach's alpha coefficient, alpha if item deleted, interitem, and item-total correlation coefficients. Cronbach's alpha values >0.6, item-total correlation coefficients >0.20, and interitem correlations coefficients <0.80 and higher than zero were regarded as acceptable. Cronbach's alpha values <0.5 were regarded as unacceptable. An item was considered for removal if its item-total correlation coefficient was lower than 0.2, provided that its deletion led to an increase of more than 0.1 in Cronbach's alpha coefficient [21].

Exploratory factor analysis (EFA) was conducted utilizing principal component analysis with varimax rotation. Criteria for retaining factors and items were having eigenvalues >1 [22] and item loading ≥0.3 [23], respectively. Confirmatory factor analysis (CFA) was conducted by structural equation modeling. The method of estimation was weighted by the least squares. The asymptotic covariance matrix was considered as a weighted matrix. The input matrix was covariance matrix of data. Relative chi-squares <5.00, a CFI value >0.90, a RMSEA value of <0.08 [24], and a SRMR value of <0.08 [25] were considered as acceptable model fit. RMSEA and SRMR values greater than 0.10 justify rejecting the model [26].

Concurrent validity was examined by calculating Pearson's correlation coefficients between the BES and GHQ28. Correlation coefficients higher than 0.50 were considered indicative of good concurrent validity in similar instruments. For known group comparison, we compared the mean score of the BES in primiparous and multiparous mothers. For predictive validity, we compared the mean score of the BES in exclusive, predominant, and partial breastfeeding mothers using ANOVA test. Paired t-test was performed to compare the BES scores in primiparous and multiparous mothers.

2.3. Process of Translation and Cultural Adaptation. First, two specialists in English language translated the BES separately. Then, we discussed differences between the two translated versions and created the final version. Finally, a Ph.D. in English language who had not read the original version of the instrument translated the Farsi version into English. We compared the two English versions and found no discrepancy. Few minor revisions were done.

2.3.1. Content Validity. Content validity was based on the judgment of experts that items and questions in an instrument were essential, relevant, and appropriate to the target culture. Therefore, the purpose of this step was to ensure that the Farsi version of the BES was clear and culturally relevant. Both qualitative and quantitative methods were applied [27]. In the qualitative phase, an expert panel consisted of 10 faculty members and specialists of reproductive health and pediatrics, gynecologists, nutritionists, epidemiologists, psychologists, and midwives who had paper in breastfeeding and evaluated grammar, wording, and scaling of the questionnaire. Four experts argued that the rate of introduction of water-based fluids was high in our population. Therefore, we added one question and changed two questions to cover the introduction of different water-based fluids. The Q22 "are you using any fluids (boiled water, sugar water, herbal teas) to feed your baby?" was added and Q23 was changed to assess how often they used fluids. In order to determine content validity ratio (CVR), we chose Lawshe approach [28]. Experts assessed essentiality of each item for the Iranian culture. They assessed the necessity of the items using a three-point rating scale: (a) not necessary, (b) useful, but not essential, and (c) essential. The CVR for every item was calculated using formula CVR = $[n - (N/2)] \div (N/2)$ (N = the total number of experts and n = the number of experts who had chosen the (c) option for each particular item). We computed a CVR for the total scale. According to the Lawshe table, an acceptable CVR value for 10 experts is 0.62. No item had a CVR less than 0.62. The mean CVR for the total scale was 0.96, indicating a satisfactory content validity.

Then, the BES was given again to the experts to express their ideas about clarity, simplicity, and relevancy of each item in a 4-point Likert scale (from a: not relevant, not simple, and not clear to d: very relevant, very simple, and very clear). The content validity index for every item was calculated by dividing the total number of experts by the number of experts

who had chosen the (c) or (d) option for each particular item (15). We calculated the CVI for relevancy, clarity, and simplicity of every item, according to the 10 experts' views for each item. Polit and Beck recommended 0.80 as the acceptable lower limit for the CVI value [29]. The mean CVI for the total scale was 0.87.

2.3.2. Pilot Study. In the pilot study, we asked 20 low educated breastfeeding multiparas visiting two health centers to fill out the translated BES to assess how understandable are the items and questions and how long the BES takes to be completed. After the mothers individually completed the BES, we conducted face-to-face interviews to determine if they felt difficulty or ambiguity in responding to the items. Most mothers indicated that the questionnaire was easy to read and understand. However, some suggested changing item "difficulty in combining work and breastfeeding" to "difficulty in combining homemaking or work outside and breastfeeding" and suggested a better idiomatic equivalence for cracked nipple.

3. Results

3.1. Subjects. The median age, educational level, and monthly family income of mothers were 26.1 years, 11 years, and 4 million RLS, respectively. Mode of delivery for 49% of mothers was vaginal. At the end of the first months postpartum the number of mothers who were on exclusive, predominant, and partial breastfeeding was 115 (33.1%), 202 (58.2%), and 30 (8.6%), respectively. Among mothers who were on partial breastfeeding, seven mothers started introducing formula within the first week postpartum and 20 mothers introduced formula every day. Among mothers who were on predominant breastfeeding, 153 mothers started introducing fluids within the first three days postpartum and 36 mothers introduced fluids every day. There was no early weaning at the end of the first month postpartum. All items of the scale have been answered.

3.2. Validity

3.2.1. Exploratory Factor Analysis. Exploratory factor analysis (EFA) was used to investigate factor structure of the BES within the sample. The Kaiser-Meyer-Olkin (KMO) measure of sampling adequacy was 0.817 and Bartlett's test of sphericity was significant ($\chi^2 = 1856$, $P < 0.001$), indicating that the variables correlated with one another. Factor analysis yielded five factors ((1) mother concern, (2) insufficient milk concern, (3) baby concern, (4) breast concern, and (5) process concern) with eigenvalues ≥ 1, which explained 58.57% of total variance. Only "insufficient milk concern" factor was the same factor that the BES developer found. Factors 1 and 3 emerged. One item was added to the "breast concern" factor and 3 items were excluded from the "process concern" factor which Wambach found. The percentage variance and eigenvalues explained for rotated factors as well as the factor loading after rotation of each item are presented in Table 1. All items had factor loadings more than 0.396.

TABLE 1: Results of exploratory factor analysis (EFA).

Item	Factors				
	1	2	3	4	5
Q16: feeling tense and overwhelmed	**0.819**	0.178	0.095	0.045	0.089
Q18: difficulty in combining work and breastfeeding	**0.751**	0.171	0.105	0.067	0.163
Q12: feeling very tired	**0.716**	0.247	0.207	0.026	0.257
Q14: difficulty in positioning baby	**0.488**	0.236	0.352	0.177	−0.250
Q17: feeling embarrassed when nursing	**0.440**	0.117	0.302	−0.075	−0.304
Q10: worry of not having enough milk	0.189	**0.821**	0.137	0.038	0.073
Q13: worry that baby was not getting enough milk	0.195	**0.772**	0.204	0.059	−0.016
Q15: worry about baby's weight gain	0.209	**0.630**	0.117	0.085	−0.006
Q5: baby reluctant to nurse due to sleepiness	0.107	0.108	**0.738**	−0.039	0.119
Q6: baby reluctant to nurse due to fussiness	0.134	0.079	**0.711**	−0.040	0.003
Q11: baby having difficulty in sucking	0.351	0.242	**0.574**	0.221	−0.052
Q4: baby having difficulty in latching on	0.198	0.313	**0.568**	0.330	0.086
Q1: sore nipple	0.106	0.050	−0.145	**0.866**	0.028
Q2: cracked nipple	0.041	0.178	0.011	**0.844**	−0.023
Q3: breast engorgement	0.161	0.002	0.132	**0.553**	0.294
Q7: breast infection	−0.165	−0.030	0.241	**0.397**	0.083
Q8: leaking breasts	0.176	−0.233	0.196	0.198	**0.689**
Q9: baby nursing too frequently	0.078	0.351	−0.037	0.068	**0.688**
Eigenvalue[b]	2.592	2.246	2.191	2.186	1.327
Variance[b]	14.402	12.478	12.171	12.145	7.374

Factors: 1: mother concern, 2: insufficient milk concern, 3: baby concern, 4: breast concern, and 5: process concern.

Item numbers refer to question numbers in the original questionnaire. [b]The percentage variance and eigenvalues explained for rotated factor matrices. Extraction method: principal component analysis, and rotation method: varimax with Kaiser normalization.

TABLE 2: Results of confirmatory factor analysis (CFA) with 18 items.

Model	Chi-square	P	Chi-square/df	RMSEA	SRMR	CFI
As originally assigned by Wambach	476	0.00	3.8	**0.09**	0.072	0.90
The model of this study	301	0.00	2.4	0.064	0.064	0.95

Observation below the recommended value is shown in bold character. Chi-square/df: minimum fit function/degree of freedom; RMSEA: root mean square error of approximation; SRMR: standardized root mean square residual; CFI: comparative fit index.

3.2.2. Confirmatory Factor Analysis. We used CFA to assess how well the model extracted by EFA and the factor structure suggested by previous study fitted the observed data. The results of the CFA for the two five-factor structures for the BES indicated a marginally acceptable fit for the proposed model and acceptable fit for the new model (RMSEA = 0.064, SRMR = 0.064, χ^2/df = 2.4, and CFI = 0.95). All parameters were significant (T value > 2). Results are shown in Table 2 and Figure 1. Factor load of items was 0.23 to 0.85.

3.2.3. Concurrent Validity. We assumed that the mothers with breastfeeding difficulties would experience psychological problems. The correlation coefficients between the BES and GHQ-28 were 0.54, indicating moderate relationships ($P < 0.001$). In addition, we expected that maternal education and intention to breastfeed were negatively correlated with the BES scores. The results showed that mothers with higher education experienced higher breastfeeding difficulties ($R = 0.26$ and $P = 0.037$). As we had been expecting, mothers who were more determined to breastfeed in late pregnancy had

lower breastfeeding difficulties ($R = -0.146$ and $P = 0.006$). However, both correlation coefficients were low.

3.2.4. Known Group Comparison. In this study, we assumed that multiparous mothers had lower BES scores than primiparous mothers. There were 200 multiparas and 147 primiparas in our sample. Results showed that the mean BES score in multiparous mothers (30.1 ± 6.4) was lower than that of primiparous mothers (32.3 ± 9.7) ($t = 2.53$ and $P = 0.012$).

3.2.5. Predictive Validity. We also evaluated the construct validity by determining the predictive validity of the instrument. We assumed that mothers with less breastfeeding difficulties would exclusively breastfeed their baby. Scores were compared by infant-feeding method at the first month postpartum. There were significant differences in breastfeeding difficulties score between mothers who were exclusively breastfeeding (30.3 ± 7.6), predominant breastfeeding (31.3 ± 8.3), and partial breastfeeding (36.7 ± 11.3) ($F = 6.79$, $P < 0.001$). The Scheffe testrevealed that mothers who were

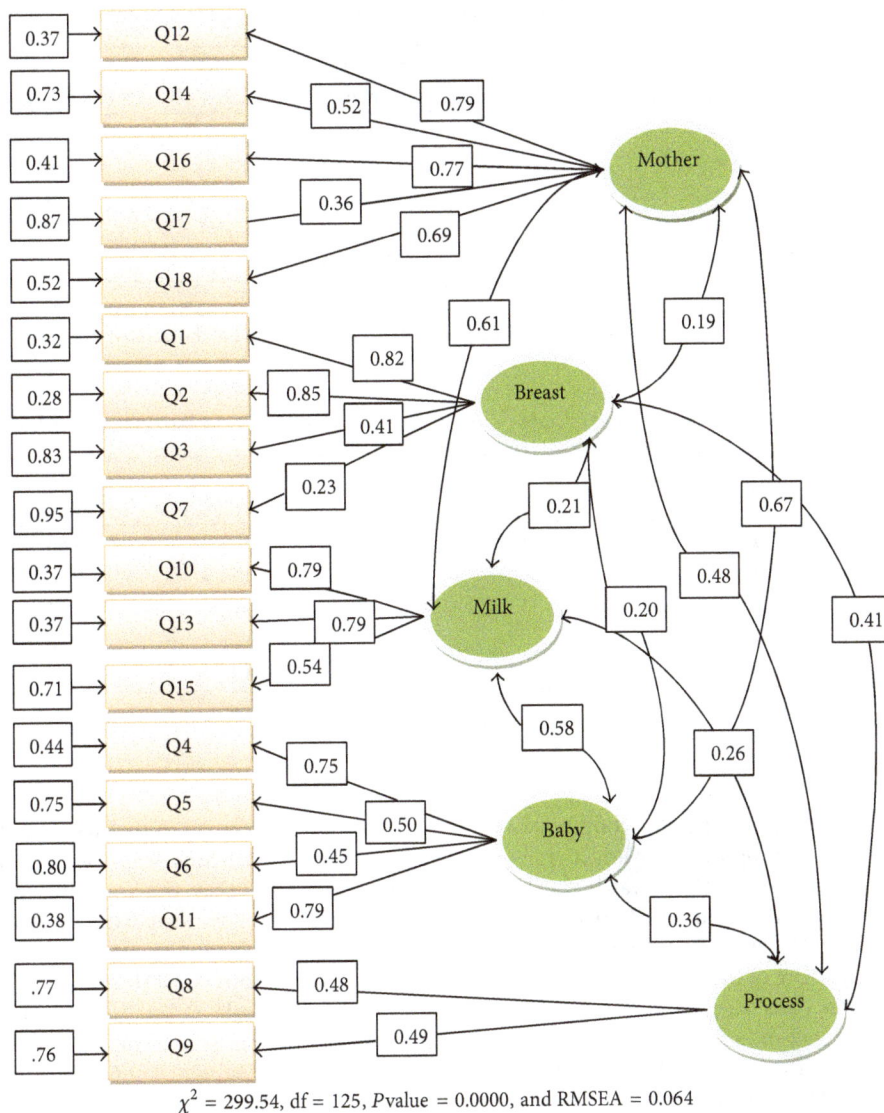

$\chi^2 = 299.54$, df $= 125$, Pvalue $= 0.0000$, and RMSEA $= 0.064$

FIGURE 1: CFA of the new five-factor model of the BES (the item numbers refer to question numbers in the original questionnaire).

exclusively breastfeeding had less breastfeeding difficulties scores than mothers who were on partial breastfeeding.

3.3. Reliability. Table 3 shows Cronbach's alpha coefficients for the five subscales of the BES as originally assigned by Wambach [13]. Table 4 shows descriptive statistics and alpha Cronbach coefficients for the BES subscales as extracted by the EFA. The values of alpha Cronbach coefficients for subscales of the BES were higher for primiparas than for multiparas for both five-factor models. Both models had one factor, which did not meet the Cronbach's alpha criteria for reliability. Interitem correlation coefficients for each subscale as assigned by this study were 0.06 to 0.71. All corrected item-total correlation coefficients for each subscale were 0.22 to 0.63. Deleting each item only resulted in a slight reduction in Cronbach's alpha coefficient (0.01–0.05) except item 7 (breast infection) and item 15 (worry about baby's weight gain) that increased Cronbach's alpha coefficient (0.05 and 0.04, resp.).

4. Discussion and Conclusions

This study was the first to describe the validity and reliability of this instrument in mothers in another language. The BES assesses the breastfeeding difficulties, practices, and outcomes. Both CVR and CVI were satisfactory, indicating that the content of the BES is congruent with the Iranian culture. All items have been answered. This demonstrates that the instrument was understandable to the mothers in this study. The results indicate that the Farsi version of the first 18 items of the BES is a reliable and valid instrument for measuring and quantifying breastfeeding difficulties in mothers.

The EFA extracted five factors, which jointly explained 58.57% of variances. These factors were not completely the same factors, which Wambach found [15]. Two new factors (mother concern and baby concern) emerged and the number of items of two factors (breast concern and

TABLE 3: Cronbach's alpha of the BES subscales as originally assigned by Wambach.

Subscales[†]	Cronbach's alpha			
	Wambach's study [13]	As originally assigned by Wambach	Primiparas	Multiparas
Mechanic	0.60 (5 items)	0.73 (5 items)	0.79	0.53
Insufficient milk	0.86 (3 items)	0.74 (3 items)	0.78	0.68
Breast	0.68 (3 items)	0.66 (3 items)	0.70	0.53
Social	0.48 (2 items)	0.40 (2 items)	0.50	0.16
Process	0.56 (5 items)	0.54 (5 items)	0.58	0.49
Total	0.77	0.83	0.86	0.71

[†]Subscales as originally assigned by Wambach (1998) [13]; the order of the subscales is based on the order of the factors extracted by Wambach.

TABLE 4: Descriptive statistics and Cronbach's alpha for the BES subscales as extracted by the EFA.

Subscales	Mean (SD)	Minimum	Maximum	Cronbach's alpha		
				All	Primiparas	Multiparas
Mother	8.52 (3.26)	5	21	0.76	0.80	0.71
Insufficient milk	5.53 (2.52)	3	14	0.74	0.78	0.68
Baby	5.85 (2.42)	4	19	0.72	0.75	0.60
Breast	6.21 (2.65)	4	20	0.65	0.68	0.60
Process	5.29 (1.73)	2	10	0.38	0.38	0.38
Total scale	31.40 (8.51)	18	74	0.83	0.86	0.71

The order of the subscales is based on the order of the factors extracted by the EFA.

process concern) changed. CFA marginally confirmed the five-factor structure of the BES proposed by Wambach in our population. Although the value of RMSEA was higher than 0.08, it was lower than 0.1 which did not justify rejecting the model proposed by Wambach [26]. The results of the CFA for the new five-factor structure of the BES were satisfactory, indicating a good fit to the data. The standardized loadings represent the correlation between each observed variable and the corresponding factors. There was only one item with factor load lower than 0.3. Assessment of parameters revealed that all of them are significant (T value > 2), indicating that each item is significantly relevant to its factor and all five factors are significantly relevant to each other and to the conceptual structure.

In terms of discriminant validity, the BES performed well. In agreement with previous study [7], we found a higher prevalence of breastfeeding difficulties in primiparous mothers.

Concurrent validity was also confirmed by the moderate correlations between the scores of BES and GHQ-28. Previous study revealed that among mothers who experienced poor support, breastfeeding difficulties might lead to depression during the first 6 months postpartum [7]. Surprisingly, mothers with higher education were more likely to experience breastfeeding difficulties. Qualitative studies are needed to answer why mothers with higher education express more breastfeeding difficulties than others in Iran.

Considering the predictive validity of the BES, we found that the BES could predict the continuation of EBF at the first month postpartum, which is in agreement with the results of previous studies, which were not using the BES to measure breastfeeding difficulties [6, 10, 11].

Internal consistency of the first 18 items of the BES was satisfactory (0.83) which was comparable with Wambach's study that found that the α-coefficient for the 18 items at 3, 6, and 9 weeks postpartum was 0.77, 0.77, and 0.81, respectively [13]. However, our results showed that the α-coefficient for the one subscale of the new BES was lower than 0.6 (process subscale, 0.38). These results were comparable to those in the study of Wambach [13] in which the α-coefficient for two subscales at 6 weeks postpartum was lower than 0.6. Since the value of alpha depends on the number of items on a scale, it is a common observation that α-coefficient decreases when the number of items decreases [30]. The item-subscale analysis showed that there was no item-subscale correlation coefficient lower than 0.2 and all interitem correlation coefficients were less than 0.80 and higher than zero, indicating satisfactory reliability.

In this study, we adapted the original English version of the BES to Farsi. The results of this study show that the Farsi version of the BES is a reliable and valid instrument for measuring breastfeeding difficulties in Iranian mothers. We recommend that further studies be designed to identify cutoff point for the BES in the first weeks postpartum for the task of screening for breastfeeding discontinuation. In addition, we recommend that in future studies the two five-factor models be tested to examine and compare their structures.

4.1. Implications for Practice and Policy. Providers of obstetric care should pay more attention to mothers having difficulty with breastfeeding during early postpartum period and consider screening for breastfeeding difficulties in early postpartum period. The Farsi version of the BES can be used as a part of routine assessments in the postpartum period and will fill an important gap in measuring breast feeding difficulties in mothers in the postpartum period in Iran.

4.2. Limitations. We did not assess reliability through test-retest analysis because the nature of breastfeeding difficulties is transient during the first months postpartum. Our sample consisted of multiparas and primiparas. Since parity is an important factor to express breastfeeding difficulties, it is likely that results improved if we made study on a larger sample of primiparas. The results are limited to mothers in early postpartum period and cannot be generalized to late postpartum period.

5. Conclusion

The present study confirmed the content validity of the BES. In addition, reliability and construct validity of the Farsi version of the first 18 items of the BES were confirmed. Although a new five-factor model was proposed, the original structure was not rejected. Further studies are needed to compare the two five-factor structures of the BES.

Conflict of Interests

The authors declare that there is no conflict of interests regarding the publication of this paper.

Authors' Contribution

Forough Mortazavi was the main investigator and wrote the proposal, collected the data, wrote the first draft, and contributed to the statistical analysis. Seyed Abbas Mousavi contributed to the study design. Reza Chaman contributed to the interpretation of the findings. Ahmad Khosravi revised the final draft.

Acknowledgments

The authors wish to thank Professor Wambach who kindly guides them to use the breastfeeding experience scale. This work is part of a Ph.D. degree thesis on the relationship between maternal QOL and breastfeeding attrition prediction tools and breastfeeding duration and was partially financed by Shahroud University of Medical Sciences (approval no. 9004).

References

[1] S. Ip, M. Chung, G. Raman et al., "Breastfeeding and maternal and infant health outcomes in developed countries," *Evidence Report/Technology Assessment*, no. 153, pp. 1–186, 2007.

[2] World Health Organization, "Infant and young child nutrition; global strategy for infant and young child feeding," Tech. Rep. EB 109/12 2002, 2002.

[3] B. Olang, K. Farivar, A. Heidarzadeh, B. Strandvik, and A. Yngve, "Breastfeeding in Iran: prevalence, duration and current recommendations," *International Breastfeeding Journal*, vol. 4, article 8, 2009.

[4] Unicef. Iran, Islamic Republic of, statistics, Nutrition, 2011, http://www.unicef.org/infobycountry/iran_statistics.html.

[5] S. Mehrparvar and M. Varzandeh, "Investigation of decreasing causes of exclusive breastfeeding in children below six months old, in Kerman City during 2008-2009," *Journal of Fasa University of Medical Sciences*, vol. 1, pp. 45–51, 2011.

[6] A.-T. Gerd, S. Bergman, J. Dahlgren, J. Roswall, and B. Alm, "Factors associated with discontinuation of breastfeeding before 1 month of age," *Acta Paediatrica, International Journal of Paediatrics*, vol. 101, no. 1, pp. 55–60, 2012.

[7] K. H. Chaput, *The effect of breastfeeding difficulty and associated factors on postpartum depression [Ph.D. thesis]*, University of Calgary, Calgary, Canada, 2013.

[8] E. R. J. Giugliani, "Common problems during lactation and their management," *Jornal de Pediatria*, vol. 80, no. 5, pp. S147–S154, 2004.

[9] J. N. Mozingo, M. W. Davis, P. G. Droppleman, and A. Merideth, "It wasn't working: women's experiences with short-term breastfeeding," *MCN. The American Journal of Maternal Child Nursing*, vol. 25, no. 3, pp. 120–126, 2000.

[10] L. Palmer, G. Carlsson, M. Mollberg, and M. Nystrom, "Severe breastfeeding difficulties: existential lostness as a mother-women's lived experiences of initiating breastfeeding under severe difficulties," *International Journal of Qualitative Studies on Health and Well-Being*, vol. 7, Article ID 10846, 2012.

[11] J. A. Scott, C. W. Binns, W. H. Oddy, and K. I. Graham, "Predictors of breastfeeding duration: evidence from a cohort study," *Pediatrics*, vol. 117, no. 4, pp. e646–e655, 2006.

[12] K. Wambach, S. H. Campell, S. L. Gill, J. E. Dodgson, T. C. Abiona, and M. J. Heinig, "Clinical lactation practice: 20 years of evidence," *Journal of Human Lactation*, vol. 21, no. 3, pp. 245–258, 2005.

[13] K. A. Wambach, "Maternal fatigue in breastfeeding primiparae during the first nine weeks postpartum," *Journal of Human Lactation*, vol. 14, no. 3, pp. 219–229, 1998.

[14] E. M. Taveras, A. M. Capra, P. A. Braveman, N. G. Jensvold, G. J. Escobar, and T. A. Lieu, "Clinician support and psychosocial risk factors associated with breastfeeding discontinuation," *Pediatrics*, vol. 112, no. 1 I, pp. 108–115, 2003.

[15] K. Wambach, "Development of an instrument to measure breastfeeding outcomes: The Breastfeeding Experience Scale," The University of Arizona, Tucson, USA, 1990.

[16] K. A. Wambach, "Lactation mastitis: a descriptive study of the experience experiencia," *Journal of Human Lactation*, vol. 19, no. 1, pp. 24–34, 2003.

[17] K. A. Wambach, "Breastfeeding intention and outcome: a test of the theory of planned behavior," *Research in Nursing & Health*, vol. 20, pp. 51–59, 1997.

[18] D. P. Goldberg and V. F. Hillier, "A scaled version of the general health questionnaire," *Psychological Medicine*, vol. 9, no. 1, pp. 139–145, 1979.

[19] A. Ebrahimi, H. Molavi, G. Moosavi, A. Bornamanesh, and M. Yaghobi, "Psychometric properties and factor structure of general health questionnaire 28 (GHQ-28) in Iranian psychiatric patients," *Journal of Research in Behavioural Sciences*, vol. 5, pp. 5–11, 2007 (Persian).

[20] J. Gross, K. Wambach, and L. Aaronson, "Perceived Behavioral Control of Breastfeeding [BSN Honors Research1:1]," University of Kansas, Kansas, Kan, USA, 2008.

[21] D. Streiner and G. Norman, *Health Measurement Scales: A Practical Guide To Their Development and Use*, Oxford University Press, Oxford, UK, 1995.

[22] J. Dixon, "Factor analysis," in *Statistical Methods for Health Care Research*, B. H. Monro, Ed., pp. 303–331, Lippincott Williams & Wilkins, Philadelphia, Pa, USA, 4th edition, 2001.

[23] C. F. Waltz, O. L. Strickland, and E. R. Lenz, *Measurement in Nursing and Health Research*, Springer, 4th edition, 2010.

[24] P. M. Bentler and D. G. Bonett, "Significance tests and goodness of fit in the analysis of covariance structures," *Psychological Bulletin*, vol. 88, no. 3, pp. 588–606, 1980.

[25] L.-T. Hu and P. M. Bentler, "Cutoff criteria for fit indexes in covariance structure analysis: conventional criteria versus new alternatives," *Structural Equation Modeling*, vol. 6, no. 1, pp. 1–55, 1999.

[26] R. B. Kline, "Exploratory and confirmatory factor analysis," in *Applied Quantitative Analysis in the Social Sciences*, Y. Petscher and C. Schatsschneider, Eds., pp. 171–207, Routledge, New York, NY, USA, 2013.

[27] D. Colton and R. W. Covert, *Designing and Constructing Instruments for Social Research and Evaluation*, John Wiley & Sons, San Francisco, Calif, USA, 2007.

[28] C. Lawshe, "A quantitative approach to content validity," *Personnel Psychology*, vol. 28, pp. 563–575, 1975.

[29] D. Polit and C. Beck, *Nursing Research: Principles and Methods*, Lippincott Williams & Wilkins, Philadelphia, Pa, USA, 46th edition, 2004.

[30] A. Field, *Discovering Statistics Using SPSS*, Sage, 3rd edition, 2009.

22

Impact of an Educational Film on Parental Knowledge of Children with Cerebral Palsy

Shilpa Khanna Arora,[1] **Anju Aggarwal,**[2] **and Hema Mittal**[2]

[1] *Department of Pediatrics, Vardhman Mahavir Medical College and Safdarjung Hospital, New Delhi 110029, India*
[2] *Department of Pediatrics, University College of Medical Sciences and GTB Hospital, Delhi 110095, India*

Correspondence should be addressed to Shilpa Khanna Arora; drshilpakhanna@yahoo.co.in

Academic Editor: Tonse N. K. Raju

Parents of children with cerebral palsy (CP) must have knowledge about the disease and its management to improve the outcome. This uncontrolled interventional trial was carried out to evaluate the parental knowledge of CP and assess the impact of an educational programme on it. Preset questionnaires were filled before and 1 week after a single session educational programme using an educational film. Out of a total of 53 subjects, majority (75.5%) were from lower socioeconomic status. Initially, none knew the correct name of child's illness; afterwards 45.3% could name it. When compared to previous status, there occurred significant improvement in the knowledge of parents after viewing the film with regard to knowing the cause of CP, knowing that motor involvement was predominant in CP, knowledge regarding curability of the disease, and knowledge about special schooling ($P < 0.05$). Change in knowledge was not related to socioeconomic or educational status ($P > 0.05$). Majority (94.3%) found the film useful and 96.2% learned how they could help in the management of their children. Parental knowledge of CP is inadequate which can be improved by incorporating such educational programmes in special clinics to improve management.

1. Introduction

Cerebral palsy (CP) is the most common physical disability in childhood [1]. Incidence of CP has been estimated to be 2–2.8 per 1000 live births [2]. CP cannot be cured but early intervention therapy can help achieve functional abilities that facilitate independence and improve quality of life [3]. It is known that a supportive home environment is one of the factors that can favourably determine the outcome of CP in a child. Parental involvement is vital in the process of rehabilitation and care of such children [4]. Thus parents of children with cerebral palsy must have knowledge about the disease and its management. This would help in planning therapy to achieve functional abilities and improve quality of life. At present there are very few studies available regarding parental knowledge on cerebral palsy. Review of the current literature shows that majority of the parents of children with CP lack the basic knowledge regarding the disease, its causation, prognosis, treatment modalities, and the outcome [3, 5–9]. Also there is paucity of studies carrying out any

intervention and evaluating the response of that intervention on the parental knowledge regarding CP. Thus this study was carried out to determine the present knowledge of parents of their child's cerebral palsy and to evaluate the impact of a single session educational programme on their knowledge.

2. Material and Methods

This uncontrolled interventional trial was carried out in a tertiary care hospital from August 2010 to March 2011. Approval was obtained from the institutional ethical committee. A written informed consent was obtained from the parents. Subjects were parents (either mother or father or both) of recently diagnosed (≤1 month) cases of CP presenting to the clinic. Guardians/caretakers other than biological parents and the parents who had already watched the educational film were excluded from the study. The parental knowledge regarding CP was assessed by filling a questionnaire by the investigator in the language they understood. It included questions about the name of the disease, its probable aetiology, treatment options, and rehabilitation of the child.

Following that, the subjects were shown an educational film and asked to follow up after one week. The film which is in Hindi language talks about the aetiology, management, and the role of parents in managing CP. It also describes briefly the eight spheres of development and how they are involved in CP as language, play, social communication, and so forth, as well as the fact that motor involvement was predominant in cerebral palsy. It emphasized the fact that a child with cerebral palsy can be rehabilitated to do activities of daily living and some of them are mentally normal. No two children of cerebral palsy are the same. Film explained the role of parental involvement in training of the child. The same questionnaire was filled up by the investigator again with a few additional questions based on the film on the follow-up visit.

The impact of the educational film on the parental knowledge of CP was assessed by comparing the responses before and after watching the educational film. Knowledge about various aspects of cerebral palsy was classified as correct or incorrect/know or do not know. Knowledge about the various aspects of the film was assessed as percentages. Statistical analysis was done using SPSS Version 14.0, SPSS Inc., Chicago. The change in parental responses to the questionnaire before and after showing the film was analysed using the McNemar test. P value of <0.05 was taken as significant. Chi-square test/Fisher exact test was used to compare the response to individual questions with each of the demographic parameters.

3. Results

Parents of a total of 53 children (35 males and 18 females) who were recently diagnosed with cerebral palsy were included. The age of the children ranged from 6 to 72 months. Majority (30/53 or 56.6%) were of first birth order. There was history of significant perinatal events in 45/53 (84.9%) children. The type of CP from which the children suffered was spastic quadriplegic (71.7%), diplegic (18.9%), hemiplegic (5.7%), and dyskinetic (3.8%). Associated comorbidities in children were drooling (66.0%), behavioural problems (64.2%), seizures (60.4%), visual disability (32.1%), contractures (17.0%), and hearing disability (11.3%). The age at which parents noted symptoms in their children ranged from 1 to 36 months (mean ± SD = 10.02 ± 6.72) whereas age at which diagnosis of CP was established ranged from 2 to 72 months (mean ± SD = 19.64 ± 15.40).

Majority (77.4%) of the parents belonged to upper-lower or lower socioeconomic strata according to modified Kuppuswamy scale [10]. The age of the fathers ranged from 23 to 64 years (mean ± SD = 31.02 ± 7.42) and that of mothers ranged from 20 to 55 years (mean ± SD = 27.11 ± 6.46). The educational status of fathers was illiterate (15.1%), primary (9.4%), intermediate (58.5%), and graduate (17%). The educational status of mothers was illiterate (37.7%), primary (9.4%), intermediate (45.3%), and graduate (7.5%). The interviewees were mothers in majority of the cases (31/53

or 58.5%) whereas fathers constituted 15.1% (8/53) and both parents were interviewed in 26.4% (14/53) of cases.

The parents' responses to the questions before and after viewing the film have been tabulated in Table 1. In the first interview 60.4% of parents answered correctly when asked about their knowledge regarding the aspect of development involved in CP by saying that the child had difficulty in holding neck/sitting/standing or walking. This figure rose significantly to 79.2% after watching the film. Thirteen (24.5%) of the parents were not aware of any of the treatment modalities of CP prior to watching of the film. After the film almost all knew about at least one treatment modality. The most common treatment modality which the parents knew of was physiotherapy.

The responses to a set of additional questions related to the film and its content which were asked in the follow-up interview have been tabulated in Table 2. The film described that child development is divided into 8 parts; 64% could recall that correctly and 69.8% remembered that the main part involved in CP was motor development. Majority (96.2%) could tell how they can contribute to better rehabilitation of their child.

There was no significant relation between the sex of the child; socioeconomic status; previous treatment or follow up at some other institutions; perinatal events; type of CP; or educational status of the parents on the change in parental knowledge of CP as assessed by chi-square/Fisher's exact test (P > 0.05).

4. Discussion

The majority of the subjects in the present study were unaware of basic knowledge of the disease like the correct name of the illness, its causation, the aspect of development involved, progression/course, curability, treatment modalities, and possibility of schooling. Thus there is lack of parental knowledge regarding cerebral palsy which is in accordance with previous studies [3, 5–9].

It has been seen that the parents of patients suffering from CP receive very little information from the treating physicians, nurses, and therapists and have many queries about the disease which tend to remain unanswered [8, 9]. This leads to lack of confidence interfering with the process of decision making [5, 7]. Also there is lack of educational activities to improve the parental knowledge; hence it leads to poor compliance with the treatment and interferes with the process of rehabilitation. There is need to better inform and educate family about the diagnosis, treatment, and prognosis so that the parents can make better decisions about their children and alleviate the stress that arises from ignorance and uncertainty [5, 8]. The best method of rehabilitative training of the child is to make the training activities part of the child's daily routine activities which can be accomplished only with parental involvement [4]. Greater understanding would form a relationship of trust between the families and the health professionals resulting in provision of better care and hence an improved outcome. In a study evaluating the knowledge of parents about child development in normal

TABLE 1: Parents response before and after viewing the educational film ($n = 53$).

Question	Response	Before	After	P value McNemar
What is the name of the illness from which your child suffers?	Correct	0 (0%)	24 (45.3%)	<0.001
	Incorrect	53 (100%)	29 (54.7%)	
What do you think is the cause of this disorder "cerebral palsy"?	Correct	14 (26.4%)	48 (90.6%)	<0.001
	Incorrect	39 (74.5%)	5 (9.4%)	
What aspect of child development is involved in cerebral palsy?	Correct	32 (60.4%)	42 (79.2%)	<0.001
	Incorrect	21 (39.6%)	11 (20.8%)	
Do you think that this disease will increase in severity?	Correct	19 (35.8%)	53 (100%)	<0.001
	Incorrect	34 (64.2%)	0 (0%)	
Will this disease be totally cured?	Correct	21 (39.6%)	50 (94.3%)	<0.001
	Incorrect	32 (60.4%)	3 (5.7%)	
Do you think that such children can get schooling or not?	Correct	33 (62.3%)	52 (98.1%)	<0.001
	Incorrect	20 (37.8%)	1 (1.9%)	
Are you aware of special schools for such children?	Yes	12 (22.6%)	35 (66.0%)	<0.001
	No	41 (77.4%)	18 (34.0%)	
Do you think that this disorder is preventable?	Correct	13 (24.5%)	48 (90.6%)	<0.001
	Incorrect	40 (75.5%)	5 (9.4%)	
How can CP be prevented?	Correct	11 (20.8%)	44 (83.0%)	<0.001
	Incorrect	42 (79.2%)	9 (17.0%)	

TABLE 2: Parents responses regarding the film and its content ($n = 53$).

Question	Yes/Correct	No/Incorrect
Was the film useful?	50 (94.3%)	3 (5.7%)
Did you acquire any additional knowledge about the disease?	46 (86.8%)	7 (13.2%)
Did you acquire any additional knowledge about the treatment?	44 (83.0%)	9 (17.0%)
Did you acquire any additional knowledge about the trainability of the child?	51 (96.2%)	2 (3.8%)
In the film child's development was divided into how many parts?	34 (64.2%)	19 (35.8%)
What are the main parts involved in cerebral palsy?	37 (69.8%)	16 (30.2%)
How can you contribute to better training of your child?	51 (96.2%)	2 (3.8%)

children, it was observed that the parents who have better knowledge about the stages of child's development can take better care of their children and this positively affects the child's development [11]. The same would be true for parents of disabled children as well.

There is paucity of studies carrying out any intervention like showing an educational film to improve the parental knowledge. In this study there occurred significant improvement in parental knowledge of CP after watching the educational film. Karande et al. carried out a single session structured educational programme comprising flash cards which also significantly improved the parental knowledge of CP [3]. In our study parents' knowledge about the disease, its probable aetiology and the fact that disease is not totally curable increased significantly. This is likely to have significant impact on parents' behaviour and help in management of the child.

The study population comprised almost double the number of male children as compared to female children which is greater than the usually observed sex ratio of 1.4 : 1 [12]. This disparity could be due to the preferential health seeking behaviour of parents for the male child. The mean age around which parents noticed their child's symptoms was 10 months, whereas mean age at diagnosis was around 20 months. This gap could probably be due to the fact that majority of the children were first in birth order hence parents being unaware of normal developmental milestones, due to delay in referral or establishment of definitive diagnosis of CP by doctors. It was observed that the majority of the interviewees were mothers. This is in accordance with previous literature which shows that more mothers than fathers are the primary care takers for their disabled children [3, 13, 14].

This study has the limitation of a brief period of follow-up, that is, 1 week, to assess the impact of the educational programme on the parental knowledge. There is need to carry out further studies to assess the long term impact of such an educational programme preferably as repeated sessions on the parental knowledge. The intervention that is the educational film used in this study was devised for Indian, Hindi speaking subjects; hence the results of the impact of this film cannot be applied to the other populations. There is need to develop similar educational films in local languages in accordance with the regional cultures and ethos in order to facilitate the understanding and improve the therapeutic outcome in CP children in other regions of the world.

As there was no significant correlation between socioeconomic and educational status of parents to the change in parental knowledge of CP hence such an educational film can help in improving parental knowledge of CP irrespective of parents' educational or socioeconomic background.

Thus we conclude that parental knowledge of CP is lacking and an intervention such as an educational film will have a positive impact on the parents' knowledge; hence measures such as educational film viewing should be a part of the management of cerebral palsy in special clinics.

Disclosure

The paper has been read and approved by all the authors and requirement for authorship of this document has been met. Each author believes that the paper represents honest work. They did not receive grants from any commercial entity in support of this work.

Conflict of Interests

There is no conflict of interests.

Authors' Contribution

Anju Aggarwal conceptualised the study. Anju Aggarwal, Shilpa Khanna Arora, and Hema Mittal designed the protocol. Shilpa Khanna Arora collected data. Anju Aggarwal, Shilpa Khanna Arora, and Hema Mittal analysed and interpreted data, searched the literature, and drafted the paper. Anju Aggarwal will act as guarantor for the study.

References

[1] P. Rosenbaum, "Cerebral palsy: what parents and doctors want to know," *British Medical Journal*, vol. 326, no. 7396, pp. 970–974, 2003.

[2] M. Gladstone, "A review of the incidence and prevalence, types and aetiology of childhood cerebral palsy in resource-poor settings," *Annals of Tropical Paediatrics*, vol. 30, no. 3, pp. 181–196, 2010.

[3] S. Karande, S. Patil, and M. Kulkarni, "Impact of an educational program on parental knowledge of cerebral palsy," *Indian Journal of Pediatrics*, vol. 75, no. 9, pp. 901–906, 2008.

[4] World Health Organisation, *Promoting the Development of Young Children with Cerebral Palsy*, 1993, http://whqlibdoc.who .int/hq/1993/WHO_RHB_93.1.pdf.

[5] M. F. M. Ribeiro, M. A. Barbosa, and C. C. Porto, "Cerebral palsy and down syndrome: level of parental knowledge and information," *Ciencia e Saude Coletiva*, vol. 16, no. 4, pp. 2099–2106, 2011.

[6] G. Baird, H. McConachie, and D. Scrutton, "Parents' perceptions of disclosure of the diagnosis of cerebral palsy," *Archives of Disease in Childhood*, vol. 83, no. 6, pp. 475–480, 2000.

[7] E. Sen and S. Yurtsever, "Difficulties experienced by families with disabled children," *Journal for Specialists in Pediatric Nursing*, vol. 12, no. 4, pp. 238–252, 2007.

[8] Y.-P. Huang, U. M. Kellett, and W. St John, "Cerebral palsy: experiences of mothers after learning their child's diagnosis," *Journal of Advanced Nursing*, vol. 66, no. 6, pp. 1213–1221, 2010.

[9] T. J. Donovan, D. S. Reddihough, J. M. Court, and L. W. Doyle, "Health literature for parents of children with cerebral palsy," *Developmental Medicine and Child Neurology*, vol. 31, no. 4, pp. 489–493, 1989.

[10] D. Mishra and H. P. Singh, "Kuppuswamy's socioeconomic status scale—a revision," *Indian Journal of Pediatrics*, vol. 70, no. 3, pp. 273–274, 2003.

[11] M. L. S. Moura, R. C. J. Ribas, C. A. Picinini et al., "Knowledge of child development in primiparous mothers from different urban centers," *Studies of Psychology*, vol. 9, pp. 421–429, 2004.

[12] M. V. Johnston, "Cerebral palsy," in *Nelson Textbook of Pediatrics*, R. M. Kliegman, B. F. Stanton, J. W. St Geme, N. F. Schor, R. E. Behrman, and H. B. Jenson, Eds., pp. 2061–2065, Saunders Elsevier, Philadelphia, Pa, USA, 19th edition, 2011.

[13] S. E. Green, ""What do you mean 'what's wrong with her?'" stigma and the lives of families of children with disabilities," *Social Science and Medicine*, vol. 57, no. 8, pp. 1361–1374, 2003.

[14] P. Raina, M. O'Donnell, P. Rosenbaum et al., "The health and well-being of caregivers of children with cerebral palsy," *Pediatrics*, vol. 115, no. 6, pp. e626–e636, 2005.

23

Genotyping of Methicillin Resistant *Staphylococcus aureus* Strains Isolated from Hospitalized Children

Mouna Ben Nejma,[1] **Abderrahmen Merghni,**[1] **and Maha Mastouri**[1,2]

[1] *Laboratoire des Maladies Transmissibles et Substances Biologiquement Actives "LR99ES27", Faculté de Pharmacie de Monastir, Avenue Avicenne, 5000 Monastir, Tunisia*
[2] *Laboratoire de Microbiologie, CHU Fattouma Bourguiba, 5000 Monastir, Tunisia*

Correspondence should be addressed to Mouna Ben Nejma; mounabennejma@yahoo.fr

Academic Editor: Francesco Porta

Community associated methicillin resistant *Staphylococcus aureus* (CA-MRSA) is an emerging pathogen increasingly reported to cause skin and soft tissue infections for children. The emergence of highly virulencet CA-MRSA strains in the immunodeficiency of young children seemed to be the basic explanation of the increased incidence of CA-MRSA infections among this population. The subjects of this study were 8 patients hospitalized in the Pediatric Department at the University Hospital of Monastir. The patients were young children (aged from 12 days to 18 months) who were suffering from MRSA skin infections; two of them had the infections within 72 h of their admission. The isolates were classified as community isolates as they all carried the staphylococcal cassette chromosome *mec* (SCC*mec*) IV and *pvl* genes. Epidemiological techniques, pulsed-field gel electrophoresis (PFGE) and multilocus sequence typing (MLST), were applied to investigate CA-MRSA strains. Analysis of molecular data revealed that MRSA strains were related according to PFGE patterns and they belonged to a single clone ST80. Antimicrobial susceptibility tests showed that all strains were resistant to kanamycin and 2 strains were resistant to erythromycin.

1. Introduction

Methicillin resistant *Staphylococcus aureus* (MRSA) was initially reported as a nosocomial pathogen responsible for adult infections [1]. However, MRSA strains have emerged in the community causing community-acquired infections. CA-MRSA has been recognized as a pathogen in adults and children without traditional risk factors for MRSA acquisition. Children colonized with MRSA are potential reservoirs for the spread of MRSA in the community [2, 3]. Furthermore, the infants and newborns with immunological immaturity, especially those born prematurely and those requiring specialized care, remained the major group susceptible to CA-MRSA infections.

Most CA-MRSA strains were associated with skin and soft tissue infections (SSTI) and necrotizing pneumonia [4]. The incidence of pediatric SSTI has increased rapidly in the previous decade [5–7].

Notably, community isolates differ significantly from nosocomial strains by the antimicrobial pattern and virulence profile. It is known that resistance to beta-lactams is mediated by the *mec*A gene carried by a mobile genetic element called staphylococcal cassette chromosome *mec* (SCC*mec*). CA-MRSA have been described as strains harboring the SCC*mec* type IV, type V, or type VII [8, 9] and remained susceptible to the majority of antimicrobial agents other than beta-lactams. Furthermore, these strains have been found to carry virulence genes encoding a leukocyte-killing toxin called the Panton-Valentine leukocidin (PVL) determinant [4].

In this report, we characterize clinical MRSA strains isolated from children hospitalized in the Pediatric Department at the University Hospital of Monastir, Tunisia. We are interested to investigate the phenotypic and genotypic markers of these isolates including antimicrobial resistance, SCC*mec* type, *pvl* genes, pulsed-field gel electrophoresis (PFGE) patterns, and multilocus sequence typing (MLST) of seven unlinked housekeeping genes (*arc*C, *aro*E, *glp*F, *gmk*, *pta*, *tpi*, and *yqil*).

2. Materials and Methods

2.1. Bacterial Strains. Eight MRSA strains were collected from clinical specimens of hospitalized children in the Pediatric Department at the University Hospital of Monastir, Tunisia, during a three-month period (from June to August 2013). The subjects were 6 boys and 2 girls, aged from 12 days to 18 months. The isolates were associated with skin infections: cutaneous abscesses (7 cases) and facial cellulites (1 case).

2.2. Identification. S. aureus were identified according to standard bacteriological procedures: Gram strain reactions, colony morphology, catalase, the ability to coagulate the rabbit plasma, and latex agglutination test (Bio-Rad).

2.3. Antimicrobial Susceptibility Tests. Susceptibility to the following antibiotics penicillin G, cefoxitin, moxalactam, kanamycin, amikacin, tobramycin, gentamicin, erythromycin, lincomycin, tetracycline, pristinamycin, furans, ofloxacin, trimethoprim-sulfamethoxazole, rifampicin, fusidic acid, fosfomycin, mupirocin, high mupirocin, vancomycin, teicoplanin, and linezolid was determined according to the recommendations of the Committee for Antimicrobial Testing of the French Society of Microbiology (CASFM) (http://www.sfm-microbiologie.org/) [10].

Methicillin resistance was determined by the disk diffusion method testing oxacillin disk (30 μg) on Mueller-Hinton agar supplemented with 2% sodium chloride.

2.4. Molecular Typing. Multiplex polymerase chain reaction (PCR) was applied to determine the SCC*mec* types according to a previous method described by Oliveira and de Lencastre [11]. *pvl* genes (*luk*S-PV, *luk*F-PV) were detected by PCR as previously described [12].

2.5. PFGE. The isolates were genotyped by pulsed-field gel electrophoresis (PFGE) using the restriction enzyme *Sma*I according to the method previously described [13]. Pulsotypes findings were interpreted according to the criteria proposed by Tenover et al. [14]. The patterns were designated by capital letter. A chromosomal DNA digest of *S. aureus* strain NCTC 8325 was used as the reference strain.

2.6. MLST Typing. MLST typing was performed as described by Enright et al. [15]. Allelic profiles and sequence type (ST) were designated using the MLST database (http://www.mlst.net).

2.7. Nucleotide Sequence Accession Numbers. The GenBank accession numbers of staphylococcal gene sequences, *arc*C, *aroe*, *glpf*, *gmk*, *pta*, *tpi*, and *yqil*, determined in this study were, respectively, JF495119, JF495120, JF495121, JF495122, JF495123, JF495124, and JF495125.

3. Results

In this study we investigate 8 MRSA strains isolated from patients hospitalized in the pediatric department. All isolates were identified as MRSA strains by the determination of methicillin resistance using oxacillin disk diffusion method. Antimicrobial susceptibility showed that all isolates were susceptible to the majority of 22 antibiotics tested (see Section 2) with the exception of the beta-lactams (oxacillin, penicillin G, and cefoxitin). All strains were resistant to kanamycin and only two of them were resistant to erythromycin.

For all clinical isolates the detection of *mec*A gene and the identification of SCC*mec* type were performed by amplification from genomic DNA, using multiplex PCR method according to Oliveira and de Lencastre method [11]. For each isolate, 2 amplified fragments were obtained: a 162 bp fragment and a 342 bp fragment. These two PCR products correspond to the amplification of *mec*A gene and specific SCC*mec* type IV locus (DCS), respectively.

Amplification of *pvl* genes (*luk*S-PV and *luk*F-PV) was performed also on the genomic DNA extracted from all strains. For each strain, the amplicon obtained has 433 bp; thus all MRSA strains harbor *pvl* genes. These results revealed that our clinical isolates have the peculiarities of CA-MRSA: susceptibility to the majority of antimicrobial agents and carrying SCC*mec* IV and *pvl* genes. To investigate the clonality of these CA-MRSA isolates, PFGE typing method was performed. PFGE pattern analysis demonstrated that they are distributed on three pulsotypes arbitrary designated A, B, and C (Figure 1). Six isolates carried the pulsotype A and two isolates carried the pulsotypes B and C, respectively. CA-MRSA strains were also characterized by multilocus sequencing of internal fragments of seven housekeeping genes (*arc*C, *aro*E, *glp*F, *gmk*, *pta*, *tpi*, and *yqil*). Nucleotide sequence analysis revealed that all isolates possess the same unique sequence type designated ST80.

4. Discussion and Conclusion

MRSA strain is known as a main cause of infections for children and young adults. MRSA strains investigated in this study are isolated from patients aged from 12 days to 18 months. Six children have been admitted with MRSA skin infections; hence, these data indicate that these infections were community-acquired but were not necessarily caused by community MRSA strains. However, the real site of MRSA acquisition is not readily determined because the community MRSA may designate MRSA colonization or a strain responsible for community infection detected in the community but not necessary acquired in the community. Two other ones are an 18-month-old child admitted with immunodeficiency and a 12-day-old child admitted with fever. They had cutaneous abscesses within 72 hours after their hospitalization. As referred to the definition of community MRSA infection, these isolates may be transmitted to these two patients from community.

Indeed, neonates are highly susceptible to MRSA colonization. CA-MRSA strains have been reported as a cause of

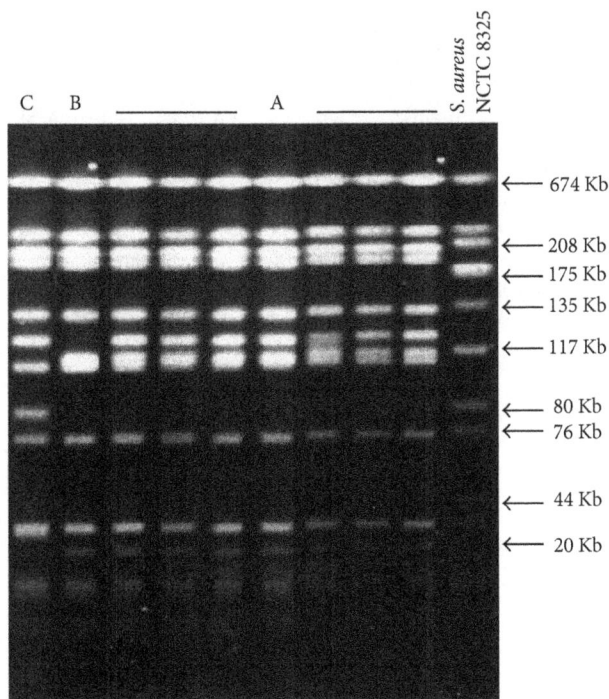

FIGURE 1: Representative PFGE patterns of MRSA strains isolated from children hospitalized in the pediatric department. A: pulsotype A; B: pulsotype B; C: pulsotype C; NCTC 8325: molecular weight marker.

colonization and infection in neonatal intensive care units in many countries [16, 17].

Furthermore, nasal carriage may be a possible explanation of the transmission of MRSA among these patients. The same observation was reported by Frazee et al. who considered that CA-MRSA is a common pathogen in cutaneous abscesses due to nasal carriage preceding infections [5]. It is interesting to note that newborns and young children, due to their immature immune systems, are easily infected by MRSA. Several similar studies reported that the majority of patients with MRSA infections were young children [6, 18]. For all strains antimicrobial resistance showed that they were resistant to oxacillin and susceptible to all non-beta-lactams. However the resistance to kanamycin and erythromycin has been also observed.

Molecular characterization of MRSA isolates by the identification of SCCmec type and the detection of lukS-PV and lukF-PV genes revealed that all strains harbored the SCCmec type IV and pvl genes. According to these results, our strains have been classified as community-acquired strains. Vandenesch et al. and Tenover et al. described SCCmec IV and pvl genes as markers for CA-MRSA [8, 19]. It has been reported that the cassette type IV and pvl genes have been found in some nosocomial MRSA strains [20–22].

PFGE analysis showed that CA-MRSA strains belonged to the same clone according to criteria of Tenover et al. [14]. MLST method revealed that all isolates have the same sequence type "ST80." Full analyses of molecular typing results suggest that isolates belong to the CA-MRSA ST80

clone. In fact, this clone is being increasingly reported in the community worldwide and mainly detected in Europe [8].

Our CA-MRSA strains display the resistance to kanamycin and to erythromycin. This antibiotic resistance pattern seems to be different from European strains "ST80," which were resistant to tetracycline and fusidic acid [23, 24].

MRSA is known as a nosocomial and a community pathogen. However, CA-MRSA has emerged within the hospital setting, posing a significant public health threat. So, what is most worrying is that these strains affect frequently newborns and young children and eventually cause potentially serious infections. In fact some MRSA epidemic clones have been reported to cause skins and soft tissue infections as well as severe diseases. Notably, "ST80" clone is recognized as a predominant clone in Europe, the United States, and Tunisia. This clone could become a health problem worldwide particularly that CA-MRSA strains were associated mainly with the presence of pvl genes which have an important impact on virulence. These observations urge emphasizing infection control measures to monitor the transmission of highly virulent CA-MRSA in our hospital.

Conflict of Interests

The authors have declared that there is no conflict of interests.

References

[1] W. R. Jarvis, C. Thornsberry, J. Boyce, and J. M. Hughes, "Methicillin-resistant Staphylococcus aureus at children's hospitals in the United States," Pediatric Infectious Disease, vol. 4, no. 6, pp. 651–655, 1985.

[2] H. F. Wertheim, D. C. Melles, M. C. Vos et al., "The role of nasal carriage in Staphylococcus aureus infections," The Lancet Infectious Diseases, vol. 5, no. 12, pp. 751–762, 2005.

[3] C. J. Chen, K. H. Hsu, T. Y. Lin, K. P. Hwang, P. Y. Chen, and Y. C. Huang, "Factors associated with nasal colonization of methicillin-resistant Staphylococcus aureus among healthy children in Taiwan," Journal of Clinical Microbiology, vol. 49, no. 1, pp. 131–137, 2011.

[4] G. Lina, Y. Piémont, F. Godail-Gamot et al., "Involvement of Panton-Valentine leukocidin-producing Staphylococcus aureus in primary skin infections and pneumonia," Clinical Infectious Diseases, vol. 29, no. 5, pp. 1128–1132, 1999.

[5] B. W. Frazee, J. Lynn, E. D. Charlebois, L. Lambert, D. Lowery, and F. Perdreau-Remington, "High prevalence of methicillin-resistant Staphylococcus aureus in emergency department skin and soft tissue infections," Annals of Emergency Medicine, vol. 45, no. 3, pp. 311–320, 2005.

[6] S. L. Kaplan, K. G. Hulten, B. E. Gonzalez et al., "Three-year surveillance of community-acquired Staphylococcus aureus infections in children," Clinical Infectious Diseases, vol. 40, no. 12, pp. 1785–1791, 2005.

[7] T. E. Zaoutis, P. Toltzis, J. Chu et al., "Clinical and molecular epidemiology of community-acquired methicillin-resistant Staphylococcus aureus infections among children with risk factors for health care-associated infection 2001–2003," Pediatric Infectious Disease Journal, vol. 25, no. 4, pp. 343–348, 2006.

[8] F. Vandenesch, T. Naimi, M. C. Enright et al., "Community-acquired methicillin-resistant Staphylococcus aureus carrying

panton-valentine leukocidin genes: worldwide emergence," *Emerging Infectious Diseases*, vol. 9, no. 8, pp. 978–984, 2003.

[9] R. H. Deurenberg and E. E. Stobberingh, "The evolution of *Staphylococcus aureus*," *Infection, Genetics and Evolution*, vol. 8, no. 6, pp. 747–763, 2008.

[10] Comité de l'Antibiogramme de la Société Française de Microbiologie, Communiqué, 2013, http://www.sfm-microbiologie .org/.

[11] D. C. Oliveira and H. de Lencastre, "Multiplex PCR strategy for rapid identification of structural types and variants of the mec element in methicillin-resistant Staphylococcus aureus," *Antimicrobial Agents and Chemotherapy*, vol. 46, no. 7, pp. 2155–2161, 2002.

[12] S. Jarraud, C. Mougel, J. Thioulouse et al., "Relationships between *Staphylococcus aureus* genetic background, virulence factors, agr groups (alleles), and human disease," *Infection and Immunity*, vol. 70, no. 2, pp. 631–641, 2002.

[13] D. S. Blanc, M. J. Struelens, A. Deplano et al., "Epidemiological validation of pulsed-field gel electrophoresis patterns for methicillin-resistant *Staphylococcus aureus*," *Journal of Clinical Microbiology*, vol. 39, no. 10, pp. 3442–3445, 2001.

[14] F. C. Tenover, R. D. Arbeit, R. V. Goering et al., "Interpreting chromosomal DNA restriction patterns produced by pulsed-field gel electrophoresis: criteria for bacterial strain typing," *Journal of Clinical Microbiology*, vol. 33, no. 9, pp. 2233–2239, 1995.

[15] M. C. Enright, N. P. J. Day, C. E. Davies, S. J. Peacock, and B. G. Spratt, "Multilocus sequence typing for characterization of methicillin-resistant and methicillin-susceptible clones of *Staphylococcus aureus*," *Journal of Clinical Microbiology*, vol. 38, no. 3, pp. 1008–1015, 2000.

[16] M. Giuffrè, C. Bonura, D. Cipolla, and C. Mammina, "MRSA infection in the neonatal intensive care unit," *Expert Review of Anti-Infective Therapy*, vol. 11, no. 5, pp. 499–509, 2013.

[17] D. M. Geraci, M. Giuffrè, C. Bonura et al., "Methicillin-resistant Staphylococcus aureus colonization: a three-year prospective study in a neonatal intensive care unit in Italy," *PLoS ONE*, vol. 9, no. 2, Article ID e87760, 2014.

[18] M. C. Lee, A. M. Rios, M. F. Aten et al., "Management and outcome of children with skin and soft tissue abscesses caused by community-acquired methicillin-resistant Staphylococcus aureus," *Pediatric Infectious Disease Journal*, vol. 23, no. 2, pp. 123–127, 2004.

[19] F. C. Tenover, L. K. McDougal, R. V. Goering et al., "Characterization of a strain of community-associated methicillin-resistant *Staphylococcus aureus* widely disseminated in the United States," *Journal of Clinical Microbiology*, vol. 44, no. 1, pp. 108–118, 2006.

[20] O. Cuevas, E. Cercenado, E. Bouza et al., "Molecular epidemiology of methicillin-resistant Staphylococcus aureus in Spain: a multicentre prevalence study (2002)," *Clinical Microbiology and Infection*, vol. 13, no. 3, pp. 250–256, 2007.

[21] N. A. Faria, D. C. Oliveira, H. Westh et al., "Epidemiology of emerging methicillin-resistant *Staphylococcus aureus* (MRSA) in Denmark: A nationwide study in a country with low prevalence of MRSA infection," *Journal of Clinical Microbiology*, vol. 43, no. 4, pp. 1836–1842, 2005.

[22] A. S. Rossney, A. C. Shore, P. M. Morgan, M. M. Fitzgibbon, B. O'Connell, and D. C. Coleman, "The emergence and importation of diverse genotypes of methicillin-resistant *Staphylococcus aureus* (MRSA) harboring the panton-valentine leukocidin

gene (pvl) reveal that pvl is a poor marker for community-acquired MRSA strains in Ireland," *Journal of Clinical Microbiology*, vol. 45, no. 8, pp. 2554–2563, 2007.

[23] W. Witte, C. Braulke, C. Cuny et al., "Emergence of methicillin-resistant Staphylococcus aureus with Panton-Valentine leukocidin genes in central Europe," *European Journal of Clinical Microbiology and Infectious Diseases*, vol. 24, no. 1, pp. 1–5, 2005.

[24] O. Denis, A. Deplano, H. De Beenhouwer et al., "Polyclonal emergence and importation of community-acquired methicillin-resistant *Staphylococcus aureus* strains harbouring Panton-Valentine leucocidin genes in Belgium," *Journal of Antimicrobial Chemotherapy*, vol. 56, no. 6, pp. 1103–1106, 2005.

24

SNAP II and SNAPPE II as Predictors of Neonatal Mortality in a Pediatric Intensive Care Unit: Does Postnatal Age Play a Role?

Mirta Noemi Mesquita Ramirez, Laura Evangelina Godoy, and Elizabeth Alvarez Barrientos

Hospital General Pediátrico "Niños de Acosta Ñú", Avenida de la Victoria and Bacigalupo, Reducto, 2160 San Lorenzo, Paraguay

Correspondence should be addressed to Mirta Noemi Mesquita Ramirez; mirtanmr@gmail.com

Academic Editor: Ju Lee Oei

Introduction. In developing countries, a lack of decentralization of perinatal care leads to many high-risk births occurring in facilities that do not have NICU, leading to admission to a PICU. *Objective.* To assess SNAP II and SNAPPE II as predictors of neonatal death in the PICU. *Methodology.* A prospective study of newborns divided into 3 groups according to postnatal age: Group 1 (G1), of 0 to 6 days; Group 2 (G2) of 7 to 14 days; and Group 3 (G3), of 15 to 28 days. Variables analyzed were SNAP II, SNAPPE II, perinatal data, and known risk factors for death. The Hosmer-Lemeshow test and the receiver operating characteristics (ROC) curve were used with SPSS 17.0 for statistical analysis. An Alpha error <5% was considered significant. *Results.* We analyzed 290 newborns, including 192 from G1, 41 from G2, and 57 from G3. Mortality was similar in all 3 groups. Median SNAP II was higher in newborns that died in all 3 groups ($P < 0.05$). The area under the ROC curve for SNAP II for G1 was 0.78 (CI 95% 0.70–0.86), for G2 0.66 (CI 95% 0.37–0.94), and for G3 0.74 (CI 95% 0.53–0.93). The area under the ROC curve for SNAPPE II for G1 was 0.76 (CI 95% 0.67–0.85), for G2 0.60 (CI 95% 0.30–0.90), and for G3 0.74 (CI 95% 0.52–0.95). *Conclusions.* SNAP II and SNAPPE II showed moderate discrimination in predicting mortality. The results are not strong enough to establish the correlation between the score and the risk of mortality.

1. Introduction

Birth weight has classically been considered as the most significant predictor of neonatal mortality. In developed countries, improvement of neonatal care, advances in neonatal ventilation, and in particular the use of pulmonary surfactant have not only reduced preterm neonatal mortality, but also increased survival for extremely premature infants. Other factors have been found to affect morbidity and mortality, among them the severity of disease upon hospitalization [1–3].

In the 1990s, Richardson et al. developed a system of assessment for the most important physiological variables affecting mortality in the first hours following admission. Each variable was assigned points based on the values found, and the result was the Score for Neonatal Acute Physiology (SNAP) [4].

SNAP assesses the worst clinical status found in the first 24 hours after admission using points assigned to 26 physiological variables: the higher the score, the greater the risk of death. With the Score for Neonatal Acute Physiology Perinatal Extension (SNAPPE), 3 additional variables were added: birth weight, the Apgar score, and being small for gestational age [4]. Due to the time needed to complete scoring, the authors subsequently developed a simplified version of the score, using only 5 variables to be measured within 12 hours of admission. The simplified scoring system was designated SNAP II and its perinatal extension SNAPPE II. These scoring systems have been validated in studies with large numbers of patients and have been shown to be good predictors of mortality in newborns in neonatal intensive care units (NICU). Use of the scoring systems has also allowed comparison of mortality rates from NICUs of different perinatal hospitals adjusted by severity of the disease at admission [5].

The clinical and epidemiological characteristics of newborns admitted to intensive therapy units in specialized hospitals present different clinical and epidemiological characteristics: they frequently of greater birth weight and are subjected to transfer procedures and show generally higher mortality [6]. Among risk factors cited for mortality of newborns managed in the NICU of pediatric hospitals are the transfer from other NICUs, presence of congenital malformations, and a requirement for surgery [6, 7]. It could be said that newborns entering polyvalent pediatric intensive care units (PICU) constitute a special subgroup of newborns. In developing countries, a lack of decentralization of perinatal care leads to many high-risk births occurring in facilities that do not have NICU, meaning that sick newborns must be transferred to specialized hospitals that may not possess an NICU, or may be overloaded with patients, leading to admission to a PICU. A group of newborns also exist who present with disease between the third and fourth weeks of life and require neonatal intensive care. Transfer of these newborns from one hospital to another is frequently done by means that are not adequate.

Our prospective study was done with the object of assessing whether SNAP II and SNAPPE II can predict mortality in this newborn population.

2. Material and Methods

We performed a prospective, observational, cohort study to assess SNAP II and SNAPPE II in a newborn population admitted to the PICU of the *Niños de Acosta Ñu* general pediatric hospital in Asunción, Paraguay. We included newborns with gestational ages between 28 and 42 weeks admitted to the PICU between January 2010 and December 2011. The newborns were divided into 3 groups according to postnatal age at admission: Group 1 (G1) was newborns with postnatal ages of from a few hours to 6 days, Group 2 (G2) were between 7 and 14 days of age, and Group 3 (G3) was from 15 to 28 days of age. Division of the population into 3 postnatal age groups at admission was decided based on the particular characteristics of each age group. Group 1 was comprised of the youngest newborns, who presented predominantly respiratory disease and symptoms of perinatal asphyxia. Group 2 was generally more stable newborns who had been hospitalized in less-well equipped hospitals and were transferred to the pediatric hospital by the reference counterreference system (including exchange of less seriously ill patients to less specialized institutions to avoid overloading), or due to complications and a requirement for mechanically assisted ventilation. Group 3 was comprised of newborns of more than 2 weeks of life who were admitted largely due to symptoms of severe bronchiolitis or late-onset neonatal sepsis.

The transfer of newborns from rural areas of the country to hospitals in the city is not always performed under appropriate conditions, for example, ambulance equipped with transport incubator and trained health workers. This is due to the small number of ambulances with proper equipment and lack of trained personnel. Many of the infants hospitalized in the pediatric hospital "Children of Acosta Nu" come from rural areas.

Variables for SNAP II and SNAPPE II scoring were taken from the patient medical records on a form created for this purpose within 12 hours of hospitalization. We excluded newborns who died within 12 hours of admission and those with congenital malformations incompatible with life. To determine the SNAPPE II score, newborns were excluded who did not receive immediate care at a health care institution (home childbirth), due to their lack of birth weight figures and Apgar tests.

Variables other than the scores analyzed were birth weight, gestational age, sex, Apgar test at 1 min. and 5 min., place and type of parturition, postnatal age at admission, intrauterine growth restriction, transfer from other hospitals, and congenital malformations. The clinical progress of patients was analyzed according to surgical intervention, entry to mechanically assisted ventilation (MV), and hospital discharge (living or dead).

For data analysis, the contingency table, Chi Square test, proportions, comparison of medians, and parametric and nonparametric means were used according to type, distribution, and variance of the variables. Analyses of true and false positives for each scoring value were done by calculating the area under the curve (AUC) using the receiving operating characteristic curve (ROC) and Hosmer-Lemeshow goodness-of-fit test for calibration of scoring using SPSS 17.0. An Alpha error of less than 5% was considered significant.

Ethical Considerations. Confidentiality of data was maintained at all times. Patient identifiers, for example, names, addresses, and so forth, were removed after data acquisition and subjects were then identified by study numbers. The protocol was approved by the hospital research and ethics committee (approval number 0022).

3. Results

In the period from January 2010 to December 2011, 350 newborns were admitted to the polyvalent PICU of our hospital, of which 60 were excluded: 2 due to congenital malformations incompatible with life, 3 due to death prior to 12 hours after admission, and 55 due to the score having not been provided prospectively. We analyzed 290 newborns. Of the 290, 192 (66%) were assigned to Group 1 (G1), 41 (14%) to Group 2 (G2), and 57 (20%) to Group 3 (G3).

No difference was found in perinatal data between the 3 groups in birth weight or percentage of low birth weight (LBW), very low birth weight (VLBW), gestational age, Apgar score at 1 min. and at 5 min., sex, place and type of parturition, or presence of intrauterine growth restriction (IUGR). Apgar score and birth weight were obtained for 232 newborns (data for 58 newborns, 39 from G1, 5 from G2, and 14 from G3 were unavailable due to home births or inability to verify data with the perinatal birth record) (Table 1).

Differences were found between groups for known risk factors in our population, including transfer from other hospitals (prior hospitalization) in the G2 group of 30 of 41 (73%); in the G1 group of 109 of 192 (57%:); and the G3 group of 19 of 57 (33%) ($P < 0.01$). The largest percentage of perinatal asphyxia was found in the G1 group, with 20%

TABLE 1: Perinatal data of the three groups $n = 290$. LBW (low birth weight); VLBW (very low birth weight) IUGR (intrauterine growth restriction).

	Group 1	Group 2	Group 3	P
Birth weight (g) Medians (range) ($n = 232$)	2900 (670–5100)	3000 (1050–4710)	2900 (1070–4500)	NS
LBW (%)	36	42	27	NS
VLBW (%)	12	15	5	NS
Gestational age Medians (range) ($n = 232$)	37 (27–42)	37 (27–40)	38 (28–40)	NS
Apgar score 1 min	6 (1–9)	7 (2–9)	7 (2–9)	NS
Apgar score 5 min Medians (range) ($n = 232$)	9 (3–10)	8 (2–9)	9 (5–9)	NS
Male sex (%)	64	54	51	NS
Delivery (%)				
Vaginal	66	73	79	NS
Caesarean	34	27	21	NS
Hospital birth (%) ($n = 232$)	80	88	68	NS
Home birth ($n = 58$)	20	12	22	NS
IUGR (%)	27	24	28	NS

TABLE 2: Mortality risk factors in each group studied. MV (mechanical ventilation).

	Group 1	Group 2	Group 3	P
SNAP II ($n = 290$) (median)	10	5	6	<0.05
SNAPPE II ($n = 232$) (median)	13	7	8	<0.05
Prior hospitalization (%)	57	73	33	<0.05
Congenital malformations (%)	30	24	26	NS
Surgery (%)	29	19,5	21	NS
Perinatal asphyxia (%)	20	10	2	<0.05
Nosocomial infection (%)	33	19,5	21	NS
MV (%)	60	37	40	NS

(39/192), compared to 10% (9/41) in the G2 group, and 2% (1/57) in the G3 group ($P < 0.05$). No differences were found in other risk factors analyzed (Table 2).

Overall mortality was 71 of 290 (24%). Mortality by age group was G1 52 of 192 (27%); G2 7 of 41 (17%); and G3 12 of 57 (21%). Although Group G1 had the highest mortality rate, the difference compared to other groups was not significant (OR 1.45 [CI 95% 0.8–2.2] $P > 0.05$).

Analysis of severity at admission measured by SNAP II ($n = 290$) scores showed higher values for newborns who died compared to those discharged alive in all 3 groups. Median SNAPPE II scoring (taken in 232 newborns) was also higher for newborns who died compared to those who survived in Groups 1 and 3, but not in Group 2, for which analysis did not show statistical significance (Table 3).

Analysis using the ROC curve showed that the area under the curve using SNAP II scores for G1 was 0.78 (CI 95% 0.71–0.86) Figure 1. While for SNAPPE II ($n = 153$) it was 0.75 (CI 95% 0.67–0.84). The Hosmer-Lemeshow goodness-of-fit test result was 0.7.

For G2, the SNAP II score was 0.66 (CI 95% 0.37–0.94), while for SNAPPE II ($n = 36$) it was 0.60 (CI 95% 0.30–0.90). For G3, the SNAP II score was 0.74 (0.53–0.93), while for SNAPPE II ($n = 43$) it was 0.74 (0.52–0.95).

4. Discussion

No significant differences in severity scores were found between the 3 groups of newborns of different postnatal ages. The median SNAP II score was significantly higher in newborns who died compared to those who survived in all 3 groups. The SNAPPE II score was also higher in newborns who died from Groups 1 and 3, but not in Group 2, which we attribute to the small number of patients. Analysis of the ROC curve for both SNAP II and SNAPPE II showed an area under

TABLE 3: Median of SNAP II and SNAPPE II score of the three groups and the condition at discharge.

Group	Condition at discharged	SNAP II	P	SNAPPE II	P
G1	Alive	5	<0.05	5	<0.05
	Deceased	16		22	
G2	Alive	0	<0.05	0	>0.05
	Deceased	10		8	
G3	Alive	0	<0.05	0	<0.05
	Deceased	13		17	

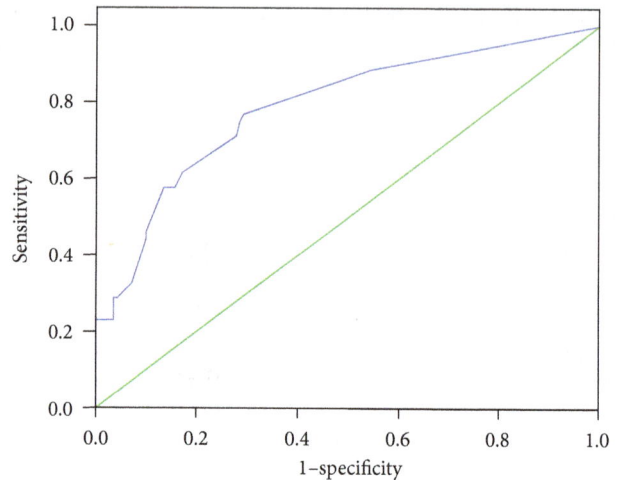

FIGURE 1: Analysis using the ROC curve showed that the area under the curve using SNAP II scores for Group 1 was 0.78 (CI 95% 0.71–0.86).

the curve with moderate values in Groups 1 and 3, but not for Group 2, as due to the small number of patients analyzed, with 7 deaths, a good curve could not be generated. These results are similar to those found by the authors of a study carried out at the same polyvalent pediatric intensive care unit of the hospital from 2006 to 2009, and in which the SNAP II and SNAPPE II scores were determined retrospectively in a group of 288 newborns with characteristics similar to those of our patients but analyzed as a single group without considering postnatal age. We found that both scores in that study showed higher values for newborns who died compared to survivors, with analysis of the ROC curve showing an area under the curve for SNAP II of 0.79 (CI 95% 0.72–0.85) and for SNAPPE II of 0.77 (CI 95% 0.69–0.86) [8]. Those findings were similar to those of the newborns in Group 1 of our study.

We have not found studies validating SNAP II and SNAPPE II scoring in populations of newborns with characteristics similar to our sample. Vasudenan et al. carried out a study using SNAP scoring in India in a population of newborns with an average postnatal age of 13 days who had been admitted to a polyvalent PICU similar to our own. In the 97 newborns analyzed scoring was significantly higher in patients who died compared to survivors and the ROC curve showed an area under the curve of 0.77 (CI 95% 0.68–0.87) [9]. These results are comparable to ours despite the use of a more complex scoring system with a larger number of physiological variables and greater time required for completion.

In another study, with a population comparable to ours in terms of postnatal age and being carried out in a developing country, although in a neonatal intensive care unit (NICU) and using different analyses, a high SNAP II score and low Apgar at 5 min. were associated with neonatal mortality in regression analysis [10].

Use of SNAP II and SNAPPE II in newborns with postnatal ages greater than 24 hours has been assessed in various studies and in specific situations in neonatal units, with varied results. In some, they did not predict mortality, sepsis, or enterocolitis [11]. In others, such as that carried out at a NICU in India, SNAP II scoring was analyzed as a predictor of mortality in very low birth weight (VLBW) newborns within average postnatal age of 4 days and diagnosis of severe septicemia. SNAP II scoring was done within 12 hours of onset of signs and symptoms. Patients who died showed a significantly higher score than those who survived. The cutoff

point was 40, with a positive predictive value of 88% [12]. A similar cutoff point was used by Nakwan et al., who assessed SNAP II in patients with persistent pulmonary hypertension. Although it showed moderate discrimination in the study population (0.71 [CI 95% 0.56–0.88]), patients with a score ≥43 showed higher risk of death [7]. In our study the very low birth weight (VLBW) population was not analyzed as a group due to the small number of such patients.

The high percentage of congenital malformations observed in our study population is explained by our hospital being a neonatal surgery hospital of reference. It has also been a cardiovascular surgery hospital of reference for the last two years, leading to increased admission of newborns with congenital cardiopathies, who however were not included in our study as they are managed by the intensive care unit of the pediatric cardiology department. Published reports exist of validation of SNAP and SNAP II in newborns with congenital cardiopathies and other malformations such as congenital diaphragmatic hernia, for which they were not very good predictors of mortality [13, 14].

As a specialized pediatric hospital, 100% of newborns admitted are transported, whether from their homes or other hospitals. One very important variable is neonatal transport, which can influence clinical deterioration of the patient at admission [15]. In the population we studied, transport of the majority of patients is not done appropriately or with prior referral, meaning that the transport risk index of physiologic stability (TRIPS) cannot be done due to a lack of pretransport data.

In our study, SNAP II and SNAPPE II scoring showed better discrimination as predictors of mortality in the group of newborns of lowest postnatal age at admission (Group 1), but this was much lower than that reported in newborns in perinatal hospitals. This group of newborns comprised the group with the largest number of patients, thereby permitting better analysis. The newborns in this group had higher severity scores at admission compared to those from Groups 2 and 3, and mortality among them was also higher, although not reaching significance.

It is possible that mortality in the newborn population we studied is associated with other factors aside from severity at admission, such as neonatal transport and nosocomial infections.

Conflict of Interests

The authors declare that there is no conflict of interests regarding the publication of this paper.

References

[1] J. E. Gray, D. K. Richardson, M. C. McCormick, K. Workman-Daniels, and D. A. Goldmann, "Neonatal therapeutic intervention scoring system: a therapy-based severity-of-illness index," *Pediatrics*, vol. 9, pp. 561–567, 1992.

[2] J. Dorling, D. J. Field, and M. Manketelow, "Neonatal diseases severity scoring system," *Archives of Disease in Childhood—Fetal and Neonatal Edition*, vol. 90, pp. F11–F16, 2005.

[3] D. K. Richardson, C. S. Phibbs, J. E. Gray, M. C. McCormick, K. Workman-Daniels, and D. A. Goldmann, "Birth weight and illness severity: independent predictors of neonatal mortality," *Pediatrics*, vol. 91, pp. 969–975, 1993.

[4] D. K. Richardson, J. E. Gray, M. C. McCormick, K. Workman, and D. A. Goldman, "Score for neonatal acute physiology: a physiologic severity index for neonatal intensive care," *Pediatrics*, vol. 91, pp. 617–623, 1993.

[5] D. K. Richardson, J. D. Corcoran, and G. J. Escobar, "SNAP II and SNAP—PE II simplifies newborn illness severity and mortality risk scores," *Journal of Pediatrics*, vol. 138, pp. 92–100, 2001.

[6] M. A. Berry, P. S. Shah, R. T. Brouillette, and J. Hellmann, "Predictors of mortality and length of stay for neonates admitted to children's hospital neonatal intensive care units," *Journal of Perinatology*, vol. 28, no. 4, pp. 297–302, 2008.

[7] N. Nakwan and J. Wannaro, "Predicting mortality in infants with persistent pulmonary hypertension of the newborn with the score for neonatal acute physiology. Version II, (SNAPII) in Thai neonates," *Journal of Perinatal Medicine*, vol. 39, pp. 311–315, 2011.

[8] M. Mesquita, E. Alvarez, L. Godoy, and S. Avalos, "Scores de gravedad SNAP II y SNAPE II en la determinación de riesgo de mortalidad neonatal en una unidad de cuidados intensivos polivalente," *Pediatría*, vol. 38, pp. 93–100, 2011.

[9] A. Vasudevan, A. Malhotra, R. Lodha, and S. K. Kabra, "Profile of neonates admitted in pediatric ICU validation of score for neonatal acute physiology (SNAP)," *Indian Pediatrics*, vol. 43, pp. 344–348, 2006.

[10] M. Kadivar, S. Saghed, S. Bavafa, F. Moghadan, and B. Eshrati, "Neonatal mortality risk assessment in a neonata intensive care unit," *Iranian Journal of Pediatrics*, vol. 17, pp. 325–331, 2007.

[11] L. Lim and H. J. Rozycki, "Postnatal SNAP II score in neonatal intensive care unit patients : relationship to sepsis, necrotizing enterocolitis and death," *Journal of Maternal—Fetal and Neonatal Medicine*, vol. 21, pp. 415–419, 2008.

[12] S. Venkataseshan, Sourabh, J. Ahluwalia, and N. Anil, "Score for neonatal acute physiology II predicts mortality and persistent organ dysfunction in neonates with severe septicemia," *Indian Pediatrics*, vol. 46, pp. 775–780, 2009.

[13] E. D. Skarsgard, Y. C. McNab, R. Little, and S. K. Lee, "SNAP II predicts mortality among infants with congenital diaphragmatic hernia," *Journal of Perinatology*, vol. 25, pp. 315–319, 2005.

[14] L. L. Simpson, K. Harvey-Wilkes, and M. E. DÁlton, "Congenital heart diseases: the impact of delivery in a tertiary care center on SNAP scores (score for neonatal acute physiology)," *The American Journal of Obstetrics & Gynecology*, vol. 182, pp. 184–191, 2000.

[15] G. Golsmitt, C. Rabasa, S. Rodriguez et al., "Factores de reiego asociados al deterioro clínico en el traslado de recién nacidos enfermos," *Archivos Argentinos de Pediatria*, vol. 110, pp. 304–310, 2012.

25

Interplay of T Helper 17 Cells with $CD4^+CD25^{high}$ $FOXP3^+$ Tregs in Regulation of Allergic Asthma in Pediatric Patients

Amit Agarwal,[1] Meenu Singh,[1] B. P. Chatterjee,[2] Anil Chauhan,[1] and Anuradha Chakraborti[3]

[1] *Advanced Pediatric Centre, Post Graduate Institute of Medical Education and Research, Sector 12, Chandigarh 160012, India*
[2] *Department of Natural Science, West Bengal University of Technology, Kolkata 700064, India*
[3] *Department of Experimental Medicine and Biotechnology, Post Graduate Institute of Medical Education and Research, Chandigarh 160012, India*

Correspondence should be addressed to Meenu Singh; meenusingh4@gmail.com

Academic Editor: Emmanuel Katsanis

Background. There is evidence that Tregs are important to prevent allergic diseases like asthma but limited literature exists on role of T_H17 cells in allergic diseases. *Methods.* Fifty children with asthma and respiratory allergy (study group) and twenty healthy children (control group) were recruited in this study. Total IgE levels and pulmonary function tests were assessed. The expression of Tregs and cytokines was determined by flow cytometry. *Results.* The average level of total IgE in study group (316.8 ± 189.8 IU/mL) was significantly higher than controls (50 ± 17.5 IU/mL, $P < 0.0001$). The frequency of T_H17 cells and culture supernatant level of IL-17 in study group (12.09 ± 8.67 pg/mL) was significantly higher than control group (2.01 ± 1.27 pg/mL, $P < 0.001$). Alternatively, the frequency of FOXP3 level was significantly lower in study group [(49.00 ± 13.47)%] than in control group [(95.91 ± 2.63)%] and $CD4^+CD25^+FOXP3^+$ to $CD4^+CD25^+$ ratio was also significantly decreased in study group [(6.33 ± 2.18)%] compared to control group [(38.61 ± 11.04)%]. The total serum IgE level is negatively correlated with FOXP3 level ($r = -0.5273$, $P < 0.0001$). The FOXP3 expression is negatively correlated with the IL-17 levels ($r = -0.5631$, $P < 0.0001$) and IL-4 levels ($r = -0.2836$, $P = 0.0460$). *Conclusions.* Imbalance in T_H17/Tregs, elevated IL-17, and IL-4 response and downregulation of FOXP3 were associated with allergic asthma.

1. Introduction

Asthma, characterized by T_H2 immune response, is a chronic inflammatory disorder, affecting children worldwide [1]. It is now universally accepted that T_H2 cytokines play a critical role in amplifying asthma [2] whereas T_H1 cytokines prevent this allergic inflammation [3, 4]. In recent years, it has been shown that the manifestation of asthma in humans is beyond the control of T_H1 and T_H2 cells. Some studies have suggested that other T cell subsets like T_H17 and Treg also play a role in regulating asthma [5]. Treg cells play a key role in the maintenance and tolerance of immune regulation [6] by suppression of T_H1, T_H2, T_H17, and allergen specific IgE. They have also been found to suppress basophils, eosinophils, and mast cells but induce levels of specific IgG4 [7]. Different types of Treg cells are classified as natural and adaptive [8]. Natural Treg cells possess high levels of CD25 ($CD25^{high}$) present on the surface of T cells and the expression of FOXP3 required for the generation and maintenance of their suppressive activity [6, 8, 9]. FOXP3 appears to be a key marker for $CD4^+CD25^+$ T cells and is considered as a master switch for development and function of natural Treg cells [10–13]. Recent studies suggest that Treg cells adopt different mechanisms to suppress immune responses: directly via cell contact and indirectly via reducing the capacity of antigen presentation on antigen presenting cells [14] or via anti-inflammatory cytokines [15, 16]. Some studies have suggested that pulmonary $CD4^+CD25^{high}$ Tregs are impaired in pediatric asthma [17]. A new subset of $CD4^+$ T cells, termed as T_H17, produces IL-17 [18]. T_H17 cells are now considered the key mediator in development of asthma [19]. T_H17 cells enhance both neutrophilic and eosinophilic airway inflammation in mouse model of asthma [20, 21]. T_H17 cells play a key role in filling the gap between T_H1 and T_H2 by secreting IL-17A and IL-17F and also contributing to immunity against certain extracellular bacteria and fungi [22]. IL-17, a proinflammatory cytokine mainly derived from $CD4^+$ T cells and also from monocytes, mast cells, macrophages, and neutrophils [23, 24], has been suggested in modulating various inflammatory diseases like asthma in humans [24–26]. T_H1 and T_H2 cells as well as T_H17 differentiation are suppressed by Tregs [27]. However, Treg cells do not suppress T_H17 cells *in vitro* [28, 29]. Recent evidence indicates that $CD4^+CD25^{high}FOXP3^+$ Tregs and T_H17 cells play an important role in mediating asthma.

Hypothesis. The null hypothesis states that T regulatory cells do not play any role in bronchial asthma. We hypothesize that T regulatory cells play a protective role in asthma. T regulatory cells, which regulate the balance between T_H1 and T_H2 cells, are downregulated in cases of asthma and allergy.

2. Materials and Methods

2.1. Subjects. Fifty children with asthma (study group) and twenty healthy children (control group) who were matched for age (in months) (control (88.86 ± 38.67); study group, (85.95 ± 35.55)) attended the Advanced Pediatric Centre in Post Graduate Institute of Medical Education and Research (PGIMER), Chandigarh, and were diagnosed as asthma and were recruited in this study with their informed consent. The sera of age and sex matched nonallergic patients were taken as controls. The Ethics Committee of PGIMER approved this study (Micro/2006/754/8th May 2006).

2.2. Methods. The diagnosis of asthma was made by clinical history, physical examination, FEV1 measurement, positive response to bronchodilators, positive skin prick test, and elevated total IgE. The asthma of all patients was under control with inhaled corticosteroids. Blood samples were collected for evaluation of T_H1, T_H2, and T_H17 expression and T_{reg} cells.

2.3. Estimation of Total IgE. The total IgE of allergic patients was measured using PATHOZYME immunoglobulin E OD 417 kit. The absorbance was measured at 450 nm after addition of tetramethyl benzidine hydrochloride (TMB) substrate and dilute hydrochloric acid. The concentration of IgE is directly proportional to the color intensity of the test samples. This test was calibrated to WHO 2nd International Reference Preparation 75/502 (1981).

2.4. Sample Preparation. Five milliliters of heparinized blood was obtained from 20 healthy subjects and 50 asthmatic patients. For cytokine analysis, plasma was isolated from peripheral blood and stored at $-80°C$ until it was used. Peripheral blood mononuclear cells (PBMC) were isolated from heparinized blood sample by density gradient centrifugation (250 g for 20 minutes at room temperature) using Histopaque (Sigma-Aldrich, Saint Louis, MO, USA).

2.5. Flow Cytometric Analysis. The serum levels of cytokines Th1 (IFN-γ), Th2 (IL-2, IL-4, IL-6, IL-10, IL-12, and IL-13), and Th17 (IL-17) were assessed using BD CBA flex set. Tests were performed according to manufacturer's instructions (BD Cytometric Bead Array, San Diego, CA). The analysis was carried out using flow cytometry (FACSCanto (Becton Dickinson, Mountain View, CA, USA) with FACS Diva Software).

For analysis of Treg cells, the buffy coat (lymphocytes and monocytes) was separated. The cell pellet washed with PBS (Phosphate Buffer Saline) was centrifuged at 200 g for 15 minutes. PBMCs were cultured in a petri dish containing 5% CO_2 at 37°C for one and half hour. Surface phenotyping (CD4 and CD25) of the cells (peripheral blood lymphocytes) and intracellular phenotyping (FOXP3) were performed by staining, paraformaldehyde fixation, and permeabilization according to the manufacturer's instructions (BD biosciences San Diego, CA). PBMCs were determined using forward and side scatter properties based on size and granularity by FACSCanto (Becton Dickinson, Mountain View, CA, USA) with FACS Diva Software. The following mAbs (BD biosciences) were used: APC antihuman CD4, PE-Cy antihuman CD25, and PE antihuman FOXP3. To correct nonspecific binding, matched isotype controls were used.

2.6. Statistical Analysis. Data were analyzed with SPSS (v16.0; SPSS Inc, Chicago, IL, USA) and Graphpad prism (v5.0; Graphpad software Inc, Le Jolla, CA, USA). The mean values and their internal differentiation with standard deviations were calculated. The spearman's r rank correlation coefficients were used to evaluate relationship between variables. When assessing the flow cytometric data, Student's t-test was used. P values <0.05 were considered statistically significant.

3. Results

Total IgE and FEV1 levels were tested in all children diagnosed with asthma. The difference between IgE levels in study and control group was analyzed using Graphpad Prism software. The nonparametric Student's t-test was applied between study group and control group for total IgE level. The average level of total IgE in study group (316.8 ± 189.8 IU/mL, range 80–720 IU/mL) was significantly higher than in control group (50.3 ± 17.5 IU/mL, range 10–80 IU/mL, $P < 0.001$) (Figure 1(a)). FEV1 (% predicted) was significantly lower in study group (75.36 ± 14.45) compared to control group (102.3 ± 8.97, $P < 0.0001$) (Table 1). Total serum IgE and FEV1 levels were also analyzed for their correlation studies. This was analyzed using Spearman's correlation coefficient in study group only. There was a negative correlation between total IgE and FEV1% levels ($r = -0.4820$, $P = 0.0004$) (Figure 1(b)).

3.1. Expression of Cytokines in Asthmatic Children. Levels of cytokines IL-2, IL-4, IL-6, IL-10, IL-12, IL-13, IFN-γ, and IL-17 in sera were expressed as mean $\pm$ standard deviation. The average level of IL-17 expression in study group (12.09 ± 8.67 pg/mL) was significantly higher than the corresponding values in control group (2.01 ± 1.27 pg/mL, $P < 0.0001$)

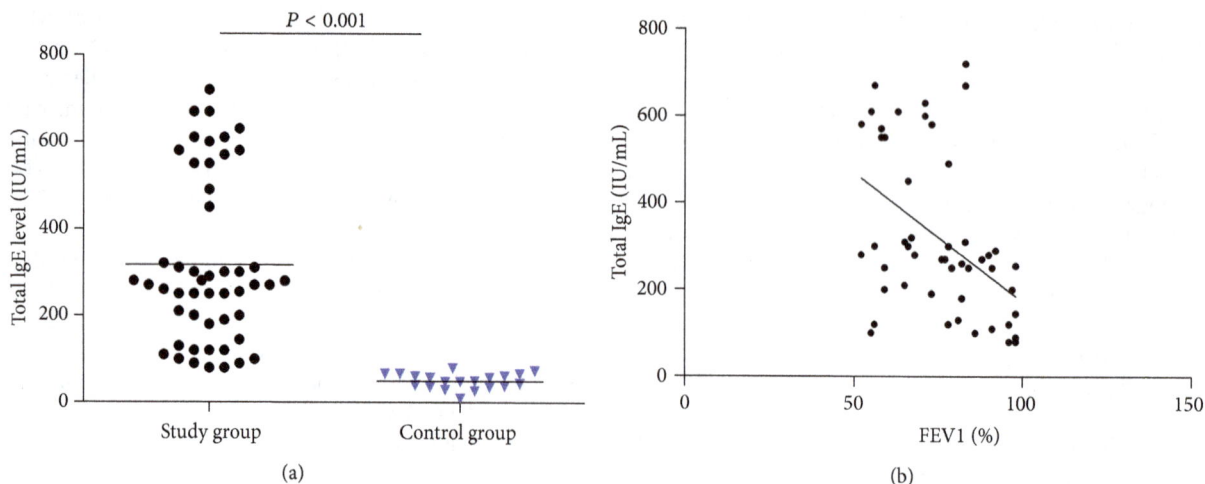

(a)

(b)

FIGURE 1: (a) Total IgE level in study and control group. (b) Correlation between total IgE and % FEV1 levels in study group.

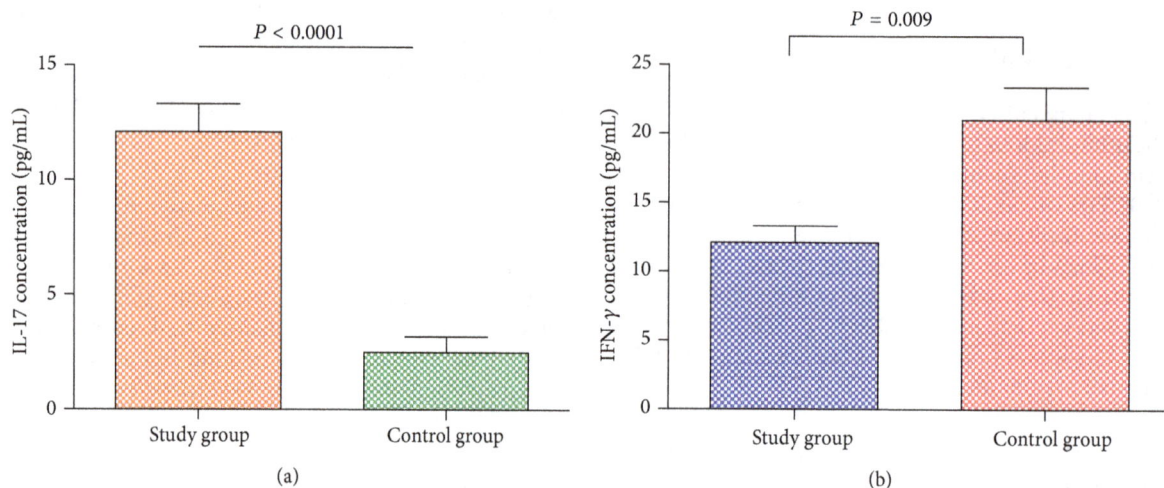

(a)

(b)

FIGURE 2: (a) IL-17 and (b) IFN-γ expression in study and control.

TABLE 1: Patients characteristics.

	Study group	Control group
Total subjects	50	20
Age (months) (mean ± SD)	88.86 ± 38.67	85.95 ± 35.55
Male; n (%)	40 (80%)	14 (70%)
Total IgE (IU/mL) (mean ± SD)	316.8 ± 189.8	50.3 ± 17.5
FEV$_1$ % (mean ± SD)	75.36 ± 14.45	102.3 ± 8.97

(Figure 2(a)) but values of IFN-γ were significantly lower in study group (12.08 ± 8.67 pg/mL) compared to control group (21.00 ± 7.53 pg/mL, $P = 0.009$) (Figure 2(b)). No significant difference was observed between study and control group for other cytokines (IL-2: 20.78 ± 9.22 pg/mL versus 18.93 ± 13.73 pg/mL ($P = 0.51$); IL-4: 21.88 ± 10.35 pg/mL versus 19.79±12.38 pg/mL ($P = 0.47$); IL-6: 18.17±10.49 pg/mL versus 15.11 ± 9.79 pg/mL ($P = 0.08$); IL-10: 22.82 ± 19.16 pg/mL

versus 18.62 ± 5.31 pg/mL ($P = 0.35$); IL-12: 17.58 ± 9.27 pg/mL versus 16.94 ± 11.00 ($P = 0.52$); IL-13: 34.55 ± 17.51 pg/mL versus 29.39±10.12 pg/mL ($P = 0.40$)) (Table 2).

The Student's t-test was done to analyze IL-17 in control and study group. The results depict a significant difference between the two groups ($P < 0.0001$). Similarly, there was also significant difference between study group and control group for IFN-γ ($P = 0.009$).

Flow cytometric analysis of FOXP3 was performed in CD4$^+$CD25$^+$ cells for both control ($n = 20$) (Figure 3) and study group ($n = 50$) (Figure 4). The percentages of FOXP3 expression were significantly lower in study group ((49.00 ± 13.47)%) than in control group ((95.91 ± 2.63)%, $P < 0.0001$) (Figure 5).

A further analysis was done to calculate CD4$^+$CD25$^+$ FOXP3$^+$ to CD4$^+$CD25$^+$ ratio, which was significantly decreased in study group ((6.33 ± 2.18)%) compared to control group ((38.61 ± 11.04)%, $P < 0.0001$) (Figure 6).

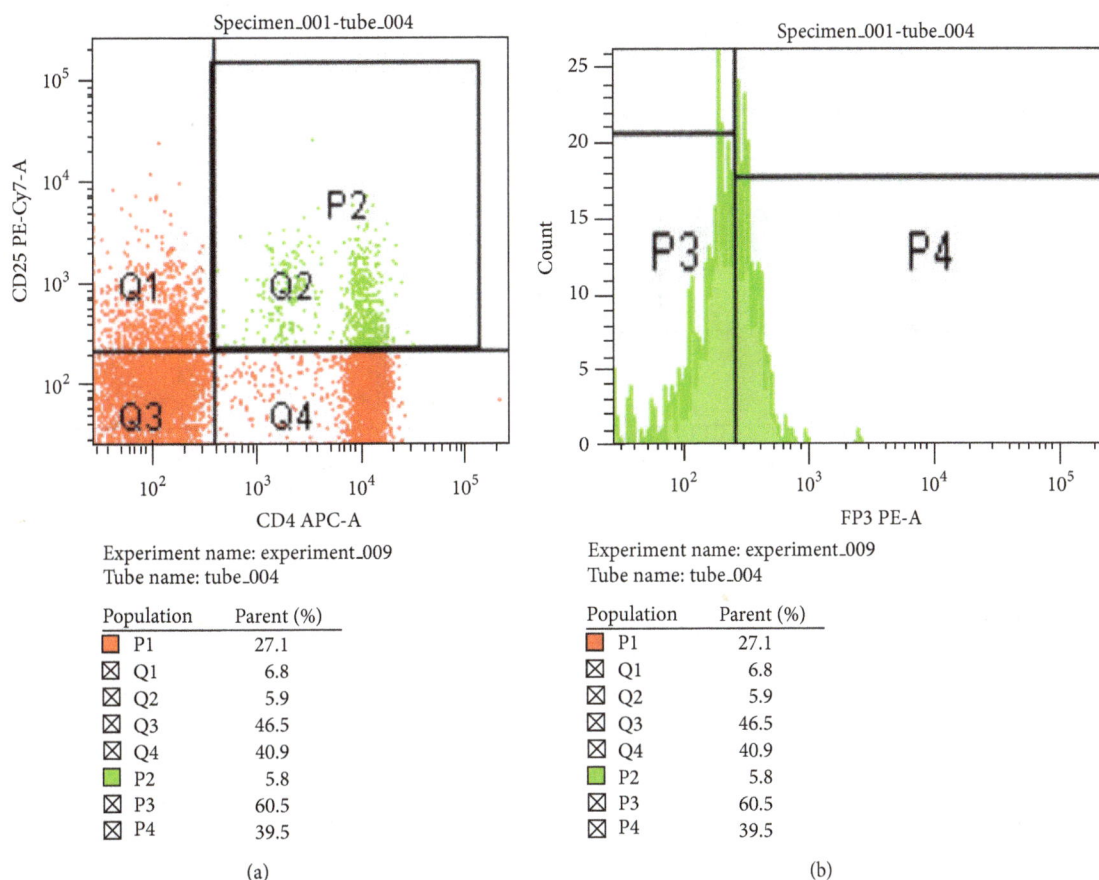

FIGURE 3: The expression level of $CD4^+CD25^+$ and FOXP3 was examined by flow cytometry in control group. (a) Representation plots of $CD4^+CD25^+$ cells (b) and FOXP3 expression in control group.

TABLE 2: Cytokine expression in study group with SPT positive for one or more food allergen and control group.

Cytokines	Study group* $N = 50$	Control group* $N = 20$	P value
IFN-γ	12.46 ± 8.88	21.00 ± 7.53	$P = 0.009$
IL-2	18.93 ± 13.73	20.78 ± 9.22	$P = 0.51$
IL-4	19.79 ± 12.38	21.88 ± 10.35	$P = 0.47$
IL-6	15.11 ± 9.79	18.17 ± 10.49	$P = 0.08$
IL-10	22.82 ± 19.16	18.62 ± 5.31	$P = 0.35$
IL-12p7	16.94 ± 11.00	17.58 ± 9.27	$P = 0.52$
IL-13	34.55 ± 17.51	29.39 ± 10.12	$P = 0.40$
IL-17A	12.09 ± 8.67	2.01 ± 1.27	$P < 0.0001$

*Values are expressed in Mean ± SD pg/mL.

3.2. Correlation Analysis

3.2.1. Relationship of Total IgE and FOXP3 Expression. There was a significant negative correlation between %FOXP3/$CD4^+CD25^{high}$ and total IgE level ($r = -0.5273$, $P < 0.0001$) (Figure 7).

3.2.2. Interaction between FOXP3 Expression and Level of IL-17 and IL-4. FOXP3 percentage and IL-17 level had a significant inverse correlation with each other ($r = -0.5631$, $P < 0.0001$)

(Figure 8(a)). There was also a significant correlation between %FOXP3 and IL-4 ($r = -0.2836$, $P = 0.0460$) (Figure 8(b)).

4. Discussion

The present work demonstrates the relationship between T_H17 and Treg cells. It is universally accepted that total IgE level is directly correlated with allergy and asthma. In our study, the average level of total IgE was significantly higher in children with bronchial asthma compared to healthy subjects. On the basis of available studies, we had hypothesized that Treg cells would be associated with lower levels of allergy markers such as IgE and T_H2 cytokines. Most studies of Treg activity come from immunotherapy studies in allergic diseases [30]. FOXP3 transcription factor has been shown as a key regulator for development of Treg cells and is expressed by these cells [10, 11, 31]. In our study, we found that FOXP3 level is significantly lower in study group compared to control group. Furthermore, there was a negative correlation between total IgE and FOXP3 expression. In this study, we also demonstrated a T_H17/Treg cytokine profile in study group. Studies have suggested that asthma is associated with chronic and recurrent inflammation [32]. T_H2 cells are associated directly with inflammation whereas T_H17 cells behave primarily as proinflammatory markers [33]. Studies suggested

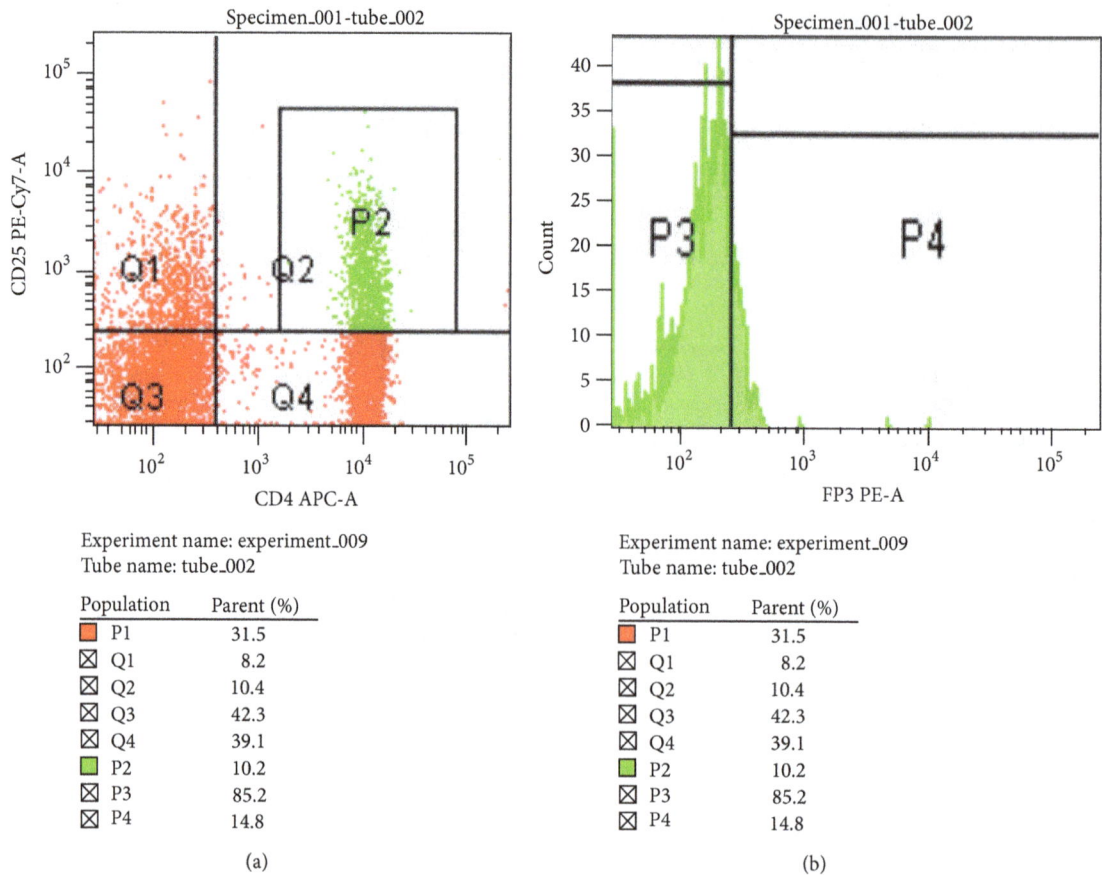

Experiment name: experiment_009
Tube name: tube_002

Population	Parent (%)
▪ P1	31.5
⊠ Q1	8.2
⊠ Q2	10.4
⊠ Q3	42.3
⊠ Q4	39.1
▪ P2	10.2
⊠ P3	85.2
⊠ P4	14.8

(a)

Experiment name: experiment_009
Tube name: tube_002

Population	Parent (%)
▪ P1	31.5
⊠ Q1	8.2
⊠ Q2	10.4
⊠ Q3	42.3
⊠ Q4	39.1
▪ P2	10.2
⊠ P3	85.2
⊠ P4	14.8

(b)

FIGURE 4: The expression level of $CD4^+CD25^+$ and FOXP3 was examined by flow cytometry in asthmatic group. (a) Representation plots of $CD4^+CD25^+$ cells (b) and FOXP3 expression in study group.

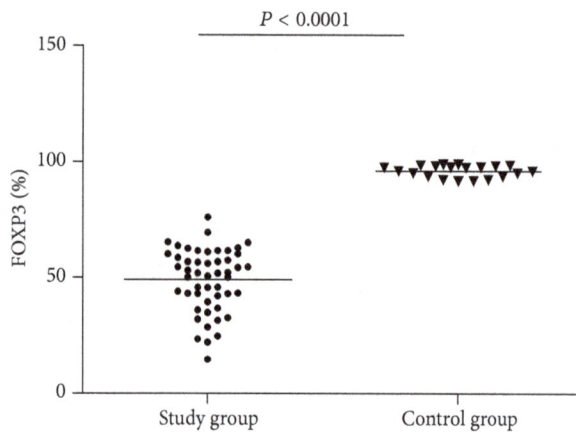

FIGURE 5: FOXP3% in study and control group.

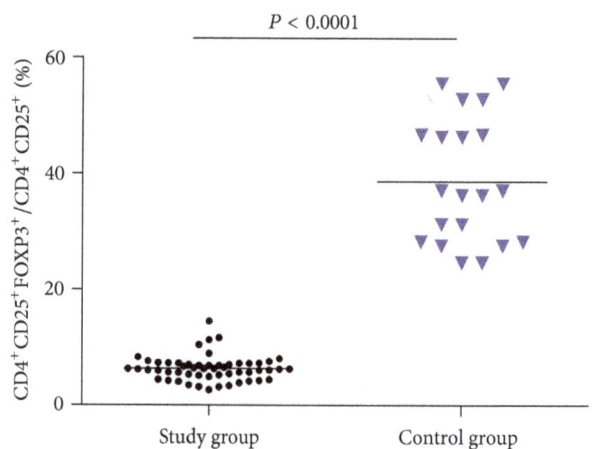

FIGURE 6: $CD4^+CD25^+FOXP3^+/CD4^+CD25^+$ (%) in study and control group.

that transcription factors and cytokines are involved in generation, differentiation, and expansion of T_H17 cells. The interaction between T_H17 cells and Tregs in various inflammatory diseases needs to be further defined [34]. The knowledge of suppressive activity of Treg cells in atopic disease is still contradictory and limited. This study supports the notion that function of Tregs is altered or impaired in

allergic patients compared to healthy individuals [13, 17, 35–40]. However, there are some studies that have shown results going the opposite way [41–43]. These alterations may be related to different allergic diseases, different environmental influences, and differences in methodology for identification of cell markers that are used in proper identification of Tregs. In our study, we found significantly higher IL-17 level in

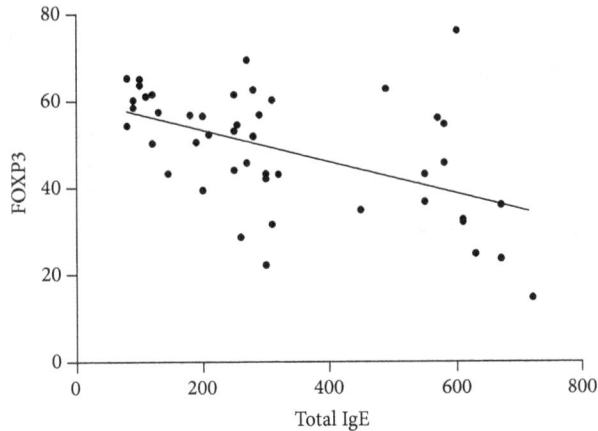

FIGURE 7: Correlation between FOXP3 and Total IgE.

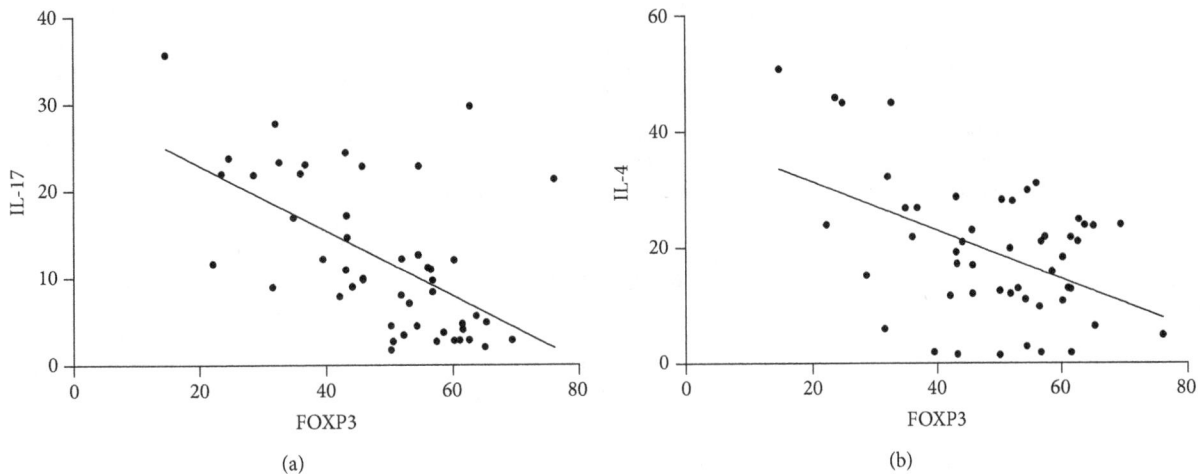

(a)

(b)

FIGURE 8: Correlation (a) between FOXP3 and IL-17 and (b) between FOXP3 and IL-4.

asthmatic patients compared to controls. Previous studies showed that IL-17 is elevated in sputum samples of patients with asthma compared to healthy controls [44–46]. Another study showed that patients with asthma had elevated IL-17 levels in serum compared with control subjects [47]. It has been suggested that IL-17 plays an important role in inflammatory and autoimmune diseases [48]. In patients with asthma, IL-17 level was significantly increased and T cell population was skewed toward T_H17 phenotype. Thus, there is a correlation of increase in IL-17 levels in patients with asthma coupled with a significant decrease in transcription factor FOXP3 Treg level when compared to controls.

We could not find a study in children with asthma reporting the relationship of T_H17 with Treg response in the milieu of T_H2 activity. These results show that there is a correlation between FOXP3 and IL-17 level and also a functional imbalance in T_H17/Treg in children with asthma. In this study, we demonstrated that IL-17 and FOXP3 are reciprocally interconnected with each other. It has already been shown that $CD4^+CD25^+FOXP3^+$ play a protective role in autoimmune disease [12]. We found that the suppressive activity of $CD4^+CD25^{high}$ T cells was variable, which is already reported

in previous studies [49, 50]. FOXP3 transcription factor plays a key role in regulation and development of $CD4^+CD25^+$ T cells and is expressed by these cells [10, 11, 31]. Our study also shows that there is a significant negative correlation between IL-4 and FOXP3.

In conclusion, the present study demonstrates that there is an imbalance between T_H17 and Tregs associated with asthma, which may play a potential role in development of asthma. Our study also shows inverse correlation between IL-17 and FOXP3. Future studies are needed to clarify these findings.

Abbreviations

FOXP3: Forkhead box P3
IL: Interleukin
Treg: Regulatory T cell
FACS: Fluorescence-activated cell sorting
IgE: Immunoglobin E
FEV1:   Forced expiratory volume 1
HRP: Horseradish peroxidase
mAbs: Monoclonal antibodies
PBMC: Peripheral blood mononuclear cell.

Conflict of Interests

The authors declare that there is no conflict of interests regarding the publication of this paper.

Acknowledgment

The research is supported by the funds from Indian Council of Medical Research, India (Grant no. 62/1/2006-BMS).

References

[1] E. von Mutius, "Influences in allergy: epidemiology and the environment," *Journal of Allergy and Clinical Immunology*, vol. 113, no. 3, pp. 373–380, 2004.

[2] H. Y. Kim, R. H. Dekruyff, and D. T. Umetsu, "The many paths to asthma: phenotype shaped by innate and adaptive immunity," *Nature Immunology*, vol. 11, no. 7, pp. 577–584, 2010.

[3] M. Larché, D. S. Robinson, and A. B. Kay, "The role of T lymphocytes in the pathogenesis of asthma," *Journal of Allergy and Clinical Immunology*, vol. 111, no. 3, pp. 450–463, 2003.

[4] S. Baraldo, K. L. Oliani, G. Turato, R. Zuin, and M. Saetta, "The role of lymphocytes in the pathogenesis of asthma and COPD," *Current Medicinal Chemistry*, vol. 14, no. 21, pp. 2250–2256, 2007.

[5] R. Afshar, B. D. Medoff, and A. D. Luster, "Allergic asthma: a tale of many T cells," *Clinical and Experimental Allergy*, vol. 38, no. 12, pp. 1847–1857, 2008.

[6] S. Sakaguchi, "Naturally arising CD4$^+$ regulatory T cells for immunologic self-tolerance and negative control of immune responses," *Annual Review of Immunology*, vol. 22, pp. 531–562, 2004.

[7] C. A. Akdis and M. Akdis, "Mechanisms and treatment of allergic disease in the big picture of regulatory T cells," *Journal of Allergy and Clinical Immunology*, vol. 123, no. 4, pp. 735–746, 2009.

[8] J. A. Bluestone and A. K. Abbas, "Natural versus adaptive regulatory T cells," *Nature Reviews Immunology*, vol. 3, no. 3, pp. 253–257, 2003.

[9] J. D. Fontenot and A. Y. Rudensky, "A well adapted regulatory contrivance: regulatory T cell development and the forkhead family transcription factor Foxp3," *Nature Immunology*, vol. 6, no. 4, pp. 331–337, 2005.

[10] J. D. Fontenot, M. A. Gavin, and A. Y. Rudensky, "Foxp3 programs the development and function of CD4$^+$CD25$^+$ regulatory T cells," *Nature Immunology*, vol. 4, no. 4, pp. 330–336, 2003.

[11] S. Hori, T. Nomura, and S. Sakaguchi, "Control of regulatory T cell development by the transcription factor Foxp3," *Science*, vol. 299, no. 5609, pp. 1057–1061, 2003.

[12] S. Sakaguchi, M. Ono, R. Setoguchi et al., "Foxp3$^+$CD25$^+$CD4$^+$ natural regulatory T cells in dominant self-tolerance and autoimmune disease," *Immunological Reviews*, vol. 212, pp. 8–27, 2006.

[13] Y. Y. Wan and R. A. Flavell, "Regulatory T-cell functions are subverted and converted owing to attenuated Foxp3 expression," *Nature*, vol. 445, no. 7129, pp. 766–770, 2007.

[14] C. Baecher-Allan, J. A. Brown, G. J. Freeman, and D. A. Hafler, "CD4$^+$ CD25^{high} regulatory cells in human peripheral blood," *Journal of Immunology*, vol. 167, no. 3, pp. 1245–1253, 2001.

[15] S. Fowler and F. Powrie, "Control of immune pathology by IL-10-secreting regulatory T cells," *Springer Seminars in Immunopathology*, vol. 21, no. 3, pp. 287–294, 1999.

[16] F. Powrie, J. Carlino, M. W. Leach, S. Mauze, and R. L. Coffman, "A critical role for transforming growth factor-beta but not interleukin 4 in the suppression of T helper type 1-mediated colitis by CD45RB(low) CD4$^+$ T cells," *The Journal of Experimental Medicine*, vol. 183, no. 6, pp. 2669–2674, 1996.

[17] D. Hartl, B. Koller, A. T. Mehlhorn et al., "Quantitative and functional impairment of pulmonary CD4$^+$CD25hi regulatory T cells in pediatric asthma," *Journal of Allergy and Clinical Immunology*, vol. 119, no. 5, pp. 1258–1266, 2007.

[18] A. Peck and E. D. Mellins, "Plasticity of T-cell phenotype and function: the T helper type 17 example," *Immunology*, vol. 129, no. 2, pp. 147–153, 2010.

[19] A. Awasthi and V. K. Kuchroo, "Th17 cells: from precursors to players in inflammation and infection," *International Immunology*, vol. 21, no. 5, pp. 489–498, 2009.

[20] H. Wakashin, K. Hirose, Y. Maezawa et al., "IL-23 and Th17 cells enhance Th2-cell-mediated eosinophilic airway inflammation in mice," *American Journal of Respiratory and Critical Care Medicine*, vol. 178, no. 10, pp. 1023–1032, 2008.

[21] R. H. Wilson, G. S. Whitehead, H. Nakano, M. E. Free, J. K. Kolls, and D. N. Cook, "Allergic sensitization through the airway primes Th17-dependent neutrophilia and airway hyper-responsiveness," *American Journal of Respiratory and Critical Care Medicine*, vol. 180, no. 8, pp. 720–730, 2009.

[22] M. M. Curtis and S. S. Way, "Interleukin-17 in host defence against bacterial, mycobacterial and fungal pathogens," *Immunology*, vol. 126, no. 2, pp. 177–185, 2009.

[23] T. Korn, E. Bettelli, M. Oukka, and V. K. Kuchroo, "IL-17 and Th17 cells," *Annual Review of Immunology*, vol. 27, pp. 485–517, 2009.

[24] S. Fujino, A. Andoh, S. Bamba et al., "Increased expression of interleukin 17 in inflammatory bowel disease," *Gut*, vol. 52, no. 1, pp. 65–70, 2003.

[25] C. E. Jones and K. Chan, "Interleukin-17 stimulates the expression of interleukin-8, growth-related oncogene-α, and granulocyte-colony-stimulating factor by human airway epithelial cells," *American Journal of Respiratory Cell and Molecular Biology*, vol. 26, no. 6, pp. 748–753, 2002.

[26] S. Ivanov and A. Lindén, "Interleukin-17 as a drug target in human disease," *Trends in Pharmacological Sciences*, vol. 30, no. 2, pp. 95–103, 2009.

[27] J. M. Kim, J. P. Rasmussen, and A. Y. Rudensky, "Regulatory T cells prevent catastrophic autoimmunity throughout the lifespan of mice," *Nature Immunology*, vol. 8, no. 2, pp. 191–197, 2007.

[28] F. Annunziato, L. Cosmi, V. Santarlasci et al., "Phenotypic and functional features of human Th17 cells," *Journal of Experimental Medicine*, vol. 204, no. 8, pp. 1849–1861, 2007.

[29] R. A. O'Connor, K. H. Malpass, and S. M. Anderton, "The inflamed central nervous system drives the activation and rapid proliferation of Foxp3$^+$ regulatory T cells," *Journal of Immunology*, vol. 179, no. 2, pp. 958–966, 2007.

[30] A. Mubeccel, "Immune tolerance in allergy," *Current Opinion in Immunology*, vol. 21, no. 6, pp. 700–707, 2009.

[31] M. R. Walker, D. J. Kasprowicz, V. H. Gersuk et al., "Induction of FoxP3 and acquisition of T regulatory activity by stimulated human CD4$^+$CD25- T cells," *Journal of Clinical Investigation*, vol. 112, no. 9, pp. 1437–1443, 2003.

[32] D. M. Murphy and P. M. O'Byrne, "Recent advances in the pathophysiology of asthma," *Chest*, vol. 137, no. 6, pp. 1417–1426, 2010.

[33] M. Veldhoen and B. Stockinger, "TGFβ1, a "Jack of all trades": the link with pro-inflammatory IL-17-producing T cells," *Trends in Immunology*, vol. 27, no. 8, pp. 358–361, 2006.

[34] J. Mai, H. Wang, and X.-F. Yang, "Th 17 cells interplay with Foxp3$^+$ Tregs in regulation of inflammation and autoimmunity," *Frontiers in Bioscience*, vol. 15, no. 3, pp. 986–1006, 2010.

[35] T. A. Chatila, "Role of regulatory T cells in human diseases," *Journal of Allergy and Clinical Immunology*, vol. 116, no. 5, pp. 949–960, 2005.

[36] M. Akdis, K. Blaser, and C. A. Akdis, "T regulatory cells in allergy: novel concepts in the pathogenesis, prevention, and treatment of allergic diseases," *Journal of Allergy and Clinical Immunology*, vol. 116, no. 5, pp. 961–969, 2005.

[37] M. A. Gavin, J. P. Rasmussen, J. D. Fontenot et al., "Foxp3-dependent programme of regulatory T-cell differentiation," *Nature*, vol. 445, no. 7129, pp. 771–775, 2007.

[38] T. Jartti, K. A. Burmeister, C. M. Seroogy et al., "Association between CD4$^+$CD25^{high} T cells and atopy in children," *Journal of Allergy and Clinical Immunology*, vol. 120, no. 1, pp. 177–183, 2007.

[39] W. G. Shreffler, N. Wanich, M. Moloney, A. Nowak-Wegrzyn, and H. A. Sampson, "Association of allergen-specific regulatory T cells with the onset of clinical tolerance to milk protein," *Journal of Allergy and Clinical Immunology*, vol. 123, no. 1, pp. 43.e7–52.e7, 2009.

[40] M. Smith, M. R. Tourigny, P. Noakes, C. A. Thornton, M. K. Tulic, and S. L. Prescott, "Children with egg allergy have evidence of reduced neonatal CD4$^+$CD25$^+$CD127lo/- regulatory T cell function," *Journal of Allergy and Clinical Immunology*, vol. 121, no. 6, pp. 1460.e7–1466.e7, 2008.

[41] M. M. Tiemessen, E. van Hoffen, A. C. Knulst, J.-A. van der Zee, E. F. Knol, and L. S. Taams, "CD4$^+$CD25+ regulatory T cells are not functionally impaired in adult patients with IgE-mediated cow's milk allergy," *Journal of Allergy and Clinical Immunology*, vol. 110, no. 6, pp. 934–936, 2002.

[42] L.-S. Ou, E. Goleva, C. Hall, and D. Y. M. Leung, "T regulatory cells in atopic dermatitis and subversion of their activity by superantigens," *Journal of Allergy and Clinical Immunology*, vol. 113, no. 4, pp. 756–763, 2004.

[43] A. L. Taylor, J. Hale, B. J. Hales, J. A. Dunstan, W. R. Thomas, and S. L. Prescott, "FOXP3 mRNA expression at 6 months of age is higher in infants who develop atopic dermatitis, but is not affected by giving probiotics from birth," *Pediatric Allergy and Immunology*, vol. 18, no. 1, pp. 10–19, 2007.

[44] S. Molet, Q. Hamid, F. Davoine et al., "IL-17 is increased in asthmatic airways and induces human bronchial fibroblasts to produce cytokines," *Journal of Allergy and Clinical Immunology*, vol. 108, no. 3, pp. 430–438, 2001.

[45] A. Barczyk, W. Pierzcha, and E. Sozañska, "Interleukin-17 in sputum correlates with airway hyperresponsiveness to methacholine," *Respiratory Medicine*, vol. 97, no. 6, pp. 726–733, 2003.

[46] D. M. A. Bullens, E. Truyen, L. Coteur et al., "IL-17 mRNA in sputum of asthmatic patients: linking T cell driven inflammation and granulocytic influx?" *Respiratory Research*, vol. 7, article 135, 2006.

[47] C. K. Wong, C. Y. Ho, F. W. S. Ko et al., "Proinflammatory cytokines (IL-17, IL-6, IL-18 and IL-12) and Th cytokines (IFN-γ, IL-4, IL-10 and IL-13) in patients with allergic asthma," *Clinical and Experimental Immunology*, vol. 125, no. 2, pp. 177–183, 2001.

[48] L. A. Tesmer, S. K. Lundy, S. Sarkar, and D. A. Fox, "Th17 cells in human disease," *Immunological Reviews*, vol. 223, no. 1, pp. 87–113, 2008.

[49] M. Jutel, M. Akdis, F. Budak et al., "IL-10 and TGF-β cooperate in the regulatory T cell response to mucosal allergens in normal immunity and specific immunotherapy," *European Journal of Immunology*, vol. 33, no. 5, pp. 1205–1214, 2003.

[50] C. M. Baecher-Allan and D. A. Hafler, "Functional analysis of highly defined, FACS-isolated populations of human regulatory CD4$^+$CD25$^+$ T cells," *Clinical Immunology*, vol. 117, no. 2, pp. 192–193, 2005.

26

Hearing and Neurological Impairment in Children with History of Exchange Transfusion for Neonatal Hyperbilirubinemia

Carlos F. Martínez-Cruz,[1] **Patricia García Alonso-Themann,**[1] **Adrián Poblano,**[2] **and Ileana A. Cedillo-Rodríguez**[1]

[1] Department of Pediatric Follow-Up, National Institute of Perinatology, 11000 Mexico City, Mexico
[2] Cognitive Neurophysiology Laboratory, National Institute of Rehabilitation, 14389 Mexico City, Mexico

Correspondence should be addressed to Adrián Poblano; drdislexia@yahoo.com.mx

Academic Editor: Ju Lee Oei

The objective was to determine frequency of sensorineural hearing loss (SNHL), identified by abnormal threshold in evoked potentials, absence of otoacoustic emissions and behavioral responses, auditory neuropathy (AN) (absence of evoked potentials, with preservation of otoacoustic emissions), and neurological comorbidity in infants with hyperbilirubinemia (HB) treated with exchange-transfusion (ET). From a total of 7,219 infants, ET was performed on 336 (4.6%). Inclusion criteria were fulfilled in 102; 234 children did not meet criteria (182 outside of the study period, 34 did not have complete audiological evaluation, and 18 rejected the followup). Thirty-five children (34%) were born at-term and 67 (66%) were preterm. Children had a mean age of 5.5 ± 3.9 years. Main causes of ET were Rh isoimmunization in 48 (47%), ABO incompatibility in 28 (27.5%), and multifactorial causes in 26 (25.5%). Fifteen (15%) children presented with SNHL. Preterm newborns presented more often with SNHL. Indirect bilirubin level was higher in children with SNHL (22.2 versus 18.7 mg/dL, $P = 0.02$). No cases of AN were documented. An increased risk of neurologic sequelae was observed in children with SNHL. In conclusion, we disclosed a high frequency of SNHL in children with neonatal HB and ET and neurological alterations. No cases of AN were observed.

1. Introduction

The auditory pathway is known as one of the most susceptible parts of the central nervous system to noxious agents. Severe neonatal hyperbilirubinemia (HB) is a common cause of sensorineural hearing loss (SNHL) and auditory neuropathy (AN) [1–4]. If not controlled, HB can lead to hyperbilirubinemic encephalopathy, or neonatal death. Moreover, surviving infants are at high risk of neurological damage, which can manifest as cerebral palsy, epilepsy, SNHL, or cognitive deficits [5–9].

Some audiological studies in children with serum bilirubin levels >20 mg/dL, have reported auditory dysfunction in 17–87% of cases [10–14]. The usual treatments for this neonatal disease are phototherapy and blood exchange transfusion (ET). Phototherapy reduces serum bilirubin levels through luminous oxidation, while ET is used primarily to maintain bilirubin levels below toxicity levels, eliminate antibodies, and correct hemolytic anemia. However, some adverse events associated with ET are asymptomatic electrolyte and other blood abnormalities, which are treatable in the neonate. Overall, 74% of ET were associated with adverse events; the most common events were thrombocytopenia (44%), hypocalcemia (29%), and metabolic acidosis (24%), of which 69%, 74%, and 44%, respectively, required treatment [15, 16].

The Joint Committee on Infant Hearing of the American Academy of Pediatrics (AAP) considers ET a risk factor for SNHL [4]. SNHL, is a severe sensory sequelae in young infants and its early diagnosis depends on systematic hearing screening. Newborn hearing screening, mainly in high-risk infants, is the most effective way of early SNHL detection. Early diagnosis and intervention are crucial for improving linguistic development and prognosis of these children [4]. Therefore the main goal of this study was to determine the frequency of SNHL, AN, and neurological comorbidity in a group of children with a history of neonatal HB and ET treated at a third-level hospital in Mexico City.

2. Material and Methods

2.1. Subjects. We designed a retrospective, case-control study, with the following inclusion criteria: having been born at the National Institute of Perinatology "Dr. Isidro Espinosa de los Reyes" (INPerIER) in Mexico City, between January 1, 2000 and December 30, 2010; a history of ET secondary to severe HB after Rh hemolytic disease; ABO incompatibility or multifactorial HB, regardless of birth gestational age or associated morbidity during the neonatal period, and belonging to the pediatric followup clinic for high-risk newborns. Severe HB was defined as a bilirubin increase >0.5 mg/dL per hour in term infants, or >0.3 mg/dL for preterm infants, requiring exchange transfusion. Rh hemolytic disease was defined as different maternal-infant antigens and a positive direct Coomb's test. ABO incompatibility was defined as an infant's blood type A or B with a type O mother. Multifactorial HB was defined as the same maternal-infant blood type and severe HB. Our clinic's characteristics have been described in previous publications [17].

Phototherapy and ET were performed according to AAP guidelines [18–21]: (1) total serum bilirubin level over threshold values for ET according to gestational age and (2) increase of bilirubin >0.5 mg/dL per hour in term infants and >0.3 mg/dL for preterm infants regardless of phototherapy. ET was performed with a double transfusion volume (160 mL/kg) for term infants and (180 mL/kg) for preterm infants using compatible reconstituted fresh whole blood units.

Two groups were defined in the followup based on their hearing status: (1) children with SNHL and (2) a control group of children, consisting of eighty-seven children (85%), who showed bilateral normal hearing (BNH) with history of exchange transfusion for severe hyperbilirubinemia. Neonatal variables and procedures were compared as follows: gestational age at birth in weeks belongs to a term (birth age between 37 and 42 weeks) or preterm (<37 weeks) infant group; birth weight, Apgar score at one and five minutes, gender, days of endotracheal ventilation, length of hospital stay, and age at time of studies. Risk variables for SNHL documented in the neonatal period were peak serum indirect bilirubin level in mg/dL at the time of ET; days of phototherapy; exposure to other potentially ototoxic drugs such as aminoglycosides [22] and diuretics [23]; severe perinatal asphyxia (Apgar < 3 at one minute, pH < 7.25, PaO_2 < 50 mmHg) [24]; intraventricular hemorrhage (determined by transfontanelar ultrasonography) during their stay in the neonatal intensive care unit (NICU) classified according to Papile et al. stages [25]. Exclusion criteria were as follows: family history of hearing loss; maternal/fetal infections in the first trimester of pregnancy (toxoplasmosis, rubella, cytomegalovirus, herpes virus, syphilis, human immunodeficiency); and congenital or metabolic diseases associated with hyperbilirubinemia such as: hereditary spherocytosis, thalassemia, Gilbert's syndrome, Crigler-Najjar disease, galactosemia, and glucose-6-phosphate dehydrogenase deficiency (diagnosis of these entities was carried out with the support of the genetics and hematology services of the hospital). Parents were informed of the importance of their child's participation, the purpose of the study, and research benefits. Causes for not participating in the pediatric followup were as follows: low economic resources, living far away from the hospital, and both parents working, among others reasons. Signed informed consent was requested when infants were recruited for the follow-up study, before hearing examinations in accordance with the institute's research committee and of the Declaration of Helsinki.

2.2. Bilirubin Determinations. Samples were obtained by peripheral venipuncture. All specimens were protected from light after they were drawn, and these were analyzed immediately. For the quantitative determination of serum bilirubin, we utilized a dichlorophenyl diazonium (DPD) reagent. Measurements were performed using a Beckman Synchron CX-9 equipment (Fullerton, CA, USA).

2.3. Brainstem Auditory Evoked Potentials (BAEP). All infants included in the study underwent determination of conventional brainstem auditory evoked potentials (BAEP) at 3 and 6 months of chronological age with a Nicolet Viking Quest (Nicolet Biomedical Inc., Madison, WI, USA) computer. The test was conducted in a soundproof room reserved for this purpose within the neurophysiology unit, with the child in physiological sleep in a regular bed. BAEP determinations were performed after skin cleaning with alcohol-acetone and to apply conductive gel, using the international 10–20 system electrode placement [26] with the following assembly A1-Cz, A2-Cz. The studied ear was (−), Cz (+), and the contralateral ear was the ground. The electrode impedance was kept <4 Kilo-ohms. The band-pass filters were placed between 300 and 3,000 Hertz. The time of analysis after the stimulation was 10 milliseconds. Stimulation was carried out with monaural clicks in rarefaction at an intensity of 80 decibels (dB) of normal hearing level (nHL). The contralateral ear was simultaneously masked with a white noise 40 dB below the intensity of the stimulus. One thousand and five hundred clicks where administered for each sweep, decreasing in 20 dB steps to search for the threshold level in each ear. The duration of the stimulus was 100 microseconds and the clicks were delivered through TDH-49P headphones (Telephonics Co., Huntington, NY, USA). A normal peripheral auditory sensitivity was considered when the infant had a response to 40 dB nHL, displaying a robust positive wave V.

2.4. Tympanometry. To rule out middle ear pathology, children were studied with a Carl Zeiss OP-MI-9 F-125 Otomicroscope (Jenna, Germany). Afterward, we used a Grason-Stadler GSI TympStar V.2 Impedanciometer (Madison, WI), with ANSI S3.6-1996 calibration. The test tone used in tympanometry was 226 Hz, 85 at dB, pressure range = −600 to 400 deca-Pascals, compliance range of 0.1 to 5.0 mL, with an accuracy of ±5%. Children should have had a Jerger type A curve [27], with pressure variation of −150 to 50 deca-Pascals (to ensure a proper audiological test of quantitative and normative function in the assessment of middle ear and Eustachian tube).

2.5. Audiometry. Children >3 years of age underwent audiometry by conditioning game technique [28]. At 3 years the child must be able to react voluntarily to sounds, if given sufficient motivation. Once the child accepted the placement of TDH-50P balanced headphones, he was conditioned to put a toy in a rack, inserting it only during the test tone stimulus; this is repeated decreasing by 10 dB steps each time until the child no longer hears the test sound. After this, the test tone was increased by steps of 5 dB until it is perceived again, thus determining hearing thresholds for frequencies between 125 and 8,000 Hz in octave steps for each ear. The decrement-increment approach is the most commonly used technique in clinical audiology for determining hearing thresholds. We used a modified Hughson-Westlake method for children from sound to silence in steps of 10 by 10 dB and silence to sound in steps of 5 by 5 dB. We used a two-channel Grason-Stadler GSI 61 clinical audiometer with ANSI S3.43-1992 ISO 389 calibration and a bone vibrator placed on the forehead. For the contralateral ear, auditory masking white noise was used with automatic synchronization 10 dB below the level of the analyzed frequency. Audiometry was performed in a 3 m^2 soundproof room.

Hearing was considered normal in conditioned audiometry when the threshold was ≤20 dB in the frequencies analyzed. The criteria for SNHL were considered when both the air and bone conduction thresholds were increased and overlapping with hearing thresholds ≥25 dB in at least two of the frequencies tested. All subjects were studied, diagnosed, and followed up by a certified pediatric audiologist (MCCF).

2.6. Evoked Otoacoustic Emissions. In order to document auditory neuropathy, automatic transient-evoked otoacoustic emissions (TEOAE) were performed in infants with abnormal BAEP result in both determinations. A Madsen otoacoustic-emission-analyzer AccuScreen GN Otometrics equipment (Copenhagen, Denmark) was utilized with the following technique: the study was conducted in a sound-proof room, placing the probe in each of the ear canals. Stimulation was performed using clicks for each ear sweep. Equipment displays automatically a "Pass" or "Refer" result. "Pass" is equivalent to normal function of outer hair cells of the cochlea in the explored ear. The criteria for diagnosing AN consisted of two abnormal BAEP determinations (flat line or only wave V at high intensity stimulation) and "Pass" otoacoustic emissions result [2, 3].

2.7. Hearing Assessment Classification. Normal binaural hearing was considered when the infant passed the first or second test of conventional BAEP study, or when the infant passed the evaluation in the audiology clinic; these children formed the control group. SNHL was identified when the infant presented two BEAP studies with thresholds >45 dB

nHL and did not pass the behavioral auditory tests. Hearing loss was classified in severity stages by averaging the hearing thresholds at 500, 1,000, and 2,000 Hz frequencies after performing the audiometric measurement for each ear. Subjects with audiometric threshold between 21 and 40 dB were classified with mild hearing loss; those between 41 and 70 dB with moderate hearing loss; children with thresholds of 71–90 dB were classified with severe hearing loss and >90 dB profound hearing loss [29].

2.8. Neurological Comorbidity. The presence of neurological sequelae (pathologic condition resulting from a disease, once the offending agent is removed) was documented by serial neurological examinations performed by a certified neuropediatrician with the help of brain imaging scans, neurophysiological recordings, laboratory studies, and with posterior appointments to the follow-up clinic to determine alterations such as cerebral palsy and/or epilepsy (according to International Classification of Diseases Tenth Edition, categories G80, and G40 resp.).

2.9. Statistical Analysis. Continuous data were presented as means and standard deviations and were analyzed using one-way analysis of variance (ANOVA) and the Mann-Whitney U test. Categorical variables are presented as percentages and were analyzed using the χ^2 test. Odds ratios (OR) were calculated for categorical variables for SNHL risk, with a statistical significance level of $P < 0.05$. For the data analysis we used the SPSS 17.0 for Windows (SPSS, Chicago, IL) [30].

3. Results

From a population of 7,219 children in the pediatric follow-up clinic for high-risk newborns, 336 (4.6%) children had undergone ET. One-hundred-two infants met inclusion criteria for this study, with a mean age of 5.5 years ±3.9 (range of 2 to 10 years), 234 children did not meet the inclusion criteria (182 were outside the study period, 34 did not have complete audiological evaluations, and 18 rejected the followup in the clinic). Causes of ET were distributed as follows: Rh isoimmunization, $n = 48$ (47%); ABO incompatibility, $n = 28$ (27.5%); and multifactorial HB, $n = 26$ (25.5%); the high number is possibly because our hospital is a referral center for high-risk pregnancies. Comparison of the mean values of indirect bilirubin and the frequency of SNHL among these three groups showed no differences (Table 1). Thirty-five children (34%) were born at term and 67 (66%) were preterm; we found fifteen patients (15%) with SNHL in our sample. We constructed a group of children with bilateral normal hearing (BNH) with 87 patients (85%) for comparison purposes.

Clinical characteristics of children with SNHL and BNH with ET are presented in Table 2. The mean Apgar score at one and five minutes was significantly lower for the group with SNHL. Children with SNHL had a lower gestational age at birth than children with BNH. Indirect serum bilirubin levels were significantly higher in the group of children with SNHL. Risk factors associated with neurological damage are presented in Table 3. Preterm birth, intraventricular

TABLE 1: Comparison of Indirect bilirubin levels in children with exchange transfusion for different causes ($n = 102$).

Causes of Exchange transfusion	SNHL			BNH			Both groups		
	n	IB mg/dL-sd	Range	n	IB mg/dL-sd	Range	n	IB mg/dL-sd	Range
Rh hemolytic disease	5	23.8 ± 7.2	16.2–35.6	43	18.0 ± 5.4	6.8–28.4	48	18.6 ± 5.8	6.8–35.6
ABO incompatibility	2	21.2 ± 9.2	14.7–27.8	26	18.7 ± 5.5	7.3–35.8	28	18.9 ± 5.6	7.3–35.8
Multifactorial hyperbilirubinemia	8	21.5 ± 4.5	16.1–29.3	18	20.2 ± 4.6	9.6–28.6	26	20.6 ± 4.5	9.6–29.3
Total	15	22.2 ± 5.7	14.7–35.6	87	18.7 ± 5.3	6.8–35.8	102	19.2 ± 5.4	6.8–35.8
P = one-way Anova		$P = 0.77$			$P = 0.34$			$P = 0.31$	

n: number of cases. Sd: standard deviation. IB: Indirect bilirubin. SNHL: sensorineural hearing loss. BNH: bilateral normal hearing. P: significance in one-way analysis of variance.

TABLE 2: Clinical characteristics of groups of children with SNHL and BNH with Exchange transfusion ($n = 102$).

Variable	SNHL group ($n = 15$)			BNH group ($n = 87$)				
	n	Average ± SD	Range	n	Average ± SD	Range	U M-W[a]	P
Gestational age (weeks)	15	33.7 ± 2.1	30–39.5	87	35.2 ± 3.3	26–40.6	425	0.03[a]
Birthweight (g)	15	1927 ± 581	910–2,975	87	2,218 ± 790	790–3795	514	0.19[a]
1 min Apgar score	15	6.4 ± 1.7	1–9	87	6.7 ± 2.2	2–9	497	0.12[a]
5 min Apgar score	15	8.3 ± 0.8	1–9	87	8.5 ± 1.0	4–9	504	0.08[a]
Mechanical ventilation (days)	5	5 ± 4	1–14	22	5 ± 2	1–20	46.5	0.58[a]
Hospital stay (days)	15	31 ± 26	7–96	87	20 ± 18	5–102	469	0.08[a]
Phototherapy (days)	15	5.5 ± 0.7	4–6	87	5.5 ± 1.4	1–10	637	0.87[a]
Indirect bilirubin (mg/dL)	15	22.2 ± 5.7	14.7–35.6	87	18.7 ± 5.3	6.8–35.8	451	0.05[a]
Age at follow-up (years)	15	6.7 ± 2.3	2–10	87	5 ± 3.7	1–10	566	0.41[a]
Male	9	60%		42	48%			0.40**
Female	6	40%		45	52%			
Term infant	1	7%		34	39%			0.01**
Premature infant	14	93%		53	61%			

SNHL: sensorineural hearing loss. BNH: bilateral normal hearing. n: number of cases. SD: standard deviation. [a]U M-W: U of Mann-Whitney test, **χ^2.

hemorrhage, and exposure to furosemide were associated with SNHL.

BAEP results in children with SNHL were as follows: three infants had hearing thresholds of 80 dB nHL, two presented only wave V at 95 dB nHL, and ten had no response to >95 dB nHL stimulation. TEOAE recordings were negative in all cases of SNHL and thus, AN was not documented in the sample. Audiometric measurements showed severe SNHL in 10 cases (hearing threshold of 82 dB) with profound SNHL in 3 cases (hearing threshold of 99 dB). In all cases the auditory alteration was bilateral and symmetrical.

The higher neurological comorbidity was observed in the group of children with SNHL. An increased frequency of cerebral palsy was documented for the group with SNHL (20%) when compared with results from those of children with BNH (3%) (OR = 7.0 [1.2–38.7], $P = 0.01$). Epilepsy also showed a significant increased frequency in the group of children with SNHL (20%), when compared to children with BNH (5%) (OR = 5.1 [1.0–26.0], $P = 0.02$).

4. Discussion

4.1. Main Findings. This paper demonstrated a higher frequency of SNHL (15%) in children with a history of ET treated in a 3rd level hospital in Mexico City. Hearing alteration was produced despite the cause of severe hyperbilirubinemia and was associated to preterm birth and low gestational age, level of indirect bilirubin, and exposure to furosemide.

4.2. Comparison with Other Studies. Comparison with other studies is limited because of the differences in methodology, severity of hyperbilirubinemia, ET criteria, and SNHL classification. The basic mechanism of bilirubin neurotoxicity remains unknown. It is unclear why some infants do not develop hearing loss or neurological injury with the serum bilirubin levels that other infants do [9].

4.2.1. Hearing Damage. Some researchers studied the effect of HB on the auditory pathway during its acute phase, with a short prospective design, assessing BAEP and otoacoustic emissions before and after phototherapy or ET [31, 32]; they found an increased risk for auditory damage in children with severe HB. Other studies have included only term infants with nonhemolytic jaundice, eliminating several risk factors and HB that cause hearing damage [33–36]. Some researchers have included the measurement of demographic or ethnic factors in their statistical analysis to weigh a multidimensional overview of the hearing damage after HB [37–39]. However, overall, their results usually coincide with our data, showing a higher frequency of auditory pathway dysfunction

TABLE 3: Odds ratio calculations for risk-factors in children with SNHL and BNH with exchange transfusion.

Variable	SNHL $n = 15$ Yes		BNH $n = 87$ Yes		OR 95% CI	P
Preterm infants	14	93%	53	61%	8.9 (1.1–71.4)	0.01
Asphyxia	2	13%	5	6%	2.5 (0.4–14.3)	0.28
Neonatal sepsis	9	60%	42	48%	1.6 (0.5–4.9)	0.40
Intraventricular hemorrhage	2	13%	2	2%	6.5 (0.8–50.5)	0.04
Amikacin exposure	7	47%	49	56%	0.6 (0.2–2.0)	0.48
Furosemide exposure	5	33%	7	8%	5.7 (1.5–21.4)	0.005

SNHL: sensorineural hearing loss. BNH: bilateral normal hearing. n: number of cases. OR: odds ratio. CI 95%: confidence interval.

in children with severe HB and reports of alterations ranging from 17 to 87% of hearing dysfunction.

In this paper we analyzed the variable ET under usual clinical conditions present in the NICU, where newborns with severe HB usually present other associated comorbidities, therefore being difficult to document severe HB as single disease. For example, Patra et al. [15] documented in a group of infants with history of neonatal ET that 62% also had other neonatal morbidities at the time of ET. In our sample, 50% of our children had other neonatal problems at the time of ET; thus, their results are in line with our observation.

Severe HB that requires ET for its treatment is a clinical variable that cannot be accurate or measured objectively, since it is not easy to precisely define a serum bilirubin value that indicates the need for ET or that is directly associated with neural or auditory damage. Thus, ET is a strong qualitative variable associated as a risk factor to SNHL. This paper demonstrates the need to pay special attention to the increased risk of SNHL among infants treated with ET for severe HB. However, not all cases of severe neonatal HB with ET result in hearing or neurological deficits, and the exact threshold in which bilirubin becomes dangerous is not uniform among populations.

HB is more prevalent and severe in preterm infants, and its course is more prolonged than in term infants as a result of the red blood cells, liver, and gastrointestinal system immaturity. As consequence of these facts, in this study we found an increased risk for SNHL in preterm infants.

Loop diuretics cause SNHL by inhibiting ion transport of within the stria vascularis, reducing the electrochemical gradients that create the Endocochlear potential. More important is the fact that loop diuretics enhance the rate of permanent hearing loss induced by aminoglycosides. The mechanism for interaction between aminoglycosides and loop diuretics implies alterations in the blood labyrinth barrier, which facilitates aminoglycoside entry to the endolymphatic compartment [23]. We do not know if this auditory

lesion may include other ototoxic agents like indirect bilirubin. In this study we found that exposure to furosemide was associated with SNHL. Given the previous findings we suggest avoiding the use of aminoglycosides and furosemide combination in neonates undergoing ET to minimize the risk of SNHL.

4.2.2. Auditory Neuropathy. The incidence of AN in infants with severe HB and ET has been reported as high [2, 12]. Nonetheless, our study did not document cases of AN, which could be due to the small number of children studied or to regional or ethnic considerations of the sample. Thus, the finding warrants future research to ascertain the nature of these differences.

The pathophysiology of SNHL secondary to severe HB is not well defined, although its toxicity can affect cochlear hair cells and neurons of the basal nuclei and of the central auditory pathways. A recent report of 30 infants with hearing loss and exposure to severe HB suggests that damage to the outer hair cells of the cochlea is very common; twenty-six infants (87%) out of 30 had cochlear damage and in four cases (13%) an AN was documented [40]. Audiological findings in the present study using BAEP, otoacoustic emissions and audiometry documented bilateral severe and profound SNHL with similar affection to both ears. Audiometry suggests damage to inner hair cells in the cochlea with greater injury to the basal turn (high tones) and manifestations of loss of sensitivity to sound stimuli. Abnormal results of otoacoustic emissions in our children with ET suggest also damage of the outer hair cells. This locates the auditory damage at the cochlear level and specifically at both: inner and outer hair cells of the organ of corti. As a secondary result, one of the main manifestations in neurodevelopment in these children may be a delay in language acquisition.

4.2.3. Neurologic Comorbidity. Unfortunately the damage to the auditory pathway is not the only sequelae of severe HB. As we observed in our study, Ogunlesi et al. reported cerebral palsy in 86.4% of 22 infants with bilirubin encephalopathy, seizures in 40.9%, and deafness in 36.4% [8]. In our paper, we documented an increased risk of cerebral palsy and epilepsy for the SNHL group. Mechanisms for the alteration comprise the loss of neurons of the basal nuclei that result in motor disorders, death of cells, and formation of scars of the cerebral cortex manifested as seizures. Unfortunately, children with SNHL are frequently accompanied by other neurological or sensory deficits which may have a more difficult rehabilitation.

4.3. Study Limitations. The size of the sample was small, and therefore we must have caution in the interpretation of these results. In infants with HB treated with ET we reported here a higher frequency of SNHL and neurological comorbidity; however, we were unable to find AN. This fact merits more research in the future by our work team. These results deserve a continuous long-term pediatric followup of infants with greater number of patients.

5. Conclusions

The frequency of SNHL in children with a history of ET treated at a 3rd level hospital in Mexico City was high (15%). No cases of AN were documented. The preterm newborns have higher risk for SNHL. Moreover, children with SNHL and history of HB-ET have an increased risk of cerebral palsy and epilepsy. Thus, the early diagnosis and early intervention are very important actions for a better outcome of these patients.

Conflict of Interests

The authors declare that there is no conflict of interests.

References

[1] S. M. Shapiro and H. Nakamura, "Bilirubin and the auditory system," *Journal of Perinatology*, vol. 21, no. 1, pp. S52–S55, 2001.

[2] S. Saluja, A. Agarwal, N. Kler, and S. Amin, "Auditory neuropathy spectrum disorder in late preterm and term infants with severe jaundice," *International Journal of Pediatric Otorhinolaryngology*, vol. 74, no. 11, pp. 1292–1297, 2010.

[3] C. Madden, M. Rutter, L. Hilbert, J. H. Greinwald, and D. I. Choo, "Clinical and audiological features in auditory neuropathy," *Archives of Otolaryngology—Head and Neck Surgery*, vol. 128, no. 9, pp. 1026–1030, 2002.

[4] J. Busa, J. Harrison, J. Chappell et al., "Year 2007 position statement: principles and guidelines for early hearing detection and intervention programs," *Pediatrics*, vol. 120, no. 4, pp. 898–921, 2007.

[5] G. Mazeiras, J.-C. Rozé, P.-Y. Ancel et al., "Hyperbilirubinemia and neurodevelopmental outcome of very low birthweight infants: results from the lift cohort," *PLoS ONE*, vol. 7, no. 1, article e30900, 2012.

[6] N. Duman, H. Özkan, B. Serbetçioglu, B. Ögün, A. Kumral, and M. Avci, "Long-term follow-up of otherwise healthy term infants with marked hyperbilirubinaemia: should the limits of exchange transfusion be changed in Turkey?" *Acta Paediatrica, International Journal of Paediatrics*, vol. 93, no. 3, pp. 361–367, 2004.

[7] J. F. Watchko and M. J. Maisels, "Jaundice in low birthweight infants: pathobiology and outcome," *Archives of Disease in Childhood*, vol. 88, no. 6, pp. F455–F458, 2003.

[8] T. A. Ogunlesi, I. O. Dedeke, A. F. Adekanmbi, M. B. Fetuga, and O. B. Ogunfowora, "The incidence and outcome of bilirubin encephalopathy in Nigeria: a bi-centre study," *Nigerian Journal of Medicine*, vol. 16, no. 4, pp. 354–359, 2007.

[9] E. Hankø, R. Lindemann, and T. W. R. Hansen, "Spectrum of outcome in infants with extreme neonatal jaundice," *Acta Paediatrica*, vol. 90, no. 7, pp. 782–785, 2001.

[10] N. Y. Boo, M. Oakes, M. S. Lye, and H. Said, "Risk factors associated with hearing loss in term neonates with hyperbilirubinaemia," *Journal of Tropical Pediatrics*, vol. 40, no. 4, pp. 194–197, 1994.

[11] N. Y. Boo, A. J. Rohani, and A. Asma, "Detection of sensorineural hearing loss using automated auditory brainstem-evoked response and transient-evoked otoacoustic emission in term neonates with severe hyperbilirubinaemia," *Singapore Medical Journal*, vol. 49, no. 3, pp. 209–214, 2008.

[12] M. H. Baradaranfar, S. Atighechi, M. H. Dadgarnia et al., "Hearing status in neonatal hyperbilirubinemia by auditory brain stem evoked response and transient evoked otoacoustic emission," *Acta Medica Iranica*, vol. 49, no. 2, pp. 109–112, 2011.

[13] D. P. C. Da Silva and R. H. G. Martins, "Analysis of transient otoacoustic emissions and brainstem evoked auditory potentials in neonates with hyperbilirubinemia," *Brazilian Journal of Otorhinolaryngology*, vol. 75, no. 3, pp. 381–386, 2009.

[14] A. Nickisch, C. Massinger, B. Ertl-Wagner, and H. Von Voss, "Pedaudiologic findings after severe neonatal hyperbilirubinemia," *European Archives of Oto-Rhino-Laryngology*, vol. 266, no. 2, pp. 207–212, 2009.

[15] K. Patra, A. Storfer-Isser, B. Siner, J. Moore, and M. Hack, "Adverse events associated with neonatal exchange transfusion in the 1990s," *Journal of Pediatrics*, vol. 144, no. 5, pp. 626–631, 2004.

[16] S. Sanpavat, "Exchange transfusion and its morbidity in ten-year period at King Chulalongkorn Hospital," *Journal of the Medical Association of Thailand*, vol. 88, no. 5, pp. 588–592, 2005.

[17] C. F. Martínez-Cruz, A. Poblano, and L. A. Fernández-Carrocera, "Risk factors associated with sensorineural hearing loss in infants at the neonatal intensive care unit: 15-year experience at the National Institute of Perinatology (Mexico City)," *Archives of Medical Research*, vol. 39, no. 7, pp. 686–694, 2008.

[18] American Academy of Pediatrics Subcommittee on Neonatal Hyperbilirubinemia, "Neonatal jaundice and kernicterus," *Pediatrics*, vol. 108, no. 3, pp. 763–765, 2001.

[19] American Academy of Pediatrics Subcommittee on Hyperbilirubinemia, "Management of hyperbilirubinemia in the newborn infant 35 or more weeks of gestation," *Pediatrics*, vol. 114, no. 1, pp. 297–316, 2004.

[20] M. Kaplan and C. Hammerman, "American Academy of Pediatrics guidelines for detecting neonatal hyperbilirubinaemia and preventing kernicterus," *Archives of Disease in Childhood*, vol. 90, no. 6, pp. F448–F449, 2005.

[21] S. Ip, M. Chung, J. Kulig et al., "An evidence-based review of important issues concerning neonatal hyperbilirubinemia," *Pediatrics*, vol. 114, no. 1, pp. e130–e153, 2004.

[22] W.-J. Wu, S.-H. Sha, and J. Schacht, "Recent advances in understanding aminoglycoside ototoxicity and its prevention," *Audiology and Neuro-Otology*, vol. 7, no. 3, pp. 171–174, 2002.

[23] K. Rais-Bahrami, M. Majd, E. Veszelovszky, and B. L. Short, "Use of furosemide and hearing loss in neonatal intensive care survivors," *American Journal of Perinatology*, vol. 21, no. 6, pp. 329–332, 2004.

[24] E. Borg, "Perinatal asphyxia, hypoxia, ischemia and hearing loss: an overview," *Scandinavian Audiology*, vol. 26, no. 2, pp. 77–91, 1997.

[25] L. A. Papile, J. Burstein, R. Burstein, and H. Koffler, "Incidence and evolution of subependymal and intraventricular hemorrhage: a study of infants with birth weights less than 1,500 gm," *Journal of Pediatrics*, vol. 92, no. 4, pp. 529–534, 1978.

[26] H. H. Jaspers, "The ten twenty electrode system of the international federation," *Electroencephalography and Clinical Neurophysiology*, vol. 10, no. 3, pp. 371–375, 1958.

[27] J. Jerger, "Clinical experience with impedance audiometry," *Archives of Otolaryngology*, vol. 92, no. 4, pp. 311–324, 1970.

[28] M. Buren, B. S. Solem, and E. Laukli, "Threshold of hearing (0.125–20 kHz) in children and youngsters," *British Journal of Audiology*, vol. 26, no. 1, pp. 23–31, 1992.

[29] D. Stephens, "Audiological terms," in *Definitions, Protocols and Guidelines in Genetic Hearing Imparirment*, A. Martini, Ed., pp. 9–16, Whurr Publishers, London, UK, 2001.

[30] J. Camacho-Rosales, *Statistics with SPSS for Windows*, Alfa-Omega, Madrid, Spain, 2001, [Spanish].

[31] C. M. Smith, G. P. Barnes, C. A. Jacobson, and D. G. Oelberg, "Auditory brainstem response detects early bilirubin neurotoxicity at low indirect bilirubin values," *Journal of Perinatology*, vol. 24, no. 11, pp. 730–732, 2004.

[32] C. E. Ahlfors and A. E. Parker, "Unbound bilirubin concentration is associated with abnormal automated auditory brainstem response for jaundiced newborns," *Pediatrics*, vol. 121, no. 5, pp. 976–978, 2008.

[33] A. Poblano, N. Ballesteros, C. Arteaga, B. Flores, and T. Flores, "Otoacoustic emissions and evoked potentials in infants after breast-feeding jaundice," *Neuroscience and Medicine*, vol. 3, no. 3, pp. 270–274, 2012.

[34] B. Öğün, B. Şerbetçioğlu, N. Duman, H. Özkan, and G. Kirkim, "Long-term outcome of neonatal hyperbilirubinaemia: subjective and objective audiological measures," *Clinical Otolaryngology and Allied Sciences*, vol. 28, no. 6, pp. 507–513, 2003.

[35] I. Soorani-Lunsing, H. A. Woltil, and M. Hadders-Algra, "Are moderate degrees of hyperbilirubinemia in healthy term neonates really safe for the brain?" *Pediatric Research*, vol. 50, no. 6, pp. 701–705, 2001.

[36] V. Wong, W.-X. Chen, and K.-Y. Wong, "Short- and long- term outcome of severe neonatal nonhemolytic hyperbilirubinemia," *Journal of Child Neurology*, vol. 21, no. 4, pp. 309–315, 2006.

[37] F. Ebbesen, C. Andersson, H. Verder et al., "Extreme hyperbilirubinaemia in term and near-term infants in Denmark," *Acta Paediatrica, International Journal of Paediatrics*, vol. 94, no. 1, pp. 59–64, 2005.

[38] F. Núñez-Batalla, P. Carro-Fernández, M. E. Antuña-León, and T. González-Trelles, "Incidence of hypoacusia secondary to hyperbilirubinaemia in a universal neonatal auditory screening programme based on otoacoustic emissions and evoked auditory potentials," *Acta Otorrinolaringologica Espanola*, vol. 59, no. 3, pp. 108–113, 2008.

[39] B. O. Olusanya, A. A. Akande, A. Emokpae, and S. A. Olowe, "Infants with severe neonatal jaundice in Lagos, Nigeria: incidence, correlates and hearing screening outcomes," *Tropical Medicine and International Health*, vol. 14, no. 3, pp. 301–310, 2009.

[40] C. Oysu, I. Aslan, A. Ulubil, and N. Baserer, "Incidence of cochlear involvement in hyperbilirubinemic deafness," *Annals of Otology, Rhinology and Laryngology*, vol. 111, no. 11, pp. 1021–1025, 2002.

27

Population-Based Placental Weight Ratio Distributions

Erin M. Macdonald,[1,2,3] **John J. Koval,**[1] **Renato Natale,**[2,4]
Timothy Regnault,[2,3,5] **and M. Karen Campbell**[1,2,3,4]

[1] *Department of Epidemiology and Biostatistics, The University of Western Ontario, London, ON, Canada N6A 5C1*
[2] *Department of Obstetrics and Gynecology, The University of Western Ontario, London, ON, Canada N6A 5C1*
[3] *Children Health Research Institute, London, ON, Canada N6C 2V5*
[4] *Department of Paediatrics, The University of Western Ontario, London, ON, Canada N6A 5C1*
[5] *Department of Physiology and Pharmacology, The University of Western Ontario, London, ON, Canada N6A 5C1*

Correspondence should be addressed to M. Karen Campbell; karen.campbell@schulich.uwo.ca

Academic Editor: Dharmapuri Vidyasagar

The placental weight ratio (PWR) is a health indicator that reflects the balance between fetal and placental growth. The PWR is defined as the placental weight divided by the birth weight, and it changes across gestation. Its ranges are not well established. We aimed to establish PWR distributions by gestational age and to investigate whether the PWR distributions vary by fetal growth adequacy, small, average, and large for gestational age (SGA, AGA, and LGA). The data came from a hospital based retrospective cohort, using all births at two London, Ontario hospitals in the past 10 years. All women who delivered a live singleton infant between 22 and 42 weeks of gestation were included (n = 41441). Nonparametric quantile regression was used to fit the curves. The results demonstrate decreasing PWR and dispersion, with increasing gestational age. A higher proportion of SGA infants have extreme PWRs than AGA and LGA, especially at lower gestational ages. On average, SGA infants had higher PWRs than AGA and LGA infants. The overall curves offer population standards for use in research studies. The curves stratified by fetal growth adequacy are the first of their kind, and they demonstrate that PWR differs for SGA and LGA infants.

1. Background

Placental weight is a measure which reflects many aspects of placental growth including the laterally expanding growth of the chorionic disc, increased placental thickness with arborization of the chorionic villi, and increased surface area for vascular nutrient exchange. Thus, the growth of the chorionic disc, beginning early in pregnancy, is the main determinant of its transfer capacity, which supports the fetus in achieving its genetic growth potential [1].

Fetal growth depends on placental growth. Fetal growth restriction (FGR) is the failure of a fetus to reach his/her biological growth potential and small for gestational age (SGA) is widely used as a statistical indicator of FGR. SGA is defined as birth weight < 10th percentile for gestational age and sex based on a population standard [2]. Placental weight is generally lowered in SGA infants than in average for gestational age (AGA) and generally larger in large for

gestational age infants (LGA) [3–5]. The placental weight ratio (PWR) reflects whether the relative growth of the placenta and fetus is proportionate and is a common measure of the balance between placental and fetal growth. The PWR is defined as the placental weight divided by the birth weight and decreases across gestation as the placental growth slows and fetal growth accelerates [6]. Placental hypertrophy and reduced fetal growth have been postulated to be an adaptation to maintain placental function in pregnant women with complications such as malnutrition [7]. If this is true, a pregnancy with impaired fetal growth, resulting in a SGA infant, should have an increased PWR compared to those infants who are AGA or LGA [1, 8].

Placental weight and the PWR have been found to vary with maternal conditions and, to be predictive of obstetrical outcomes, perinatal morbidity and mortality, childhood growth and development, and fetal origins of adult onset disease [9–14]. Previous studies that have looked at the relationships between PWRs and outcomes have not used a population standard to objectively identify abnormal PWRs [15–17]. It is important to have population percentile standards in order to objectively differentiate a normal from abnormal PWR. Accordingly, the first objective of this study was to develop standard curves for the PWR across gestational ages in a population-based birth cohort. Since literature evidence suggests that placental weights differ between SGA, AGA, and LGA infants, a second objective was to examine this in order to refine the potential applications of the PWR trajectories. Having normative PWR standards by gestational age and an understanding of how these differ for under grown and overgrown fetuses will provide a useful standard for further research.

2. Methods

The study included all in-hospital singleton births in the city of London, Ontario. Research ethics board approval from Western University was obtained. Data arose from a perinatal database including all births occurring at St. Joseph's Health Care and Victoria Hospital in London, Ontario, between April 1, 2001 and March 31, 2011. A dedicated research assistant collected the information in the database from the medical charts, delivery records, and neonatal records. Placentas and infants were weighed by nursing assistants with an electronic weight scale. Placentas were weighed with the membranes and umbilical cord, including the segment of cord used for cord blood sampling. No attempt was made to remove placental blood before weighing. Anomalies (n = 881), stillbirths (n = 422), and multiple gestations (n = 2876) were excluded from the analyses. Placental weight was not available for 13,084 records, largely because one hospital did not collect placental weight for the entire study period. However, examination of the placental weights across gestational ages between the two hospitals revealed no significant differences. Therefore, total sample size consisted of 21,255 males and 20,186 females (total n = 41,441), as detailed in sample flow chart in Figure 1. Of these, 33,582 were residents of London-Middlesex while 7,859 were regional referrals. Only births between 22 and 42 weeks of gestation were included. Gestational age was truncated to the number of completed weeks based on the recommendations from World Health Organization and International Classification for Disease and was based on ultrasound or last menstrual period. Birth weight was categorized into SGA, AGA, and LGA based on Kramer et al. standards [18].

Descriptive analyses were performed on all study variables. Implausible values and potential errors were excluded including birth weights above or below the mean by three SDs, placental weights that were ≤100 g or ≥2500 g, maternal age, maternal height, prepregnancy weight below the 1st and above 99th percentiles, and any unknown or ambiguous genders.

Placental and birth weight distribution curves, and PWR curves, by gestational age were produced stratified by sex. The primary analysis estimated PWR curves for the total population, including referrals from outside the London-Middlesex. A sensitivity analysis was performed excluding

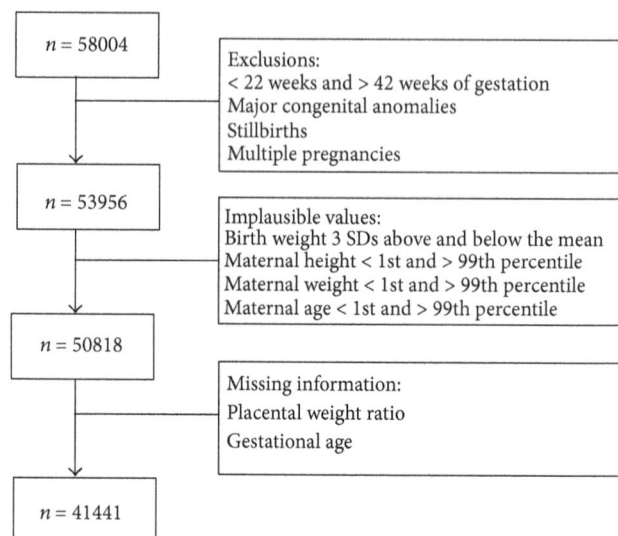

FIGURE 1: Flow chart illustrating the process by which the study population was obtained.

regional referrals from outside London-Middlesex. This sample, hereinafter referred to as the "city-wide" sample, would be expected to produce estimates with high internal validity because they represent a "whole population" perspective. The citywide PWR distributions were compared to the total population PWR distributions inclusive of referrals in order to assess their similarity. Due to its larger size, particularly at earlier gestational ages, the sample including regional referrals was used to create PWR distribution curves separately for SGA, AGA, and LGA infants.

We created growth charts at the 3rd, 5th, 10th, 25th, 50th, 75th, 90th, 95th, and 97th percentiles using quantile regression with quadratic terms on gestational age for the PWR. Quantile regression was also used for the placental and birth weight distributions, but quadratic splines at 22, 32, and 42 weeks of gestation were used as opposed to a quadratic term for gestational age, as it allowed for a better fit of the model. Quantile regression does not impose any parametric assumptions on the response distributions, which makes it appropriate for the anthropometric measures [19].

3. Results

3.1. Placental Weight, Birth Weight, and PWR Distributions. Figures 2(a) and 2(b) present placental weight and birth weight distributions for males and females, respectively. Because these curves are for the last half of gestation, placental growth has to some degree leveled off while fetal growth continues at an accelerated pace. Changes in birth weight and placental weight across the study period were examined and we found no differences (data not shown).

Additional file 1.xlsx and Additional file 2.xlsx in Supplementary Material available online at http://dx.doi.org/10.1155/2014/291846 present the PWR standards when inclusion criteria are relaxed to include regional referrals in the sample. All of the percentiles achieved a good fit across the range of gestational ages and reached a statistical significance of

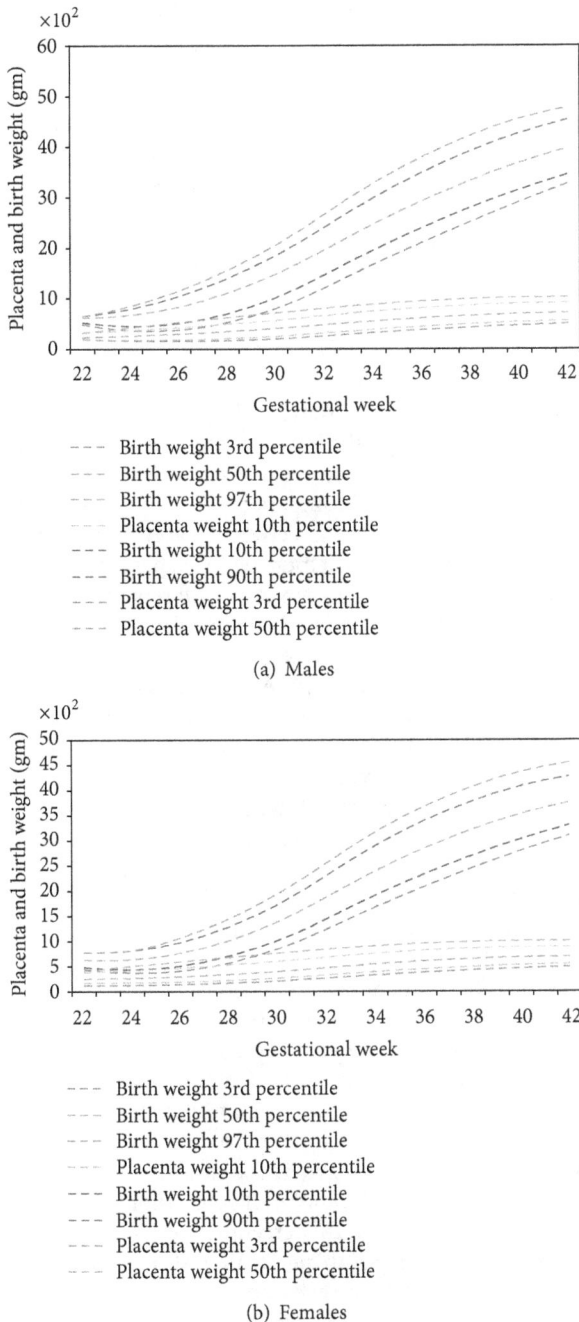

FIGURE 2: Inclusive of regional referrals placenta and birth weight percentile distributions by gestational age.

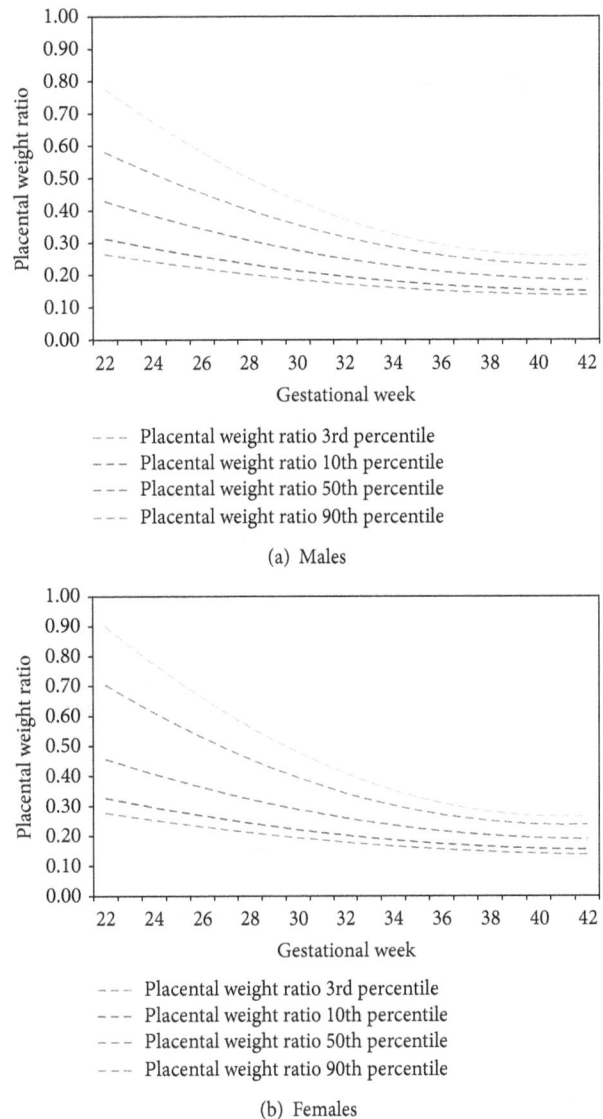

FIGURE 3: Inclusive of regional referrals PWR distributions by gestational age.

$P < 0.001$. Comparing the citywide population to the total sample revealed them to be similar, with minute differences presenting themselves at the extreme percentiles at the earlier gestational ages. Furthermore, comparing the 10th and 90th percentiles, which are often used as cut-off points, revealed almost no differences, even at the earlier gestational ages. The distributions of the PWR curves for males and females are illustrated in Figures 3(a) and 3(b), for the total population including regional referrals. The PWR decreases as gestational increases. In general, the females have higher PWRs than males. The slightly higher PWR in females than in males is consistent across percentiles. The ranges for the PWR are greatest at the highest percentiles. For both males and females, the ranges at the 90th percentile are more than 2 times as wide as at the 10th percentile.

3.2. Placental Weight Ratio Distribution Curves Stratified by SGA, AGA, and LGA Status. PWR distributions for the entire sample, inclusive of regional referrals, were used in an analysis of SGA, AGA, and LGA. The proportion with PWRs <10th percentile between the 10th and the 90th percentile and >90th percentile are presented in Table 1. There are a higher proportion of SGA infants for both males and females in the extreme PWR groups. Furthermore, there are fewer LGA infants in the lowest PWR group. The median PWR curves for each of SGA, AGA, and LGA are presented in Figures 4(a) and 4(b). At the earlier gestational ages both male and female SGA infants have higher PWRs than male and female AGA

TABLE 1: Placenta weight ratio distributions for SGA, AGA, and LGA infants based upon the inclusive of regional referrals standards.

Inclusive of regional referrals standards	Expected %	Males			Females		
		SGA	AGA	LGA	SGA	AGA	LGA
>90th	10%	13.18%	9.74%	9.82%	11.68%	9.66%	11.69%
10–90th	80%	74.42%	80.22%	81.64%	77.56%	80.22%	80.14%
<10th	10%	12.10%	10.04%	8.53%	10.76%	10.12%	8.16%

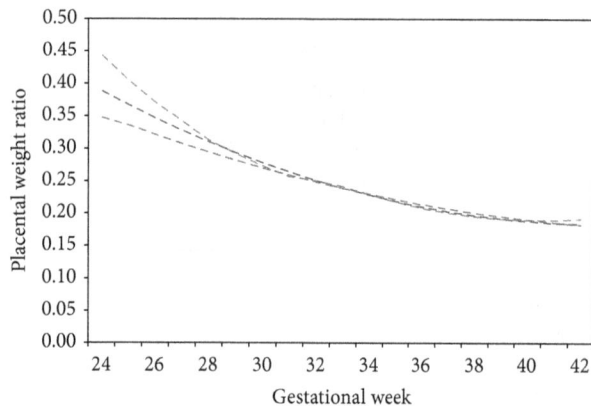

(a) Males

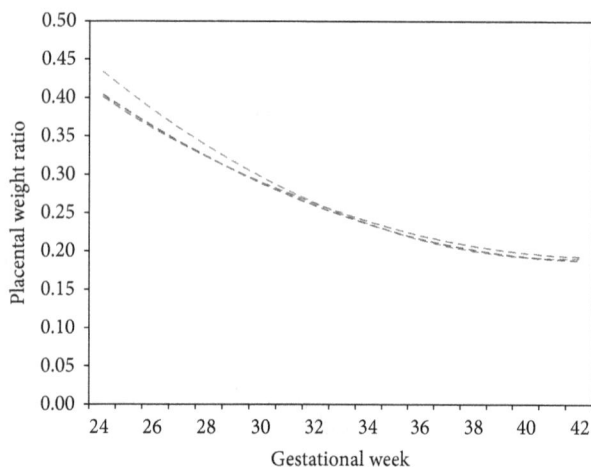

(b) Females

FIGURE 4: Inclusive of regional referrals SGA, AGA, and LGA median PWR distributions by gestational age.

and LGA infants. However, the PWRs at term gestations are nearly identical in both SGA and LGA infants. In fact, LGA infants have slightly higher median ratios at term than both SGA and AGA infants.

4. Discussion

The results of this study contribute to the current literature by creating gender-specific PWR percentile standards. While PWR is an important indicator of fetal health, there are few population standards for comparison. A few previous studies have presented the relation between placental weight and birth weight and only two of these reported percentiles curves for the PWR [6, 20]. Thompson et al. [20] reported placental percentile curves for a Norwegian population, and Almog et al. [6] presented PWR curves for a Canadian population. Comparison of our results with Almog's Canadian standards reveals close resemblance between the two populations, such as median 40-week PWRs (0.1938 and 0.19 for males and 0.1981 and 0.20 for females, resp.). Dombrowski et al. [21] published data on placental weight and PWR in North American population. However, their study is based on data from 1984 to 1991, over two decades ago and contained data mostly on a black population (81.4%), so the results cannot reasonably be compared. Compared to the only other available set of PWR percentiles in a Canadian population, [6] our results complement this literature and now provide more precise PWR predictions, particularly at the extreme percentiles, due to our larger sample size.

Our standards include earlier gestational ages than both of the aforementioned studies. Both of the abovementioned studies have gestational age standards starting at 24 weeks; however, our standards provide estimates starting at 22 weeks. Comparison of our results to Thompson et al.'s [20] shows that our <10th percentile estimates are lower than theirs, but our >90th percentile estimates are higher than their standards. However, comparisons of our results inclusive of regional referrals to Almog's curves reveal very similar standards. Our results have slightly lower PWRs at all gestational ages and percentiles [6].

A declining PWR with increasing gestational age reported here is similar to that described by others [21–23]. The placenta and fetus follow different growth patterns during gestation [3]. The placenta follows an S-shaped growth curve whereas fetal growth follows an exponential pattern in mid pregnancy, with most growth occurring in a linear fashion during the third trimester [3]. In the earlier gestational ages the birth weight is low in comparison to the placental weight as a result of the higher growth rate of the placenta earlier in gestation. Moreover, our placental growth curves show how the majority of placental growth occurs before 33 weeks of gestation. This accounts, at least in part, for the higher PWRs at earlier gestations. Previous authors have shown that the placenta responds to the interruption of the fetal villous circulation in the first half of gestation by initiating compensatory hyperplasia [24]. The majority of placental growth occurs at the earlier gestational ages; therefore, this is where the greatest differentiation of PWRs is expected.

Our birth weight distributions differ from the Kramer et al. [18] birth weight distributions in that our birth weights are somewhat larger. This might be expected since our population included more recent data and birth weight is increasing over time due to increases in maternal anthropometry, reduced cigarette smoking, and changes in sociodemographic factors [25]. Also, Kramer's curves did not include the Ontario population [18]; therefore, the reference populations are somewhat different.

Our PWR curves are similar whether inclusive or exclusive of the referral population. This may be because, at earlier gestations, the vast majority of regional births occur in this tertiary referral center. Thus, the lower gestations represent a "whole population." At later gestational ages, where one might expect the referral population to represent a biased sample of higher risk births, the actual numbers contributed by regional referrals are much smaller and would not substantially affect the percentile estimates for term and near-term births. Thus, the results are not unduly biased by inclusion of regional births. This is important because their inclusion had a sample size advantage, as it allowed us to use the total population for analyses stratified by fetal growth adequacy.

4.1. Stratification by Fetal Growth Adequacy. An additional novelty is the examination of percentile curves stratified by fetal growth adequacy, specifically focusing upon how PWRs change across gestational age between SGA, AGA, and LGA infants.

The literature suggests that a higher proportion of LGA infants have placenta weights above the 90th percentile and a lower share of placental weights below the 10th percentile than SGA and AGA infants [26]. Furthermore, PWRs have been found to be the lower in LGA infants than in AGA and SGA infants [27]. Our results show that, at earlier gestational ages in male infants, LGA infants generally have lower PWRs than AGA infants. This pattern holds true across all percentiles until the 33rd week of gestation, when the LGA and AGA standards become more similar. However, the differences between the LGA and AGA standards are not as pronounced as the differences between the SGA and AGA standards.

Previous studies have indicated that overall SGA infants have higher PWRs [3, 5] and that SGA infants have a higher proportion of placental weights at both extremes, but none of these studies have looked at the relationships across gestation or between percentiles [4, 16, 26, 28, 29].

Our curves show that as gestational age advances, the PWRs become more similar between SGA, AGA, and LGA infants, yet the PWR is still higher in female SGA infants. At earlier gestational ages the SGA standards are much higher than the AGA standards. This suggests that SGA may be detectable early in pregnancy. Therefore, the SGA infant is generally under grown in relation to placental size, suggesting placental function, rather than size, constrains

for fetal growth. Salafia et al. [1] showed that an elevated PWR might be an indication of an inefficient placenta with a reduced ability to maintain fetal growth. Indeed Kingdom and Kaufmann [30] report that preplacental or uteroplacental hypoxia with adaptive placental growth is a primary cause for growth restriction at term. However, the nonplacental chorion and amnion also contribute to overall placental weight, and more so for SGA infants; [23] this may also account, at least in part, for the higher PWR of infants in the SGA group. On the other hand, low PWRs are indicative of an increased efficiency of the placentas of the smaller fetuses, whereas, high PWRs are indicative of a potential failed compensation [17, 31–36]. The adaptive response in the placenta enhances transfer of substrates from the mother to fetus and improves efficiency of substrate utilization. The placenta compensates to minimize fetal growth restriction. However, placental function is not always improved with increases in weight. This may be due in part to the increase in syncytial knots especially in hypertensive pregnancies, which is an attempt at placental hyperplasia. The difference being that there is no associated functional angiogenesis, and therefore, no functional placental tissue in terms of oxygen and nutrient transfer [1, 37–41]. Therefore, it is suggested that the PWR can be used as a predictor for placental functional efficiency. Based on these suggestions, and the fact that our results show that SGA infants have a higher PWR than AGA and LGA infants, we propose that this may be due to a failed compensation of the placenta in SGA infants, whereas the lower PWRs seen in the SGA infants are indicative of either a biological tendency to smaller stature or an adaptive increase in placental efficiency.

A major strength of the study is the available sample size. The perinatal database provided a large number of observations with matching placental weight, birth weight, and gestational age. This allowed for the creation of accurate standards, and for the resulting percentile curves to be stratified by fetal growth adequacy standard.

Birth weights vary widely from country to country [18, 42] and as such it might be considered appropriate that birth weight percentiles should be based on data from the actual country or at least from a comparable country. This is often not the case and can lead to inappropriate use of the percentiles in a population where the distribution of birth weight is shifted, particularly to the left. Therefore, our results may be considered generalizable to other urban centers in Western based cultures. Also, the study of placental weight at the time of delivery is a crude measure of placental growth and development. However, when it is collected in a routine manner and related to birth weight, it provides information of biological importance.

5. Conclusions

The PWR distribution curves provide a standard that researchers can apply as a reference to identify infants who have abnormal PWRs. Identifying infants with high PWRs is important for patient care in both the short and long term. These analyses have included birth weight, placental weight, and even the PWR; however, the relative magnitude of the latter, in terms of percentiles, has not been previously available for all gestational ages in a Canadian population.

Abbreviations

PWR: Placental weight ratio
SGA: Small for gestational age
AGA: Average for gestational age
LGA: Large for gestational age.

Conflict of Interests

The authors declare that there is no conflict of interests regarding the publication of this paper.

Authors' Contribution

Erin M. Macdonald performed the literature search, conceptualized the study framework along with her MSc thesis supervisory committee, and performed the analyses. She also drafted the paper. John Koval assisted in the analyses plan and performed some analyses. He also reviewed, revised, and approved the final paper as submitted. Renato Natale assisted in conceptualizing the study framework and interpretation of results. He reviewed, revised, and approved the final paper as submitted. Timothy Regnault assisted in conceptualizing the study framework and interpreting the results. He also reviewed, revised, and approved the final paper as submitted. M. Karen Campbell oversaw all aspects of the work, as EMM's thesis supervisor, including conceptualizing the study framework and design, interpreting the results, and drafting the paper. She also reviewed, revised, and approved the final paper as submitted.

References

[1] C. M. Salafia, A. K. Charles, and E. M. Maas, "Placenta and fetal growth restriction," *Clinical Obstetrics and Gynecology*, vol. 49, no. 2, pp. 236–256, 2006.

[2] "Expert Committee Report: physical status: the use and interpretation of anthropometry," Tech. Rep. 854, WHO, Geneva, Switzerland, 1995, http://www.ncbi.nlm.nih.gov/pubmed/8594834.

[3] S. Heinonen, P. Taipale, and S. Saarikoski, "Weights of placentae from small-for-gestational age infants revisited," *Placenta*, vol. 22, no. 5, pp. 399–404, 2001.

[4] Y.-F. Lo, M.-J. Jeng, Y.-S. Lee, W.-J. Soong, and B. Hwang, "Placental weight and birth characteristics of healthy singleton newborns," *Acta Paediatrica Taiwanica*, vol. 43, no. 1, pp. 21–25, 2002.

[5] F. Lackman, V. Capewell, R. Gagnon, and B. Richardson, "Fetal umbilical cord oxygen values and birth to placental weight ratio in relation to size at birth," *American Journal of Obstetrics and Gynecology*, vol. 185, no. 3, pp. 674–682, 2001.

[6] B. Almog, F. Shehata, S. Aljabri, I. Levin, E. Shalom-Paz, and A. Shrim, "Placenta weight percentile curves for singleton and twins deliveries," *Placenta*, vol. 32, no. 1, pp. 58–62, 2011.

[7] J. M. Wallace, R. P. Aitken, J. S. Milne, and W. W. Hay, "Nutritionally mediated placental growth restriction in the growing adolescent: consequences for the fetus," *Biology of Reproduction*, vol. 71, no. 4, pp. 1055–1062, 2004.

[8] C. M. Salafia, J. Zhang, R. K. Miller, A. K. Charles, P. Shrout, and W. Sun, "Placental growth patterns affect birth weight for given placental weight," *Birth Defects Research A: Clinical and Molecular Teratology*, vol. 79, no. 4, pp. 281–288, 2007.

[9] K. R. Risnes, P. R. Romundstad, T. I. L. Nilsen, A. Eskild, and L. J. Vatten, "Placental weight relative to birth weight and long-term cardiovascular mortality: findings from a cohort of 31,307 men and women," *American Journal of Epidemiology*, vol. 170, no. 5, pp. 622–631, 2009.

[10] D. J. P. Barker, P. D. Gluckman, K. M. Godfrey, J. E. Harding, J. A. Owens, and J. S. Robinson, "Fetal nutrition and cardiovascular disease in adult life," *The Lancet*, vol. 341, no. 8850, pp. 938–941, 1993.

[11] D. J. P. Barker, C. N. Hales, C. H. D. Fall, C. Osmond, K. Phipps, and P. M. S. Clark, "Type 2 (non-insulin-dependent) diabetes mellitus, hypertension and hyperlipidaemia (syndrome X): relation to reduced fetal growth," *Diabetologia*, vol. 36, no. 1, pp. 62–67, 1993.

[12] D. J. Barker, C. Osmond, J. Golding, D. Kuh, and M. E. Wadsworth, "Growth in utero, blood pressure in childhood and adult life, and mortality from cardiovascular disease," *British Medical Journal*, vol. 298, no. 6673, pp. 564–567, 1989.

[13] S. Frankel, P. Elwood, P. Sweetnam, J. Yarnell, and G. D. Smith, "Birthweight, body-mass index in middle age, and incident coronary heart disease," *The Lancet*, vol. 348, no. 9040, pp. 1478–1480, 1996.

[14] A. D. Nyongo and P. B. Gichangi, "Placental weights: do they have clinical significance?" *East African Medical Journal*, vol. 68, no. 3, pp. 239–240, 1991.

[15] R. E. Little, T. D. Zadorozhnaja, O. P. Hulchiy et al., "Placental weight and its ratio to birthweight in a Ukrainian city," *Early Human Development*, vol. 71, no. 2, pp. 117–127, 2003.

[16] M. Janthanaphan, O. Kor-Anantakul, and A. Geater, "Placental weight and its ratio to birth weight in normal pregnancy at Songkhlanagarind Hospital," *Journal of the Medical Association of Thailand*, vol. 89, no. 2, pp. 130–137, 2006.

[17] R. A. Molteni, S. J. Stys, and F. C. Battaglia, "Relationship of fetal and placental weight in human beings: fetal/placental weight ratios at various gestational ages and birth weight distributions," *Journal of Reproductive Medicine*, vol. 21, no. 5, pp. 327–334, 1978.

[18] M. S. Kramer, R. W. Platt, S. W. Wen et al., "A new and improved population-based Canadian reference for birth weight for gestational age," *Pediatrics*, vol. 108, no. 2, p. E35, 2001.

[19] C. Chen, "An introduction to quantile regression and the QUANTREG procedure," Tech. Rep. 213-30, SAS Institute, Cary, NC, USA, 2003.

[20] J. M. D. Thompson, L. M. Irgens, R. Skjaerven, and S. Rasmussen, "Placenta weight percentile curves for singleton deliveries," *BJOG*, vol. 114, no. 6, pp. 715–720, 2007.

[21] M. P. Dombrowski, S. M. Berry, M. P. Johnson, A. A. A. Saleh, and R. J. Sokol, "Birth weight-length ratios, ponderal indexes, placental weights, and birth weight-placenta ratios in a large population," *Archives of Pediatrics and Adolescent Medicine*, vol. 148, no. 5, pp. 508–512, 1994.

[22] R. A. Molteni, "Placental growth and fetal/placental weight (F/P) ratios throughout gestation—their relationship to patterns of fetal growth," *Seminars in Perinatology*, vol. 8, no. 2, pp. 94–100, 1984.

[23] J. G. Sinclair, "Significance of placental and birthweight ratios," *The Anatomical Record*, vol. 102, no. 2, pp. 245–258, 1948.

[24] M. J. Novy, M. L. Aubert, S. L. Kaplan, and M. M. Grumbach, "Regulation of placental growth and chorionic somatomammotropin in the rhesus monkey: effects of protein deprivation, fetal anencephaly, and placental vessel ligation," *American Journal of Obstetrics and Gynecology*, vol. 140, no. 5, pp. 552–562, 1981.

[25] M. S. Kramer, I. Morin, H. Yang et al., "Why are babies getting bigger? Temporal trends in fetal growth and its determinants," *The Journal of Pediatrics*, vol. 141, no. 4, pp. 538–542, 2002.

[26] A. Eskild, P. R. Romundstad, and L. J. Vatten, "Placental weight and birthweight: does the association differ between pregnancies with and without preeclampsia?" *American Journal of Obstetrics and Gynecology*, vol. 201, no. 6, pp. 595.e1–595.e5, 2009.

[27] R. Bortolus, L. Chatenoud, E. di Cintio et al., "Placental ratio in pregnancies at different risk for intrauterine growth," *European Journal of Obstetrics & Gynecology and Reproductive Biology*, vol. 80, no. 2, pp. 157–158, 1998.

[28] M. Thame, C. Osmond, F. Bennett, R. Wilks, and T. Forrester, "Fetal growth is directly related to maternal anthropometry and placental volume," *European Journal of Clinical Nutrition*, vol. 58, no. 6, pp. 894–900, 2004.

[29] M. Thame, C. Osmond, R. Wilks, F. I. Bennett, and T. E. Forrester, "Second-trimester placental volume and infant size at birth," *Obstetrics and Gynecology*, vol. 98, no. 2, pp. 279–283, 2001.

[30] J. C. Kingdom and P. Kaufmann, "Oxygen and placental villous development: origins of fetal hypoxia," *Placenta*, vol. 18, no. 8, pp. 613–621, 623–626, 1997.

[31] J. C. Ross, P. V. Fennessey, R. B. Wilkening, F. C. Battaglia, and G. Meschia, "Placental transport and fetal utilization of leucine in a model of fetal growth retardation," *The American Journal of Physiology—Endocrinology and Metabolism*, vol. 270, no. 3, part 1, pp. E491–E503, 1996.

[32] J. M. Wallace, D. A. Bourke, R. P. Aitken, J. S. Milne, and W. W. Hay, "Placental glucose transport in growth-restricted pregnancies induced by overnourishing adolescent sheep," *The Journal of Physiology*, vol. 547, part 1, pp. 85–94, 2003.

[33] R. Ain, L. N. Canham, and M. J. Soares, "Dexamethasone-induced intrauterine growth restriction impacts the placental prolactin family, insulin-like growth factor-II and the Akt signaling pathway," *Journal of Endocrinology*, vol. 185, no. 2, pp. 253–263, 2005.

[34] N. Jansson, J. Pettersson, A. Haafiz et al., "Down-regulation of placental transport of amino acids precedes the development of intrauterine growth restriction in rats fed a low protein diet," *The Journal of Physiology*, vol. 576, part 3, pp. 935–946, 2006.

[35] W. Allen, "The influence of maternal size on placental, fetal and postnatal growth in the horse. II. Endocrinology of pregnancy," *Journal of Endocrinology*, vol. 172, no. 2, pp. 237–246, 2002.

[36] P. M. Coan, O. R. Vaughan, Y. Sekita et al., "Adaptations in placental phenotype support fetal growth during undernutrition of pregnant mice," *The Journal of Physiology*, vol. 588, part 3, pp. 527–538, 2010.

[37] F. Barut, A. Barut, B. D. Gun et al., "Intrauterine growth restriction and placental angiogenesis," *Diagnostic Pathology*, vol. 5, article 24, 2010.

[38] C. Pfarrer, L. Macara, R. Leiser, and J. Kingdom, "Adaptive angiogenesis in placentas of heavy smokers," *The Lancet*, vol. 354, no. 9175, p. 303, 1999.

[39] J. Kingdom, B. Huppertz, G. Seaward, and P. Kaufmann, "Development of the placental villous tree and its consequences for fetal growth," *European Journal of Obstetrics & Gynecology and Reproductive Biology*, vol. 92, no. 1, pp. 35–43, 2000.

[40] T. Todros, A. Sciarrone, E. Piccoli, C. Guiot, P. Kaufmann, and J. Kingdom, "Umbilical doppler waveforms and placental villous angiogenesis in pregnancies complicated by fetal growth restriction," *Obstetrics and Gynecology*, vol. 93, no. 4, pp. 499–503, 1999.

[41] A. Ahmed and J. Perkins, "Angiogenesis and intrauterine growth restriction," *Best Practice & Research Clinical Obstetrics & Gynaecology*, vol. 14, no. 6, pp. 981–998, 2000.

[42] J. M. Thompson, E. A. Mitchell, and B. Borman, "Sex specific birthweight percentiles by gestational age for New Zealand," *New Zealand Medical Journal*, vol. 107, no. 970, pp. 1–3, 1994.

28

Female Genital Mutilation in Infants and Young Girls: Report of Sixty Cases Observed at the General Hospital of Abobo (Abidjan, Cote D'Ivoire, West Africa)

Kouie Plo,[1,2] Kouadio Asse,[1] Dohagneron Seï,[1] and John Yenan[1]

[1] *Department of Pediatrics, General Hospital of Abobo, 14 PB 125 Abidjan 14, Cote D'Ivoire*
[2] *Department of Pediatrics, University Teaching Hospital of Bouake, 01 BP 1174 Bouake 01, Cote D'Ivoire*

Correspondence should be addressed to Kouie Plo; plo.kouie@yahoo.fr

Academic Editor: Hans Juergen Laws

The practice of female genital mutilations continues to be recurrent in African communities despite the campaigns, fights, and laws to ban it. A survey was carried out in infants and young girls at the General Hospital of Abobo in Cote D'Ivoire. The purpose of the study was to describe the epidemiological aspects and clinical findings related to FGM in young patients. Four hundred nine (409) females aged from 1 to 12 years and their mothers entered the study after their consent. The results were that 60/409 patients (15%) were cut. The majority of the young females came from Muslim families (97%); the earlier age at FGM procedure in patients is less than 5 years: 87%. Amongst 409 mothers, 250 women underwent FGM which had other daughters cut. Women were mainly involved in the FGM and their motivations were virginity, chastity, body cleanliness, and fear of clitoris similar to penis. Only WHO types I and II were met. If there were no incidental events occurred at the time of the procedure, the obstetrical future of these young females would be compromised. With FGM being a harmful practice, health professionals and NGOs must unite their efforts in people education to abandon the procedure.

1. Introduction

Female genital mutilation or clitoris cutting (FGM) is defined as the partial or total removal of clitoris and labia. Well known since antiquity in Egypt, this practice is widespread in the world but mainly in Africa [1–7]. Many factors related to tradition, sexual behavior in the males, and religious beliefs impact on FGM [8–11]. The clinical observation of three cases: first in female newborn twins aged three weeks and second in an 8-year girl led us to carry out a prospective study on FGM in infants and young girls. We studied the prevalence and etiologic factors in the pediatric ward at the General Hospital of Abobo, a suburb of Abidjan. Our study also aimed to influence the parents of girls and the traditional circumcisers and practitioners to abandon the practice. Not only are there laws prohibiting FGM, but there are later gynecological and obstetrical consequences of FGM.

Our objectives were (1) to identify FGM in infants and young girls seen in our clinic, (2) to describe the sociocultural context of young girls who had undergone FGM, (3) to assess the mothers' FGM status and attitudes regarding the practice, (4) and to determine the clinical issues in terms of immediate or later complications.

2. Patients and Methods

The General Hospital of Abobo is the premier public health entity that takes care of many patients of Abobo and others from periurban areas of Abidjan. This includes about 1,500,000 inhabitants or 20% of the population of the city of Abidjan. The pediatric ward enrolls 8,000 outpatients and hospitalizes about 2,500 inpatients a year. Eligible for the survey were infants and young girls seen at the hospital for any reason and whose mothers agreed verbally or by written consent to enter the survey and answer the questionnaire items.

From 16 April to 16 December, 2007, during eight months, 409 infants and young girls aged from 1 to 14 years and

TABLE 1: Main characteristics of patients' parents.

Parents' characteristics	Number (%)	
Nationality		
Cote d'Ivoire	35 (58.3)	
Mali	18 (30.0)	
Burkina Faso	5 (8.3)	
Benin and Niger	2 (3.4)	
Ethnic groups		
Malinke and Senoufo (Cote d'Ivoire)	35 (58.3)	
Malinke, Bambara, Dogon, and Peulh (Mali)	18 (30.0)	
Senoufo (Burkina Faso)	5 (8.3)	
Hausas (Benin and Niger)	2 (3.4)	
Religion		
Muslim	59 (98.3)	
Christian	1 (1.7)	
Level of education	Mothers	Fathers
Analphabets	40 (66.7)	33 (55.0)
Primary school	9 (15.0)	19 (31.7)
Secondary school	6 (10.0)	5 (8.3)
High school	5 (8.3)	3 (5.0)
Decision makers		
Grandmothers	43 (71.6)	
Mothers and aunts	15 (25.0)	
Fathers	2 (3.4)	
Parents' motivations		
Virginity and chastity	60 (100.0)	
Body cleanliness	38 (63.3)	
Clitoris: male organ and harmful	38 (63.3)	

their mothers entered the prospective study. The FGM status of girls was recorded during in- or outpatient visits. These examinations were complemented by a questionnaire comprising four groups of items: (1) patient's identification with age, native region (north, south, east, west, and center of the country), ethnic group, religion, and nationality; (2) history and circumstances of FGM practice, age at FGM procedure, observance of ritual ceremony or not, the individuals behind the decision of FGM practice, and the motivations; the circumciser (childbirth attendant or matron), tools used for FGM, and the occurrence of immediate complications such as bleeding, the medicines used to heal the wounds, the rituals observed during the FGM ceremony, time elapsing before full wound healing, and the FGM status of the mothers themselves; (3) evidence of FGM by a physical general examination including the genitalia and classification of FGM, when present, according to the World Health Organization's (WHO) classification [12]: these are type I: Sunna partial or total removal of the clitoris and/or the prepuce or excision, type II: partial or total removal of the clitoris and the labia minora, with or without excision of the labia majora (clitoredectomy), type III: narrowing of the vaginal orifice with creation of a covering seal by cutting and apposing the labia minora and/or the labia majora with or without excision of the clitoris (infibulations or pharaonic circumcision), and type IV: all other harmful procedures to the female genitalia for nonmedical purposes piercing, pricking, incising, scraping, and cauterization of the genitalia area (unclassifiable).

Ethics of Our Study. The General Hospital Consultative Committee that evaluates the relevance, feasibility, confidentiality of the information obtained, and ethnical aspects of clinical research reviewed our protocol of research and gave its permission. Once the mother's oral or written consent was obtained, the same female physician organized the questionnaire, performed the physical examinations, and filled out the data sheets during both inpatients and outpatients consultations.

3. Results

Sixty of 409 infants and young girls (15%) were diagnosed as having undergone FGM. Their age distribution at the time of consultation or hospitalization was between 1 and 5 years: 19, (32%) between 5 and 10 years: 29 (48%) and between 10 and 15 years: 12 (20%). The baseline characteristics on epidemiological aspects were the earlier age at FGM practice, 19 infants under one-year old; women were the individuals behind the decision of FGM practice (96.60%); several West

TABLE 2: Characteristics of infants and young girls undergone FGM.

Patients' characteristics	Number (%)
Age at FGM practice (years)[1]	
<1	19 (31.7)
(1–5)	29 (48.3)
(5–10)	12 (20.0)
FGM classification (WHO)	
Type I	8 (13.3)
Type II	52 (86.7)
Symptoms reported after FGM[2]	
Pain	60 (100.0)
Fever	47 (78.3)
Minimal bleeding	60 (100.0)

[1] Areas where FGM took place: Abobo and Adjamé (35 or 58% in Abidjan); Korhogo, Ferkessedougou, Odienne, and Boundiali: 11 (Northern region of Cote d'Ivoire); Kaye, Mopti, Boroni, and Bonangoro 14 (23%) in Mali. All the FGMs were performed in circumcisers' home with knives, razors, or blades.
[2] Each girl could have one or more symptoms.

TABLE 3: Distribution of patients according to the age at FGM practice and FGM types.

Age at FGM practice (years)	FGM classification (WHO)		
	Type I	Type II	Total
<1	0	19	19
1–5	1	28	29
5–10	7	5	12
Total	8	52	60

There is a high risk to have undergone FGM type II between 1–5 years (IC 95% P value < 0.05).

African ethnic groups from Cote d'Ivoire, Mali, Burkina Faso, Benin, and Niger were implicated; Muslim families 59/60 and the illiterate or low educational level of the parents 81% and 87%, respectively in mothers and fathers were found as major factors. The practitioners were traditional circumcisers; no nurses, midwives, or physicians were involved.

About the clinical findings, only FGM types I and II were diagnosed. Pain, fever, and minimal bleeding were the main symptoms and signs disclosed by the mothers surveyed. There was a potential relative risk of undergoing type II mutilation for those under five years of age. Amongst the mothers, 250 women out of 409 had had FGM (61.1%). Among them, 151 had their daughters (60.4%) undergone the procedure. The details of sociocultural characteristics of our samples and the clinical findings of our patients are reported on the Tables 1, 2, and 3 and Figure 1 shows a FGM type II in a 1-year-old Peulh female.

4. Discussion

4.1. Epidemiology. The prevalence of FGM among our patients population was 15%. The main associated factors were as follows: women were the decision makers relative to FGM; in 97% of cases, it was a grandmother, mother, or aunt who

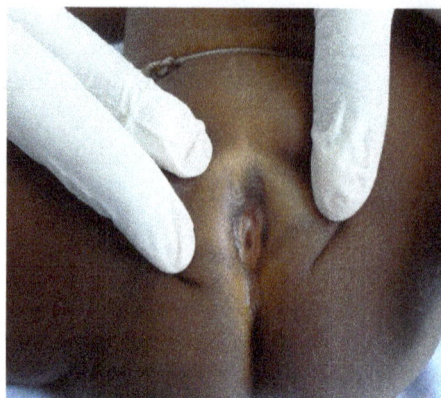

FIGURE 1: FCM type II in a 1-year-old Peulh female (picture photographed in our ward of pediatrics).

initiated the operation. Their chief motivations encompassed chastity (100%) and esthetics (68%).

FGM was encountered most often in the communities of three countries with a relative high rate in some ethnic groups as the Malinke and Senoufo. Most families were Muslim (98.3%) and most parents were illiterate, 81% and 87% in mothers and fathers, respectively.

Previous reports on FGM in West African women [13–17] gave rates varying from 45 to 60% in the general population and 20 up to 87% in northern and western regions of the country. Rates were high among the Dan, Malinke, Wè, and Senoufo ethnic groups. The proportion of young girls has been estimated by Oulaï in his report to be about 500 females. Those were 31% for 155 children between 0 and 5 years; 31.4% for 157 between 12 and 16 years of age; and 38.6% in 193 women.

The majority were of the Dan group (80.12%); 94.6% were illiterate. Only 5.4% had had a primary and secondary school level of education. The religions were distributed in this way: Christians: 55.91%, Muslims: 43.34%, and animists 0.75% [18]. The decision makers were mainly women: grandmothers (71.6%), mothers (25.0%), and fathers (3.4%). In a survey carried out in 38,816 Egyptian young school girls the prevalence of FGM was 50.3% (19,543). The motivations were religion: 33.4%, cleanliness for girls: 18.9%, cultural and ancient tradition: 17.9%, and chastity 15%. Compared to the study of Snow et al. in Nigeria, similar characteristics had been found amongst young girls and women between 15 and 49 years victims of FGM and interviewed: age at FGM prior one year 371 (68.3%), between one and ten years 43 (7.9%), and ten to twenty years 88 (16.3%) [19]. The religious context in this study was Pentecostals: 562 (33.1%), Protestants 277 (16.3%), Catholics 613 (36.1%), Muslim 100 (5.9%), and others 146 (8.6%). On the other hand educational level of the surveyed girls was distributed as follows: primary: 330 (19.3%), secondary: 533 (32.2%), tertiary 767 (44.9%), and none 77 (4.5%) showing the inhomogeneous and spatial distribution of sociocultural factors in the practice of FGM. The commonest basis would be the ancient and tradition beliefs [20, 21]. These observations are similar to those in data from Burkina Faso, Mali, Guinea, and Gambia in West Africa [22].

4.2. Clinical Findings and FGM Classification. About the clinical findings, FGM types I and II accounted for 100% of cases whereas in Somalia, Sudan and Egypt, Mali, and Burkina Faso types III and IV were mentioned up to 89% [23–25]. The immediate complications, such as pain, fever, and minimal or incidental bleeding as short period of bleeding (if it is severe) could be catastrophic, were probably underestimated. Hemorrhages, infections, and death have been reported together with the posttraumatic stress disorders and memory problems [26, 27]. What is the future of our patients? Most did not have major long-term complications, after the fear and the psychological trauma of FGM, finding similar to those of Althaus [28].

These infants and young girls, once adults, could nonetheless face the late consequences of FGM. These include psychological, gynecological, and obstetrical difficulties. Painful intercourse, bleeding, dystocia, long labor, and episiotomy needed at the time of labor have been reported by gynecologists and many nongovernmental organizations fighting for the abandonment of FGM [29, 30].

Although in our study no major psychological troubles were encountered, posttraumatic stress disorders have been reported in patients similar to ours [31–35].

4.3. Elimination of FGM. Many African countries and elsewhere in the world have laws prohibiting FGM. Nongovernmental organizations (NGOs) campaigns against FGM continue to fight for its abandonment [36–40]. Despite these laws and campaigns to eliminate it, FGM continues in urban and rural areas, as our study and other recent reports have shown [41, 42].

5. Conclusion

Our study has shown the current reality of FGM in earlier age. It resulted from traditional and religious beliefs. Women, having a past history of FGM, play the key role in the occurrence of FGM in their daughters. Only types I and II mutilations have been met.

There were few immediate complications. The combination of law-enforcement together with information and education activities by NGO's aimed at female populations has curtailed FGM in most countries. Continuing efforts are needed to eliminate FGM as a threat to the health and wellbeing of women.

Conflict of Interests

On behalf of all the authors of this paper Kouie Plo states and certifies that there is no conflict of interests in the publication of this report. The authors did not receive any finance for this survey.

Acknowledgments

The authors would like to thank the Head of the General Hospital of Abobo and the members of the Consultative Committee for its approval, Professor Emeritus Giulio John D'Angio, formerly at the Department of Radiation Oncology at the University of Pennsylvania, Philadelphia, PA, USA, for the prereview and improvement of the final manuscript.

References

[1] E. Herieka and J. Dhar, "Female genital mutilation in the Sudan: survey of the attitude of Khartoum University students towards this practice," *Sexually Transmitted Infections*, vol. 79, no. 3, pp. 220–223, 2003.

[2] L. Morison, C. Scherf, G. Ekpo et al., "The long-term reproductive health consequences of female genital cutting in rural Gambia: a community-based survey," *Tropical Medicine and International Health*, vol. 6, no. 8, pp. 643–653, 2001.

[3] M. A. Tag-Eldin, M. A. Gadallah, M. N. Al-Tayeb, M. Abdel-Aty, E. Mansour, and M. Sallem, "Prevalence of female genital cutting among Egyptian girls," *Bulletin of the World Health Organization*, vol. 86, no. 4, pp. 269–274, 2008.

[4] P. S. Yoder and M. Mahy, *Female Genital Cutting in Guinea: Qualitative and Quantitative Research Strategies*, vol. 5 of *DHS Analytical Studies*, DHS, Calverton, Md, USA, 2001.

[5] P. S. Yoder and S. Khan, "Numbers of women circumcised in Africa: the production of a total," Demographic Health Research, DHS Working Papers no. 39, Macro, 2008.

[6] G. A. O. Magoha and O. B. Magoha, "Current global status of female genital mutilation: a review," *East African Medical Journal*, vol. 77, no. 5, pp. 268–272, 2000.

[7] D. Dubourg, F. Richard, R. Eggermont et al., "Etudes des femmes excisées et des filles à risque d'excision en Belgique," Institut de Médecine Tropicale, 2010.

[8] S. Faizang, "Circoncision, excision et rapports de domination," *Anthropologie Et Société*, vol. 9, no. 1, pp. 117–127, 1985.

[9] R. A. Shweder, "What about female genital mutilation? And why understanding culture matters the first place," in *Engaging Cultural Differences: The Multicultural Challenge in Liberal Democracies*, R. Shweder, M. Minow, and H. Markus, Eds., pp. 216–225, Russell Sage Foundation, New York, NY, USA, 2002.

[10] C. Ibe and C. Johnson-Agbakwu, "Female genital cutting: addressing the issues of culture and ethics," *The Female Patient*, vol. 36, pp. 28–31, 2011.

[11] J. Whitehorn, O. Ayonrinde, and S. Maingay, "Female genital mutilation: cultural and psychological implications," *Sexual and Relationship Therapy*, vol. 17, no. 2, pp. 161–170, 2002.

[12] World Health Organization, "Female genital mutilation," Report of a WHO Technical Working Group, World Health Organization, Geneva, Switzerland, 1995.

[13] UNICEF, "History and estimated prevalence among women aged 15–49 years," MICS, 2006, http://www.orchildproject.org/category/resources/country-pages/page3.

[14] MICS, WHO, DHS, and UNICEF Côte d'Ivoire, "Overview of female genital mutilation/cutting," Unicef DHS 1994, 1998/1999, http://www.childinfo.org/files/CotedIvoire_FGC_profile_English.pdf.

[15] J. C. Oulai, *La pratique de l'excision dans la région de Logoualé (Côte-d'Ivoire) [Ph.D. thesis]*, Université d'Abidjan, 2006.

[16] UNICEF, Benin DSH, "Overview of female genital mutilation/cutting. FGM/country profile," 2001, http://www.childinfo.org/files/Benin_FGC_profile_English.pdf.

[17] UNICEF, Niger DSH, "Overview of female genital mutilation/cutting," 1998, http://www.childinfo.org/files/Niger_FGC_profile_English.pdf.

[18] N. J. Diop, Z. Congo, A. Ouédraogo et al., "Analysis of the evolution of the practice of female genital mutilation/cutting in Burkina Faso," Population Council Frontiers Reproductive Health, USAID, 2008.

[19] R. C. Snow, T. E. Slanger, F. E. Okonofua, F. Oronsaye, and J. Wacker, "Female genital cutting in southern urban and peri-urban Nigeria: delf-reported validity, social determinants and secular decline," Tropical Medicine and International Health, vol. 7, no. 1, pp. 91–100, 2002.

[20] C. Feldman-Jacobs and D. Clifton, "Female genital mutilation/cutting: data and trends," Population Reference Bureau, USAID, 2010.

[21] P. S. Yoder, N. Abderrahim, and A. Zhuzhuni, "Female genital cutting in the demographic and health surveys: a critical and comparative analysis," DHS Comparative Reports no. 7, ORC Macro, Calverton, Md, USA, 2004.

[22] P. S. Yoder and S. Khan, "Numbers of women circumcised in Africa: the production of a total," Demographic Health Research, DHS Working Papers no. 39, Macro, 2008.

[23] D. M. Westley, "Female circumcision and infibulation in Africa," Electronic Journal of Africana Bibliography, vol. 4, pp. 1–50, 1999.

[24] L. Almroth, Genital Mutilation of Girls in Sudan: Community and Hospital-Based Studies on Female Genital Cutting and Its Sequelae, Karolinska University Press, Stockholm, Sweden, 2005.

[25] H. Jones, N. Diop, I. Askew, and I. Kaboré, "Female genital cutting practices in Burkina Faso and Mali and their negative health outcomes," Studies in Family Planning, vol. 30, no. 3, pp. 219–230, 1999.

[26] D. O. Osifo and I. Evbuomwan, "Female genital mutilation among Edo people: the complications and pattern of presentation at a pediatric surgery unit, Benin City," African Journal of Reproductive Health, vol. 13, no. 1, pp. 17–25, 2009.

[27] A. R. Oduro, P. Ansah, A. Hodgson et al., "Trends in the prevalence of female genital mutilation and its effect on delivery outcomes in Kassena-Nankana district of Northern Ghana," Ghana Medical Journal, vol. 40, no. 3, pp. 87–92, 2006.

[28] F. A. Althaus, "Female circumcision: rite of passage or violation of rights?" International Family Planning Perspectives, vol. 23, no. 3, pp. 130–133, 1997.

[29] M. Brady, "Female genital mutilation: complications and risk of HIV transmission," AIDS Patient Care and STDs, vol. 13, no. 12, pp. 709–716, 1999.

[30] A. Behrendt and S. Moritz, "Posttraumatic stress disorder and memory problems after female genital mutilation," The American Journal of Psychiatry, vol. 162, no. 5, pp. 1000–1002, 2005.

[31] J. I. Kizilhan, "Impact of psychological disorders after female genital mutilation among Kurdish girls in Northern Iraq," European Journal of Psychiatry, vol. 25, no. 2, pp. 92–100, 2011.

[32] American Academy of Pediatrics Committee on Bioethics, "Ritual genital cutting of female minors," Pediatrics, vol. 125, no. 5, pp. 1088–1093, 2010.

[33] D. M. Elsayed, R. M. Elamin, and S. M. Sulaiman, "Female genital mutilation and ethical issue," Sudanese Journal of Public Health, vol. 6, no. 2, pp. 63–67, 2011.

[34] UNICEF, "The impact of a harmful traditional practice on child girl," Ras-Work B UNICEF, Innocenti Research Centre, Florence, Italy, 2006.

[35] A. Rahman and N. Toubia, Female Genital Mutilation: A Guide to Laws and Policies Worldwide, Center for Reproductive Law & Policy Rainbo, Zed, London, UK, 2000.

[36] E. Finke, "Genital mutilation as an expression of power structures: ending FGM through education, empowerment of women and removal of taboos," African Journal of Reproductive Health, vol. 10, no. 2, pp. 13–17, 2006.

[37] OHCHR, UNAIDS, UNDP et al., "Eliminating female genital mutilation: an interagency statement," 2008.

[38] I. Askew, "Methodological issues in measuring the impact of interventions against female genital cutting," Culture, Health & Sexuality, vol. 7, no. 5, pp. 463–477, 2005.

[39] W. Zuckerman, "Female genital mutilation becomes less common in Egypt," New Scientist, vol. 17, article 22, 2011.

[40] E. Denison, R. C. Berg, S. Lewin et al., "Effectiveness of interventions designed to reduce the prevalence of female genital mutilation/cutting," Systematic Report no. 25, Kunnskapssenteret Norwegian Knowledge Center for the Health Sciences, Oslo, Norway, 2005.

[41] E. Dorkenoo and S. Elworthy, "Female genital mutilation: proposals for change," Health and Medicine, Minority Rights, London, UK, 1992.

[42] UNICEF Innocenti Research Centre, "Changing a harmful social convention: female genital mutilation/cutting," Innocenti Digest, Florence, Italy, 2005.

29

Parental Involvement in the Preoperative Surgical Safety Checklist Is Welcomed by Both Parents and Staff

Martin T. Corbally[1,2] and Eamon Tierney[3,4]

[1] Our Lady's Hospital for Sick Children, Crumlin, Dublin 12, Ireland
[2] Paediatric Surgery, Royal College of Surgeons, Dublin 2, Ireland
[3] King Hamad University Hospital, Busaiteen, P.O. Box 24343, Bahrain
[4] Anaesthesia and Intensive Care, RCSI Medical University of Bahrain, Al Sayh, Bahrain

Correspondence should be addressed to Eamon Tierney; estjmt@gmail.com

Academic Editor: Samuel Menahem

We involved the parents of paediatric patients in the first part of the three-stage WHO Surgical Safety Checklist (SSC) process. Forty-two parents took part in the study. They came to the theatre suite with their child and into the induction room. Immediately before induction of anaesthesia they were present at, and took part in, the first stage of the three-stage SSC process, confirming with staff the identity of their child, the procedure to be performed, the operating site, and the consent being adequately obtained and recorded. We asked parents and theatre staff later whether they thought that parental involvement in the SSC was beneficial to patient safety. Both parents and staff welcomed parental involvement in the WHO Surgical Safety Checklist and felt that it improved patient safety.

1. Introduction

The past thirty years have witnessed major technological advances in medicine and surgery that have in turn generated an expectation that all aspects of care should be delivered faultlessly and without negative consequence to the patient.

However the latent marriage of human error and systems failure continues to contribute to shortfalls in care delivery and this is especially evident in the continuing risks involved in anaesthesic and surgical practice. These risks are not insignificant and are reported to be as high as 22% in all surgical procedures, with an overall mortality approaching 1% [1–3].

Arising from this reported negative outcome, the World Health Organisation (WHO) introduced the Surgical Safety Checklist in 2008 to reduce the risk of adverse events during surgery. The checklist is in three parts consisting of

(i) an initial check (time in) by the anaesthetist and his assistant;

(ii) a "time out" checklist before incision by the surgeon anaesthetist and nurse;

(iii) a final check by the surgeon, anaesthetist, and nurse before the patient leaves theatre.

These checks are designed to ensure the following.

(i) The patient is the correct patient.

(ii) The planned surgery is the correct surgery for the patient.

(iii) The surgical site is marked on the correct side.

(iv) All equipment, both anaesthetic and surgical, is available.

(v) The anaesthetist is prepared for any patient allergy, airway problem, and blood loss.

(vi) Prophylactic antibiotics are given if considered appropriate.

(vii) The surgeon has essential imaging displayed, performs the correct operation, and anticipates duration of surgery and blood loss.

(viii) All specimens are labeled correctly.

(ix) Surgical, anaesthetic, and nursing concerns for recovery are expressed before leaving theatre.

In paediatric surgical practice the parent is usually omitted from the safety check. Parental involvement in the Surgical Safety Checklist process has been recommended by WHO but is not universally accepted. This may reflect local concerns that parents are already stressed and that their involvement in the first stage of the Surgical Safety Checklist may add to their anxiety. There is also an unwritten concern that parental involvement will cause delay and add to staff anxiety in an already stressful environment.

2. Objectives

This prospective study was conducted to establish how theatre staff and parent(s) would accept parental involvement in the first stage of the three-stage WHO Surgical Safety Checklist performed in theatre before anaesthetic induction. We explored the question of whether parents and staff agreed with and welcomed parental involvement in the first stage of the three-stage WHO Surgical Safety Checklist.

3. Method

Following institutional approval at Our Lady's Children's Hospital, Crumlin, parents were given a leaflet detailing the nature of the normal Surgical Safety Checklist. Their approval to be involved was sought and they were asked to complete a survey before their child was discharged. The parents of all consecutive day-case patients with laterality issues were asked to participate in this study over a defined 6-week period. The patients ranged in age from two years to twelve years of age. Patients where laterality was not an issue, for example, umbilical hernia repair, excluded from the study. There were no other exclusions, as all patients with laterality issues had an accompanying parent. In the first of the three stages of the WHO Surgical Safety Checklist a change was made. This was the standard first-stage check before induction of anaesthesia but this time with the parent present to assist in the confirmation of the child's identity, the operation to be performed, and the site of surgery and to confirm the correct consent. The parents were also asked to express any concern they may have. No parent refused to be involved in the checklist.

The parent remained with the child until after anaesthesia had been induced and was then accompanied out of the theatre suite by a theatre orderly.

Postoperatively, parents were asked the following questions.

(1) Rate your involvement in the Surgical Safety Checklist.

Poor Average Good Excellent

(2) Do you believe that your involvement improves patient safety? Yes No

(3) Do you believe that the correct surgery was to be performed? Yes No

(4) Should parental involvement in the Surgical Safety Checklist be mandatory for all children undergoing surgery? Yes No

All staff (nurses, anaesthetists, and surgeons) were also briefed as to the nature of the study and its objectives and asked to complete a questionnaire.

For staff the questions were as follows.

(1) Rate the benefit of parental involvement in the Surgical Safety Checklist.

Poor Average Good Excellent

(2) Do you believe that parental involvement in the Surgical Safety Checklist improves patient safety during surgery? Yes No

(3) Do you feel that parental involvement in the Surgical Safety Checklist adds to the complexity of the process? Yes No

4. Results

4.1. Parents. A total of 46 patients were admitted to the study. Four patients were omitted due to survey completion errors. 31% (13/42) and 69% (29/42) of parents rated their involvement in the Surgical Safety Checklist as good or excellent, respectively. All parents (100%, 42/42) considered their involvement as improving patient safety and 97.6% (41/42) considered that the site and procedure were correct. One parent expressed concern as the surgical team appropriately changed the consent prior to the operation to reflect a change of procedure. All parents (42/42) considered that parental involvement should be mandatory for all children undergoing surgery and none expressed any concern of added anxiety.

4.2. Staff. 52.4% (22/42), 73.8% (31/42), and 28.6% (12/42) of nurses, surgeons, and anaesthetists rated parental involvement in the Surgical Safety Checklist as excellent while 47.6% (20/42) 26.2% (11/42) and 69% (29/42) rated it as good. 2.4% (1 anaesthetist) rated it as average. All staff believed that it improved patient safety and 100% of surgeons, 88% of nurses, and 76% of anaesthetists considered that parental involvement in the Surgical Safety Checklist did not add to the complexity of the process while the remainder felt that it was a justifiable addition.

5. Discussion

Risk management structures are now embedded in hospital practice and are accepted as a vital component of our efforts to prevent inadvertent surgical outcomes and wrong site surgery. The Surgical Safety Checklist is a relatively new concept aimed at ensuring that the correct patient is in theatre to have the correct procedure on the correct side and also to enable any team member to voice concerns about the planned procedure. In paediatric surgical practice however the parent is frequently excluded from this process. Of course informed consent has already been obtained and logically it would seem impossible for any error to occur. Yet it is the case that surgical errors are often due to a failure to communicate concerns or a continuation of the classic "Plan-Continue-Fail" scenario with potentially serious negative outcomes [4]. Generally parents are fully acquainted with the planned procedure but while they may have already expressed concerns this concern may not be relayed correctly or at all to the operating surgeon especially if a different staff member had taken consent. It is at this juncture that the latent marriage of human error and reliance on hospital systems, including the Surgical Safety Checklist, places the patient at most risk. Errors in communication occur with unacceptable frequency and are generally based on an assumption that concerns will be noted, addressed, and, more importantly, acted upon. While responsibility will always rest with the operating surgeon it seems prudent to provide further safeguards and ensure that all information will be passed on. We believed that it would be better to achieve this by ensuring that parents are able to express their approval or concerns at the time of induction in the presence of the operating team.

The reasons for not involving parents at this crucial stage may however underscore a belief that the Surgical Safety Checklist and consent process are robust enough and cannot possibly fail or that the institution and its staff believe that parents are already too stressed with the prospect of their child undergoing surgery. Parental involvement allows the parent to express concerns or questions which may not have been answered preoperatively or which may have come into the parent's mind after completion of the consent process. Paternalistic attitudes to minimise parental anxiety at the time of induction may explain why the Surgical Safety Checklist has not been more widely practiced in paediatric surgery. This study clearly demonstrates that parents valued their involvement in the Surgical Safety Checklist process and did so willingly with no reported added anxiety. It also demonstrated that all theatre staff did not feel parental involvement was intrusive to the operating list and that they too felt it should be a welcome part of the process.

6. Conclusion

Our results suggest that parents consider their involvement in the Surgical Safety Checklist as worthwhile and they consider that it should be mandatory. No parent expressed added anxiety from this involvement and 97% felt reassured that that correct procedure was to be performed. Similarly, staff responses confirmed the view that parental involvement improves patient safety and does not increase the complexity of the checklist process. This small, prospective study indicates that parents and staff alike consider that parental involvement in the Surgical Safety Checklist should be welcomed and encouraged, where local conditions allow it, to minimize the risks of wrong surgery or wrong site surgery.

Ethical Approval

The Research Ethics Committee at Our Lady's Hospital, Crumlin, Dublin, granted ethical approval for this study.

Disclosure

This study was conducted as a requirement for a Higher Diploma course in Healthcare and Risk Management, at University College, Dublin, June 2011, and was presented orally by Martin T. Corbally for assessment at the Faculty of Legal Medicine, UCD, in part fulfillment of that award.

Conflict of Interests

The authors declare that there is no conflict of interests regarding the publication of this paper.

Authors' Contribution

Dr. Tierney contributed to the plan of the study. Professor Corbally carried out the study at Our Lady's Hospital for Sick Children, Crumlin, Dublin. Data were analysed and the paper was written jointly by Martin Corbally and Eamon Tierney.

References

[1] P. F. Stahel, A. L. Sabel, M. S. Victoroff et al., "Wrong-site and wrong-patient procedures in the universal protocol era: analysis of a prospective database of physician self-reported occurrences," *Archives of Surgery*, vol. 145, no. 10, pp. 978–984, 2010.

[2] L. L. Leape, "Error in medicine," *Journal of the American Medical Association*, vol. 272, no. 23, pp. 1851–1857, 1994.

[3] J. Neily, P. D. Mills, N. Eldridge et al., "Incorrect surgical procedures within and outside of the operating room," *Archives of Surgery*, vol. 144, no. 11, pp. 1028–1034, 2009.

[4] P. J. Pronovost and J. A. Freischlag, "Improving teamwork to reduce surgical mortality," *Journal of the American Medical Association*, vol. 304, no. 15, pp. 1721–1722, 2010.

30

Neonatal Thrombocytopenia after Perinatal Asphyxia Treated with Hypothermia: A Retrospective Case Control Study

N. Boutaybi,[1] **F. Razenberg,**[1] **V. E. H. J. Smits-Wintjens,**[1] **E. W. van Zwet,**[2]
M. Rijken,[1] **S. J. Steggerda,**[1] **and E. Lopriore**[1]

[1] *Division of Neonatology, Department of Pediatrics, Leiden University Medical Center, J6-S, Albinusdreef 2,*
 2333 ZA Leiden, The Netherlands
[2] *Department of Medical Statistics, Leiden University Medical Center, Albinusdreef 2, 2333 ZA Leiden, The Netherlands*

Correspondence should be addressed to E. Lopriore; e.lopriore@lumc.nl

Academic Editor: Naveed Hussain

Our objective was to estimate the effect of therapeutic hypothermia on platelet count in neonates after perinatal asphyxia. We performed a retrospective case control study of all (near-) term neonates with perinatal asphyxia admitted between 2004 and 2012 to our neonatal intensive care unit. All neonates treated with therapeutic hypothermia were included in this study (hypothermia group) and compared with a historic control group of neonates with perinatal asphyxia treated before introduction of therapeutic hypothermia (2008). Primary outcome was thrombocytopenia during the first week after birth. Thrombocytopenia was found significantly more often in the hypothermia group than in the control group, 80% (43/54) versus 59% (27/46) ($P = .02$). The lowest mean platelet count in the hypothermia group and control group was 97×10^9/L and 125×10^9/L ($P = .06$), respectively, and was reached at a mean age of 4.1 days in the hypothermia group and 2.9 days in the control group ($P < .001$). The incidence of moderate/severe cerebral hemorrhage was 6% (3/47) in the hypothermia group versus 9% (3/35) in the control group ($P = .64$). In conclusion, neonates with perinatal asphyxia treated with therapeutic hypothermia are at increased risk of thrombocytopenia, without increased risk of cerebral hemorrhage.

1. Introduction

Thrombocytopenia, defined as a platelet count below 150×10^9/L, occurs in 1 to 5% of healthy term neonates [1, 2]. The prevalence of thrombocytopenia is reported to be much higher in sick neonates, ranging from 22 to 35% in those admitted to neonatal intensive care units [1–4]. Thrombocytopenia is associated with an increased risk of pulmonary, gastrointestinal, and intraventricular hemorrhage (IVH) [5].

One of the most common causes of early-onset thrombocytopenia (<72 h of birth) in term neonates is perinatal asphyxia [2]. Perinatal asphyxia remains an important cause of morbidity and mortality of the full-term newborn and is still a major cause of death worldwide [6–10]. Therapeutic hypothermia, nowadays considered as the gold standard of treatment for perinatal asphyxia, reduces the risk of permanent brain injury and is associated with decreased rates of mortality and neurodevelopmental disability [6, 9, 11–13].

The protective effects of hypothermia are attributed primarily to a reduction of apoptosis and of inflammation [12].

In a recent Cochrane meta-analysis, therapeutic hypothermia was reported to increase the relative risk (RR) of thrombocytopenia in neonates with perinatal asphyxia (relative risk (RR): 1.21 (95% confidence interval (CI) 1.05–1.40)) compared to a control group [14]. However, research on the severity, course, and consequences of thrombocytopenia after therapeutic hypothermia is limited.

The aim of this study was to estimate the incidence, timing, and severity of thrombocytopenia during the first week after birth in neonates with perinatal asphyxia and to study the effect of therapeutic hypothermia on platelet count.

2. Methods

All (near-) term neonates (≥36 weeks' gestation) with perinatal asphyxia admitted to the tertiary neonatal intensive care

(i) Gestational age at birth ≥36 weeks

(ii) **AND** perinatal asphyxia defined as:

Apgar score at 5 minutes ≤5 **OR**

respiratory failure requiring resuscitation measures during at least 10 minutes after birth **OR**

arterial pH <7.0 and base excess ≤ −16 mmol/L in either arterial umbilical cord blood sample/arterial blood gas within one hour after birth **OR**

lactate >10 mmol/L in either arterial umbilical cord blood sample or arterial blood gas within one hour after birth

(iii) **AND** Encephalopathy with:

Thompson score >7 between 1 and 3 hours after birth **OR**

abnormal background pattern on aEEG

(iv) **AND** Start time of hypothermia as soon as possible, at least within 6 hours after birth.

Box 1: Selection criteria for therapeutic hypothermia at the Leiden University Medical Center.

unit of the Leiden University Medical Center from January 2004 to November 2012 were eligible for the study. In the hypothermia group we included all neonates with perinatal asphyxia treated with therapeutic hypothermia. In our neonatal intensive care unit treatment with hypothermia was introduced as standard management for perinatal asphyxia in September 2008. Neonates were cooled by whole-body hypothermia at a degree of 33.5°C for 72 hours. They were nursed on a cooling blanket in which fluid was circulating; the temperature of the fluid was regulated automatically (Criticool, MTRE Advanced technologies). After 72 hours we rewarmed them in intervals of 0.3°C per 60 minutes till a body temperature of 36.5°C was reached. The selection criteria for therapeutic hypothermia used in our center are shown in Box 1. Neonates with perinatal asphyxia admitted to our neonatal intensive care unit before October 2008 were not treated with therapeutic hypothermia and were included in the control group.

The primary aim of the study was to compare the incidence, severity, and course of thrombocytopenia between the hypothermia and the control group. Thrombocytopenia was defined as a platelet count below 150×10^9/L. The severity of thrombocytopenia was classified in four categories, based on the lowest platelet count in the first week after birth: mild (platelet count $100–149 \times 10^9$/L), moderate (platelet count $50–99 \times 10^9$/L), severe (platelet count $30–49 \times 10^9$/L), and very severe (platelet count $< 30 \times 10^9$/L). Data were extracted from our patient database and laboratory files. We recorded neonatal, laboratory, neurologic morbidity, and hematologic data in both groups.

2.1. Neonatal and Laboratory Data. The following neonatal and laboratory data were recorded: birth weight, gestational age at birth, gender, mode of delivery, Apgar score at 5 minutes, intubation in the delivery room, blood gas pH, base excess, and lactate level. Measurements of the laboratory data were performed either in arterial umbilical cord blood or in arterial or capillary blood gas within one hour after birth.

2.2. Hematologic Data. The following hematologic laboratory data were recorded: platelet count (at day 1 till day 7 after birth), prothrombin time (PT), activated partial thromboplastin time (APTT), international normalized ratio (INR), and fibrinogen level. As for hematologic treatment we recorded treatment with fresh frozen plasma (FFP), red blood cell transfusions, and/or platelet transfusions. In our neonatal intensive care unit, platelet transfusions are given when: (1) platelet count is below 30×10^9/L, stable infant, (2) platelet count is below 50×10^9/L, unstable infant, previous major bleeding or before planned surgery, or (3) platelet count is below 100×10^9/L in neonates with active bleeding [4].

2.3. Mortality, Neurologic Morbidity, and Other Clinical Data. The following postnatal data were recorded: mortality within 1 month after birth, neonatal seizures, treatment with anticonvulsants, neonatal sepsis (defined as a positive blood culture in a neonate with clinical signs of infection), small for gestational age (SGA, defined as a birth weight < 10th centile), days on mechanical ventilation, number of hospital days in our neonatal intensive care unit, and hemorrhage on cranial ultrasound and/or magnetic resonance imaging (MRI). Cranial ultrasound scan (CUS) results were assessed for IVH and parenchymal hemorrhage. IVH was classified according to Papile et al. [15]. MRI scans were reviewed for presence of subdural, intraparenchymal, and/or intraventricular hemorrhage.

We classified mild hemorrhage as mild IVH (grade 1), punctate parenchymal hemorrhage, and minor subdural bleeds without parenchymal compression and/or shift detected by CUS and/or MRI. Moderate/severe IVH (≥grade 2), larger parenchymal hemorrhage, and large subdural hemorrhage causing parenchymal compression and/or shift were classified as moderate/severe hemorrhage.

2.4. Statistical Analysis. We calculated that group sizes of at least 45 infants were required to demonstrate a 25% difference in incidence of thrombocytopenia (75% versus 50%) with a significance of 0.05 and a power of 80%, by one-tailed analysis. Chi-square tests or Fisher's exact tests were applied to analyze categorical variables, as appropriate. For comparison of continuous variables, independent-sample *t*-test was used. Odds ratios (OR) and 95% CI were calculated by univariate logistic regression. All reported *P* values were

TABLE 1: Baseline characteristics of the study population.

	Hypothermia group $n = 54$	Control group $n = 46$	P value
Birth weight—grams*	3446 (625)	3352 (606)	.45
Gestational age—weeks*	39.4 (1.55)	39.8 (1.85)	.28
Male gender—n (%)	27 (50%)	18 (39%)	.28
Caesarean delivery—n (%)	27 (50%)	28 (61%)	.28
Vacuum extraction—n (%)	16 (30%)	15 (33%)	.75
Forceps delivery—n (%)	2 (4%)	3 (7%)	.66
Shoulder dystocia—n (%)	4 (7%)	1 (2%)	.37
Apgar at 5 min ≤ 5—n (%)	51 (96%)	31 (67%)	.00
Arterial cord blood/blood gas			
pH <7.0—n (%)	39 (72%)	34 (74%)	.85
Base excess ≤ −16 mmol/L—n (%)	33 (61%)	24 (52%)	.37
Lactate >10 mmol/L—n (%)	33 (61%)	22 (48%)	.18

* Value given as mean (SD).

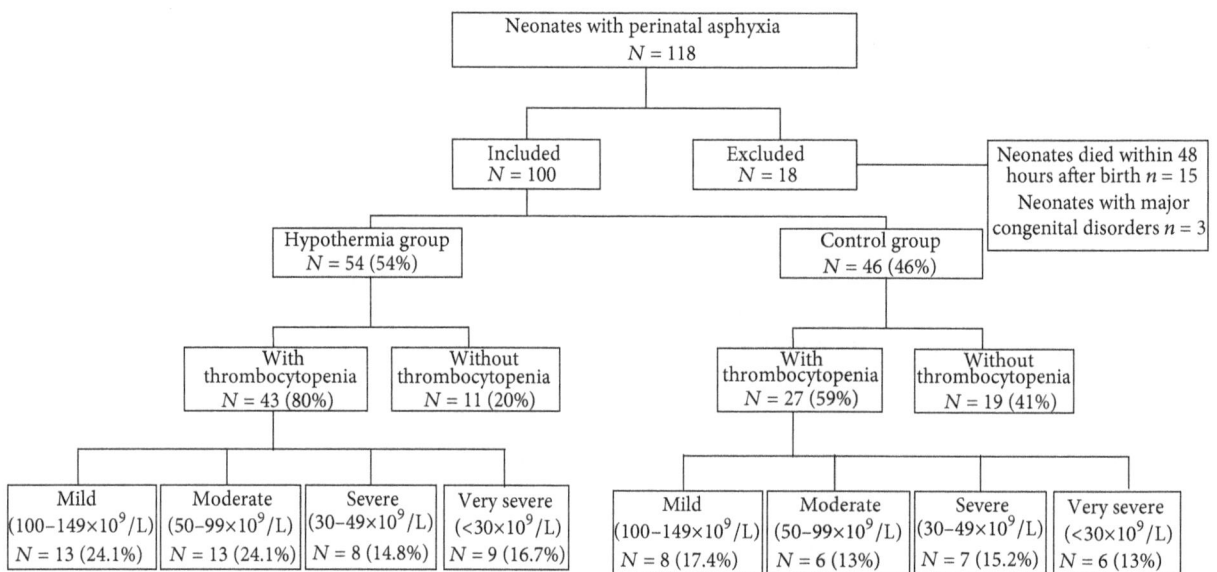

FIGURE 1: Flowchart showing the derivation of our population and the severity of thrombocytopenia.

two-sided and were considered statistically significant at $P < .05$. Data analyses were performed using SPSS Statistics software (version 20.0, SPSS Inc., Chicago, IL, USA).

3. Results

During the study period, 118 (near-) term neonates (≥36 weeks' gestation) with perinatal asphyxia were admitted to our neonatal intensive care unit. Neonates who died within 48 hours after birth ($n = 15$) and neonates with major congenital disorders ($n = 3$) were excluded. A total of 100 neonates met our inclusion criteria. In the hypothermia group 54 neonates were included and 46 neonates, born in the period before introduction of therapeutic hypothermia, were included in the control group. The criteria for perinatal asphyxia were the same in the two groups. Baseline characteristics were similar between the hypothermia group and the control group,

except for lower Apgar scores in neonates in the hypothermia group (see Table 1). The flow chart showing the derivation of our population and the severity of thrombocytopenia is shown in Figure 1.

Platelet counts were measured in 74/100 (74%) neonates at day 1 (day of birth) and at least once in the first week after birth in all neonates (100%). At day 1, the mean platelet count in the hypothermia group was 154×10^9/L compared to 156×10^9/L in the control group ($P = .90$). The lowest platelet count during the first week after birth was in the hypothermia group 97×10^9/L compared to 125×10^9/L in the control group ($P = .06$). The incidence of thrombocytopenia ($< 150 \times 10^9$/L) was significantly higher in the hypothermia group than in the control group, 80% (43/54) versus 59% (27/46), respectively (OR 2.75, 95% CI 1.14–6.66, $P = .02$). The subdivision of thrombocytopenia in mild, moderate, severe, and very severe was similar between the hypothermia group and the control

TABLE 2: Hematologic results of the study population.

	Hypothermia group $n = 54$	Control group $n = 46$	P value	OR [95% CI]
Platelet count/transfusions				
Platelet count <150 × 10^9/L*	43 (80%)	27 (59%)	.02	2.75 [1.14–6.66]
Platelet count at birth—×10^9/L*	154 (77)	157 (81)	.90	1.00 [0.99–1.01]
Lowest platelet count in the first week after birth*	97 (62)	125 (78)	.06	0.99 [0.99–1.00]
Day lowest platelet count*	4.1 (1.8)	2.9 (1.4)	<.001	1.58 [1.21–2.06]
Neonates requiring platelet transfusions—n (%)	15 (28%)	10 (22%)	.49	1.39 [0.55–3.47]
Number. of platelet transfusions per neonate**	0.00 (1)	0.00 (0)	.94	0.99 [0.74–1.32]
Coagulation disorders/FFP transfusions				
PT—seconds*	25.3 (15.0)	21.2 (16.7)	.27	1.02 [0.98–1.06]
INR*	1.8 (1.1)	1.8 (1.5)	.96	0.99 [0.69–1.43]
APTT—seconds*	50.0 (20.1)	42.6 (23.8)	.16	1.02 [0.99–1.04]
Fibrinogen—gram/L*	1.6 (0.8)	2.0 (0.9)	.08	0.60 [0.34–1.07]
Neonates requiring FFP transfusions—n (%)	13 (24%)	8 (17%)	.41	1.51 [0.56–4.03]
Number of FFP transfusions per neonate**	0.00 (0)	0.00 (0)	.81	0.95 [0.62–1.45]

PT: prothrombin time; INR: international normalized ratio; APTT: activated partial thromboplastin time; FFP: fresh frozen plasma.
**Value given as median (IQR).

group: 24% (13/54) versus 17% (8/46) (P = .41), 24% (13/54) versus 13% (6/46) (P = .16), 15% (8/54) versus 15% (7/46) (P = .96), and 17% (9/54) versus 13% (6/46) (P = .61), respectively. The lowest platelet count in the hypothermia group was reached later compared to in the control group: at a mean age of 4.1 days (at day 5) versus 2.9 days (at day 3), after birth (P < .001) (see Figure 2). Coagulation data were collected from both groups. No significant differences in mean values of PT, APTT, INR, and fibrinogen were found between both groups. Further details on hematologic outcome in the study population are shown in Table 2.

3.1. Mortality, Neurologic Morbidity, and Other Clinical Data. An overview of neurologic morbidity, clinical findings, and presence of hemorrhage on neuroimaging in both groups is presented in Table 3. Mortality rate in the hypothermia group was 31% (17/54) compared to 20% (9/46) in the control group (OR 1.89, 95% CI 0.75–4.78, P = .18). In the hypothermia group 83% (45/54) of the neonates were treated with anticonvulsants, compared to 74% (34/46) in the control group, with phenobarbital being the most commonly administered drug (alone or in combination with other drugs). The number of neonates requiring more than 2 types of anticonvulsants, number of hospital days, and number of ventilation days were similar in both groups. CUS was performed in all neonates. The incidence of IVH grades II-III was similar in both groups, 2% (1/54) in the hypothermia group and 2% (1/46) in the control group (OR 0.87, 95% CI 0.05–14.24, P = .92). On CUS no subdural and intraparenchymal bleedings were detected. MRI was performed in 82% (82/100) of neonates (hypothermia group 47/54; control group 35/46). The overall

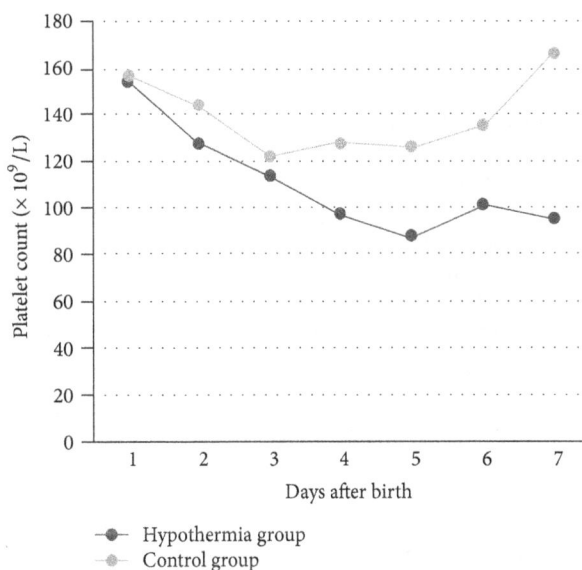

FIGURE 2: Mean platelet count during the first week after birth in our study population.

incidence of intracranial hemorrhage detected on MRI was similar in both groups, 23% (11/47) in the hypothermia group versus 23% (8/35) in the control group (OR 1.03, 95% CI 0.37–2.91, P = .95) and hemorrhages were mostly mild (Table 3). The incidence of moderate/severe hemorrhage was similar in both groups, 6% (3/47) versus 9% (3/35) (P = .64), respectively.

TABLE 3: Morbidity, clinical findings, and presence of hemorrhage on neuroimaging.

	Hypothermia group $n = 54$	Control group $n = 46$	P value	OR [95% CI]
Seizures—n (%)	45 (83%)	34 (74%)	.25	1.77 [0.67–4.67]
Treatment with >2 types of anticonvulsants—n (%)	18 (33%)	8 (18%)	.07	2.38 [0.92–6.14]
Neonatal sepsis	3 (6%)	2 (4%)	.78	1.29 [0.20–8.10]
SGA	0 (0%)	2 (4%)	.12	∞
IVH grades II-III on cranial US—n (%)	1 (2%)	1 (2%)	.92	0.87 [0.05–14.24]
Cerebral bleeding on MRI—n (%)	11 (23%)	8 (23%)	.95	1.03 [0.37–2.91]
Mild	8 (17%)	5 (14%)	.64	
Moderate/severe	3 (6%)	3 (9%)	.64	
Type of moderate/severe hemorrhage				
Subdural	0 (0%)	0 (0%)	—	
Intraparenchymal	2 (4%)	2 (6%)	.74	
Intraventricular	2 (4%)	1 (3%)	.76	
Mortality—n (%)	17 (31%)	9 (20%)	.18	1.89 [0.75–4.78]
Mechanical ventilation days*	4.8 (2.94)	3.6 (3.40)	.07	1.13 [0.99–1.28]
Hospital days*	10.7 (7.07)	10.4 (8.46)	.89	1.00 [0.95–1.06]

SGA: small for gestational age; IVH: intraventricular haemorrhage; US: ultrasound; MRI: magnetic resonance imaging; ∞: infinite (because of zero value in one group); *value given as mean (SD).

4. Discussion

This study shows that the vast majority (80%) of neonates with perinatal asphyxia treated with hypothermia develop thrombocytopenia. This is an important topic especially since there is a movement to cool babies of lower gestational age without adequate safety data. The incidence of thrombocytopenia was almost threefold higher (OR 2.75) than in the control group with perinatal asphyxia treated without therapeutic hypothermia. The higher incidence of thrombocytopenia in the hypothermic group appears to be primarily an increase in the numbers of infants with mild or moderate thrombocytopenia.

Despite the increased rate of thrombocytopenia in the hypothermia group, we found no increased risk of intracranial hemorrhage. This is in accordance with previous studies showing no association between thrombocytopenia and the occurrence of major intracranial hemorrhage [4, 5, 16].

The incidence of thrombocytopenia in neonates treated with therapeutic hypothermia reported in the literature varies greatly from 3% to 65% [6–10, 17]. Differences in reported incidence are probably related to methodological differences between the studies, including different definitions for perinatal asphyxia, differences in timing of platelet count measurement, and variations in number of included patients. We found a difference in the course of platelet count between the hypothermia group and control group (see Figure 2). The lowest platelet count in the hypothermia group was reached at a later stage compared to the control group (day 5 versus day 3). This difference suggests an additional effect of hypothermia on platelet count in infants with perinatal asphyxia.

Our findings are in agreement with recent studies reported in the literature. In a recent Cochrane review (2013), eight randomized studies comparing platelet count in the hypothermia group with a control group were identified [14]. Meta-analysis of these eight trials showed a relative risk of thrombocytopenia in the hypothermia group of 1.21 (95% CI 1.05–1.40) compared to the control group [14]. This was in accordance with another systematic review from Shah et al. in 2007 (RR 1.51, 95% CI 1.09–2.10) [12]. In this review thrombocytopenia was defined as a platelet count below 100×10^9/L and three randomized studies were analyzed [7, 8, 17]. Up to now, no individual randomized study found a difference in thrombocytopenia in the hypothermia group as compared to the control group [6–10, 17]. This correlation was only found in reviews after meta-analysis of different randomized studies [12, 14].

According to the recent Cochrane review, the mode of hypothermia (head cooling with mild systemic versus whole-body) may influence the incidence of thrombocytopenia. A slight increase (statistical) in risk of thrombocytopenia was detected in the group of infants treated with selective head cooling [14].

Hypothermia is known to decrease platelet function and platelet number [18]. The production of thromboxane B2, which has a role in clot formation, is dependent on temperature: lowering of the body temperature causes a reversible platelet dysfunction [18]. Hypothermia is also known to increase PT and APTT [19]. Enzymatic reactions of the coagulation cascade are inhibited by hypothermia [19]. However, in our study we found no differences in PT, APTT, and number of neonates requiring FFP transfusions. The occurrence of coagulation disorders was similar in both groups.

Because of the retrospective design the results of this study should be interpreted with care. Despite the fact that both groups in our study had the same criteria for perinatal asphyxia, the hypothermia group had lower Apgar scores. The higher incidence of thrombocytopenia in the hypothermia group could partly be due to the more severe degree of perinatal asphyxia. However, arterial cord blood values and other clinical parameters were similar in both groups suggesting that differences between groups were probably minimal. A further limitation of our study is the small number (n = 100) of included neonates. Larger prospective studies should be conducted to determine the exact mechanism that contributes to the occurrence of thrombocytopenia by hypothermia. Randomized controlled trials are not ethical anymore because of the proven protective effect of therapeutic hypothermia.

In conclusion, this is the first study focusing on the incidence, severity, and course of thrombocytopenia after treatment with hypothermia. We conclude that therapeutic hypothermia increases the risk of thrombocytopenia in neonates after perinatal asphyxia, without increased risk of cerebral hemorrhage. Thrombocytopenia lasts longer and the nadir of platelet count is reached a couple of days later in neonates treated with hypothermia.

Abbreviations

APTT: Activated partial thromboplastin time
CI: Confidence intervals
CUS: Cranial ultrasound scan
FFP: Fresh frozen plasma
INR: International normalized ratio
IVH: Intraventricular hemorrhage
MRI: Magnetic resonance imaging
OR: Odds ratios
PT: Prothrombin time
RR: Relative risk
SGA: Small for gestational age.

Conflict of Interests

The authors declare that there is no conflict of interests regarding the publication of this paper.

References

[1] S. Chakravorty, N. Murray, and I. Roberts, "Neonatal thrombocytopenia," *Early Human Development*, vol. 81, no. 1, pp. 35–41, 2005.

[2] I. A. G. Roberts and N. A. Murray, "Thrombocytopenia in the newborn," *Current Opinion in Pediatrics*, vol. 15, no. 1, pp. 17–23, 2003.

[3] M. C. Sola, A. Del Vecchio, and L. M. Rimsza, "Evaluation and treatment of thrombocytopenia in the neonatal intensive care unit," *Clinics in Perinatology*, vol. 27, no. 3, pp. 655–679, 2000.

[4] J. S. von Lindern, T. van den Bruele, E. Lopriore, and F. J. Walther, "Thrombocytopenia in neonates and the risk of intraventricular hemorrhage: a retrospective cohort study," *BMC Pediatrics*, vol. 11, article 16, 2011.

[5] V. L. Baer, D. K. Lambert, E. Henry, and R. D. Christensen, "Severe thrombocytopenia in the NICU," *Pediatrics*, vol. 124, no. 6, pp. e1095–e1100, 2009.

[6] D. V. Azzopardi, B. Strohm, A. D. Edwards et al., "Moderate hypothermia to treat perinatal asphyxial encephalopathy," *The New England Journal of Medicine*, vol. 361, no. 14, pp. 1349–1358, 2009.

[7] P. D. Gluckman, J. S. Wyatt, D. Azzopardi et al., "Selective head cooling with mild systemic hypothermia after neonatal encephalopathy: multicentre randomised trial," *The Lancet*, vol. 365, no. 9460, pp. 663–670, 2005.

[8] A. J. Gunn, P. D. Gluckman, and T. R. Gunn, "Selective head cooling in newborn infants after perinatal asphyxia: a safety study," *Pediatrics*, vol. 102, no. 4, pp. 885–892, 1998.

[9] S. E. Jacobs, C. J. Morley, T. E. Inder et al., "Whole-body hypothermia for term and near-term newborns with hypoxic-ischemic encephalopathy: a randomized controlled trial," *Archives of Pediatrics and Adolescent Medicine*, vol. 165, no. 8, pp. 692–700, 2011.

[10] S. Shankaran, A. R. Laptook, R. A. Ehrenkranz et al., "Whole-body hypothermia for neonates with hypoxic-ischemic encephalopathy," *New England Journal of Medicine*, vol. 353, no. 15, pp. 1574–1584, 2005.

[11] D. J. Eicher, C. L. Wagner, L. P. Katikaneni et al., "Moderate hypothermia in neonatal encephalopathy: efficacy outcomes," *Pediatric Neurology*, vol. 32, no. 1, pp. 11–17, 2005.

[12] P. S. Shah, A. Ohlsson, and M. Perlman, "Hypothermia to treat neonatal hypoxic ischemic encephalopathy: systematic review," *Archives of Pediatrics and Adolescent Medicine*, vol. 161, no. 10, pp. 951–958, 2007.

[13] G. Simbruner, R. A. Mittal, F. Rohlmann et al., "Systemic Hypothermia after Neonatal Encephalopathy: outcomes of neo .nEURO.network RCT," *Pediatrics*, vol. 126, no. 4, pp. e771–e778, 2010.

[14] S. E. Jacobs, M. Berg, R. Hunt, W. O. Tarnow-Mordi, T. E. Inder, and P. G. Davis, "Cooling for newborns with hypoxic ischaemic encephalopathy," *The Cochrane Database of Systematic Reviews*, vol. 1, Article ID CD003311, 2013.

[15] L. A. Papile, J. Burstein, R. Burstein, and H. Koffler, "Incidence and evolution of subependymal and intraventricular hemorrhage: a study of infants with birth weights less than 1,500 gm," *Journal of Pediatrics*, vol. 92, no. 4, pp. 529–534, 1978.

[16] S. J. Stanworth, "Thrombocytopenia, bleeding, and use of platelet transfusions in sick neonates.," *The American Society of Hematology. Education Program*, vol. 2012, pp. 512–516, 2012.

[17] D. J. Eicher, C. L. Wagner, L. P. Katikaneni et al., "Moderate hypothermia in neonatal encephalopathy: safety outcomes," *Pediatric Neurology*, vol. 32, no. 1, pp. 18–24, 2005.

[18] C. R. Valeri, G. Cassidy, and S. Khuri, "Hypothermia-induced reversible platelet dysfunction," *Annals of Surgery*, vol. 205, no. 2, pp. 175–181, 1987.

[19] M. J. Rohrer and A. M. Natale, "Effect of hypothermia on the coagulation cascade," *Critical Care Medicine*, vol. 20, no. 10, pp. 1402–1405, 1992.

31

What Parents Think about Giving Nonnutritive Sweeteners to Their Children: A Pilot Study

Allison C. Sylvetsky,[1,2] Mitchell Greenberg,[1] Xiongce Zhao,[3] and Kristina I. Rother[1]

[1] Section on Pediatric Diabetes & Metabolism, NIDDK, NIH, 9000 Rockville Pike, Building 10, Room 8C432A, Bethesda, MD 20892, USA

[2] Department of Exercise and Nutrition Sciences, The George Washington University, 950 New Hampshire Avenue NW, Room 204, Washington, DC 20052, USA

[3] Diabetes, Endocrinology, and Obesity Branch, NIDDK, NIH, 9000 Rockville Pike, Building 10, Room 7C432B, Bethesda, MD 20892, USA

Correspondence should be addressed to Allison C. Sylvetsky; asylvets@gwu.edu

Academic Editor: Alessandro Mussa

Objective. To evaluate parental attitudes toward providing foods and beverages with nonnutritive sweeteners (NNS) to their children and to explore parental ability to recognize NNS in packaged foods and beverages. *Methods.* 120 parents of children ≥ 1 and ≤ 18 years of age completed brief questionnaires upon entering or exiting a grocery store. Parental attitudes toward NNS were assessed using an interviewer-assisted survey. Parental selection of packaged food and beverages (with and without NNS) was evaluated during a shopping simulation activity. Parental ability to identify products with NNS was tested with a NNS recognition test. *Results.* Most parents (72%) disagreed with the statement "NNS are safe for my child to consume." This was not reflected during the shopping simulation activity because about one-quarter of items selected by parents contained NNS. Parents correctly identified only 23% of NNS-containing items presented as foods or beverages which were sweetened with NNS. *Conclusions.* The negative parental attitudes toward providing NNS to their children raise the question whether parents are willing to replace added sugars with NNS in an effort to reduce their child's calorie intake. Our findings also suggest that food labeling should be revised in order for consumers to more easily identify NNS in foods and beverages.

1. Introduction

Sugar-sweetened foods and beverages contribute to weight gain in children and adults [1]. As a result, lower calorie alternatives have become widely available and many of these products contain nonnutritive sweeteners (NNS), such as acesulfame potassium, aspartame, saccharin, and sucralose. While NNS are chemically diverse compounds, they are all sweet-tasting and contribute no or few calories. At present, it remains unclear whether substitution of caloric sugars with NNS can ameliorate weight gain [2, 3]. Many physiological and psychological explanations for the inconsistent effects on weight have been proposed [4, 5] (for a detailed review, see Pepino and Bourne 2011) and recent data has suggested that NNS may affect weight and weight-related chronic diseases

through altering glycemia [6–8], satiety and food intake [9], taste preferences [10], and/or the composition of the gut microbiota [6, 11]. However, the clinical relevance of these findings in humans has not been well studied and little is known about the long-term effects of NNS consumption beginning in childhood [3].

A recent survey conducted by the International Food Information Council Foundation (IFIC) found that 20% of adult participants reported consciously avoiding NNS, though specific concerns about their use were not detailed [12]. Similarly, many consumers reported specifically avoiding NNS in the Sweetener360 study (http://www.cornnaturally.com/Sweetener-360), yet these same consumers were found to purchase foods and beverages sweetened with NNS. Given these findings in adults, the current pilot study aimed to evaluate parental attitudes toward providing NNS-containing items to their children and to explore parents' ability to identify commercially available products containing NNS.

2. Materials and Methods

The Office of Human Subjects Research (OHSR) at the National Institutes of Health (NIH) approved the content of the questionnaires and the procedure. The management of the national grocery chain granted permission to conduct the project on store premises. No written consent was obtained, as all data were obtained anonymously.

2.1. Sample. This survey-based study was conducted in a convenience sample of 125 adults recruited upon entering or exiting a grocery store in Kensington, Maryland, a suburb of Washington, DC. Given the exploratory nature of this study, a sample size calculation was not performed prior to the start of the study. Individuals were eligible to participate if they were ≥18 years of age, if they had a child aged ≥1 year and ≤18 years, and if they spoke and understood English. Volunteers were excluded if they indicated that they were employees of a food or a beverage company, nutritionists, or health policy specialists.

2.2. Procedure. Parents were surveyed throughout the summer of 2012 at varying times of the day and on various days of the week to avoid selection bias. Members of the study team approached parents as they entered or exited the grocery store and asked parents if "they would be willing to complete a brief interview about their family's grocery preferences?" After providing verbal informed consent, participants were asked to partake in 4 components of our study: (1) to complete an 11-item interviewer-assisted demographic questionnaire, (2) to indicate which products they would like to purchase for their families during a grocery shopping simulation activity, (3) to identify NNS in foods and beverages as part of an NNS recognition test, and (4) to indicate their agreement with statements related to NNS in their children's diet. Commercially available food and beverage items ($n = 142$) were displayed on a large table and were arranged in the same order each day. Forty-four of the 142 items contained NNS. The NNS products were selected to include a wide range of low-calorie beverages, no-calorie beverages, low-calorie condiments, low-calorie desserts, and low-calorie grains and cereals. Non-NNS-containing products (up to three per NNS-containing item) were chosen which most closely resembled an NNS-containing food or beverage. Fresh fruits, vegetables, and other perishable, nonpackaged foods were not displayed. Presentation of foods and beverages was such that the front of the package was easily visible and all items were numerically coded.

Parents were asked to indicate which items they would hypothetically purchase for their family by stating the numeric code of each item selected and were instructed to assume that price was not an issue. Next, study team members explained what was meant by the term NNS and provided

examples of the chemical names of NNS (e.g., aspartame, sucralose) as well as examples of the tabletop packets that contain NNS (e.g., Equal, Splenda). Before being asked to identify NNS-containing items by their numeric codes, participants had the opportunity to ask study team members for clarification about what constituted NNS. Finally, participants completed a 28-item questionnaire to assess their attitudes toward providing foods and beverages with NNS to their child. Parents were asked to provide answers that applied to a single child (if they had more than 1 child in the home) and individuals were only eligible to complete the survey once. After completing the survey, study team members disclosed which of the items presented in the grocery shopping simulation activity contained NNS. Participants received a $20 grocery store gift card as compensation for their participation in the study.

2.3. Measures

2.3.1. Sociodemographic Characteristics. Sociodemographic variables included gender, age group (18–25, 26–35, 36–45, 46–55, or >55 years), race and ethnicity (non-Hispanic white, non-Hispanic black, Hispanic, or other), self-reported weight and height, perceived weight category (underweight, normal weight, overweight, and obese), number of children in the household, occupation, and educational attainment (≤high school, some college, Bachelor's degree, Master's degree, and Doctorate degree). Body mass index (BMI) was calculated (weight in kg ÷ height in m^2) using self-reported height and weight.

2.3.2. Grocery Shopping Simulation Activity. The percentage of NNS-containing items out of the total number of groceries selected was calculated for each participant. For example, if a participant selected 24 items and 12 of these items contained NNS, this participant's *NNS grocery score* would be 50% (12 out of 24×100).

2.3.3. Nonnutritive Sweetener Recognition Test. An *NNS recognition score* was calculated based on how many of the 44 NNS-containing items were identified out of the 142 presented products. For example, if a participant correctly identified 15 NNS-containing items, this participant's NNS recognition score would be 34% (15 out of 44×100).

2.3.4. Nonnutritive Sweetener Attitudes. NNS attitudes were measured using a 28-item questionnaire. The wording and items in the NNS-attitude questionnaire were developed based upon the expertise of the study team. Members of the study team read the statements out loud and parents indicated their level of agreement with each statement using a 5-point Likert scale, where "1" was strongly disagree and "5" was strongly agree.

2.4. Statistical Analysis. Descriptive statistics were calculated for NNS-grocery and NNS-recognition scores. *P* values were calculated using *t*-tests, ANOVA, and chi-square test as

TABLE 1: Sociodemographic characteristics of sample based on NNS recognition ($n = 120$).

	N (% of total)
All participants	
n	120 (100%)
Gender	
Male	26 (22%)
Female	94 (78%)
Age group	
18–25	8 (7%)
26–35	23 (19%)
36–45	44 (37%)
46–55	34 (28%)
55+	11 (9%)
Race	
Non-Hispanic white	53 (44%)
Non-Hispanic black	41 (34%)
Hispanic	18 (15%)
Other	8 (6%)
BMI (kg/m^2)^a	26.4 ± 5.5
Education	
≤High school	20 (17%)
Some college	21 (18%)
Bachelor's	39 (33%)
Master's/Doctorate	40 (33%)

^{a}BMI was calculated based on self-reported height and weight.

appropriate. A P value < 0.05 was considered statistically significant.

3. Results

The sociodemographic characteristics of our sample are shown in Table 1. Of approximately 450 parents approached, 125 (28%) agreed to participate in the study, and 120 were included in the analyses. Two individuals were excluded because their child was less than 1 year old, while three parents were excluded due to lack of compliance with study procedures. Seventy-eight percent of participants were female and most self-identified as either non-Hispanic white (44%) or non-Hispanic black (34%). Fifty-one percent of participants perceived themselves as having a normal weight, and the mean parental BMI (based on self-reported weight and height) was 26.4 ± 5.5 kg/m^2.

3.1. Grocery Choices. The average number of groceries that the participants indicated they would hypothetically buy was 22 items (16%) out of the 142 packaged foods and beverages presented. On average, 22% of the groceries selected by parents contained NNS. Parent BMI was not a significant predictor of the number of groceries selected.

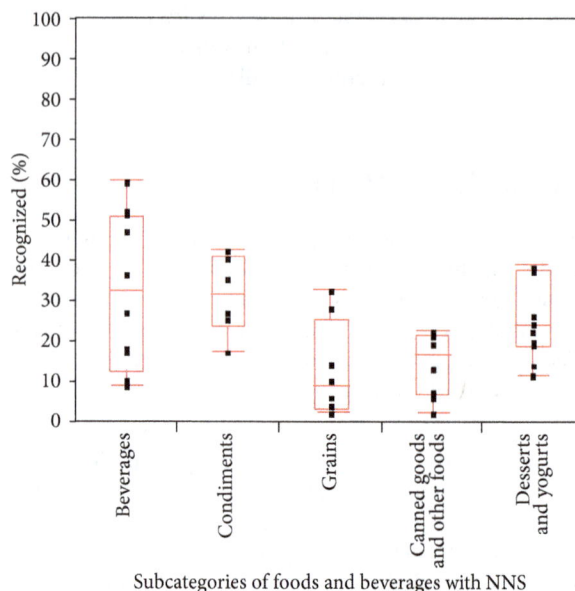

FIGURE 1: Parental ability to recognize foods and beverages ($n = 44$) containing nonnutritive sweeteners. Recognition of NNS varied based on the type of food and beverage presented ($P = 0.02$). Participants generally recognized NNS with higher frequency in beverages, condiments, desserts, and yogurts, while NNS in grains, canned goods, and other foods were more frequently overlooked. Each black dot corresponds to individual food or beverage items within each category.

3.2. NNS Recognition. The mean NNS-recognition score was $23 \pm 14\%$. As shown in Figure 1, recognition of NNS depended on the type of food and beverage presented ($P = 0.02$). Participants generally recognized NNS with higher frequency in beverages, condiments, desserts, and yogurts while NNS in grains, canned goods, and other foods were more frequently overlooked. NNS recognition was inversely associated with BMI ($P < 0.002$).

3.3. Nonnutritive Sweetener Attitudes. Parental agreement with survey items assessing NNS acceptance is shown in Table 2. Seventy-two percent of parents disagreed with the statement "NNS are safe for my child to use," while an additional 12% neither agreed nor disagreed. Fifty-eight percent of participants indicated that they looked for NNS in the ingredients lists on foods and beverages because they wanted to avoid purchasing items that contained NNS. These parents were significantly more accurate in recognizing foods and beverages with NNS ($P = 0.003$). However, the mean NNS-grocery score did not differ between parents who reported avoiding foods and beverages with NNS and those who did not.

Parents indicated a preference for items labeled "reduced sugar" and "no sugar added" (53% and 52%, resp.). Fewer indicated that they sought out items labeled "light," "low carb," or "sugar-free" (37%, 33%, and 22%, resp.). Definitions of relevant food claims are available on the US Food and Drug Administration (FDA) website [13].

TABLE 2: Percent agreement with questionnaire items related to NNS, sugar-related nutrient content claims, and parental concern regarding specific macronutrients.

Statement	Percent agreement (%)
I seek out items labeled "reduced sugar"	53
I seek out items labeled "no sugar added"	52
I seek out items labeled light	37
I seek out items labeled low carb	33
I seek out items labeled sugar-free	22
I read the ingredients in the packaged items that I purchase	64
I look for NNS in packaged foods and beverages because I want to avoid them	58
I am concerned with the calorie content of the items that I select	52
I am concerned with the sugar content of the items that I select	73
I am concerned with the fat content of the items that I select	68
Nonnutritive sweeteners (i.e., Splenda, Sweet N Low, and Equal) are safe for my child to use	16
I recommend that my child use diet (NNS) foods and beverages because I am concerned about his/her sugar intake	14
I recommend that my child use diet (NNS) foods and beverages because I am concerned about his/her weight	13

4. Discussion

The findings of the current pilot study indicate that the majority of parents do not believe that NNS are safe for their children to consume. We found that parental recognition of NNS in commercially available foods and beverages was limited, as parents were unable to identify NNS in 77% of the NNS-containing products presented. The negative parental views observed in this pilot study raise the question as to whether parents are willing to replace sources of added sugars in children's diets with foods and beverages containing NNS.

Over half of parents reported a preference for foods and beverages with "no sugar added" nutrient content claims. These items frequently contain NNS. Meanwhile, the "sugar-free" and "light" nutrient content claims, which may more obviously convey the replacement of caloric sugars with NNS, were perceived less favorably. This suggests that certain food label claims (e.g., "no sugar added") inadvertently encourage parents to select grocery items with NNS. This discrepancy between reported parental attitudes toward NNS and their selection of items that contain them draws attention to issues in parental nutrition literacy.

Our findings are particularly important because the consumption of NNS has increased in the United States over the last decade [14] and NNS consumption is likely to continue to increase. For example, school beverage guidelines [15], taxation of sugar-sweetened beverages [16], and alterations to the food label to highlight added sugar content [17] have been proposed, which may encourage sugar-sweetened beverage consumers to switch to NNS-containing beverages. While NNS have the potential to serve as a valuable dietary tool in reducing caloric intake from added sugars, their safety remains a topic of debate and conclusive evidence of their safety for children specifically is lacking. Epidemiological studies support an association between NNS, weight gain, and other cardiometabolic abnormalities, but prospective, interventional studies are inconclusive. Two recent clinical trials in children and adolescents have shown less weight gain upon replacing sugar-sweetened sodas with NNS sweetened beverages [18, 19], but these trials did not include a control arm with unsweetened beverages (e.g., water). It is therefore necessary to elucidate the long-term metabolic and health effects of NNS in order to appropriately educate parents about the use of NNS among children.

Limitations of our study include a relatively small convenience sample at a single grocery store. While the use of a diverse population of parents representing various race/ethnicity groups added strength to our study, the high level of educational attainment in our sample challenges the generalizability of our findings to the general population. However, given that parental ability to recognize NNS-containing foods and beverages was low despite the high level of educational attainment, we expect that recognition of NNS would be even lower among less educated parents. We also used nonvalidated survey instruments and activities and did not collect qualitative data or information about the parents' habitual NNS consumption habits to further explain our findings. Our participants were required to choose products in a setting which simulated grocery shopping in a free-living population.

5. Conclusions

Our study clearly demonstrates that parents generally do not perceive NNS as safe for their children and frequently do not recognize common NNS-containing foods and beverages. Our findings support the need to identify and implement simple approaches to food labeling in order to facilitate informed dietary choices among consumers and to improve parental knowledge about foods and beverage composition. Considering the recently proposed changes in food labeling [17] and heightened consumer awareness about the health effects of added sugars [20], parents may increasingly seek foods with lower added sugar content, while failing to recognize that many of these foods and beverages will instead contain NNS.

The results of this study also challenge the extent to which parents may be willing to provide their children with NNS and emphasize the need to identify other strategies to reduce added sugar intake and mitigate excessive weight gain in children. The low parental recognition of NNS and strikingly negative parental attitudes towards consumption of NNS-containing foods and beverages should also be considered by pediatricians and other practitioners when counseling parents to reduce their child's sugar intake. Furthermore, our findings call attention to the need to elucidate the long-term health effects of NNS in order to confirm their safety and appropriately educate both clinicians and parents.

Conflict of Interests

None of the authors have any conflict of interests to report.

Acknowledgments

This work was supported by the Intramural Research Program of the National Institute of Diabetes and Digestive and Kidney Diseases. The authors would like to thank Safeway Inc. for allowing them to conduct this study on their premises in Kensington, Maryland. The authors are grateful to Dr. Rebecca J. Brown for her assistance in the design and implementation of this project and critical review of the paper and they would like to acknowledge Marisa Abegg, Alexandra Gardner, and Vik Jayadeva who assisted in the data collection and critically reviewed the paper.

References

[1] V. S. Malik, A. Pan, W. C. Willett, and F. B. Hu, "Sugar-sweetened beverages and weight gain in children and adults: a systematic review and meta-analysis," *American Journal of Clinical Nutrition*, vol. 98, no. 4, pp. 1084–1102, 2013.

[2] R. J. Brown, M. A. de Banate, and K. I. Rother, "Artificial sweeteners: a systematic review of metabolic effects in youth," *International Journal of Pediatric Obesity*, vol. 5, no. 4, pp. 305–312, 2010.

[3] A. Sylvetsky, K. I. Rother, and R. Brown, "Artificial sweetener use among children: epidemiology, recommendations, metabolic outcomes, and future directions," *Pediatric Clinics of North America*, vol. 58, no. 6, pp. 1467–1480, 2011.

[4] S. E. Swithers, "Artificial sweeteners produce the counterintuitive effect of inducing metabolic derangements," *Trends in Endocrinology and Metabolism*, vol. 24, no. 9, pp. 431–441, 2013.

[5] M. Y. Pepino and C. Bourne, "Non-nutritive sweeteners, energy balance, and glucose homeostasis," *Current Opinion in Clinical Nutrition and Metabolic Care*, vol. 14, no. 4, pp. 391–395, 2011.

[6] J. Suez, T. Korem, D. Zeevi et al., "Artificial sweeteners induce glucose intolerance by altering the gut microbiota," *Nature*, vol. 514, no. 7521, pp. 181–186, 2014.

[7] M. Y. Pepino, C. D. Tiemann, B. W. Patterson, B. M. Wice, and S. Klein, "Sucralose affects glycemic and hormonal responses to an oral glucose load," *Diabetes Care*, vol. 36, no. 9, pp. 2530–2535, 2013.

[8] J. A. Mennella, M. Y. Pepino, S. M. Lehmann-Castor, and L. M. Yourshaw, "Sweet preferences and analgesia during childhood: effects of family history of alcoholism and depression," *Addiction*, vol. 105, no. 4, pp. 666–675, 2010.

[9] S. E. Swithers, A. F. Laboy, K. Clark, S. Cooper, and T. L. Davidson, "Experience with the high-intensity sweetener saccharin impairs glucose homeostasis and GLP-1 release in rats," *Behavioural Brain Research*, vol. 233, no. 1, pp. 1–14, 2012.

[10] G.-H. Zhang, M.-L. Chen, S.-S. Liu et al., "Effects of mother's dietary exposure to acesulfame-K in pregnancy or lactation on the adult offspring's sweet preference," *Chemical Senses*, vol. 36, no. 9, pp. 763–770, 2011.

[11] M. B. Abou-Donia, E. M. El-Masry, A. A. Abdel-Rahman, R. E. McLendon, and S. S. Schiffman, "Splenda alters gut microflora and increases intestinal P-glycoprotein and cytochrome P-450 in male rats," *Journal of Toxicology and Environmental Health A: Current Issues*, vol. 71, no. 21, pp. 1415–1429, 2008.

[12] Food & Health Survey, Consumer Attitudes toward Food Safety, Nutrition and Health, http://www.foodinsight.org/Resources/Detail.aspx?topic=2012_Food_Health_Survey_Consumer_Attitudes_toward_Food_Safety_Nutrition_and_Health.

[13] United States Food and Drug Administration, *Guidance for Industry: A Food Labeling Guide*, 2009.

[14] A. C. Sylvetsky, J. A. Welsh, R. J. Brown, and M. B. Vos, "Low-calorie sweetener consumption is increasing in the United States," *The American Journal of Clinical Nutrition*, vol. 96, no. 3, pp. 640–646, 2012.

[15] American Beverage Association, *Alliance School Beverage Guidelines Final Progress Report*, 2010, http://www.ameribev.org/nutrition-science/school-beverage-guidelines/.

[16] T. Andreyeva, F. J. Chaloupka, and K. D. Brownell, "Estimating the potential of taxes on sugar-sweetened beverages to reduce consumption and generate revenue," *Preventive Medicine*, vol. 52, no. 6, pp. 413–416, 2011.

[17] D. A. Kessler, "Toward more comprehensive food labeling," *The New England Journal of Medicine*, vol. 371, pp. 193–195, 2014.

[18] J. C. de Ruyter, M. R. Olthof, J. C. Seidell, and M. B. Katan, "A trial of sugar-free or sugar-sweetened beverages and body weight in children," *The New England Journal of Medicine*, vol. 367, no. 15, pp. 1397–1406, 2012.

[19] C. B. Ebbeling, H. A. Feldman, V. R. Chomitz et al., "A randomized trial of sugar-sweetened beverages and adolescent body weight," *The New England Journal of Medicine*, vol. 367, no. 15, pp. 1407–1416, 2012.

[20] M. Boles, A. Adams, A. Gredler, and S. Manhas, "Ability of a mass media campaign to influence knowledge, attitudes, and behaviors about sugary drinks and obesity," *Preventive Medicine*, 2014.

32

The Relation between *Helicobacter pylori* Infection and Acute Bacterial Diarrhea in Children

Maryam Monajemzadeh,[1,2] **Ata Abbasi,**[3] **Parin Tanzifi,**[4]
Sahar Taba Taba Vakili,[5] **Heshmat Irani,**[6] **and Leila Kashi**[6]

[1] *Clinical and Surgical Pathology, Department of Pathology, Children Medical Center Hospital,*
  Tehran University of Medical Sciences, Tehran 14161351, Iran
[2] *Pediatric Infectious Disease Research Center, Children Medical Center Hospital,*
  Tehran University of Medical Sciences, Tehran 14161351, Iran
[3] *Department of Pathology, Tehran University of Medical Science, Tehran 1439665663, Iran*
[4] *Department of Pathology, Children Medical Center Hospital, Tehran University of Medical Science, Tehran 14161351, Iran*
[5] *Department of Gastroenterology, Tehran University of Medical Science, Tehran 1419733141, Iran*
[6] *Children Medical Center Hospital, Tehran University of Medical Sciences, Tehran 14161351, Iran*

Correspondence should be addressed to Ata Abbasi; ata.abasi@gmail.com

Academic Editor: Alessandro Mussa

Background. H. pylori infection leads to chronic gastritis in both children and adults. But recently, there are arising theories of its protective effect in diarrheal diseases. *Aim.* To explore the prevalence of H. pylori infection in children with bacterial diarrhea and compare it with healthy controls. *Patients and Methods.* Two matched groups consisted of 122 consecutive children, aged 24–72 months old, with acute bacterial diarrhea, who had Shigellosis ($N = 68$) and Salmonellosis ($N = 54$) as patients group and 204 healthy asymptomatic children as control group enrolled in this study. *Results.* The prevalence of H. pylori infection in healthy control children was significantly higher than in patients group, (odds ratio = 3.6, 95% CI: 1.33–9.5, $P = 0.007$). In our study, only 2/54 Salmonella infected patients and 3/68 of Shigellosis had evidence of H. pylori infection, while normal control children had 27/204 infected individuals. *Conclusion.* H. pylori infection may play a protective role against bacterial diarrhea in children. So it is important to consider all of the positive and negative aspects of H. pylori infection before its eradication.

1. Introduction

Helicobacter pylori (*H. pylori*) is one of the most important factors in the gastroduodenal diseases. The infection is most commonly acquired in early childhood and leads to chronic gastritis in both children and adults and is the leading cause of peptic ulcer disease in humans [1–4]. It is a challenging matter for many physicians due to lack of knowledge about its life cycle and low rate of bacterial eradication. *H. pylori* has been shown to play a major role in the pathogenesis of gastric atrophy, chronic diarrhea, and growth retardation in children, intestinal metaplasia, dysplasia, and the development of gastric carcinoma and lymphoma subsequently [5–7]. Besides, some benefits are also noted such as reducing prevalence of esophageal adenocarcinoma by decreasing the periods

of gastroesophageal reflux disease [8]. Fecal-oral or oral-oral routes are the main candidate ways of its transmission, although much is unknown in this regard [9].

Gastroenteritis is another important disease in children caused by a variety of bacterial and viral agents and the exact responsible organisms are different from one area to another but generally, *E. coli*, *Shigella*, and *Salmonella* are the most common enteric bacterial pathogens [10, 11].

Recently, there are arising theories of protective effect of *H. pylori* infection on diarrheal diseases, showing the low prevalence of diarrhea in children infected by *H. pylori* [12–14], although there is still a living debate about it. On the other hand, it has been shown that *H. pylori* infection is associated with *Vibrio cholerae* and *Salmonella* infection possibly through hypochlorhydria resulting from acute or chronic *H. pylori* infection [9, 14].

As *Salmonella* and *Shigella* entritis and also *H. pylori* infection are common gastrointestinal problems in children, especially in developing and underdeveloped countries, we designed this study to investigate the association between *H. pylori* infection and this bacterial gastroenteritis in children.

2. Patients and Methods

2.1. Patients. The study is a case control study performed during 2009–2011 in the Children Medical Center Hospital, the major children's hospital of Iran affiliated to Tehran University of Medical Sciences, Tehran, Iran.

Two matched groups were studied as follows: (1) group of children with acute bacterial gastroenteritis due to *Salmonella* or *Shigella* consisted of 122 consecutive children (55 females and 67 males), aged 24–72 months old, 68 with Shigellosis and 54 with Salmonellosis; (2) control group consisted of two hundred and four healthy children (100 males and 104 females) with no history of diarrhea and no bacterial growth in their stool cultures. Age parameter was matched between both genders ($P > 0.05$).

Healthy children with history of diarrhea within 2 weeks before sampling and any child in each group with history of antibiotic therapy within 4 weeks prior to stool collection were excluded from study. None of the participants were treated with a proton-pump inhibitor or bismuth preparations. No underlying medical disease or immunodeficiency was detected in enrolled groups.

Personal data including age (1–3 years and 3–6 years), gender, and address was also obtained from parents using a structured questionnaire. Cases were from urban area but parents defer to get information about the exact socioeconomic level but as the hospital is governmental and located in the middle part of the city and the admitted children were from nearby areas, one can conclude that cases belonged to medium socioeconomic level. The study was approved by the Tehran University of Medical Sciences Ethics Committee.

2.2. Determination of H. pylori Status. Stool samples were collected in the hospital and immediately frozen and stored at $-70°$C. Solid and semisolid stool specimens were tested for *H. pylori* antigen by the GA Generic Assays GmbH kit, *H. pylori* sandwich enzyme immunoassay (Germany), in accordance with the manufacturer's instructions. In summary frozen specimens were immediately thawed and 100 mg (2-3 mm in diameter of a solid specimen) of feces was suspended thoroughly. Then the specimens were treated with anti-*H. pylori* antibody (antibiotin conjugate) and incubated at room temperature for 60 minutes. After washing, streptavidin-HRP conjugate (included in the kit) was added and the solution was incubated for 30 min at room temperature, then substrate F (included in the kit) was added, and after 15 min of incubation stop solution was added and finally the OD was read at 450 nm and interpreted according to the manufacturer's guideline.

TABLE 1: *H. pylori* prevalence in different groups.

	HP* positive	HP negative	Total	P value
Bacterial diarrhea				
Shigella	3	65	68	
Salmonella	2	52	54	
Control	27	177	204	0.007

*HP: *H. pylori.*

2.3. Media for the Isolation of Bacteria from Stools. Bacteria from stool samples were cultivated on eight different selective agar plates in order to isolate the microorganisms. MacConkey agar was used for the detection of *E. coli*, *Salmonella*, and *Shigella* species. Thiosulfate-citrate-bile salts-sucrose (TCBS) agar was used for the detection of Vibrio species, mannitol-malt agar (MSA) for *Staphylococcus aureus*, and SS and XLD for *Shigella* and *Salmonella*. The growth pattern of each organism on the specific agar including color and also biochemical tests were also used for organism detection.

2.4. Statistical Analysis. The results are expressed as mean ± SD. Statistical analyses were performed using SPSS version 16.0.1 (SPSS Inc., Chicago, IL, USA). The statistical differences between proportions were determined by χ^2 analysis. Numerical data were evaluated using analysis of variance, followed by Tukey's post hoc test. P values less than 0.05 were considered to be statistically significant.

3. Results

Among 112 patients enrolled in this study, 68 had *Shigella* infection and 54 had *Salmonella* infection. The prevalence of *H. pylori* infection in control group was significantly higher than in acute bacterial diarrhea group ($P = 0.007$), in which two of fifty-four cases of *Samonella* infection and three of sixty-eight cases of Shigellosis were infected by *H. pylori* while 27 out of 204 control children were infected. The risk of positive *H. pylori* infection in control group was 3.6 (odds ratio = 3.6, 95% CI: 1.33–9.5, $P = 0.007$) times higher than bacterial infection group (Table 1). There was no statistical difference in prevalence of *H. pylori* infection in variable age groups in control versus patients groups (data not shown).

4. Discussion

Diarrheal disease is recognized as a globally burdensome disease, associated with considerable children's mortality and morbidity specifically in developing countries where most of the complications occur and can cause up to three million deaths per year [3, 15, 16].

The cause of diarrhea differs from one country to another and generally one can expect higher rates of bacterial infections in underdeveloped and developing countries in comparison with developed countries [15]. Several pathogenic microorganisms are incriminated as the etiologic agents of acute diarrhea such as rotavirus, adenoviruses, caliciviruses, and astroviruses, *Salmonella*, *Shigella*, enteropathogenic and enterotoxigenic *E. coli* (EPEC and ETEC, resp.), *Aeromonas*, *Plesiomonas* spp. *Campylobacter jejuni*, *Yersinia enterocolitica*, *Vibrio cholerae*, protozoa, and helminthes [17, 18].

Gastroenteritis, especially bacterial gastroenteritis, mostly occurs in developing areas where *H. pylori* infection is more prevalent and it has been proposed that there may be a common rout for both *H. pylori* and *Shigella* transmission by houseflies [3]. Previous studies have shown conflicting results on association of *H. pylori* infection with other gastrointestinal pathogens [3, 7, 9, 14].

In this study we evaluated the *H. pylori* status in children with gastroenteritis and compared it with normal controls. We focused on *Shigella* and *Salmonella* as they are the most frequent isolates from stool cultures of children in our area.

Our results revealed that the prevalence of *H. pylori* infection in healthy children was higher than in patients with bacterial diarrhea indicating that bacterial infected patients are less infected with *H. pylori*. These findings are in line with other studies showing protective role of *H. pylori* infection and reporting a reduced frequency of diarrheal illness in *H. pylori* infected children [12, 14]. It can be due to either increase in gastric acid production in individuals infected by *H. pylori* which leads to bacterial pathogens damage [19] or activation of immune system as a result of *H. pylori* infection and increased IgA production, which is fatal for enteric pathogens [20–23]. As a matter of fact, gastric acid and peptides are necessary for activation of some enteric pathogens especially that viruses and *H. pylori* infection can disrupt this process [24–27]. Previous studies have shown that children's response to *H. pylori* infection is more severe than adults so this observation may be in part due to the natural response of immune system of children.

Contradictorily, some studies have shown *H. pylori* infection to be a risk factor of some bacterial gastroenteritis [28, 29]. According to the fact that the pathogenesis and etiology of *H. pylori* infection are not fully understood and there are very few studies considering the relation between *H. pylori* infection and other bacterial pathogens causing gastroenteritis, further investigations, considering different aspects including *H. pylori* life cycle, products, and cytotoxins are needed. Considering lack of correlation between prevalence of *H. pylori* infection and gender or age, it can be suggested that the difference in *H. pylori* prevalence in the two examined groups would be due to the organism itself. This hypothesis was previously noted by Perry et al. [13].

Our study has some limitations, such as having rather small number of enrolled patients in this study which may to some extent weaken our results. Another issue is about the method. Parenthetically, it should be mentioned that the specificity and sensitivity of the used kit were 100% and 91%, respectively, according to its manual. In the literature review, we found some conflicting data about this test but many of the articles indicated it as a good alternative in children [30–34].

There are different complications in *H. pylori* infection such as gastritis, gastric lymphoma, and carcinoma, but in contrast *H. pylori* infection decreases the risk of esophageal adenocarcinoma [6, 35, 36]. There are many studies showing association or protective role of *H. pylori* infection in different disease groups, for example, reducing Barrett's esophagitis [37], decreasing risk of esophageal cancer [38], decreasing risk of gastric cardiac cancer [39], or decreasing the bleeding risk of esophageal varices in cirrhotic patients [40]. According to our findings, *H. pylori* infection may be candidate agent which plays a protective role in gastroenteritis in children. So it is important to consider all of the positive and negative aspects of *H. pylori* infection before its eradication; however, because of the current debate and considering the fact that knowledge about *H. pylori* life cycle and its pathogenesis is not explicitly defined more comprehensive research is recommended. Searching for viral gastroenteritis and determining the Cag A status of *H. pylori* by means of PCR method are also suggested.

Conflict of Interests

The authors declare that there is no conflict of interests regarding the publication of this paper.

Acknowledgment

This study was supported by grants from Tehran University of Medical Sciences Research Fund.

References

[1] N. Gallo, C.-F. Zambon, F. Navaglia et al., "Helicobacter pylori infection in children and adults: a single pathogen but a different pathology," *Helicobacter*, vol. 8, no. 1, pp. 21–28, 2003.

[2] A. E. Whitney, J. Guarner, L. Hutwagner, and B. D. Gold, "Helicobacter pylori gastritis in children and adults: comparative histopathologic study," *Annals of Diagnostic Pathology*, vol. 4, no. 5, pp. 279–285, 2000.

[3] H. Shmuely, Z. Samra, S. Ashkenazi, G. Dinari, G. Chodick, and J. Yahav, "Association of Helicobacter pylori infection with Shigella gastroenteritis in young children," *American Journal of Gastroenterology*, vol. 99, no. 10, pp. 2041–2045, 2004.

[4] F. Mansour-Ghanaei, N. Taefeh, F. Joukar, S. Besharati, M. Naghipour, and R. Nassiri, "Recurrence of Helicobacter pylori infection 1 year after successful eradication: a prospective study in Northern Iran," *Medical Science Monitor*, vol. 16, no. 3, pp. CR144–CR148, 2010.

[5] P. M. Sherman, "Peptic ulcer disease in children—diagnosis, treatment, and the implication of Helicobacter pylori," *Gastroenterology Clinics of North America*, vol. 23, no. 4, pp. 707–725, 1994.

[6] P. Correa, "Human gastric carcinogenesis: a multistep and multifactorial process—first American Cancer Society award lecture on cancer epidemiology and prevention," *Cancer Research*, vol. 52, no. 24, pp. 6735–6740, 1992.

[7] D. J. Passaro, D. N. Taylor, R. Meza, L. Cabrera, R. H. Gilman, and J. Parsonnet, "Acute Helicobacter pylori infection is followed by an increase in diarrheal disease among Peruvian children," *Pediatrics*, vol. 108, no. 5, article E87, 2001.

[8] J. Parsonnet, G. D. Friedman, D. P. Vandersteen et al., "Helicobacter pylori infection and the risk of gastric carcinoma," *The New England Journal of Medicine*, vol. 325, no. 16, pp. 1127–1131, 1991.

[9] M. Monajemzadeh, M. T. H. Ashtiani, A. M. Ali et al., "Helicobacter pylori infection in children: association with giardiasis," British Journal of Biomedical Science, vol. 67, no. 2, pp. 86–87, 2010.

[10] A. Raghunath, A. P. S. Hungin, D. Wooff, and S. Childs, "Prevalence of Helicobacter pylori in patients with gastro-oesophageal reflux disease: systematic review," British Medical Journal, vol. 326, no. 7392, pp. 737–739, 2003.

[11] F. Jafari, M. Hamidian, M. Rezadehbashi et al., "Prevalence and antimicrobial resistance of diarrheagenic Escherichia coli and Shigella species associated with acute diarrhea in Tehran, Iran," Canadian Journal of Infectious Diseases and Medical Microbiology, vol. 20, no. 3, pp. e56–e62, 2009.

[12] R. Ranjbar, M. M. Soltan Dallal, M. Talebi, and M. R. Pourshafie, "Increased isolation and characterization of Shigella sonnei obtained from hospitalized children in Tehran, Iran," Journal of Health, Population and Nutrition, vol. 26, no. 4, pp. 426–430, 2008.

[13] S. Perry, L. Sanchez, S. Yang, T. D. Haggerty, P. Hurst, and J. Parsonnet, "Helicobacter pylori and risk of gastroenteritis," The Journal of Infectious Diseases, vol. 190, no. 2, pp. 303–310, 2004.

[14] M. K. Bhan, R. Bahl, S. Sazawal et al., "Association between Helicobacter pylori infection and increased risk of typhoid fever," The Journal of Infectious Diseases, vol. 186, no. 12, pp. 1857–1860, 2002.

[15] D. Antoš, J. Crone, N. Konstantopoulos, and S. Koletzko, "Evaluation of a novel rapid one-step immunochromatographic assay for detection of monoclonal Helicobacter pylori antigen in stool samples from children," Journal of Clinical Microbiology, vol. 43, no. 6, pp. 2598–2601, 2005.

[16] F. Jafari, L. Shokrzadeh, M. Hamidian, S. Salmanzadeh-Ahrabi, and M. R. Zali, "Acute diarrhea due to enteropathogenic bacteria in patients at hospitals in Tehran," Japanese Journal of Infectious Diseases, vol. 61, no. 4, pp. 269–273, 2008.

[17] S. M. El-Sheikh and S. M. El-Assouli, "Prevalence of viral, bacterial and parasitic enteropathogens among young children with acute diarrhoea in Jeddah, Saudi Arabia," Journal of Health Population and Nutrition, vol. 19, no. 1, pp. 25–30, 2001.

[18] A. M. K. Al Jarousha, M. A. El Jarou, and I. A. El Qouqa, "Bacterial enteropathogens and risk factors associated with childhood diarrhea," Indian Journal of Pediatrics, vol. 78, no. 2, pp. 165–170, 2011.

[19] M. F. Dixon, "Pathology of gastritis and peptic ulceration," in Helicobacter Pylori: Physiology and Genetics, H. L. T. Mobley, G. L. Mendz, and S. L. Hazell, Eds., chapter 38, ASM Press, Washington, DC, USA, 2001.

[20] R. Goll, F. Gruber, T. Olsen et al., "Helicobacter pylori stimulates a mixed adaptive immune response with a strong T-regulatory component in human gastric mucosa," Helicobacter, vol. 12, no. 3, pp. 185–192, 2007.

[21] H. A. Haeberle, M. Kubin, K. B. Bamford et al., "Differential stimulation of interleukin-12 (IL-12) and IL-10 by live and killed Helicobacter pylori in vitro and association of IL-12 production with gamma interferon-producing T cells in the human gastric mucosa," Infection and Immunity, vol. 65, no. 10, pp. 4229–4235, 1997.

[22] R. Srivastava, A. Kashyap, M. Kumar, G. Nath, and A. K. Jain, "Mucosal IgA & IL-1β in Helicobacter pylori infection," Indian Journal of Clinical Biochemistry, vol. 28, no. 1, pp. 19–23, 2013.

[23] A. Mattsson, A. Tinnert, A. Hamlet, H. Lönroth, I. Bölin, and A.-M. Svennerholm, "Specific antibodies in sera and gastric aspirates of symptomatic and asymptomatic Helicobacter pylori-infected subjects," Clinical and Diagnostic Laboratory Immunology, vol. 5, no. 3, pp. 288–293, 1998.

[24] C. J. L. Murray and A. D. Lopez, "Mortality by cause for eight regions of the world: Global Burden of Disease study," The Lancet, vol. 349, no. 9061, pp. 1269–1276, 1997.

[25] A. Mattsson, H. Lönroth, M. Quiding-Järbrink, and A.-M. Svennerholm, "Induction of B cell responses in the stomach of Helicobacter pylori—infected subjects after oral cholera vaccination," Journal of Clinical Investigation, vol. 102, no. 1, pp. 51–56, 1998.

[26] J. E. Crabtree, "Immune and inflammatory responses to Helicobacter pylori infection," Scandinavian Journal of Gastroenterology, vol. 31, no. 215, pp. 3–10, 1996.

[27] R. Ranjbar, M. M. Soltan-Dallal, M. R. Pourshafie, and C. Mammina, "Antibiotic resistance among Shigella serogroups isolated in Tehran, Iran (2002–2004)," Journal of Infection in Developing Countries, vol. 3, no. 8, pp. 647–648, 2009.

[28] M. Feldman, B. Cryer, K. E. McArthur, B. A. Huet, and E. Lee, "Effects of aging and gastritis on gastric acid and pepsin secretion in humans: a prospective study," Gastroenterology, vol. 110, no. 4, pp. 1043–1052, 1996.

[29] J. Clemens, M. J. Albert, M. Rao et al., "Impact of infection by Helicobacter pylori on the risk and severity of endemic cholera," The Journal of Infectious Diseases, vol. 171, no. 6, pp. 1653–1656, 1995.

[30] N. Konstantopoulos, H. Rüssmann, C. Tasch et al., "Evaluation of the Helicobacter pylori stool antigen test (HpSA) for detection of Helicobacter pylori infection in children," American Journal of Gastroenterology, vol. 96, no. 3, pp. 677–683, 2001.

[31] S. Kato, K. Ozawa, M. Okuda et al., "Accuracy of the stool antigen test for the diagnosis of childhood Helicobacter pylori infection: a multicenter Japanese study," American Journal of Gastroenterology, vol. 98, no. 2, pp. 296–300, 2003.

[32] M. P. Dore, R. Negrini, V. Tadeu et al., "Novel monoclonal antibody-based Helicobacter pylori stool antigen test," Helicobacter, vol. 9, no. 3, pp. 228–232, 2004.

[33] S. Kato, K. Nakayama, T. Minoura et al., "Comparison between the 13C-urea breath test and stool antigen test for the diagnosis of childhood Helicobacter pylori infection," Journal of Gastroenterology, vol. 39, no. 11, pp. 1045–1050, 2004.

[34] D. Rothenbacher, M. J. Blaser, G. Bode, and H. Brenner, "Inverse relationship between gastric colonization of Helicobacter pylori and diarrheal illnesses in children: results of a population-based cross-sectional study," The Journal of Infectious Diseases, vol. 182, no. 5, pp. 1446–1449, 2000.

[35] A. Guarino, "Enterotoxic effect of the vacuolating toxin produced by Helicobacter pylori in caco-2 cells," The Journal of Infectious Diseases, vol. 178, no. 5, pp. 1373–1378, 1998.

[36] Y. Abe, T. Koike, K. Iijima et al., "Esophageal adenocarcinoma developing after eradication of Helicobacter pylori," Case Reports in Gastroenterology, vol. 5, no. 2, pp. 355–360, 2011.

[37] G. W. Falk, B. C. Jacobson, R. H. Riddell et al., "Barrett's esophagus: prevalence-incidence and etiology-origins," Annals of the New York Academy of Sciences, vol. 1232, no. 1, pp. 1–17, 2011.

[38] F. J. Xie, Y. P. Zhang, Q. Q. Zheng et al., "Helicobacter pylori infection and esophageal cancer risk: an updated meta-analysis," World Journal of Gastroenterology, vol. 19, no. 36, pp. 6098–6107, 2013.

[39] F. Kamangar, S. M. Dawsey, M. J. Blaser et al., "Opposing risks of gastric cardia and noncardia gastric adenocarcinomas

associated with *Helicobacter pylori* seropositivity," *Journal of the National Cancer Institute*, vol. 98, no. 20, pp. 1445–1452, 2006.

[40] Y. Sakamoto, K. Oho, A. Toyonaga, M. Kumamoto, T. Haruta, H. Inoue et al., "Effect of *Helicobacter pylori* infection on esophagogastric variceal bleeding in patients with liver cirrhosis and portal hypertension," *Journal of Gastroenterology and Hepatology*, vol. 28, no. 9, pp. 1444–1449, 2013.

33

The Effects of Skin-to-Skin Contact on Temperature and Breastfeeding Successfulness in Full-Term Newborns after Cesarean Delivery

Shourangiz Beiranvand,[1] Fatemeh Valizadeh,[2] Reza Hosseinabadi,[3] and Yadollah Pournia[4]

[1]*Faculty of Nursing, School of Nursing and Midwifery, Lorestan University of Medical Sciences, Khorramabad, Iran*
[2]*Faculty of Nursing, Jondishapour Ahvaz University of Medical Sciences, Ahvaz, Iran*
[3]*Faculty of Nursing, Social Determinants of Health Research Center, Lorestan University of Medical Sciences, Khorramabad, Iran*
[4]*Faculty of Medicine, School of Medicine, Lorestan University of Medical Sciences, Khorramabad, Iran*

Correspondence should be addressed to Reza Hosseinabadi; reza_hosseinabadi@yahoo.com

Academic Editor: Namık Yaşar Özbek

Background. The skin-to-skin contact (SSC) of mother and newborn is uncommon full-term newborns after delivering via cesarean section due to the possibility of hypothermia in the infants. The aim of this study was to compare mothers' and infant's temperatures after delivering via cesarean section. *Material and Methods.* In this randomized clinical trial, 90 infant/mothers dyads delivered via cesarean section were randomized to SSC ($n = 46$) and routine care ($n = 44$). In experimental group, skin-to-skin contact was performed for one hour and in the routine group the infant was dressed and put in the cot according to hospital routine care. The newborns' mothers' temperatures in both groups were taken at half-hour intervals. The data was analyzed using descriptive statistics, t-tests, and chi-square tests. *Results.* The means of the newborns' temperatures immediately after SSC ($P = 0.86$), half an hour ($P = 0.31$), and one hour ($P = 0.52$) after the intervention did not show statistically significant differences between the two groups. The mean scores of the infants' breastfeeding assessment in SSC (8.76 ± 3.63) and routine care (7.25 ± 3.5) groups did not show significant differences ($P = 0.048$). *Conclusion.* Mother and infant's skin-to-skin contact is possible after delivering via cesarean section and does not increase the risk of hypothermia.

1. Introduction

One of the most important needs of infants at birth is the maintenance of temperature because an infant is not able to generate heat due to lack of shivering mechanism, and this leads to a rapid decline in its temperature [1]. Currently, the routine care to prevent hypothermia is to put the infant under a warmer, causing the separation of the mother and newborn. One of the most important roles of a nurse is to facilitate a close bonding relationship between the mother and infant. To fulfill this role and to treat hypothermia, nurses apply an efficient, accessible, and applicable method called mother and newborn skin-to-skin contact [2]. The movement of the infant's hands over the mother breasts in kangaroo care leads to increased secretion of oxytocin, which results in increased secretion of breast milk and breast heat. The heat is transferred from the mother to the baby because the mother's body temperature activates the baby's sensory nerves, and it results in the baby's relaxation, reduction in the tone of the sympathetic nerves, dilation of the skin vessels, and increase in the baby's body temperature [3].

Mother and infant skin-to-skin contact is well-known in full-term infants with natural deliveries [4]. However, it is believed that infants delivered via cesarean section are predisposed to hypothermia due to low temperature in the operation room, mother's unconsciousness, spread of mother's heat from the center to the environment, and reduction in mother's central temperature. Therefore, mother and infant skin-to-skin contact is potentially limited in infants after born via cesarean deliveries [5]. However, cesarean section surgery has increased dramatically, so that it has increased four times over the last 30 years [6]. The statistics by the Iranian Ministry of Health and Medical Education in 2004 obtained from different areas in Iran reported an estimation of 40 to 60% of caesarean sections in the country. Numerous studies have been conducted on the physiological effects of mother's skin-to-skin contact with preterm and full-term infants after natural deliveries, but few studies have been done on full-term newborns after being delivered via cesarean section [7].

Although mother and infant skin-to-skin contact immediately after birth and the start of breastfeeding during the first hour of birth are considered the top fourth measures to obtain baby friendly status within hospitals, these measures are still not done effectively in Iran and there has been no endeavor to initiate SSC in the country so that the mean of breastfeeding starting is 3.5 hours in natural deliveries and 6.9 hours in delivering via cesarean section, and only 1.5% of infants are breastfed during the first hour of birth [8]. According to the Center for Disease Prevention, only 32 percent of American's hospitals were doing skin-to-skin contact of mother and newborn for two hours after birth and the usual method is to take the baby under a radiant heating in the operating room and nursery word while the World Health Organization recommends that skin-to-skin contact for mothers and newborn should be done regardless of age, birth weight, and the clinical status [9]. The results of a study by Huang et al. (2006) showed that cesarean infants in skin-to-skin contact group had higher mean temperatures compared to the controls who received the routine care under the warmer [10]. Therefore, this study was conducted to determine the effect of skin-to-skin contact on infants' temperatures and breastfeeding successfulness in full-term infants after delivering via cesarean section.

2. Materials and Methods

This study was designed as a Randomized Clinical Trial (RCT) conducted in Asali Hospital (west of Iran). The inclusion criteria for the mothers included singleton pregnancy, gestational age of 38–42 weeks, age range of 18–40 years old, and elective cesarean section surgery under spinal anesthesia. The exclusion criteria for the mothers included problems such as severe bleeding, uterine inertia, gestational diabetes and hypertension, and heart disease. The inclusion criteria for the infants included being full-term and having first- and fifth-minute Apgar above seven. The study excluded the infants with high risks and abnormalities or any other problems which needed hospitalization, according to the doctor's advice. According to sample size formula and considering the loss of samples 96 mother-infant dyads were selected. Then the samples were randomized to skin-to-skin ($n = 48$) and routine care ($n = 48$) groups via a random number table.

The data collection tools consisted of four parts. The first part included the demographic data of the mothers including age, weight, and gestational age, number of miscarriages, number of children, history of lactation, and history of problems during pregnancy, along with the demographic data

of the infants including height, weight, head circumference, chest circumference, and first and fifth-minute Apgar. The second part was a form to record temperatures of the mothers and infants infrared ray thermometer on the forehead, IN4K8210 model. The third part was the standard Infant Breastfeeding Assessment Tool (IBAT), which included four subscales of sucking, rooting, readiness, and latching, each having 0–3 scores and 0–12 scores in total, which were completed through direct observation of infant breastfeeding. IBAT is a reliable tool for assessing infant success in first breastfeeding which has been used in several studies [11, 12]. The questionnaire was prepared from authentic scientific resources. Its validity was confirmed through the content validity based on the expert viewpoints of faculty members in the Faculty of Nursing and Midwifery in Khorramabad (west of Iran), and its reliability was confirmed through direct observation in a random sample of 20 cases of breastfeeding in the pilot study in which correlation coefficient was 0.95.

The fourth part was a form of maternal satisfaction with skin-to-skin contact, which consisted of 11 questions (yes, no, and not know) and was completed as a self-report with a confirmed validity in previous studies.

To perform the study, the researcher first arranged with the authorities of the Obstetrics Ward of Asalaian Hospital of Lorestan University of Medical Sciences (west of Iran) and then attended the hospital. The samples were selected from July 2011 to September 2011, according to the inclusion criteria of the study and their informed consent to participate in the study. Subsequently, the mothers' temperatures in the two groups before and after of surgery were recorded via the forehead infrared thermometer; infants temperatures were recorded on arrival at the operating room after their umbilical cords were cut and a general assessment of the infants then their first and fifth-minute Apgar scores were measured. The infants were then wrapped in blankets and taken to the nursery ward. In this unit, their temperatures were recorded after anthropometric measurements and vitamin K injections were performed. Then the babies were delivered to their mothers when mother back from operation room, and in the experimental group the naked infants in diapers were positioned between their mother breasts in a prone position. To preserve the infants' temperatures, their heads were covered with hats and their backs with suitable covers. The mothers and infants' temperatures were measured and recorded at the start of skin-to-skin contact, half an hour, and one hour after with infrared ray thermometer on the forehead. In the control group, the infants were dressed and embraced by their mothers to be breastfed, and their temperatures were measured at the time they were delivered to their mothers, after half an hour, and after one hour. Also, the mothers in the two groups were trained how to breastfeed. Then the Infant Breastfeeding Assessment Tool (IBAT) was applied to assess breastfeeding in the two groups, and the satisfaction form was completed by the mothers in the skin-to-skin contact group. Moreover, the temperatures of the nursery ward, the operation room, and the mother's ward were measured and recorded in all the steps.

To analyze the data, descriptive statistics including frequencies, means, standard deviations, t-tests, chi-square

TABLE 1: The relationship between demographic characteristics of mothers and infants in the skin-to-skin contact and routine care groups.

Variable	Group		P	t
	Skin-to-skin contact	Routine care		
Mother's age	27.66 ± 9.32	27.28 ± 6.88	0.83	0.22
Mother's weight (kg)	79 ± 12.95	81.3 ± 11.73	0.37	−0.9
Mother's gestational age (week)	39 ± 0.92	38.8 ± 1.017	0.66	0.44
Infant's weight	3240 ± 287.8	3220 ± 339.9	0.78	0.28
Infant's head circumference (cm)	35.5 ± 1.03	35.7 ± 1.12	0.42	−0.8
Infant's chest circumference (cm)	34.2 ± 1.07	34.3 ± 1.3	0.6	−5.3
Infant's height (cm)	49.8 ± 3.52	49.8 ± 3.10	0.83	−0.2
First-minute Apgar	9 ± 0	9 ± 0	—	—
Fifth-minute Apgar	10 ± 0	10 ± 0	—	—
Number of miscarriages				
0	39 (84.8%)	39 (88.6%)		
1	6 (13%)	4 (9.1%)	0.83	$\chi^2 = 0.35$
2	1 (2.2%)	1 (2.3%)		
Number of pregnancies				
1, 2	37 (73%)	37 (79.5%)	0.67	$\chi^2 = 3.2$
3 and more	9 (26.1%)	8 (20.5%)		
Number of children				
1	23 (50%)	27 (61.4%)	0.27	$\chi^2 = 1.2$
More than 1	23 (50%)	17 (38.8%)		
Educational level				
Lower than high school diploma	19 (41.3%)	13 (29.5)		
High school diploma	22 (48.8%)	23 (52.3%)	0.59	$\chi^2 = 1.92$
Bachelor's degree and higher	5 (10.9%)	8 (18.2%)		
Infant's gender				
Female	23 (50%)	26 (59.1%)	0.38	$\chi^2 = 0.75$
Male	23 (50%)	18 (40.9%)		
History of lactation				
Yes	22 (48.8%)	13 (29.5%)	0.14	$\chi^2 = 3.8$
No	24 (52.2%)	31 (70.5%)		
Problems during pregnancy				
Yes	26 (56.5%)	27 (61.4%)	0.64	$\chi^2 = 0.22$
No	20 (43.5%)	17 (38.6%)		

tests, and Kolmogorv-Smirnov tests were applied. The analyses were done and considered as blind and the analyst of the data was not aware of the classifications. To follow the ethical considerations, the researchers provided the participants with necessary information, and the secrecy of their personal data was followed. Therefore, the participants' names were not recorded in the forms. The study was approved by the Ethics Committee of Lorestan University of Medical Sciences (west of Iran).

3. Results

90 infant/mother dyads completed the study. Two infant/mother dyads in the skin-to-skin group and 4 infant/mother dyads in the routine group were excluded from the study due to neonatal respiratory distress syndrome.

The results showed no significant differences between the two groups concerning the means and standard deviations

of the mothers' demographic data including age, weight, and gestational age, along with the infants' data including height, weight, head circumference, chest circumference, and first and fifth-minute Apgar. Moreover, the results of chi-square tests showed no significant differences between the two groups in terms of mother's educational level, number of miscarriages, number of children, history of lactation, history of problems during pregnancy, and infant's gender (Table 1).

The results also showed no significant differences between the two groups concerning the means and standard deviations related to mother's temperatures before and after the surgery, infant's temperatures on arrival at the operating room and the nursery room, and temperatures of the operation room and mother's and infants' rooms after arriving at the ward (Table 2).

In addition, the analysis of the data concerning the means and standard deviations of mother and infant's temperatures at the start of skin-to-skin contact, half an hour, and one hour

TABLE 2: Comparison of the means and standard deviations related to the general situations of the mothers and infants in the skin-to-skin contact and routine care groups.

Variable	Group		t	P
	Skin-to-skin contact	Routine care		
Preoperative maternal temperature	36.44 ± 0.38	36.42 ± 0.48	0.13	0.9
Postoperative maternal temperature	36.48 ± 0.37	36.4 ± 0.41	0.98	0.32
Infant's temperature in the operating room	36.2 ± 0.62	36 ± 0.58	0.83	0.4
Infant's temperature on arrival at the nursery unit	36.7 ± 0.4	36.8 ± 0.5	-1.6	0.11
Temperature of the operating room	28 ± 1.2	28 ± 1.52	0.3	0.75
Temperature of the nursery unit	28.1 ± 0.96	28 ± 0.61	0.035	0.97
Temperature of the mother's room	29.9 ± 0.64	29.7 ± 1.63	0.8	0.42

TABLE 3: Comparison of the means and standard deviations related to the mothers and infants' temperatures in the skin-to-skin contact and routine care group.

Variable	Group		t	P
	Skin-to-skin contact	Routine care		
Maternal temperature at the start of the intervention	36.56 ± 0.46	36.4 ± 0.41	1.6	0.11
Maternal temperature half an hour after the intervention	36.56 ± 0.46	36.4 ± 0.52	1.6	0.11
Maternal temperature one hour after the intervention	36.43 ± 0.46	36.2 ± 0.67	1.6	0.11
Infant's temperature at the start of the intervention	36.35 ± 0.46	36.32 ± 0.46	0.16	0.86
Infant's temperature half an hour after the intervention	36.25 ± 0.5	36.4 ± 0.48	-1.01	0.31
Infant's temperature one hour after the intervention	36.44 ± 0.45	36.4 ± 0.48	0.63	0.52

after the contact did not show significant differences between the two groups of skin-to-skin and routine care (Table 3).

In general, repeated measure tests showed that the infants' temperatures repeated over time, namely, at the start of skin-to-skin contact, half an hour, and one hour after the contact, did not show significant differences in the two groups of skin-to-skin contact ($P = 0.201$, $F = 1.68$) and routine care ($P = 0.4$, $F = 0.59$).

Moreover, repeated measure tests showed significant differences in terms of the mothers' temperatures in the skin-to-skin contact group ($P = 0.01$, $F = 0.002$), but the differences in the routine care group were not statistically significant ($P = 0.11$, $F = 2.74$). The disturbing effects of maternal and neonatal temperatures before the intervention were not significant in any of the cases ($P > 0.05$).

Regarding the breastfeeding assessment of the infants after delivered via cesarean section, 52.2% of the infants in the skin-to-skin contact group and 25% in the routine care group showed readiness to breastfeed without doing any attempts, and the chi-square test showed the difference between the two groups to be statistically significant ($P = 0.021$).

In terms of sucking, 50% and 37% of the infants in the skin-to-skin contact group showed good and moderate sucking, respectively. In the routine care group, 36.4% and 27.3% of the infants showed good and moderate sucking, respectively. The chi-square test showed statistically significant differences ($P = 0.03$).

Concerning latching, 39/1% of the infants in the skin-to-skin contact group and 20/5% in the routine care group held mothers' breasts immediately, and chi-square test did not show a statistically significant difference between the groups ($P = 0.21$).

In relation to rooting, 47.8% in the skin-to-skin contact group and 29.5% the routine care group, respectively, immediately started looking for mothers' breasts to suck, and the chi-square test did not show significant difference between the two groups ($P = 0.19$) (Table 4).

The means and standard deviations of the total score of breastfeeding assessment related to the infants in the skin-to-skin contact group and in the routine care group were 8.76 ± 3.63 and 7.25 ± 3.5, respectively, and the t-test did not show a significant difference between the two groups ($P = 0.048$). Most of the mothers gave "yes" answers to the questions related to their satisfaction with skin-to-skin contact.

4. Discussion

The findings of the present study showed that skin-to-skin contact between mother and infant after delivering via cesarean section did not cause a drop in infants' temperatures and that it was effective in their breastfeeding successfulness. Gouchon et al., 2010, compared infants' temperatures after delivering via cesarean section in two groups of skin-to-skin and routine care. They measured infants' temperatures every half an hour for two hours after skin-to-skin contact, and did not report significant difference between the two groups. In their study, the infants in the skin-to-skin group started the initial breastfeeding sooner than the infants in the routine care group [5].

Infant skin temperature rises after birth in relation to an increased metabolic rate and the mechanism by which skin-to-skin contact influences the infant's temperature is not fully

TABLE 4: Breastfeeding assessment of the cesarean infants in the skin-to-skin contact and routine care groups.

Variable	Group		χ^2	P
	Skin-to-skin contact	Routine care		
Readiness				
With no attempts	24 (52.2%)	11 (25%)		
Needing weak stimulation	13 (28.3%)	19 (43.2%)	9.68	0.021
Needing more stimulation	4 (8.7%)	11 (25%)		
Sleepiness	5 (10.9%)	3 (6.8%)		
Sucking				
Good	23 (50%)	16 (36.4%)		
Moderate	17 (37%)	12 (27.3%)	8.42	0.03
Weak	2 (4.3%)	11 (25%)		
No sucking	4 (8.7%)	5 (11.4%)		
Latching				
Immediately	18 (39.1%)	9 (20.5%)		
After 3–10 minutes	15 (32.6%)	15 (34.1%)	4.44	0.21
After more than 10 minutes	9 (19.6%)	14 (31.8%)		
Not start breastfeeding	4 (8.7%)	6 (13.6%)		
Rooting				
Immediately	22 (47.8%)	13 (29.5%)		
Needing stimulation	17 (37%)	18 (40.9%)	4.68	0.19
Weak rooting	3 (6.5%)	8 (18.2%)		
No rooting	4 (8.7%)	5 (11.4%)		

known. It has been suggested that the touch, light pressure, and, in particular, the warmth received by the infant during the skin-to-skin contact activate sensory nerves, leading to cutaneous vasodilation and increased skin temperature. The increase in maternal breast skin temperature occurring in the postpartum period is probably on expression of an inborn psychophysiological pattern which aimed at helping the mother in her interaction with the baby after birth. The maternal giving of warmth diminishes the risk for development of hypothermia in the infant in the postpartum period [13].

Chiu and Anderson (2009) also investigated newborns' temperatures with breastfeeding difficulties during skin-to-skin contact with their mothers and found that the newborns' temperatures reached the normal rate of 36.5 to 37.6° Celsius and became fixed at that level, showing that mothers were able to regulate the newborns' temperatures in kangaroo care [14].

A study by Keshavarz and Haghighi which investigated the effects of kangaroo contact on physiological variables in term neonates after cesarean section included 160 neonates and assigned them randomly to skin-to-skin contact and routine care groups. The newborns' temperatures in the skin-to-skin group were measured half an hour and an hour after the contact and half an hour after the cessation of contact. Moreover, the newborns' temperatures in the routine care group were measured half an hour, an hour, and one and a half hour after they were placed in cots. The mean temperature in the skin-to-skin group was 36.8 compared to the mean temperature of 36.6 in the routine care group ($P = 0.05$), and the mean temperature one hour after skin-to-skin contact was 36.9, which was higher than the mean temperature of 36.6 in

the control group ($P = 0.001$). In total, the mothers in the skin-to-skin contact group had more satisfaction [15]. These results are consistent with the results of our study. In these studies that were conducted, mothers' temperatures were not measured but in our study were measured and did not show significant differences between the two groups of skin-to-skin and routine care.

This study showed that infants in the skin-to-skin group were more successful in rooting reflex and the scores of the investigated breastfeeding indicators were higher in the skin-to-skin contact group. In the study of Bystrova et al., 2009, the infants in skin-to-skin contact with their mothers after birth soon started to search for the mother's breast, found the breast, and started sucking without the help of the mother or care staff [16].

Also infants sucking reflexes the scores of the investigated breastfeeding indicators that were higher in the skin-to-skin contact group. Some studies have shown that term newborns placed skin to-skin on the mother's abdomen immediately after birth spontaneously start moving toward the breasts and onto the nipple, but these behaviors are less likely to occur if infants are first placed under a radiant warmer [17].

Concerning latching, although there was not a statistically significant difference between the two groups, greater number of the infants in the skin-to-skin contact group held mothers' breasts immediately. In the first hours postpartum, the mother and infant learn to breastfeed together. In the first phase called self-attached breastfeeding, the baby latches to the breast without assistance and self-attaches to the breast using the stepping-crawling reflex. In the second phase, called collaborative breastfeeding, the mother and baby work together to achieve the latch and feeding. If the infant has been placed skin-to-skin without separation until self-attachment has been accomplished, although each type of latch and suckling deviation from optimal is associated with maternal pain, beginning to breastfeed without prefeeding behavior in the infant is associated with the highest levels of pain [18].

In this study breastfeeding successfulness in the skin-to-skin contact group was higher than in the routine care group. Moore and Anderson in their study reported stronger readiness, sucking, and quicker readiness in the infants in the skin-to-skin contact group compared to those in the routine care group [11]. Khadivzadeh and Karimi (2009) also reported higher breastfeeding successfulness in the skin-to-skin contact group compared to the routine care group [19].

Newborn babies should not be separated from their mothers except for significant medical reasons but should be placed skin-to-skin as soon as possible after birth to have the ability to start self-regulation [16].

In the present study, most of the mothers were satisfied with the skin-to-skin contact with their infants and were willing to continue this type of care. In a study by Carfoot et al. (2005) 90% of the mothers were satisfied with mother and neonate skin-to-skin contact and 86% were willing to continue the care in the future. Moreover, 90% and 81% of the infants, in the skin-to-skin contact and the routine care groups, respectively, had successful breastfeeding, showing no significant differences between the groups [12].

This care was performed for the first time in Asali Hospital of Khorramabad (west of Iran). This method of caring is simple, safe, economical, practical, and applicable. It is also a therapeutic method to prevent hypothermia in term neonates. Therefore, it is necessary to standardize nursing workforce to implement this method routinely after cesarean sections. To implement the method, it is recommended that extensive research on it should be performed.

5. Conclusion

According to the results of the present study, it is concluded that skin-to-skin contact after delivering via cesarean section was possible, maternal satisfaction level with skin-to-skin contact was higher, and cesarean neonates were not prone to hypothermia and improve breastfeeding initiation and facilitate the first successful experience of breastfeeding compared to routine method of infant care in delivered via cesarean section. The results of this study can be applied in various areas of nursing including nursing management, nursing education, and nursing research.

Conflict of Interests

The authors declare that there is no conflict of interests regarding the publication of this paper.

Acknowledgments

This study was approved by Lorestan University of Medical Sciences (Iran) and the record code of IRCT was 201110037697N1. The authors hereby appreciate the support of Vice Chancellor for Research of Lorestan University of Medical Sciences. Moreover, the authors are sincerely grateful to the staff of the cesarean ward, the nursery unit, and the operation room of Asali Hospital in Khorramabad (city of Iran).

References

[1] L. Debra, F. P. Jolie, and G. Win, *Thompsons Pediatric Nursing*, Elsevier, Philadelphia, Pa, USA, 9th edition, 2006.

[2] M. Galligan, "Proposed guidelines for skin-to-skin treatment of neonatal hypothermia," *The American Journal of Maternal/Child Nursing*, vol. 31, no. 5, pp. 298–306, 2006.

[3] W. Jonas, I. Wiklund, E. Nissen, A.-B. Ransjö-Arvidson, and K. Uvnäs-Moberg, "Newborn skin temperature two days postpartum during breastfeeding related to different labour ward practices," *Early Human Development*, vol. 83, no. 1, pp. 55–62, 2007.

[4] K. Erlandsson, A. Dsilna, I. Fagerberg, and K. Christensson, "Skin-to-skin care with the father after cesarean birth and its effect on newborn crying and prefeeding behavior," *Birth*, vol. 34, no. 2, pp. 105–114, 2007.

[5] S. Gouchon, D. Gregori, A. Picotto, G. Patrucco, M. Nangeroni, and P. di Giulio, "Skin-to-skin contact after cesarean delivery: an experimental study," *Nursing Research*, vol. 59, no. 2, pp. 78–84, 2010.

[6] J. Dickinson, D. K. James, C. P. Weiner, P. J. Steer, and B. Gonik, *High Risk Pregnancy in Cesarean Section*, Saunders Elsevier, Philadelphia, Pa, USA, 3th edition, 2006.

[7] M. Keshavarz, N. W. Cheung, G. R. Babaee, H. K. Moghadam, M. E. Ajami, and M. Shariati, "Gestational diabetes in Iran: incidence, risk factors and pregnancy outcomes," *Diabetes Research and Clinical Practice*, vol. 69, no. 3, pp. 279–286, 2005.

[8] F. Nahidi, F. Dori, M. Davari, and A. Akbarzadeh, "Effect of early skin-to-skin contact of mother and newborn on mother's satisfaction," *Journal of Nursing and Midwifery*, vol. 20, no. 4, pp. 1–5, 2010.

[9] World Health Organization and Department of Reproductive Health and Research, *Kangaroo Mother Care: A Practical Guide*, Department of Reproductive Health and Research, World Health Organization, Geneva, Switzerland, 2003.

[10] Y.-Y. Huang, C.-Y. Huang, S.-M. Lin, and S.-C. Wu, "Effect of very early kangaroo care on extrauterine temperature adaptation in newborn infants with hypothermia problems," *The Journal of Nursing*, vol. 53, no. 4, pp. 41–48, 2006.

[11] E. R. Moore and G. C. Anderson, "Randomized controlled trial of very early mother –infant skin to skin contact and breastfeeding status," *Journal of Midwifery and Women's Health*, vol. 52, no. 2, pp. 116–125, 2007.

[12] S. Carfoot, P. Williamson, and R. Dickson, "A randomised controlled trial in the North of England examining the effects of skin-to-skin care on breast feeding," *Midwifery*, vol. 21, no. 1, pp. 71–79, 2005.

[13] K. Bystrova, A. S. Matthiesen, I. Vorontsov, A. M. Widström, A.-B. Ransjö-Arvidson, and K. Uvnäs-Moberg, "Maternal axillar and breast temperature after giving birth: effects of delivery

ward practices and relation to infant temperature," *Birth*, vol. 34, no. 4, pp. 291–300, 2007.

[14] S.-H. Chiu and G. C. Anderson, "Effect of early skin-to-skin contact on mother-preterm infant interaction through 18 months: randomized controlled trial," *International Journal of Nursing Studies*, vol. 46, no. 9, pp. 1168–1180, 2009.

[15] M. Keshavarz and N. B. Haghighi, "Effects of kangaroo contact on some physiological parameters in term neonates and pain score in mothers with cesarean section," *Journal of Semnan University of Medical Sciences*, vol. 11, no. 2, pp. 91–98, 2010.

[16] K. Bystrova, V. Ivanova, M. Edhborg et al., "Early contact versus separation: effects on mother-infant interaction one year later," *Birth*, vol. 36, no. 2, pp. 97–109, 2009.

[17] M. W. Walters, K. M. Boggs, S. Ludington-Hoe, K. M. Price, and B. Morrison, "Kangaroo care at birth for full term infants: a pilot study," *MCN The American Journal of Maternal/Child Nursing*, vol. 32, no. 6, pp. 375–381, 2007.

[18] K. Cadwell, "Latching-on and suckling of the healthy term neonate: breastfeeding assessment," *Journal of Midwifery & Women's Health*, vol. 52, no. 6, pp. 638–642, 2007.

[19] T. Khadivzadeh and A. Karimi, "The effects of post-birth mother-infant skin to skin contact on first breastfeeding," *Iranian Journal Nursing and Midwifery Research*, vol. 14, no. 3, pp. 111–117, 2009.

34

Neonatal Meningitis by Multidrug Resistant *Elizabethkingia meningosepticum* Identified by 16S Ribosomal RNA Gene Sequencing

V. V. Shailaja,[1] **Ashok Kumar Reddy,**[2] **M. Alimelu,**[3] **and L. N. R. Sadanand**[1]

[1] *Department of Microbiology, Niloufer Hospital for Women and Children, Hyderabad 500004, India*
[2] *GHR Micro Diagnostics, Hyderabad 500082, India*
[3] *Department of Pediatrics, Niloufer Hospital for Women and Children, Hyderabad 500004, India*

Correspondence should be addressed to V. V. Shailaja; shailajavv@yahoo.co.in

Academic Editor: Lavjay Butani

Clinical and microbiological profile of 9 neonates with meningitis by *Elizabethkingia meningosepticum* identified by 16S ribosomal gene sequencing was studied. All the clinical isolates were resistant to cephalosporins, aminoglycosides, trimethoprim-sulfamethoxazole, β-lactam combinations, carbapenems and only one isolate was susceptible to ciprofloxacin. All the isolates were susceptible to vancomycin. Six of nine neonates died even after using vancomycin, based on susceptibility results. *E. meningosepticum* meningitis in neonates results in high mortality rate. Though the organism is susceptible to vancomycin in vitro, its efficacy in vivo is questionable and it is difficult to determine the most appropriate antibiotic for treating *E. meningosepticum* meningitis in neonates.

1. Introduction

Elizabethkingia meningosepticum (formerly known as *Chryseobacterium meningosepticum/Flavobacterium meningosepticum*) is a nonfermentative gram negative bacillus, ubiquitous in nature [1, 2]. *E. meningosepticum* causes meningitis, pneumonia, bacteremia, and sepsis in infants and pneumonia, endocarditis, postoperative bacteremia, and meningitis in adults [1–3]. Among the different infections, a high mortality and severe postinfection sequelae including hydrocephalus, deafness, and developmental delay have been reported in neonates with meningitis due to *E. meningosepticum* [2]. Infections caused by *E. meningosepticum* are difficult to treat because of its resistance to extended spectrum β-lactam agents and aminoglycosides [1–3]. In this study we report the clinical profile, antibiotic susceptibility, and treatment outcome of meningitis caused by multidrug resistant *Elizabethkingia meningosepticum* in neonates.

2. Materials and Methods

Nine neonates with *E. meningosepticum* meningitis who presented to the Neonatal Intensive Care Unit of Niloufer Hospital for Women and Children, Hyderabad, India, between January 2009 and December 2010, were included in the study. Cerebrospinal fluid collected from the neonates was subjected to direct microscopic examination, inoculated on to blood agar, chocolate agar, and MacConkey's agar, and incubated overnight at $37°C$. Blood cultures were done by automated blood culture systems (Bact/Alert, Biomerieux, France). The isolates were identified by conventional biochemical reactions and Vitek 2 (Biomerieux, France). The identity of the isolates was further confirmed by 16S rRNA gene sequencing. Sequencing was performed (forward primer, 5′-TTGGAGAGTTTGATCCTGGCTC-3′; reverse primer, 5′-GGACTACCAGGGTATCTAA-3′) with fluorescence-labeled dideoxynucleotide terminators using an ABI 3130 Xl automated sequencer, following the

TABLE 1: Antibiotic susceptibility and GenBank accession numbers of isolates.

S. number	GenBank accession number	Antibiotic susceptibility								
		AK/G	CIP/OF	CZ/CTX/CFP	IM/MP	PC	PTB	AC	V	SXT
1	HM042305	R	R	R	R	R	R	R	S	R
2	HM042306	R	S	R	R	R	R	R	S	R
3	HM130055	R	R	R	R	R	R	R	S	R
4	HM130056	R	R	R	R	R	R	R	S	R
5	HM130057	R	R	R	R	R	R	R	S	R
6	HM130058	R	R	R	R	R	R	R	S	R
7	HM130059	R	R	R	R	R	R	R	S	R
8	NS	R	R	R	R	R	R	R	S	R
9	NS	R	R	R	R	R	R	R	S	R

PC: piperacillin; PTB: piperacillin-tazobactam; AK: amikacin; G: gentamicin; CZ: ceftazidime; CTX: cefotaxime; CFP: cefepime; MP: meropenem; IM: imipenem; CP: ciprofloxacin; OF: ofloxacin; SXT: trimethoprim-sulfamethoxazole; V: vancomycin; R: resistant; S: sensitive; NS: not submitted in the GenBank.

manufacturer's instructions (PE Applied Biosystems). The sequences were analysed and identified using the Megablast search program of the GenBank database. The sequence of the isolate perfectly (100%) matched the sequences of E. meningosepticum deposited in GenBank. The gene sequences of the isolates were deposited in the GenBank. Antibiotic susceptibility of the isolates was done by Kirby Bauer's disk diffusion method and also by Vitek 2.

3. Results and Discussion

Gram's stain of CSF showed polymorphonuclear leukocytes and Gram negative bacilli in all the nine patients. Confluent growth of moist raised colonies was seen on blood and chocolate agar in all patients. Blood culture was collected in only one patient apart from CSF culture. Blood culture was positive and showed the growth of moist raised colonies on subculture on blood and chocolate agar. There was no growth on MacConkey's agar in all patients. All the isolates were non motile, and catalase and oxidase positive, indole positive, citrate and urease negative, ortho-nitrophenyl-beta-galactoside positive, gelatin was liquefied after 48 hours; oxidative fermentative test was positive after 72 hours. All the isolates were identified as E. meningosepticum by Vitek 2. Antibiotic susceptibility and GenBank accession numbers of the isolates were shown in Table 1. Clinical features and treatment outcome of the nine patients with E. meningosepticum meningitis are shown in Table 2.

The data on antibiotic susceptibility of E. meningosepticum is limited because it is rarely isolated from clinical specimen and there are no standard guidelines on antibiotic susceptibility testing and reporting and interpretation of the susceptibility data. According to the published literature E. meningosepticum is known to be resistant to β-lactams, extended spectrum cephalosporins, carbapenems, and gentamicin, susceptible to vancomycin, trimethoprim-sulfamethoxazole, rifampicin, and ciprofloxacin, and moderately susceptible to piperacillin [2]. In the present study we have noted that all the isolates are resistant to β-lactams, extended spectrum cephalosporins, β-lactam combinations, carbapenems, aztreonam, aminoglycosides, tetracyclines,

and trimethoprim-sulfamethoxazole and only one isolate has been susceptible to ciprofloxacin. All the isolates are susceptible to vancomycin by disk diffusion method. Determination of antibiotic susceptibility by disk diffusion is not a recommended method, but there is no option in Vitek to check the susceptibility of nonfermenting Gram negative bacilli to vancomycin. There is no discrepancy between the susceptibility results of the isolates by Vitek and disk diffusion to the remaining antibiotics. Antibiotic susceptibility data of our study highlights that the majority of isolates (8/9) are multidrug resistant (resistant to all drugs except vancomycin).

The underlying host factors associated with E. meningosepticum meningitis in neonates are prematurity and low birth weight and we also observed the same risk factors [4, 5]. Based on the susceptibility of the isolates only to vancomycin, we have used vancomycin in 7/9 neonates and one neonate received combination of vancomycin and ciprofloxacin antibiotics. One neonate succumbed before the susceptibility results were available. Only two neonates recovered from infection after using vancomycin and the remaining 7 expired. According to the previous reports vancomycin is not an effective antimicrobial agent to treat the E. meningosepticum meningitis [2, 6, 7]. Based on our study findings and other reports the efficacy of vancomycin in treating E. meningosepticum meningitis in neonates is questionable. Previous authors treated neonates with E. meningosepticum meningitis successfully with piperacillin in combination with rifampicin [5]. All our study isolates were resistant to piperacillin and piperacillin-tazobactam. The limitation of our study is that susceptibility to rifampicin is not determined. The mortality rate (6/9) in our study is high compared to other studies [5].

Several outbreaks of E. meningosepticum meningitis in neonates have been reported [8, 9]. The outbreaks reported in the literature occurred within few weeks to months except in one study, where the authors reported an outbreak with one strain of E. meningosepticum for 2 years [8]. All the nine cases reported in the present study occurred over a period of one year. We have tried to identify the source of infection in the present study by collecting environmental

TABLE 2: Clinical features and treatment outcome of nine neonates with meningitis.

S. number	Age (days)/sex	Underlying condition	Clinical features at presentation	Clinical diagnosis	Initial antibiotic used before collection of specimen	Modified antibiotic therapy after microbiological diagnosis	Outcome
1	2/F	Preterm baby	Fever, seizures	Meningitis	Cefotaxime and amikacin	Vancomycin	Recovered
2	17/F	Preterm baby	Seizures, neck rigidity	Meningitis	Cefotaxime and amikacin	Vancomycin and ciprofloxacin	Recovered
3	15/F	Preterm baby	Fever, icterus, seizures	Septicemia and meningitis	Cefotaxime and Amikacin	Vancomycin	Left against medical advise
4	7/F	Low birth weight	Seizures, icterus, vomiting	Septicemia	Cefotaxime and amikacin	Vancomycin	Expired
5	21/M	Low birth weight, preterm baby	Seizures, fever, neck rigidity	Septicemia and meningitis	Cefotaxime and amikacin	Vancomycin	Expired
6	16/F	Low birth weight, preterm baby	Seizures, fever, neck rigidity	Meningitis	Cefotaxime and amikacin	Vancomycin	Expired
7	30/M	Low birth weight, preterm baby	Seizure, vomiting, neck rigidity	Meningitis	Cefotaxime and amikacin	Vancomycin	Expired
8	22/M	Preterm baby	Seizure, neck rigidity	Meningitis	Cefotaxime and amikacin	Vancomycin	Expired
9	10/F	Low birth weight, preterm baby	Not accepting feeds, seizures, neck rigidity	Meningitis	Cefotaxime and amikacin	Expired before the susceptibility results were available	Expired

specimens like water from incubators, tap water, suction fluids, the disinfectants and healthy babies were also screened for asymptomatic carriage by collecting rectal and umbilical swabs. All the environmental specimens and healthy babies were negative for *E. meningosepticum*. We also carried out the gene sequencing of the isolates from seven patients and phylogenetic tree was constructed to see the genetic relatedness of the isolates (gene sequences of the isolates deposited in the GenBank) and found that none of the isolates are genetically related to each other. In the present study we could not identify the source of infection.

4. Conclusion

E. meningosepticum meningitis in neonates results in high mortality rate. Though the organism shows susceptibility in vitro to vancomycin, its efficacy in vivo is questionable and it is difficult to determine the most appropriate antibiotic for treating *E. meningosepticum* meningitis in neonates.

Conflict of Interests

The authors declare that there is no conflict of interests regarding the publication of this paper.

Acknowledgments

The authors thank Hyderabad Eye Research Foundation, L. V. Prasad Eye Institute, Hyderabad, India, for allowing them to use the sequencing facility, and Mr. Praveen Kumar Balne for technical help.

References

[1] P.-Y. Lin, C. Chu, L.-H. Su, C.-T. Huang, W.-Y. Chang, and C.-H. Chiu, "Clinical and microbiological analysis of bloodstream infections caused by *Chryseobacterium meningosepticum* in nonneonatal patients," *Journal of Clinical Microbiology*, vol. 42, no. 7, pp. 3353–3355, 2004.

[2] J. T. Kirby, H. S. Sader, T. R. Walsh, and R. N. Jones, "Antimicrobial susceptibility and epidemiology of a worldwide collection of *Chryseobacterium* spp.: report from the SENTRY antimicrobial surveillance program (1997–2001)," *Journal of Clinical Microbiology*, vol. 42, no. 1, pp. 445–448, 2004.

[3] N. Ozkalay, M. Anil, N. Agus, M. Helvaci, and S. Sirti, "Community-acquired meningitis and sepsis caused by *Chryseobacterium meningosepticum* in a patient diagnosed with thalassemia major," *Journal of Clinical Microbiology*, vol. 44, no. 8, pp. 3037–3039, 2006.

[4] J. R. Dooley, L. J. Nims, and V. H. Lipp, "Meningitis of infants caused by *Flavobacterium meningosepticum*. Report of a patient

and analysis of 63 infections," *Journal of Tropical Pediatrics*, vol. 26, no. 1, pp. 24–30, 1980.

[5] M. I. Issack and Y. Neetoo, "An outbreak of *Elizabethkingia meningoseptica* neonatal meningitis in mauritius," *Journal of Infection in Developing Countries*, vol. 5, no. 12, pp. 834–839, 2011.

[6] M. C. Di Pentima, E. O. Mason Jr., and S. L. Kaplan, "In vitro antibiotic synergy against *Flavobacterium meningosepticum*: implications for therapeutic options," *Clinical Infectious Diseases*, vol. 26, no. 5, pp. 1169–1176, 1998.

[7] S. L. Fraser and J. H. Jorgensen, "Reappraisal of the antimicrobial susceptibilities of *Chryseobacterium* and *Flavobacterium* species and methods for reliable susceptibility testing," *Antimicrobial Agents and Chemotherapy*, vol. 41, no. 12, pp. 2738–2741, 1997.

[8] S. N. Hoque, J. Graham, M. E. Kaufmann, and S. Tabaqchali, "*Chryseobacterium (Flavobacterium)* meningosepticum outbreak associated with colonization of water taps in a neonatal intensive care unit," *Journal of Hospital Infection*, vol. 47, no. 3, pp. 188–192, 2001.

[9] S. Maraki, E. Scoulica, A. Manoura, N. Papageorgiou, C. Giannakopoulou, and E. Galanakis, "A *Chryseobacterium meningosepticum* colonization outbreak in a neonatal intensive care unit," *European Journal of Clinical Microbiology and Infectious Diseases*, vol. 28, no. 12, pp. 1415–1419, 2009.

35

Evaluation of Heart Rate Assessment Timing, Communication, Accuracy, and Clinical Decision-Making during High Fidelity Simulation of Neonatal Resuscitation

Win Boon,[1] **Jennifer McAllister,**[1] **Mohammad A. Attar,**[1] **Rachel L. Chapman,**[1] **Patricia B. Mullan,**[2] **and Hilary M. Haftel**[1,2]

[1] *Department of Pediatrics and Communicable Diseases, University of Michigan, Ann Arbor, MI 48109, USA*
[2] *Department of Medical Education, University of Michigan, Ann Arbor, MI 48109, USA*

Correspondence should be addressed to Mohammad A. Attar; mattar@med.umich.edu

Academic Editor: Patrick Brophy

Objective. Accurate heart rate (HR) determination during neonatal resuscitation (NR) informs subsequent NR actions. This study's objective was to evaluate HR determination timeliness, communication, and accuracy during high fidelity NR simulations that house officers completed during neonatal intensive care unit (NICU) rotations. *Methods.* In 2010, house officers in NICU rotations completed high fidelity NR simulation. We reviewed 80 house officers' videotaped performance on their initial high fidelity simulation session, prior to training and performance debriefing. We calculated the proportion of cases congruent with NR guidelines, using chi square analysis to evaluate performance across HR ranges relevant to NR decision-making: <60, 60–99, and ≥100 beats per minute (bpm). *Results.* 87% used umbilical cord palpation, 57% initiated HR assessment within 30 seconds, 70% were accurate, and 74% were communicated appropriately. HR determination accuracy varied significantly across HR ranges, with 87%, 57%, and 68% for HR <60, 60–99, and ≥100 bpm, respectively ($P < 0.001$). *Conclusions.* Timeliness, communication, and accuracy of house officers' HR determination are suboptimal, particularly for HR 60–100 bpm, which might lead to inappropriate decision-making and NR care. Training implications include emphasizing more accurate HR determination methods, better communication, and improved HR interpretation during NR.

1. Introduction

Timely and accurate heart rate (HR) assessments are central to effective neonatal resuscitation [1]. The International Liaison Committee on Resuscitation's recent consensus statement reaffirms that HR should determine the adequacy of resuscitation and guide medical decision-making and that an increase in HR remains the most sensitive indicator of effective resuscitative measures [2].

Incorrect HR determination may lead providers to initiate inappropriate treatment or fail to implement warranted intervention. This is particularly important for HR between 60 and 100 beats per minute (bpm), due to the need to provide positive pressure ventilation (PPV) for HR below 100 bpm and chest compressions for HR below 60 bpm in the setting of effective PPV [1].

Deficiencies in communication of HR have been documented among neonatologists, fellows, house officers, nurse practitioners, nurses, and respiratory therapists [3, 4]. Studies also show clinical HR determinations can be inaccurate; however, most studies were performed on low risk newborns who did not require resuscitation at the time of their assessment and had heart rates greater than 100 bpm [5, 6]. Other studies evaluated HR assessment accuracy across various ranges using manikins, but these assessments included prompts for when the heart rates should be checked and were not performed during full resuscitation scenarios [7, 8]. A recent study using high fidelity simulation (HFS), in which subjects were instructed to assess and verbalize their HR determination before and after any interventions, also found deficiencies in HR accuracy that could lead to inappropriate actions [9].

This study evaluated the timeliness, communication, and accuracy of house officers' HR determination and their subsequent resuscitation decision-making in the context of neonatal resuscitations during required HFS exercises.

2. Methods

We designed standardized simulation scenarios, based on the Neonatal Resuscitation Program (NRP) 5th edition curriculum, by adapting scenarios associated with the SimNewB Advanced high fidelity neonatal simulator (Laerdal Medical, Stavanger, Norway). Features of our standardized cases included the need to assess HR and respiratory effort and required house officers to make decisions regarding performing PPV, endotracheal intubation, and chest compressions. Initial HR for all scenarios varied between 0 and 80 bpm. Participants were oriented to the SimNewB Advanced high fidelity neonatal simulator prior to their sessions. HFS scenarios were then conducted during these sessions, using the simulator as an assessment tool.

Each scenario was recorded digitally via a webcam placed on the resuscitation cot to facilitate review. Participants were aware of recording and their faces were not in the field of view. Participants were informed prior to participation in this educational curriculum that these recordings might be reviewed for educational purposes, quality improvement, and research. Our Institutional Review Board provided exempt status for this educational intervention.

The NRP Megacode checklist and a previously established scoring instrument have both been cited in the literature, with several reports evaluating their validity [10, 11]. Elements from this checklist and scoring tool were combined and used to track defined house officer performance characteristics during these resuscitations, including measures related to the timing, accuracy, and communication of HR determination. Two of the instructors (WB and JM) underwent a process to confirm interrater reliability. This process included review and discussion of HR scoring definitions, followed by independent scoring of 5 resuscitation scenarios. The two raters agreed on 117 of 120 (97%) of HR scores. Videos of all recorded scenarios from January through December 2010 were then reviewed by one of these instructors. Data were subsequently deidentified for statistical analysis.

All trainees rotating through the University of Michigan's level 4 NICU from January through December 2010 participated in 1-2 simulated resuscitation sessions per month as part of the monthly rotation curriculum. A session was composed of two different NRP scenarios, in which each HO played the role of NRP team leader in one scenario and the role of the assistant in the other scenario. All house officers were NRP trained and certified prior to their NICU rotations. 82 house officers participated in this study. We analyzed data from 80 of these house officers after limiting the dataset to scenarios that (1) represented the participants' first HFS (in order to represent performance prior to training and performance debriefing) and (2) were not affected by simulation, equipment or video malfunctions, or other participants (Table 1). All house officers (including emergency medicine residents) at the University of Michigan

TABLE 1: Medical training level and specialty of house officer participants in the baseline high fidelity neonatal resuscitation simulation exercises.

Residency training level	HO 1	HO 2	HO 3	HO 4	Total
Pediatrics	28	9	12	—	49
Medicine/pediatrics	7	6	3	1	17
Emergency medicine	0	14	0	0	14

are NRP certified at the start of residency and undergo an NRP recertification process every two years thereafter while in training.

We evaluated HR assessments at three key time points during NR: (1) heart rate assessment #1: initial HR check at birth, (2) heart rate assessment #2: HR check to assess response to resuscitative measures beyond the initial steps of warming/drying/stimulating the infant (i.e., after initiation of PPV), and (3) heart rate assessment #3: HR check after continued resuscitative measures. The simulator's actual HR, trainee's method of HR assessment (auscultation, palpation, or both), timeliness, communication to the lead resuscitator, and accuracy of each HR check were tracked. The appropriateness of decision-making based on NRP defined guidelines was evaluated for each HR assessment. Subsequent HR determination trends and associated decision-making beyond these initial three checkpoints were reported in aggregate when appropriate.

HR checks were defined as timely if they were performed within the first 30 seconds of life (for initial HR checks) or performed after 30 seconds of subsequent intervention based on NRP guidelines (for all subsequent HR checks). HR communication was deemed appropriate if it was reported as a specific numerical rate or within one of the NRP defined HR ranges. HR communication was deemed inappropriate if a specific HR or HR range was not explicitly stated (e.g., stating that the HR was "okay" was not acceptable) or if there was a delay >15 seconds in reporting the HR to the lead resuscitator. HR checks were defined as accurate only if they were communicated as either a specific numerical rate or NRP defined HR range and if the HR the resident reported matched the simulator's set HR. HR checks were deemed inaccurate if they were not communicated as a specific HR or HR range or if the stated HR or range did not conform to the simulator's set HR. Decision-making was deemed correct if the appropriate intervention (per NRP 5th edition guidelines) was performed, based on the simulator's set HR and clinical status at the time of the HR assessment.

The proportion of cases congruent with NR guidelines was calculated for HR determination timing, communication, accuracy, and subsequent decision-making. We further evaluated HR ranges relevant to decision-making in NR: <60, 60–99, and ≥100 bpm. Chi square analysis examined the distribution of correct performance across HR ranges with significance set at $P < 0.05$.

3. Results

Table 2 summarizes trainees' performance on the defined HR assessments. 72% of all HR assessments were performed via

TABLE 2: House officers' percentage of correct performance on heart rate (HR) assessments and clinical decision-making on neonatal high fidelity simulation resuscitations.

	Overall	First heart rate assessment	Second heart rate assessment	Third heart rate assessment	Subsequent heart rate assessment
HR assessment method					
Palpation	72%	66%	72%	71%	77%
Auscultation	13%	8%	14%	15%	14%
Both	15%	25%	14%	14%	9%
Timely HR assessment	82%	57%	90%	94%	82%
HR communicated appropriately	74%	81%	75%	74%	65%
HR accurate	70%	74%	70%	64%	70%
Clinical decision-making for HR	81%	91%	81%	73%	80%

TABLE 3: House officers' performance on high fidelity neonatal simulation heart rate assessment measures according to actual heart rate.

	HR < 60 bpm	HR 60–99 bpm	HR ≥ 100 bpm	P value
Heart rate assessed in a timely manner	90%	75%	91%	$P < 0.001$
Heart rate communicated appropriately	85%	76%	70%	$P = 0.002$
Heart rate accurate	87%	57%	68%	$P < 0.001$
Correct decision-making	82%	80%	86%	$P = 0.357$

palpation of the umbilical cord, with 13% via auscultation. Both methods were used in 15% of HR assessments. 82% of all HR checks occurred in a timely manner. The first HR assessment was initiated within 30 seconds in 57% of cases, with an average initiation time of 37 seconds. Timing of the first HR check was as early as 4 seconds and as delayed as 115 seconds. 74% of all HR assessments were communicated appropriately to the team leader. 10% of trainees communicated HR with nonspecific language (i.e., without explicit numerical values or ranges).

70% of all HR determinations were accurate within the appropriate NRP defined range. For the first HR assessment, medical decisions consistent with NRP guidelines occurred in 91% of cases. Decision-making was correct with 81% of all HR checks. Excluding the first HR assessment, appropriate decisions were made 75% of the time.

Chi square analysis (Table 3) revealed statistically significant differences in the timeliness, communication, and assessments among the three NRP defined HR ranges: <60 bpm (range 1), 60–99 bpm (range 2), and at least 100 bpm (range 3). In contrast, the appropriateness of decision-making did not vary significantly among the defined HR ranges.

HR was assessed in a timely manner: 90% of the time for HR range 1 (<60 bpm), 75% of the time for HR range 2 (60–99 bpm), and 91% of the time for HR range 3 (≥100 bpm). 87% of HR in range 1 was determined accurately, while HR in range 2 was accurately assessed 57% of the time, and HR in range 3 was accurate in 68% of cases.

Certain performance metrics appeared to be worse in PGY2 residents, who would have been the furthest from initial training or NRP renewal. For example, HR was measured correctly by first-year residents 78% of the time and by third-year residents 69% of the time but by second-year residents only 61% of the time. Appropriateness of medical decision-making improved slightly with increased years of training, with 83%, 87%, and 89% of first-, second-, and third-year residents, respectively. making the correct next step. There were otherwise no statistically or clinically significant differences in any of the measured categories when compared across HO training programs, by residency year, or number of months of NICU experience.

4. Discussion

Timely and accurate heart rate determination, communication, and interpretation are central to effective neonatal resuscitation. Our study of residents' observed behavior with HFS in the neonatal setting provides empirical insights into important limitations of their practice with direct implications for training. Auscultation of the HR with a stethoscope is more accurate than palpation of the umbilical cord [5, 6]. In our study of house officers participating in HFS of neonatal resuscitations, 72% of HR checks were done via palpation only, while 13% were auscultated with a stethoscope only and 15% used both auscultation and palpation.

We analyzed the first and subsequent HR evaluations separately because of the possibility of improved HR assessment with subsequent HR evaluations and because the required intervention may vary between the first and subsequent measured HRs. Despite delays in the first HR check, we found that 91% of cases still provided correct initial medical intervention. This discrepancy suggests that, in practice, the first HR check may not be as integral to initial decision-making in the resuscitation scenarios, particularly if the infant appears depressed to the resuscitation team (e.g., the infant is apneic). Correct decisions were made 75% of the time in association with all HR checks when excluding the initial HR check. This latter figure may more accurately reflect the assessment and use of HR during ongoing neonatal resuscitation.

Our findings that HR checks were not consistently communicated are congruent with existing research [3, 4, 12]. Communicating HR with nonspecific terms such as "good" or "okay" may be misinterpreted by other team members, leading to incorrect interventions that are range specific.

Among HR visibly tapped in video review, only 56% were accurate. There were also instances in which tapping was performed correctly (i.e., it matched the simulator's programmed HR) but the stated HR was inaccurate. HR determination in the midst of a stressful resuscitation is prone to error; this may be complicated by the need to multitask counting the heart beat while keeping track of the time spent counting, followed by calculations to derive an actual rate. Trainees inconsistently used the 6-second method of counting HR recommended by the NRP. Counting devices have been proposed to help simplify this process, but they are not widely available [7, 13].

70% of all HR assessments in our sample were accurate within NRP defined ranges. We found clinical HR determination least accurate between 60 and 100 bpm (57% accuracy rate). Errors in HR determination, particularly in the critical range between 60 and 100 bpm, may lead to inappropriate resuscitative measures, such as the provision of chest compressions when they are not indicated or failure to provide PPV when it is indicated. Our findings corroborate the results reported by Chitkara et al. [9] on NRP trained subjects, in which 22 out of the 67 subjects were pediatric residents. Their randomized controlled study using simpler full resuscitation scenarios, which evaluated the accuracy of HR determination, found an error rate of 36% to 48% for rates of 90 bpm, which is similar to the 43% rate our study identified. Junior residents take the task of HR evaluation in most of the neonatal resuscitations in our institution. Neonatology fellows and attending physicians quickly take up this task when the HR is reported to be lower than 100 bpm, given the potential inaccuracy of trainees' HR determinations.

Previous studies [7, 8] evaluating the accuracy of HR assessments using manikins found deficiencies in HR assessment accuracy. However, those assessments were performed in limited scenarios (i.e., not full neonatal resuscitation), and participants in those studies received prompts to assess and communicate HR appropriately. Our study builds on this existing research through the use of full resuscitation scenarios, during which HR assessments were not prompted.

The 6th edition of the NRP recommends use of pulse oximetry (PO) during neonatal resuscitation [14]. In addition to providing saturation values, PO allows continuous HR assessments for infants receiving prolonged resuscitation [15]. More recent studies have found that electrocardiogram (ECG) provides accurate HR information faster than PO [16, 17]. The ability to obtain accurate HR assessments quickly with technology such as ECG or PO may in part ameliorate the deficiencies in clinical HR assessments we have found in this study. Regardless of which technology is used, the ability to have ongoing HR assessments during resuscitation would allow members of the team to perform other tasks

and possibly lead to better outcomes. Our findings support the NRP's 6th edition recommendation to utilize objective heart rate monitoring technology early in resuscitation. If the recommendations change practice, this may render this study's findings less relevant in the years to come with the increased use of PO or ECG early during resuscitation. However, both the common finding that medical practice does not always quickly adopt recommended practices and the potential for limited access to the recommended technology in all delivery situations suggest that clinical assessment remains an important skill.

There was a tendency towards worse performance metrics in the PGY-2 group. Almost half of that group (14/29) were emergency medicine residents. However, these emergency medicine residents had similar intervals as the other residents from their last NRP certification. Our findings suggest that reinforcement before the two-year recertification process may be beneficial. House officer training could potentially be improved with educational interventions such as a HFS curriculum. However, follow-up studies of HO performance upon repeated exposure to such a curriculum would be needed to assess this further.

This study used HFS, with data obtained via video review of resuscitation cases. While this manikin represents muscle tone, heart rate, respiratory effort, cyanosis, and cry, assessment nevertheless only approximated that of a real infant. Equipment was subject to malfunction, which was responsible for the exclusion of 7 scenarios. Audiovisual review was limited to what could be recorded clearly. Furthermore, this study does not establish a causal relationship between HR determination/accuracy and clinical decision-making but rather makes available empirical assessments of their frequency and associations.

5. Conclusion

Clinical HR determination by house officers during simulated neonatal resuscitation is suboptimal and appears to be least accurate between 60 and 100 bpm. Errors in HR determination, communication, or interpretation may lead to inappropriate resuscitative measures and adverse outcomes. Additional educational emphasis beyond what is provided in current training should be undertaken to improve the clinical acquisition and use of HR during neonatal resuscitation.

Conflict of Interests

The authors have no relevant affiliations or financial involvement with any organization or entity with financial interests or financial conflict with the subject matter or materials discussed in the paper. The authors report no external funding source for this study.

References

[1] J. Kattwinkel, Ed., *Neonatal Resuscitation Textbook*, American Academy of Pediatrics, 5th edition, 2006.

[2] J. M. Perlman, J. Wyllie, J. Kattwinkel et al., "Neonatal resuscitation: 2010 international consensus on cardiopulmonary resuscitation and emergency cardiovascular care science with treatment recommendations," *Pediatrics*, vol. 126, no. 5, pp. e1319–e1344, 2010.

[3] D. N. Carbine, N. N. Finer, E. Knodel, and W. Rich, "Video recording as a means of evaluating neonatal resuscitation performance," *Pediatrics*, vol. 106, no. 4, pp. 654–658, 2000.

[4] B. Gelbart, R. Hiscock, and C. Barfield, "Assessment of neonatal resuscitation performance using video recording in a perinatal centre," *Journal of Paediatrics and Child Health*, vol. 46, no. 7-8, pp. 378–383, 2010.

[5] C. O. F. Kamlin, C. P. F. O'Donnell, N. J. Everest, P. G. Davis, and C. J. Morley, "Accuracy of clinical assessment of infant heart rate in the delivery room," *Resuscitation*, vol. 71, no. 3, pp. 319–321, 2006.

[6] C. J. Owen and J. P. Wyllie, "Determination of heart rate in the baby at birth," *Resuscitation*, vol. 60, no. 2, pp. 213–217, 2004.

[7] D. T. Theophilopoulos and D. J. Burchfield, "Accuracy of different methods for heart rate determination during simulated neonatal resuscitations," *Journal of Perinatology*, vol. 18, no. 1, pp. 65–67, 1998.

[8] K. G. J. A. Voogdt, A. C. Morrison, F. E. Wood, R. M. van Elburg, and J. P. Wyllie, "A randomised, simulated study assessing auscultation of heart rate at birth," *Resuscitation*, vol. 81, no. 8, pp. 1000–1003, 2010.

[9] R. Chitkara, A. K. Rajani, J. W. Oehlert, H. C. Lee, M. S. Epi, and L. P. Halamek, "The accuracy of human senses in the detection of neonatal heart rate during standardized simulated resuscitation: implications for delivery of care, training and technology design," *Resuscitation*, vol. 84, pp. 369–372, 2013.

[10] J. Lockyer, N. Singhal, H. Fidler, G. Weiner, K. Aziz, and V. Curran, "The development and testing of a performance checklist to assess neonatal resuscitation megacode skill," *Pediatrics*, vol. 118, no. 6, pp. e1739–e1744, 2006.

[11] P. A. van der Heide, L. van Toledo-Eppinga, M. van der Heide, and J. H. van der Lee, "Assessment of neonatal resuscitation skills: a reliable and valid scoring system," *Resuscitation*, vol. 71, no. 2, pp. 212–221, 2006.

[12] T. A. Stavroudis, K. Frank, B. Sextin, A. Knight, L. P. Halamek, and E. A. Hunt, "Compliance with the neonatal resuscitation program timeline," Pediatric Academic Soscieties, E-PAS2008:634453.3, 2008.

[13] R. P. Lemke, M. Farrah, and P. J. Byrn, "Use of a new doppler umbilical cord clamp to measure heart rate in newborn infants in the delivery roomlow perceived social support is associated to cd8+cd57+ lymphocyte expansion and increased," *E-Journal of Neonatology Research*, vol. 1, pp. 83–88, 2011.

[14] *Textbook of Neonatal Resuscitation*, American Academy of Pediatrics, 6th edition, 2011.

[15] C. O. F. Kamlin, J. A. Dawson, C. P. F. O'Donnell et al., "Accuracy of pulse oximetry measurement of heart rate of newborn infants in the delivery room," *Journal of Pediatrics*, vol. 152, no. 6, pp. 756–760, 2008.

[16] H. Mizumoto, S. Tomotaki, H. Shibata et al., "Electrocardiogram shows reliable heart rates much earlier than pulse oximetry during neonatal resuscitation," *Pediatrics International*, vol. 54, no. 2, pp. 205–207, 2012.

[17] A. Katheria, W. Rich, and N. Finer, "Electrocardiogram provides a continuous heart rate faster than oximetry during neonatal resuscitation," *Pediatrics*, vol. 130, no. 5, pp. e1177–e1181, 2012.

36

Inflammatory Bowel Disease in Children of Middle Eastern Descent

Christina Mai Ying Naidoo,[1] Steven T. Leach,[1] Andrew S. Day,[1,2,3] and Daniel A. Lemberg[1,2]

[1] School of Women's and Children's Health, University of New South Wales, Sydney, NSW 2052, Australia
[2] Department of Gastroenterology, Sydney Children's Hospital, High Street, Randwick, Sydney, NSW 2031, Australia
[3] Department of Pediatrics, University of Otago (Christchurch), Christchurch 8140, New Zealand

Correspondence should be addressed to Daniel A. Lemberg; daniel.lemberg@health.nsw.gov.au

Academic Editor: Sandeep Gupta

Increasing rates of inflammatory bowel disease (IBD) are now seen in populations where it was once uncommon. The pattern of IBD in children of Middle Eastern descent in Australia has never been reported. This study aimed to investigate the burden of IBD in children of Middle Eastern descent at the Sydney Children's Hospital, Randwick (SCHR). The SCHR IBD database was used to identify patients of self-reported Middle Eastern ethnicity diagnosed between 1987 and 2011. Demographic, diagnosis, and management data was collected for all Middle Eastern children and an age and gender matched non-Middle Eastern IBD control group. Twenty-four patients of Middle Eastern descent were identified. Middle Eastern Crohn's disease patients had higher disease activity at diagnosis, higher use of thiopurines, and less restricted colonic disease than controls. Although there were limitations with this dataset, we estimated a higher prevalence of IBD in Middle Eastern children and they had a different disease phenotype and behavior compared to the control group, with less disease restricted to the colon and likely a more active disease course.

1. Introduction

Inflammatory bowel disease (IBD) is a chronic, relapsing, idiopathic inflammation of the gastrointestinal tract. Subtypes of IBD include Crohn's disease (CD), ulcerative colitis (UC), and inflammatory bowel disease unclassified (IBD-U). The majority of epidemiological studies on the incidence and prevalence of IBD relate to the adult population [1]. Historically, Europe and North America have been considered high incidence areas while Asia, Africa, and the Middle East have been considered low incidence areas [2, 3]. Emerging data has suggested that the incidence of IBD is increasing globally in both developed and developing countries [3]. One study from Central Saudi Arabia on the epidemiology of juvenile onset IBD estimated an incidence of 0.5 per 100 000 per year and a prevalence of 5/100 000 [4]. While this is significantly lower than the incidence rates of 11.43/100 000 per year reported in North America [5], comparison with older data nevertheless suggests an increasing incidence [4].

The emergence of chronic inflammatory diseases such as IBD has been closely linked to social and economic development [6] and it has been postulated that the "Westernisation" of society accounts for the increasing incidence of IBD in countries where it was once considered rare [3]. The importance of ethnic, racial, and geographic factors in IBD is illustrated by the considerable literature citing varying risks of developing IBD in different ethnic populations. It has been well established that the Ashkenazi Jewish population have a higher risk of developing IBD than other ethnic groups [7, 8]. Several studies also show that ethnic groups with low rates of IBD in their home country have a much higher incidence of IBD following immigration to Western countries [9]. For instance, studies on migrant populations found a higher incidence of IBD in South Asians than Non-South Asians in the pediatric population of British Columbia and the adult population of Leicester [9–11].

Recent studies have found the overall incidence rate of IBD in Australia to be among the highest reported [12].

In addition, Phavichitr et al. [13] found that the incidence of pediatric CD in Victorian children rose from 0.128 per 100 000 per year in 1971 to 2.0 per 100 000 per year in 2001. However, there are no reports on the epidemiology of IBD in specific ethnic groups in Australia. Given the fact that Australia is a multicultural society with significant emigration of families from the Middle East this may be relevant. Therefore the objectives of the current study were to examine the clinical characteristics and management of IBD in children of Middle Eastern descent diagnosed at the Sydney Children's Hospital Randwick (SCHR).

2. Methods

2.1. Patients and Data Collection. A retrospective chart review was undertaken on all patients identified as being of Middle Eastern ethnicity on the SCHR IBD database. IBD specific data collection began at SCHR in 1987 and data was complete up to the year 2011 at the time of review. At diagnosis, parents were requested to provide a familial history including familial ethnicity. Children were considered to be of Middle Eastern ethnicity if one or both parents self-identified as being of Middle Eastern ethnicity or from any of the following countries: Egypt, Iran, Iraq, Israel, Jordan, Kuwait, Lebanon, Oman, Qatar, Saudi Arabia, Syria, United Arab Emirates, West Bank and Gaza, and Yemen. Children with Israeli ancestry and Jewish ethnicity were not included in this study due to the well-defined predisposition to IBD in this population. A control group of patients of non-Middle Eastern descent was also identified from the SCHR IBD database: these were matched to patients of Middle Eastern descent according to age at diagnosis, gender, and disease type. The project was approved by the South Eastern Sydney and Illawarra Area Health Service Research Ethics Committee.

Information collected at diagnosis for the study and control groups included family history of IBD in first degree relatives, smoking exposure history, residential postal code, age at diagnosis, symptoms at presentation, duration of symptoms at presentation, specific blood tests (erythrocyte sedimentation rate (ESR), C-reactive protein (CRP), platelets, albumin, haematocrit, alanine transaminase (ALT), aspartate transaminase (AST)), disease location, extraintestinal manifestations, pediatric Crohn's disease activity index (PCDAI) or pediatric ulcerative colitis activity index (PUCAI) score, height, and weight. Disease management information was also collected including whether they received the following treatments: exclusive enteral nutrition (EEN), corticosteroids, aminosalicylates, thiopurines, methotrexate, biological, tacrolimus, or surgical intervention.

Disease location was classified according to the Montreal classification of L1 (terminal ileum), L2 (colon), L3 (ileocolonic), and L4 (upper gastrointestinal (GI)) for CD [14]. Symptoms at presentation were grouped under the following categories: abdominal pain, diarrhoea, mucus and/or blood in stools, weight loss, per rectal bleeding, and loss of appetite. Height and weight measurements at diagnosis were converted to height for age z-scores and weight for age z-scores using the Centre for Disease Control application EpiInfo, based on the CDC-2000 charts.

2.2. Estimation of Point Incidence and Point Prevalence. Point incidence and point prevalence were calculated for both the Middle Eastern study group and the control group for the SCHR catchment area. For this purpose the catchment of the SCHR was defined as the Local Government Areas (LGA) of the South Eastern Sydney and Illawarra Area Health Service, which includes Botany, Hurstville, Kogarah, Randwick, Rockdale, Sutherland, Sydney, Waverley, Wollongong, and Woollahra. Population information for the LGAs was obtained from the Australian Bureau of Statistics 2006 census data. Ancestry information in the 2006 census data was collected by similar means to data in the SCHR database, where ancestry was defined by self-reporting of familial ancestry and birthplace. The census data was sorted by ancestry, LGA, and age (0–16 years). The SCHR IBD database was used to identify patients who resided in the defined catchment area and had active inflammatory bowel disease in 2006 to calculate point prevalence. The database was also used to identify those patients within the catchment area who were diagnosed in 2006 to calculate the point incidence.

The remoteness area category was calculated for each patient from residential postal codes based on the Australian Standard Geographical Classification-Remoteness Area (ASGC-RA). The ASGC-RA is a hierarchical classification system of geographical areas developed by the Australian Bureau of Statistics (ABS) that provides a common framework of statistical geography. The categories used were RA1 (major cities of Australia), RA2 (inner regional Australia), RA3 (outer regional Australia), RA4 (remote Australia), and RA5 (very remote Australia).

2.3. Statistics. Statistical analysis was carried out using Graph Pad Prism 5. A Fisher's exact test was used to compare the two groups with regard to smoking exposure history, family history, symptoms at presentation, extraintestinal manifestations, and disease location. The management of IBD was analysed by Fisher's exact tests, with UC and CD being analysed separately. A chi-squared test was used to compare ASGC-RA scores. An unpaired t-test was used to compare platelets, albumin, haematocrit, PCDAI, height for age z-scores, and weight for age z-scores between the two groups. The Mann-Whitney test was used to compare the groups for ESR, CRP, ALT, and AST. Results were considered significant if $P < 0.05$. The relative risk (RR) was calculated for incidence and prevalence; a result was considered significant if the confidence intervals (CI) did not embrace a relative risk of one.

3. Results

3.1. Study and Control Populations, Demographics, and Disease Characteristics. Of the 441 patients on the SCHR IBD database, 35 (7.9%) were identified as being of Middle Eastern ethnicity. However, 11 of the 35 were excluded from this retrospective study as files for these patients were unavailable.

TABLE 1: Group characteristics.

	Middle Eastern	Control	P value
Males	15 (62.5%)	15 (62.5%)	1.00
UC	7 (29.2%)	7 (29.2%)	1.00
CD	14 (58.3%)	14 (58.3%)	1.00
IBD-U	3 (12.5%)	3 (12.5%)	1.00
Age at diagnosis[#]	9.8 (4.5)	9.9 (4.4)	0.98

Data presented as number of patients (%) and compared by Fisher's exact test except [#] where data is presented as mean (SD) and compared by unpaired t-test.

Therefore a final cohort of 24 patients of Middle Eastern ethnicity (both parents of Middle Eastern ethnicity) and 24 non-Middle Eastern controls were included in this study.

Of the 24 patients of Middle Eastern ethnicity, 14 (58.3%) had CD, 7 (29.2%) had UC, and the remainder had IBD-U (Table 1). Fifteen (62.5%) of the group were male: 9 of these had CD and 4 had UC and 4 had IBD-U. Twenty (83.3%) patients were born in Australia, 2 (8.3%) were born in Lebanon, and 2 were born in the USA. The mean age at diagnosis overall was 9.8 years (range, 0.7–15.7). Four patients (16.6%) were diagnosed under the age of five years and 11 patients (45.8%) were diagnosed before the age of 10 years. There was mean of 92 days (range 2–3227 days) between date of diagnosis of the Middle Eastern ethnicity patients and their matched controls. All but one of the control patients were born in Australia. Data on consanguinity was unavailable.

In those children identified as Middle Eastern ethnicity, 16 had parents identified as Lebanese, 3 Egyptian, 2 Turkish, and 1 Algerian, and 2 parents did not provide a country of birth but self-identified as Middle Eastern ethnicity. Of the controls, 18 had parents identified as Caucasian, 2 Indian, and 1 Caucasian-Jewish, and 3 did not provide a country of birth but self-identified as non-Middle Eastern ethnicity. There was no difference in family history of IBD in first-degree relatives of Middle Eastern (5/22; 2 unknown; 22.7%) and control (2/22; 2 unknown; 9.1%) patients. There was no difference in smoking exposure history between the two groups, Middle Eastern (7/21; 33.3%) and control patients (5/19; 26.3%). All Middle Eastern patients (24/24; 100%) were living in RA1 (major city), while the controls had fewer patients (17/24; 70.8%) in RA1 and a greater distribution over RA2 (4/24; 16.7% inner regional Australia) and RA3 (3/24; 12.5% outer regional Australia) areas ($P = 0.017$).

Symptom duration prior to diagnosis did not vary between the Middle Eastern (median 8, range 1–208 weeks) and control groups (median 16, range 2–104 weeks) ($P = 0.37$). Abdominal pain and diarrhoea were the most common symptoms at presentation for both groups (Table 2). Erythrocyte sedimentation rate (ESR) at diagnosis was more elevated in Middle Eastern children compared to controls ($P = 0.02$); however, all other standard blood results were similar in both groups (Table 3). ALT and AST values were lower in the Middle Eastern group compared to the control group ($P = 0.03$ and $P = 0.02$, resp.) (Table 3).

PCDAI scores at diagnosis were significantly higher in the Middle Eastern group (mean 37, SD 13) compared to

TABLE 2: Symptoms at presentation.

	Middle Eastern		Control		P value
	Yes	No	Yes	No	
Abdominal pain	13	8	13	10	0.77
Diarrhoea	16	5	18	5	1.00
Mucus or blood in stools	10	11	13	10	0.76
Weight loss	10	11	8	15	0.54
Per rectal bleeding	2	19	7	16	0.14
Loss of appetite	3	18	2	21	0.66

Data compared by Fisher's exact test. Presenting symptoms not available for 3 Middle Eastern patients and 1 control patient.

TABLE 3: Blood results at diagnosis.

	Middle Eastern	Control	P value
[^]ESR	31 (3–74)	18.5 (2–69)	0.02*
[^]CRP	5 (1–198)	6 (1–62)	0.34
Platelets	392 (96)	434 (130)	0.24
Haematocrit	0.35 (0.05)	0.35 (0.05)	0.53
Albumin	35.6 (7.1)	38.6 (8.8)	0.23
[^]ALT	12 (6–35)	18.5 (8–147)	0.03*
[^]AST	14 (5–28)	24 (6–128)	0.01*

Data presented as mean (SD) and compared by unpaired t-test except [^]where data is presented as median (range) and compared by Mann Whitney test. *indicates statistical significance.

the control group (mean 27, SD 11; $P = 0.033$) (Figure 1). There was insufficient data to analyse PUCAI scores. Height for age z-score and weight for age z-scores at diagnosis were similar between the groups. Two (8.3%) of the Middle Eastern patients and one (4.2%) control had height for age z-score indicating stunted growth (<-2 SD). There was a lower incidence of colonic disease (L2) ($P = 0.01$) in the Middle Eastern group with CD compared with the control group (Table 4). Upper GI disease was present in 10 (71%) of the controls and 13 (93%) of the Middle Eastern CD patients. Terminal ileal location (L1), ileocolonic disease (L3), and upper GI tract involvement (L4) were similar in both patient groups (Table 4). There was no difference between the groups for disease location in UC as most patients in both groups had pancolitis (E3).

3.2. Estimated Point Incidence and Point Prevalence. The incidence of IBD in the SCHR catchment area in 2006 for the Middle Eastern pediatrics population (aged 0–16 years) was higher (33.1 per 100 000 children per year) compared to the control group (4.3 per 100 000 children per year). The relative risk analysis, although indicating a high risk of IBD with Middle Eastern ethnicity, does not reach significance (RR 7.63, 95% CI 0.95–65.01) (Figure 2). However the prevalence of IBD in the Middle Eastern pediatric population was significantly higher at 165.4 per 100 000 children compared to the control prevalence rates of 28.7 per 100 000 children (RR 5.76, 95% CI 2.30–14.43) (Figure 2).

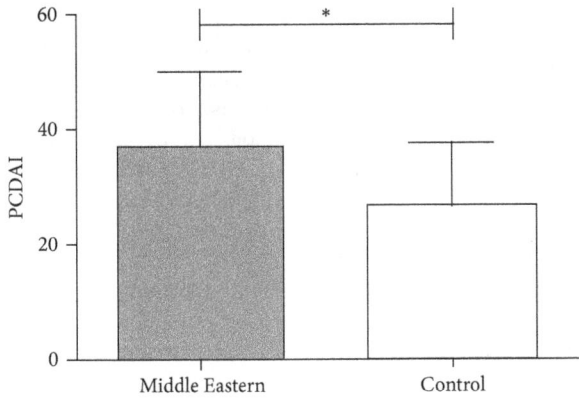

FIGURE 1: The pediatric Crohn's disease activity index (PCDAI) at diagnosis was significantly higher ($^{*}P = 0.033$) in children identified with Middle Eastern descent compared to children of non-Middle Eastern decent.

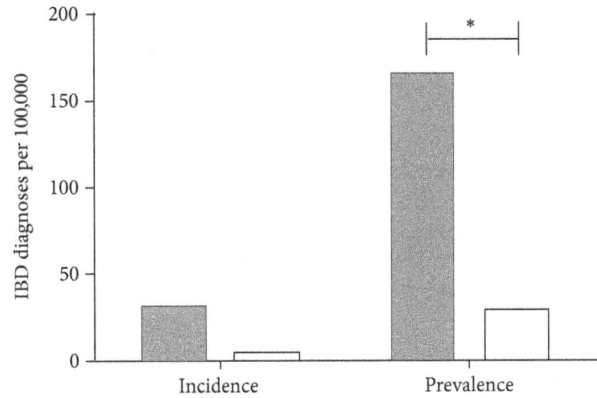

FIGURE 2: The incidence and prevalence of IBD in the pediatric population were calculated for the Sydney Children's Hospital, Randwick, catchment area for the year 2006. The prevalence of IBD amongst children with Middle Eastern ethnicity was significantly higher (*RR 5.76; CI 2.30–14.43) than prevalence amongst children with non-Middle Eastern ethnicity.

TABLE 4: Disease location CD.

	Middle Eastern	Control	P value
L1	3	0	0.22
L2	3	11	0.01*
L3	8	3	0.12
L4	13	10	0.33

Data compared by Fisher's exact test. *indicates statistical significance.

3.3. Therapy. Overall, there were no differences in the use of standard medical therapies between the groups ($P > 0.05$ for all). In addition, there was no difference in surgical management between the two groups ($P > 0.05$). However, considering the children with CD separately, the use of thiopurines was significantly higher in the Middle Eastern group for the management of CD ($P = 0.002$) (Table 5). There was no difference in use of corticosteroids, aminosalicylates, biologicals, or tacrolimus for management of CD between the groups (Table 5). There was also no difference for any of the therapies between the groups for the management of UC.

4. Discussion

This is the first study comparing the incidence, presentation, and management of IBD in a Middle Eastern pediatric population now residing in a "Western" country. The estimated incidence rate for IBD in this population in 2006 was among the highest reported in the pediatric literature and was almost 8 times higher than that observed for the non-Middle Eastern population in the same location. There is great variation in the literature on the difference in incidence between different populations. However our findings are consistent with those of other studies that have identified higher risk of IBD in specific groups such as South Asians and Ashkenazi Jews [7, 9].

Accurate prevalence and incidence rates of pediatric IBD for many Middle Eastern countries have not been reported in the literature [4]. It has been postulated that the low incidence of IBD in developing countries is attributed to poor sanitation and hygiene and greater exposure to microorganisms during

TABLE 5: Clinical management of CD.

	Middle Eastern		Control		P value
	Yes	No	Yes	No	
Corticosteroids	13	1	9	5	0.16
EEN	9	5	3	11	0.054
Aminosalicylates	10	4	13	1	0.33
Thiopurines	14	0	6	8	0.002*
Methotrexate	5	9	1	13	0.16
Biologicals	1	13	1	13	1.00
Tacrolimus	0	14	1	13	1.00
Surgery	4	10	2	12	0.65

Data compared by Fisher's exact test. *indicates statistical significance.

childhood [15]. The recent rise in incidence in both developed and developing countries has coincided with improvements in hygiene over the twentieth century and the move from a lifestyle of high microbial exposure to low microbial exposure [6, 16]. Australia is a relatively young country with high levels of migration. Previous studies have reported people who emigrate to Western industrialised countries are at higher risk of developing IBD [17]. Similar findings of increased incidence upon migration have been reported in patients of South Asian origin upon emigration to Canada and the UK [9]. Interestingly, 83.3% of the Middle Eastern patients in the current study were born in Australia, adding support to the theory that the 2nd generation of immigrants to industrialised countries is most at risk of developing IBD.

We have presented point incidence and point prevalence; however, there are a number of limitations that must be considered when assessing this data. The cohort was limited to the geographical catchment area of one pediatric centre in Sydney, Australia. Taking into consideration the limitations of this dataset, the small sample size and potential confounders due to immigration, emigration, and referrals outside of the catchment area, the results presented here may have either overestimated or underestimated the incidence of IBD in this population. Ahuja and Tandon [2] suggested studies that relying on the reporting of pediatric hospitals, such as the current study, may lead to an underestimation of incidence and an overestimation of disease severity. The control cohort were matched based on age, gender, and type of disease; therefore, 24 controls were included from 406 non-Middle Eastern patients listed in the IBD database. Several patients listed in the IBD database were excluded from the incidence and prevalence calculations as they came from outside the SCHR catchment area. Although the numbers are likely to be small, it is also possible that several pediatric IBD patients, both Middle Eastern and non-Middle Eastern, from within the catchment area were attending other hospitals or were being treated as private patients and as such were not included in the SCHR database. Therefore, we propose that these initial findings indicate that a further population based cohort study is warranted.

The gender preponderance (higher number of boys) observed among these Middle Eastern children contrasts with studies of the adult IBD population where there are a slightly greater proportion of females with CD [3], although a recent report by El Mouzan et al. [18] of childhood-onset IBD in Saudi Arabia also reports a higher predominance of males with CD at 56%. Nevertheless this pattern of disease distribution (58.3% CD, 29.2% UC, and 12.5% IBD-U) is consistent with recent British, Canadian, and American studies of pediatric CD populations [19–21].

Middle Eastern children with CD had significantly less disease restricted to the colon (L2) than the controls while there were similar levels of terminal ileal disease, ileocolonic disease, and upper gastrointestinal involvement between the groups. In contrast to this, studies in other ethnic populations have found more extensive colonic disease than the general IBD population [9]. However, this is consistent with a low incidence of colonic disease and high incidence of ileocolonic disease that has been observed in a series of Kuwaiti children with IBD [22]. In the current study, excluding upper gastrointestinal involvement (L4), ileocolonic disease (L3) was the most common presentation site affected in Middle Eastern CD patients. Studies estimate that upper gastrointestinal involvement occurs in the range of 30–80% in children and less than 10% of adults with CD [23–26]. In concordance with this, a large proportion of both groups in the current study had upper GI (L4) involvement.

The comparatively high use of thiopurines in the treatment of CD in the Middle Eastern patients is suggestive of a more severe disease requiring immunosuppressive treatment. The efficacy of thiopurines in maintaining clinical remission in CD is well established with trial data supporting the introduction of thiopurines in children with moderately severe disease at diagnosis [27]. Interestingly, in the current study, the severity of disease was not reflected in the duration of symptoms, symptoms at presentation, or surgical management, as there were no differences between the two groups. However the Middle Eastern patients had higher CD activity scores and ESR at diagnosis than the controls. This finding, along with the higher thiopurine use, is suggestive of a more active disease in Middle Eastern children.

The mean age at diagnosis for this cohort of patients was 9.8 years, which was slightly lower than reported in the literature [20]. Family history appears to be one of the most important factors that confer risk for the development of IBD. No difference was established in family history rates between the Middle Eastern (22.7%) and non-Middle Eastern patients (9.1%). Recent publications of pediatric IBD in Saudi Arabia report family history rates of 15.3% [18] and 9.4% [28]. Further, the incidence of a positive family history in the Middle Eastern patients was comparable to that observed in a series of Kuwaiti children [22]. Despite this, there is variability in the family history rates reported which likely reflects the small numbers of patients in these reports. Therefore further investigation is required to determine if Middle Eastern children are at the same or greater risk of IBD than non-Middle Eastern children. Consanguinity data was not available for either the Middle Eastern or non-Middle Eastern cohorts and could not be considered when assessing family history rates.

Altered linear growth is commonly present in children at the time of presentation with IBD [29, 30]. A pediatric study in Kuwait found that growth failure was a significant problem in their patients at presentation [22]. In contrast to this, only 8.3% of the Middle Eastern children and 4.2% of controls had height for age z-scores indicative of stunted growth. This inconsistency may be due to the small sample size or may represent shorter symptom duration prior to diagnosis and therefore less impact upon linear growth. Active IBD may also impact adversely upon pubertal development, especially in boys [31]. Although the pubertal status of the children at diagnosis in the current retrospective study was not available, many of the children were of a prepubertal age. In addition to the limitations provided by a retrospective study design, the sample size of the current study also limited more complete full data interpretation. This was especially evident in analysis of the UC subgroup. The sample size also likely influenced the interpretation of the incidence rates between the two groups: this lack of significance may reflect a type 2 error.

In conclusion, the present study indicated that Middle Eastern patients were less likely to have disease restricted to the colon than the control children. Further the Middle Eastern children had higher CD activity at diagnosis and also required a higher incidence of immunosuppressive treatment. This data is consistent with a more severe phenotype of CD in Middle Eastern children. Although there were limitations with the dataset used to calculate point incidence and prevalence, the calculated values indicated that there is a higher point incidence and prevalence of IBD in Middle Eastern children attending the SCHR. Likely these patterns of disease in an ethnic group now resident in Australia reflect the interactions between environmental and genetic factors. Further epidemiological and genetic investigations of such populations with high incidence of disease are required to better understand the aetiology of pediatric IBD.

Conflict of Interests

The authors have no conflict of interests to declare.

References

[1] M. Cosgrove, R. F. Al-Atia, and H. R. Jenkins, "The epidemiology of paediatric inflammatory bowel disease," *Archives of Disease in Childhood*, vol. 74, no. 3, pp. 460–461, 1996.

[2] V. Ahuja and R. K. Tandon, "Inflammatory bowel disease in the Asia-Pacific area: a comparison with developed countries and regional differences," *Journal of Digestive Diseases*, vol. 11, no. 3, pp. 134–147, 2010.

[3] E. I. Benchimol, K. J. Fortinsky, P. Gozdyra, M. Van Den Heuvel, J. Van Limbergen, and A. M. Griffiths, "Epidemiology of pediatric inflammatory bowel disease: a systematic review of international trends," *Inflammatory Bowel Diseases*, vol. 17, no. 1, pp. 423–439, 2011.

[4] M. I. El Mouzan, A. M. Abdullah, and M. T. Al Habbal, "Epidemiology of juvenile-onset inflammatory bowel disease in Central Saudi Arabia," *Journal of Tropical Pediatrics*, vol. 52, no. 1, pp. 69–71, 2006.

[5] E. I. Benchimol, A. Guttmann, A. M. Griffiths et al., "Increasing incidence of paediatric inflammatory bowel disease in Ontario, Canada: evidence from health administrative data," *Gut*, vol. 58, no. 11, pp. 1490–1497, 2009.

[6] J. A. Walker-Smith, E. Lebenthal, and D. Branski, *Pediatric Inflammatory Bowel Disease: Perspective and Consequences*, Karger, London, UK, 2009.

[7] H. Yang, C. McElree, M.-P. Roth, F. Shanahan, S. R. Targan, and J. I. Rotter, "Familial empirical risks for inflammatory bowel disease: differences between Jews and non-Jews," *Gut*, vol. 34, no. 4, pp. 517–524, 1993.

[8] J. I. Rotter, H. Yang, and T. Shohat, "Genteic complexitites of inflammatory bowel disease and its distribution among the Jewish people," in *Genetic Diversity Among Jews: Disease and Markers at the DNA Level*, pp. 395–411, Oxford University Press, New York, NY, USA, 1992.

[9] V. Pinsk, D. A. Lemberg, K. Grewal, C. C. Barker, R. A. Schreiber, and K. Jacobson, "Inflammatory bowel disease in the South Asian pediatric population of British Columbia," *American Journal of Gastroenterology*, vol. 102, no. 5, pp. 1077–1083, 2007.

[10] I. Carr and J. F. Mayberry, "The effects of migration on ulcerative colitis: a three-year prospective study among Europeans and first- and second-generation South Asians in Leicester (1991–1994)," *American Journal of Gastroenterology*, vol. 94, no. 10, pp. 2918–2922, 1999.

[11] C. S. J. Probert, V. Jayanthi, D. Pinder, A. C. Wicks, and J. F. Mayberry, "Epidemiological study of ulcerative proctocolitis in Indian migrants and the indigenous population of Leicestershire," *Gut*, vol. 33, no. 5, pp. 687–693, 1992.

[12] J. Wilson, C. Hair, R. Knight et al., "High incidence of inflammatory bowel disease in Australia: a prospective population-based Australian incidence study," *Inflammatory Bowel Diseases*, vol. 16, no. 9, pp. 1550–1556, 2010.

[13] N. Phavichitr, D. J. S. Cameron, and A. G. Catto-Smith, "Increasing incidence of Crohn's disease in Victorian children," *Journal of Gastroenterology and Hepatology*, vol. 18, no. 3, pp. 329–332, 2003.

[14] M. S. Silverberg, J. Satsangi, T. Ahmad et al., "Toward an integrated clinical, molecular and serological classification of inflammatory bowel disease: report of a Working Party of the 2005 Montreal World Congress of Gastroenterology," *Canadian Journal of Gastroenterology*, vol. 19, supplement A, pp. 5–36.

[15] S. Danese, M. Sans, and C. Fiocchi, "Inflammatory bowel disease: the role of environmental factors," *Autoimmunity Reviews*, vol. 3, no. 5, pp. 394–400, 2004.

[16] N. A. Koloski, L. Bret, and G. Radford-Smith, "Hygiene hypothesis in inflammatory bowel disease: a critical review of the literature," *World Journal of Gastroenterology*, vol. 14, no. 2, pp. 165–173, 2008.

[17] M. Barreiro-de Acosta, A. Alvarez Castro, R. Souto, M. Iglesias, A. Lorenzo, and J. E. Dominguez-Muñoz, "Emigration to western industrialized countries: a risk factor for developing inflammatory bowel disease," *Journal of Crohn's and Colitis*, vol. 5, no. 6, pp. 566–569, 2011.

[18] M. I. El Mouzan, M. A. Al Mofarreh, A. M. Assiri, Y. H. Hamid, A. M. Al Jebreen, and N. A. Azzam, "Presenting features of childhood-onset inflammatory bowel disease in the central region of Saudi Arabia," *Saudi Medical Journal*, vol. 33, no. 4, pp. 423–428, 2012.

[19] C. N. Bernstein, J. F. Blanchard, P. Rawsthorne, and A. Wajda, "Epidemiology of Crohn's disease and ulcerative colitis in a central Canadian province: a population-based study," *American Journal of Epidemiology*, vol. 149, no. 10, pp. 916–924, 1999.

[20] S. Kugathasan, R. H. Judd, R. G. Hoffmann et al., "Epidemiologic and clinical characteristics of children with newly diagnosed inflammatory bowel disease in Wisconsin: a statewide population-based study," *Journal of Pediatrics*, vol. 143, no. 4, pp. 525–531, 2003.

[21] A. Sawczenko, B. K. Sandhu, R. F. A. Logan et al., "Prospective survey of childhood inflammatory bowel disease in the British Isles," *The Lancet*, vol. 357, no. 9262, pp. 1093–1094, 2001.

[22] W. Al-Qabandi, E. Buhamrah, K. Hamadi, S. Al-Osaimi, A. Al-Ruwayeh, and J. Madda, "Inflammatory bowel disease in children, an evolving problem in Kuwait," *Saudi Journal of Gastroenterology*, vol. 17, no. 5, pp. 323–327, 2011.

[23] D. A. Lemberg, C. M. Clarkson, T. D. Bohane, and A. S. Day, "Role of esophagogastroduodenoscopy in the initial assessment of children with inflammatory bowel disease," *Journal of Gastroenterology and Hepatology*, vol. 20, no. 11, pp. 1696–1700, 2005.

[24] T. Ruuska, P. Vaajalahti, P. Arajarvi, and M. Maki, "Prospective evaluation of upper gastrointestinal mucosal lesions in children with ulcerative colitis and Crohn's disease," *Journal of Pediatric Gastroenterology and Nutrition*, vol. 19, no. 2, pp. 181–186, 1994.

[25] E. Schmidt-Sommerfeld, B. S. Kirschner, and J. K. Stephens, "Endoscopic and histologic findings in the upper gastrointestinal tract of children with Crohn's disease," *Journal of Pediatric Gastroenterology and Nutrition*, vol. 11, no. 4, pp. 448–454, 1990.

[26] J. Van Limbergen, R. K. Russell, H. E. Drummond et al., "Definition of phenotypic characteristics of childhood-onset inflammatory bowel disease," *Gastroenterology*, vol. 135, no. 4, pp. 1114–1122, 2008.

[27] J. Markowitz, K. Grancher, N. Kohn, M. Lesser, and F. Daum, "A multicenter trial of 6-mercaptopurine and prednisone in children with newly diagnosed Crohn's disease," *Gastroenterology*, vol. 119, no. 4, pp. 895–902, 2000.

[28] O. I. Saadah, "Childhood onset of Crohn disease: experience from a university teaching hospital in Saudi Arabia," *Annals of Saudi Medicine*, vol. 32, no. 6, pp. 596–602, 2012.

[29] R. Heuschkel, C. Salvestrini, R. M. Beattie, H. Hildebrand, T. Walters, and A. Griffiths, "Guidelines for the management of growth failure in childhood inflammatory bowel disease," *Inflammatory Bowel Diseases*, vol. 14, no. 6, pp. 839–849, 2008.

[30] A. Levine, A. Griffiths, J. Markowitz et al., "Pediatric modification of the Montreal classification for inflammatory bowel
disease: the Paris classification," *Inflammatory Bowel Diseases*,
vol. 17, no. 6, pp. 1314–1321, 2011.

[31] A. B. Ballinger, M. O. Savage, and I. R. Sanderson, "Delayed
puberty associated with inflammatory bowel disease," *Pediatric
Research*, vol. 53, no. 2, pp. 205–210, 2003.

37

Prevalence of Dental Caries in relation to Body Mass Index, Daily Sugar Intake, and Oral Hygiene Status in 12-Year-Old School Children in Mathura City: A Pilot Study

Prahlad Gupta,[1] **Nidhi Gupta,**[2] **and Harkanwal Preet Singh**[3]

[1] *Department of Public Health Dentistry, Dasmesh Institute of Research and Dental Sciences, Faridkot, Punjab 151203, India*
[2] *Department of Prosthodontics, Dasmesh Institute of Research and Dental Sciences, Faridkot, Punjab 151203, India*
[3] *Department of Oral Pathology and Microbiology, Dasmesh Institute of Research and Dental Sciences, Faridkot, Punjab 151203, India*

Correspondence should be addressed to Harkanwal Preet Singh; hkps0320@gmail.com

Academic Editor: Alessandro Mussa

Aim. To correlate the prevalence of dental caries to body mass index, daily sugar intake, and oral hygiene status of 12-year-old school children of Mathura city. *Material and Methods.* The study design was cross-sectional and included 100 school children aged 12 years (n = 50 boys and n = 50 girls) who were randomly selected from two schools based upon inclusion and exclusion criteria. Body weight/height was recorded and BMI was calculated and plotted on CDC-BMI for age growth charts/curves for boys and girls to obtain percentile ranking. Dental caries was recorded using WHO criteria. Oral hygiene status of the study subjects was assessed using oral hygiene index-simplified. Data regarding the daily sugar intake was recorded using 24-hour recall diet frequency chart. The data obtained was analysed using SPSS version 11.5 for windows. *Result.* Only 27 subjects were affected by caries. The mean DMFT/dmft was 0.37 ± 0.79 and 0.12 ± 0.60, respectively. Statistical analysis by means of a logistic regression model revealed that only oral hygiene status had a significant effect on caries prevalence (OR = 5.061, P = 0.004), whereas daily sugar intake and body mass index had no significant effect. *Conclusion.* From the analysis, it was concluded that oral hygiene status had a significant effect on caries prevalence of 12-year-old school children of Mathura city.

1. Introduction

Dental Caries is a chronic disease which can affect us at any age. If untreated, it can lead to pain and discomfort and finally loss of teeth. Caries is one of the most common diseases of childhood. The disease is not self-limiting and without adequate intervention, the process can continue until the tooth is destroyed. The term "caries" denotes both the disease process and its consequences, that is, the damage caused by the disease process [1]. The World Health Organization's report on oral health in 2003 and Global Oral Data Bank of WHO confirm the international distribution of dental caries and stated that by the age of 12 only 15 to 30% of the population were caries-free with a global DMFT of 1.74 [2–4]. The global distribution of dental caries presents a varied picture; countries with low caries prevalence are experiencing an unprecedented increase in caries prevalence and severity of dental caries. On the other hand, in developed countries a reduction of dental caries incidence and improvement of gingival health care are evident. This decline in dental caries was mainly due to appropriate use of fluorides and preventive oral health care measures. The scenario in India is not different from developing countries [5].

Dental caries has a multifactorial aetiology in which there is interplay of three principal factors: the host (saliva and teeth), the microflora (plaque), and the substrate (diet) and a fourth factor: time. There is no single test that takes into consideration all these factors and can accurately predict an individual's susceptibility to caries. The risk of dental caries can be evaluated by analysing and integrating several causative factors such as fluoride, microbial plaque, diet, bacterial and salivary activity, and social and life style related behavioural factors [1].

Excessive body weight in children is a major public health problem. According to National Family Health Survey (NFHS), obesity has reached epidemic proportions in India, affecting 5% of the country's population. India is following a trend of other developing countries that are steadily becoming more obese [6, 7]. Obesity status in children is measured by assessment of body mass index (BMI) corresponding to gender and age [6]. Consumption of soft drinks and fast foods together with less activity and exercise contributed to the increasing number of overweight people worldwide [8]. High sugar intake, for example, sugar containing snacks and soft drinks, is reported to be more common among overweight and obese children/adolescents than those with normal weight. Frequent sugar intake is also a recognized risk factor for dental caries. Thus, the eating pattern among overweight or obese children may be a common risk factor in overweight children and dental caries [9]. Given that the strong evidence supporting the relation between dental caries with indiscriminate dietary intake has been linked to the development of obesity at a young age, a link between dental caries and weight is biologically possible [6]. The role of sugar (and other fermentable carbohydrates such as highly refined flour) as a risk factor in the initiation and progression of dental caries is overwhelming. Sugar acts as a favoured substrate for the cariogenic bacteria that reside in dental plaque, particularly the mutans streptococci, and the acid byproducts of this metabolic process induce demineralization of the enamel surface. Whether this initial demineralization proceeds to clinically detectable caries or whether the lesion is remineralized by plaque minerals depends on a number of factors, of which the amount and frequency of further sugars consumption are of utmost importance [10]. Another risk factor for development of caries is the existence of bacterial plaque on the teeth. Caries can be reduced by mechanical removal of plaque from tooth surfaces; however, most children do not remove it effectively which means the deficiency of maintenance of good oral hygiene. Several studies have shown that, in countries where proper oral hygiene is followed, caries prevalence has decreased despite increases in sugar consumption, thus marking the importance of oral hygiene in caries etiology [11, 12].

Dental caries is a multifactorial disorder and it is difficult to assess all the associated risk factors simultaneously. There have been no studies documented in literature in this part of India assessing the prevalence of dental caries in relation to body mass index, daily sugar intake, and oral hygiene. So an attempt was made to assess the prevalence of dental caries in relation to body mass index, daily sugar intake, and oral hygiene status in 12-year-old school children in Mathura city. Cross-sectional study was designed to evaluate the daily sugar intake, oral hygiene status, and body mass index and to correlate each of them with the prevalence of dental caries among 12-year-old school children in Mathura city.

2. Material and Method

Ethical permission from institutions ethical committee was taken before the commencement of study. Consent from subjects, parents, and school was also taken.

Sample size was determined by the formula based on the study population:

$$n = \frac{4pqn}{e^2(N-1) + 4pq}, \qquad (1)$$

where p = prevalence 27% (prevalence of dental caries obtained from previous study), $q = (1 - p) = 100 - 27 = 73$, e = permissible error in estimation of prevalence 10%, N = study population 5000 (Department of Education Mathura), and n = sample size.

The estimated sample size for the study based on the prevalence of the dental caries came out to be 860.10% of sample size; that is, 86 was included in pilot study, but to avoid any error slightly higher sample of 100 was taken for study.

This study was planned to be conducted in high schools of Mathura city in 12-year-old children. There are 141 primary schools and 37 high schools as per the record in the District Education Departments of Mathura. Out of 37 high schools, 16 are government aided and the rest are all private institutions. Government institutions had children with similar socioeconomic and cultural background. Children do not have any specific habit such as tobacco chewing and smoking, but they were very fond of having sugar candies.

Level of fluoride ion concentration in drinking water in Mathura city is in optimum range and subjects maintained their oral hygiene by using fluoridated toothpaste.

Out of 16 government aided high schools, 2 schools were randomly selected to obtain the sample size of 100 study subjects having similar socioeconomic and cultural background. Subjects who were willing to participate, have completed 12 years of age, and were continuously residing in Mathura city right from their birth were included in the study whereas subjects who were suffering from any acute or chronic diseases and were under medication, were below 12 years of age and above 13 years of age, and did not obtain parental consent were excluded from the study. A proforma was used for collection of data in the study.

2.1. Anthropometric Measurements. Body weight of study subjects was measured using standardized digital weighing machine. The fractional weight below 500 grams and above 500 grams was rounded to the nearest whole number. Height of study subjects was measured using a measuring tape and recorded in meters. Measurement of weight and height was taken without shoes and with their school dress. From the above data, BMI was calculated and plotted on CDC-BMI for age growth charts/curves for boys and girls to obtain a percentile ranking and subjects were categorized as follows [13].

Underweight: less than 5th percentile.

Healthy weight: 5th percentile to less than 85th percentile.

At risk of overweight: 85th to less than the 95th percentile.

Overweight: equal to or greater than the 95th percentile.

TABLE 1

Form	Frequency	Points
Liquid: soft drinks, fruit drinks, cocoa, sugar and honey in beverages, nondairy creamers, ice cream, sherbet, gelatine desert, flavoured yoghurt, pudding, custard, popsicles	— × 5 =	
Solid and sticky: cake, cupcakes, donuts, sweet rolls, pastry, canned fruit in syrup, bananas, cookies, chocolate candy, caramel, toffee, jelly beans, other chewy candies, chewing gum, dried fruit, marshmallows, jelly, jam	— × 10 =	
Slowly dissolving: hard candies, breath mints, antacid tablets, cough drops	— × 15 =	
Total sweet score: —		
Interpretation sweet score: 5 or less: excellent 10: good 15 or more: "watch out" zone		

Total sweet score: —

Interpretation sweet score: 5 or less: excellent; 10: good; and 15 or more: "watch out" zone.

2.2. Dental Caries. Dental caries status was collected using Dentition Status of WHO criteria mentioned in Basic Oral Health Survey Methodology (1997) [14] and from the above data DMFT/dmft was calculated.

2.3. Oral Hygiene Status. Oral hygiene of study subjects was determined using oral hygiene index-simplified (OHI-S) by Greene and Vermilion [15]. This index is based upon two parameters: Debris and Calculus and it has been validated by other authors in 12-year-old children of different geographic region.

2.4. Daily Sugar Intake. Data regarding the daily sugar intake was recorded using 24-hour recall diet frequency chart and the subjects were grouped into excellent, good, and watch out zone based upon sugar sweet score (see Table 1) [16].

All examinations and data collection were done by a single examiner and proforma was filled by a recording assistant after standardization. The examination of study subjects was carried out in their school premises using natural light, ordinary chair, plain mouth mirror and CPI probe for dental caries, and explorer no. 5 (Shepard's hook) for OHI-S. Presterilized armamentarium was used to carry out the examinations.

2.5. Statistical Analysis. The data obtained was analysed using SPSS version 11.5 for windows. Mean and standard deviations were calculated for each clinical parameter. Differences between means were tested with one-way ANOVA followed by post hoc tukey's test. Independent effects of BMI, oral hygiene status, and daily sugar intake on caries prevalence were tested using linear multiple regression analysis. Significance for all statistical tests was predetermined at a probability (P) value of 0.05 or less.

3. Results

An epidemiological survey conducted showed that the study population consisted of 100 school children, out of which 50

TABLE 2: Distribution of various characteristics of study population.

Sociodemographic characteristics	Study subjects ($n = 100$)	
	Male ($n = 50$)	Female ($n = 50$)
Diet		
Vegetarian	41 (82%)	44 (88%)
Mixed	9 (18%)	6 (12%)
Oral hygiene means		
Toothbrush with toothpaste	45 (90%)	50 (100%)
Toothbrush with toothpowder	4 (8%)	0 (0%)
Indigenous (chewing stick)	1 (2%)	0 (0%)
Oral hygiene frequency		
Once	38 (76%)	31 (62%)
Twice	12 (24%)	19 (38%)
Body mass index categories		
Underweight**	4 (8%)	23 (46%)
Healthy weight**	40 (80%)	24 (48%)
At risk of overweight	5 (10%)	3 (6%)
Overweight**	1 (2%)	0 (0%)
Daily sugar intake		
Excellent	8 (16%)	3 (6%)
Good	12 (24%)	17 (34%)
Watch out	30 (60%)	30 (60%)
Oral hygiene status		
Good*	12 (24%)	19 (38%)
Fair	34 (68%)	31 (62%)
Poor*	4 (8%)	0 (%)

**represents that values obtained are highly statistically significant ($P < 0.001$).

*represents that values obtained are statistically significant ($P < 0.05$).

(50%) were males and 50 (50%) were females. Table 2 shows sex-wise distribution of various characteristics of study population collected by survey. One-way ANOVA was applied

TABLE 3: Multiple linear regression analysis of oral hygiene status, body mass index, and daily sugar intake on caries prevalence in 12-year-old school children.

Independent variables	Dependent variable (caries affected at 12 years of age)				
	Odd ratio	95% CI		SE	P value
		Lower	Upper		
Body mass index	0.742	0.365	1.511	0.363	0.411
Daily sugar intake	1.214	0.613	2.407	0.349	0.578
Oral hygiene status	5.061	1.669	15.347	0.566	**0.004**

to determine the association between mean DMFT and BMI categories of study population (underweight, health weight, at risk of overweight and overweight) but no significant association was found ($F = 1.145$, $P = 0.335$, N.S.) but when it was applied to determine the association between mean dmft and BMI Categories of study population (underweight, health weight, at risk of overweight and overweight), significant association was found ($F = 7.783$, $P = 0.000$, S). Similarly, one-way ANOVA was applied to determine the association between mean DMFT/dmft and daily sugar intake categories of study population (excellent, good, and watch out); no significant associations were found ($F = 1.348$, $P = 0.265$, N.S., and $F = 0.489$, $P = 0.615$, N.S.), respectively. When one-way ANOVA was applied to determine the association between mean DMFT/dmft and oral hygiene status of study population (good, fair, and poor), no significant associations were found ($F = 2.563$, $P = 0.082$, N.S., and $F = 1.051$, $P = 0.354$, N.S.). Multiple linear regression analysis was done to determine the independent effects of BMI, oral hygiene status, and daily sugar intake on caries prevalence. It was found that oral hygiene status had a significant effect on caries prevalence (OR = 5.061, $P = 0.004$, S). However, body mass index and daily sugar intake had no significant effect on caries prevalence (Table 3).

4. Discussion

The main objective of the present study was to determine the prevalence of dental caries in relation to body mass index, daily sugar intake, and oral hygiene status of 12-year-old school children of the Mathura city. Our study found a low caries prevalence (27%) with a mean DMFT of 0.37 and mean dmft of 0.12, respectively, when compared with the global DMFT for 12-year-olds [4]. Similar results were obtained in a study by David et al. (2005) [17] who reported 27% prevalence of dental caries with a mean DMFT of 0.5. Our study found no statistically significant association between DMFT and BMI ($F = 1.145$, $P = 0.335$, N.S.). Similarly, Tramini et al. [18] found no significant association between DMFT and BMI. This finding is consistent with the results from the prospective study by Pinto et al. [6], where no correlation between dental decay and BMI was detected in a multiple regression analysis. Kopycka-Kedzierawski et al. [9] even found an inverse association between BMI and caries experience: overweight children were less likely to have caries experience than normal weight children aged 6–11 years.

After having performed a systematic review of obesity and dental caries, Kantovitz et al. [19] concluded that only one study with high level of evidence showed direct association between obesity and dental caries.

Recent systematic review and meta-analysis conducted by Hayedn et al. [20] showed that, overall, there was a significant relationship between childhood obesity and dental caries. However, this relationship was not significant for newly industrialized countries similar to present study conducted in Mathura, India [20]. This might be attributed to the fact that both obesity and dental caries are multifactorial in aetiology and various genetic and environmental factors have an impact on them. Another risk factor common to both obesity and dental caries is high sugar intake. Ludwig et al. [21], in a longitudinal study, found that the increasing prevalence of obesity in children was linked to the consumption of sugar-sweetened drinks. However, our study found no significant association between dental caries (DMFT/dmft) and daily sugar intake. Even with increased consumption or high intake of sugar there was decrease in dental caries. This might be attributed to the widespread exposure to fluoride not only through drinking water but also through toothpaste, professional applications, and through fluoride's presence in processed foods and drinks [11]. This result is consistent with the findings of systematic review by Burt and Pai [11] which concluded that the relationship between sugar consumption is much weaker in modern age of fluoride exposure. Another study by Loveren [22] concluded that if good oral hygiene is maintained and fluoride is supplied frequently, teeth will remain intact even if the carbohydrate-containing food is frequently eaten. Local oral factors such as retention around the teeth and salivary functions may be factors strongly modifying caries activity [22]. Oral hygiene is a basic factor for oral health. Poor oral hygiene leads to accumulation of dental plaque which has an important role in the aetiology of dental caries [23]. The overall oral hygiene status among study population was recorded as fair in 65% and good in 31% and only 4% of the study population showed poor oral hygiene status. There was significant difference between oral hygiene status of males and females ($P = 0.037$). The OHI-S and its components showed a high mean value for males as compared to females. The probable reason for lower mean scores of OHI-S and its components in females was perhaps the increased grooming habits of girls in this age group. These findings are in accordance with the study by Sogi and Bhaskar [24]. Even though oral hygiene status of majority of the study population was between fair and good, 27% of the study subjects were affected by caries in the present study but no statistically significant difference was seen between DMFT/dmft and oral hygiene status (DMFT, $P = 0.082$; dmft, $P = 0.354$). However, multiple linear regression analysis found that oral hygiene status had a significant effect on caries prevalence (OR = 5.061, $P = 0.004$, S).

5. Conclusion

Oral hygiene status had an intricate relationship with caries prevalence whereas body mass index and daily sugar intake did not reveal any significant association in 12-year-old school children of Mathura city. The relationship between dental caries and obesity should be further explored by longitudinal studies as they both have common risk determinants.

Conflict of Interests

The authors declare that there is no conflict of interests regarding the publication of this paper.

References

[1] E. Reich, A. Lussi, and E. Newbrun, "Caries-risk assessment," *International Dental Journal*, vol. 49, no. 1, pp. 15–26, 1999.

[2] B. L. Edelstein, "The dental caries pandemic and disparities problem," *BMC Oral Health*, vol. 6, no. 1, article no. S2, 2006.

[3] P. C. Baehni and B. Guggenheim, "Potential of diagnostic microbiology for treatment and prognosis of dental caries and periodontal diseases," *Critical Reviews in Oral Biology and Medicine*, vol. 7, no. 3, pp. 259–277, 1996.

[4] Caries for 12-Year-Olds by Country/Area, 2010, http://www.whocollab.od.mah.se/countriesalphab.html.

[5] J. K. Dash, P. K. Sahoo, S. K. Bhuyan, and S. K. Sahoo, "Prevalence of dental caries and treatment needs among children of Cuttack (Orissa)," *Journal of the Indian Society of Pedodontics and Preventive Dentistry*, vol. 20, no. 4, pp. 139–143, 2002.

[6] A. Pinto, S. Kim, R. Wadenya, and H. Rosenberg, "Is there an association between weight and dental caries among pediatric patients in an urban dental school? A correlation study," *Journal of Dental Education*, vol. 71, no. 11, pp. 1435–1440, 2007.

[7] Obesity in India, 2010, http://en.wikipedia.org/wiki//Obesity_in_India.

[8] M. Sadeghi and F. Alizadeh, "Association between dental caries and body mass index-for-age among 6-11-year-old children in Isfahan in 2007," *Journal of Dental Research, Dental Clinics, Dental Prospects*, vol. 1, no. 3, pp. 119–124, 2007.

[9] D. T. Kopycka-Kedzierawski, P. Auinger, R. J. Billings, and M. Weitzman, "Caries status and overweight in 2- to 18-year-old US children: Findings from national surveys," *Community Dentistry and Oral Epidemiology*, vol. 36, no. 2, pp. 157–167, 2008.

[10] E. W. Gerdin, M. Angbratt, K. Aronsson, E. Eriksson, and I. Johansson, "Dental caries and body mass index by socioeconomic status in Swedish children," *Community Dentistry and Oral Epidemiology*, vol. 36, no. 5, pp. 459–465, 2008.

[11] B. A. Burt and S. Pai, "Sugar consumption and caries risk: a systematic review," *Journal of dental education*, vol. 65, no. 10, pp. 1017–1023, 2001.

[12] S. Petti, G. Tarsitani, P. Panfili, and A. S. D'Arca, "Oral hygiene, sucrose consumption and dental caries prevalence in adolescent systemic fluoride non-users," *Community Dentistry and Oral Epidemiology*, vol. 25, no. 4, pp. 334–336, 1997.

[13] R. J. Kuczmarski, C. L. Ogden, S. S. Guo et al., "2000 CDC Growth Charts for the United States: methods and development," *National Center for Health Statistics*, vol. 11, no. 246, pp. 1–201, 2002.

[14] World Health Organization, *Oral Health Surveys—Basic Methods*, WHO, Geneva, Switzerland, 4 edition, 1997.

[15] J. C. Greene and J. R. Vermillion, "The simplified oral hygiene index," *Journal of the American Dental Association*, vol. 68, pp. 7–13, 1964.

[16] M. L. Darby and M. M. Walsh, "Nutritional counseling," in *Dental Hygiene Theory and Practice*, pp. 567–568, Saunders, 2nd edition, 2003.

[17] J. David, N. J. Wang, A. N. Åstrøm, and S. Kuriakose, "Dental caries and associated factors in 12-year-old schoolchildren in Thiruvananthapuram, Kerala, India," *International Journal of Paediatric Dentistry*, vol. 15, no. 6, pp. 420–428, 2005.

[18] P. Tramini, N. Molinari, M. Tentscher, C. Demattei, and A. G. Schulte, "Association between caries experience and body mass index in 12-year-old French children," *Caries Research*, vol. 43, no. 6, pp. 468–473, 2009.

[19] K. R. Kantovitz, F. M. Pascon, R. M. P. Rontani, and M. B. D. Gavião, "Obesity and dental caries—a systematic review," *Oral Health & Preventive Dentistry*, vol. 4, no. 2, pp. 137–144, 2006.

[20] C. Hayedn, J. O. Bowler, S. Chambers et al., "Obesity and Dental caries in children: a systematic review and meta-analysis," *Community Dentistry and Oral Epidemiology*, vol. 41, no. 4, pp. 289–308, 2013.

[21] D. S. Ludwig, K. E. Peterson, and S. L. Gortmaker, "Relation between consumption of sugar-sweetened drinks and childhood obesity: a prospective, observational analysis," *The Lancet*, vol. 357, no. 9255, pp. 505–508, 2001.

[22] C. Loveren, "Diet and dental caries: cariogenicity may depend more on oral hygiene using fluorides than on diet or type of carbohydrates," *European Journal of Paediatric Dentistry*, vol. 1, pp. 55–62, 2000.

[23] Oral Hygiene Indices. Introduction, 2010, http://www.whocollab.od.mah.se/expl/ohiintrod.html.

[24] G. Sogi and D. J. Bhaskar, "Dental caries and oral hygiene status of 13-14 year old school children of Davangere," *Journal of the Indian Society of Pedodontics and Preventive Dentistry*, vol. 19, no. 3, pp. 113–117, 2001.

38

Peristeen© Transanal Irrigation System for Paediatric Faecal Incontinence: A Single Centre Experience

Omar Nasher, Richard E. Hill, Riyad Peeraully, Ali Wright, and Shailinder J. Singh

Department of Paediatric Surgery, Queen's Medical Centre, Nottingham University Hospital NHS Trust, Derby Road, Nottingham NG7 2UH, UK

Correspondence should be addressed to Omar Nasher; omar.nasher@nhs.net

Academic Editor: Joseph M. Croffie

Aim. To evaluate the efficacy of the Peristeen© transanal irrigation system when treating faecal incontinence in children due to chronic idiopathic constipation. *Methods.* A retrospective study was conducted of the first cohort of patients affected with faecal incontinence and referred to our centre for Peristeen© transanal irrigation treatment between January 2010 and December 2012. Patients with neurogenic bowel disturbance were excluded. A previously described and validated faecal continence scoring system was used to assess bowel function and social problems before and after treatment with Peristeen©. *Results.* 13 patients were referred for Peristeen© transanal irrigation during the study period. Mean time of using Peristeen© was 12.6 months ($\pm$0.6 months) and mean length of follow-up was 21.2 months ($\pm$0.9 months). All patients were noted to have an improvement in their faecal continence score, with a mean improvement from 9.7 ± 1.4 to 14.8 ± 2.7 ($P = 0.0008$) and a reduction in episodes of soiling and increasing in quality of life scores. *Conclusion.* In this initial study, Peristeen© appears to be a safe and effective bowel management system, which improves bowel function and quality of life in children affected with faecal incontinence as a result of chronic idiopathic constipation, Hirschsprung's disease, and anorectal malformations.

1. Introduction

Childhood constipation is a common problem worldwide with an estimated median prevalence in the general population of 8.9% [1]. It can present as difficulty passing stools associated with abdominal pain and infrequent passage of stools and may progress to faecal incontinence due to retention with overflow [2]. In 90% of children, no specific organic cause is found [3] and they are eventually diagnosed with chronic idiopathic constipation (CIC). Faecal incontinence may also occur after definitive surgery for congenital problems such as Hirschsprung's disease (HD) and anorectal malformations (ARM). Chronic constipation can also occur secondary to neuropathic bowel dysfunction due to spina bifida or traumatic spinal cord injuries. CIC has a considerable effect on a patient's psychological and emotional well-being and as such has a substantial impact on patient quality of life [4, 5]. Patients will often have long-term laxative regimes and may require suppositories, behavioural therapy, and sometimes surgical procedures such as manual evacuations,

rectal biopsies, and the Malone antegrade continence enema [6]. The Peristeen© transanal irrigation system involves water irrigation of the large intestine through a disposable balloon catheter and has been successfully employed in the treatment of faecal incontinence in patients with neuropathic bowel dysfunction secondary to spinal cord injuries [7–9]. There is no published literature on its use in treatment of faecal incontinence in children due to CIC, HD, or ARM excluding neuropathic bowel patients. We report the effective use of the Peristeen© transanal irrigation system for faecal incontinence secondary to CIC, HD, and ARM.

2. Methods

A retrospective follow-up study was conducted on the first cohort of patients affected with faecal incontinence and referred to our centre for Peristeen© transanal irrigation treatment between January 2010 and December 2012. Peristeen© was offered to all patients who were seeing no improvements on conventional medical therapy, since it became available in our unit in January 2010. Both surgical and nonsurgical management options were explained to parents and patients in depth and those who selected Peristeen© transanal irrigation treatment were enrolled in the study. These patients would have previously been offered surgery in the form of an antegrade continence enema (ACE) prior to the availability of Peristeen©. The main factor influencing the choice of transanal irrigation was the age and maturity of the patient. In particular, children had to be able to understand and cooperate with the procedure in order to achieve successful results. Patients with constipation due to neuropathic bowel dysfunction (e.g., spinal cord injuries or spina bifida) were excluded from the study. The faecal continence scoring system (Table 1) used previously and validated by Rintala and Lindahl [10] was used to assess bowel function and social issues before and after treatment with Peristeen©. The mean and standard deviation were used to analyse descriptive data and a t-test was used to analyse the difference in faecal continence scores before and after Peristeen©.

Patients and their parents were taught how to use the Peristeen© device during a trial admission onto our surgical ward by our paediatric gastroenterology nurse specialist (AW). We recommended using Peristeen© as described in the guidelines published by the manufacturing company Coloplast [11]. The families were then supported at home by the local paediatric community nurse who had been educated in the transanal irrigation system. The device was easily accessible to patients, as it is provided by the UK National Health Service on a free of charge prescription. If patients were unhappy with the procedure, they did not have to continue with it. The Peristeen© system consists of a control unit with a pump, a water bag, and a rectal catheter. Tap water is warmed (36–38°C) and introduced into the colon via the rectal catheter. Once the rectal catheter has been inserted, an inflatable balloon ensures that it remains in situ until the balloon is deflated. The water, along with the stools in the lower portion of the bowel, is then emptied into the toilet [11].

3. Results

A total of 13 patients were referred for Peristeen© during the study period, 3 of which were excluded from the study as they suffered discomfort whilst passing the rectal catheter or simply did not like passing the catheter and decided not to continue with Peristeen©. Two of these had been referred to the psychology service because they refused to take oral medications and the third patient was still continuing on maximal medical therapy, as the parents did not want surgery. The remaining 10 patients (7 males) who underwent Peristeen© transanal irrigation had underlying diagnoses of CIC in 7, HD in 2, and ARM in 1 (Table 2) and had a mean age of 11.1 ± 2.7 years (age range 10–18 years).

The presenting clinical features were abdominal discomfort, constipation, and faecal soiling in all patients. Previously attempted treatment methods included oral laxatives (both

TABLE 1: Faecal continence scoring system (Rintala and lindahl, 1995, [10]).

Ability to hold back defecation	
Always	3
Problems less than 1/week	2
Weekly problems	1
No voluntary control	0
Feels/reports the urge to defecate	
Always	3
Most of the time	2
Uncertain	1
Absent	0
Frequency of defecation	
Every other day to twice a day	2
More often	1
Less often	1
Soiling	
Never	3
Staining less than 1/week, no change of underwear required	2
Frequent staining, change of underwear often required	1
Daily soiling requires protective aids	0
Accidents	
Never	3
Fewer than 1/week	2
Weekly accidents often require protective aids	1
Daily accidents require protective aids during day and night	0
Constipation	
No constipation	3
Manageable with diet	2
Manageable with laxatives	1
Manageable with enemas	0
Social problems	
No social problems	3
Sometimes (foul odors)	2
Problems causing restrictions in social life	1
Severe social and/or psychic problems	0

TABLE 2: Patient data.

Primary diagnosis	Male	Female
Chronic idiopathic constipation (CIC)	4	3
Anorectal malformations (ARM)	1	
Hirschsprung's disease (HD)	2	
Total	7	3

osmotic and stimulant) and per rectum sodium phosphate enemas as per NICE guidelines [6], but these did not result in successful management. In addition, 3 patients required anorectal myectomy, manual evacuation, and intrasphincteric injection of Botulinum toxin.

The mean time of Peristeen© use was 12.6 months (± 0.6 months) and these patients were followed up for a mean length of 21.2 months (±0.9 months). In each patient, a symptomatic improvement was noted and measured using

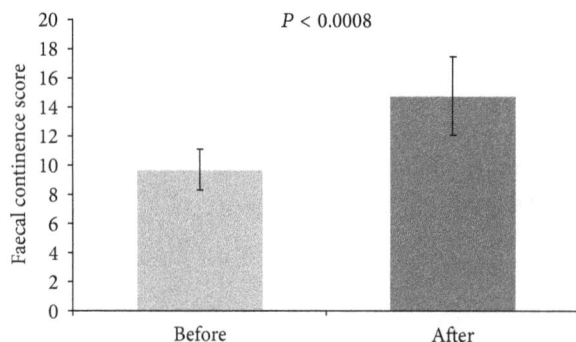

FIGURE 1: Faecal continence score before and after Peristeen© treatment.

the faecal continence scoring system [10]. Prior to Peristeen© treatment, the mean score was 9.7 ± 1.4, whereas after transanal irrigation the mean score was significantly higher at 14.8 ± 2.7 ($P < 0.0008$) (Figure 1). In addition, there was a particular improvement in the frequency of soiling scores and the restrictions in social life scores with 90% having improvement in their "social problems" or quality of life score and 60% achieving a normal score with no social problems following Peristeen© treatment. No treatment complications were recorded during the follow-up period and none of these patients needed the ACE procedure.

4. Discussion

We have demonstrated, albeit in a small study, that Peristeen© is a safe and effective bowel management system for children with chronic idiopathic constipation not caused by neuropathic bowel disturbance. We have shown a statistically significant improvement in faecal continence score after using the Peristeen© system and none of the patients who tolerated the transanal irrigation system required a further surgical procedure such as an ACE. A number of studies have looked at Peristeen© use in patients with neuropathic bowel and demonstrated the benefits of this system [7–9, 12] but we believe this is the first study to exclude neuropathic bowel patients and demonstrate an improvement in faecal continence scores in patients with CIC, HD, and ARMs.

Transanal irrigation has been known since 1500 BC and was initially used in attempts to detoxify the bowel and prevent ileus. In 1987, Shandling and Gilmour demonstrated that faecal continence could be achieved by using enema continence catheters in children with spina bifida affected with faecal incontinence [13]. More recently, the Peristeen© system has been shown to be effective in the treatment of faecal incontinence in paediatric as well as adult patients with neuropathic bowel dysfunction due to spinal cord injury and spina bifida [7]. In this randomised, controlled, multicenter trial of transanal irrigation versus conservative treatment in spinal-cord-injured patients with neurogenic bowel dysfunction, transanal irrigation improved constipation and faecal

incontinence and also ameliorated the quality of life of those patients [7]. In another study of 16 patients with bowel dysfunction secondary to myelomeningocele, transanal irrigation was evaluated by monitoring the intestinal emptying time through radiological imaging. Transanal irrigation was once again proven to be safe and effective and demonstrated to work by increasing intestinal emptying and increasing the progression of the intestinal bolus through the colon [14]. A recent study by Corbett et al. looked at quality of life scores in patients after using the Peristeen© system and demonstrated that 20 out of 21 had improved quality of life scores [12]. Their study group included patients with myelomeningocele, which our study excluded, and interestingly their median age was 6 years, which is younger than our mean age of 11.1 years. Our mean age is more similar to that reported in other studies demonstrating benefits of Peristeen© in children with neuropathic bladders: 8.4 years [9] and 12.5 years [8]. We believe that the Peristeen© is tolerated well by the older patients who are able to understand why they are performing an uncomfortable procedure and tend to be more dedicated and motivated to the task.

There are various qualitative faecal continence scoring systems and quality of life scores, which have been published in the literature. We chose the score developed by Rintala and Lindahl [10], because it had been used and validated in surgical patients. Validated, quantitative scoring systems such as the one used in this study enable a more reliable and accurate statistical analysis [15].

Malone antegrade continence enema procedure is an established surgical treatment option for children with constipation or faecal incontinence [16]. However, it is necessary for the child to undergo a general anaesthetic both to perform the procedure and to close the ACE stoma when it is eventually no longer required. In addition to potential effects on body image, there are well-recognised complications associated with the ACE procedure, with stomal problems including stenosis, leak, and granulation occurring in up to 30% of children [17]. In contrast, no surgical intervention is required for the use of Peristeen© and the only complication we have witnessed is the potential to cause a mild degree of discomfort. It is documented, however, that irrigation through rectal catheters has a less than 1 in 100,000 chances of causing rectal perforation [18] and we include this information when we have our initial discussions with patients and carers about the Peristeen© system. It is reasonable to suggest that the response to management using this retrograde irrigation method would also provide evidence of whether the antegrade management of an ACE is likely to be effective; however, as none of our patients who used Peristeen© needed a further surgical procedure, we cannot confirm this. It is certainly true that, in order for the system to work, it requires dedicated patient and carers.

We believe that this is the first study to assess the response to Peristeen© transanal irrigation in children with faecal incontinence secondary to CIC, HD, or ARM excluding those with neuropathic bowels. The positive results obtained from this small study are encouraging and point to the need for a larger trial, which we are currently planning.

Conflict of Interests

The authors declare that there is no conflict of interests regarding the publication of this paper.

References

[1] M. M. van den Berg, M. A. Benninga, and C. di Lorenzo, "Epidemiology of childhood constipation: a systematic review," *American Journal of Gastroenterology*, vol. 101, no. 10, pp. 2401–2409, 2006.

[2] American College of Gastroenterology Chronic Constipation Task Force, "An evidence-based approach to the management of chronic constipation in North America," *American Journal of Gastroenterology*, vol. 100, supplement 1, pp. S1–S4, 2005.

[3] V. Loening-Baucke, "Chronic constipation in children," *Gastroenterology*, vol. 105, no. 5, pp. 1557–1564, 1993.

[4] N. N. Youssef, A. L. Langseder, B. J. Verga, R. L. Mones, and J. R. Rosh, "Chronic childhood constipation is associated with impaired quality of life: a case-controlled study," *Journal of Pediatric Gastroenterology and Nutrition*, vol. 41, no. 1, pp. 56–60, 2005.

[5] E. P. Athanasakos, K. I. Kemal, R. S. Malliwal et al., "Clinical and psychosocial functioning in adolescents and young adults with anorectal malformations and chronic idiopathic constipation," *British Journal of Surgery*, vol. 100, no. 6, pp. 832–839, 2013.

[6] National Institute for Health and Clinical Excellence: Guidance, *Constipation in Children and Young People: Diagnosis and Management of Idiopathic Childhood Constipation in Primary and Secondary Care*, RCOG Press, London, UK, 2010.

[7] P. Christensen, G. Bazzocchi, M. Coggrave et al., "A randomized, controlled trial of transanal irrigation versus conservative bowel management in spinal cord-injured patients," *Gastroenterology*, vol. 131, no. 3, pp. 738–747, 2006.

[8] P. López Pereira, O. P. Salvador, J. A. Arcas, M. J. M. Urrutia, R. L. Romera, and E. J. Monereo, "Transanal irrigation for the treatment of neuropathic bowel dysfunction," *Journal of Pediatric Urology*, vol. 6, no. 2, pp. 134–138, 2010.

[9] M. Trbay and K. Neel, "Management of neuropathic bowel dysfunction with transanal irrigation system," *Journal of Pediatric Urology*, vol. 6, supplement 1, pp. S74–S75, 2010.

[10] R. J. Rintala and H. Lindahl, "Is normal bowel function possible after repair of intermediate and high anorectal malformations?" *Journal of Pediatric Surgery*, vol. 30, no. 3, pp. 491–494, 1995.

[11] Bowel Management Patient Guide—Your Guide to using Peristeen, February 2014, http://www.coloplast.co.uk/.

[12] P. Corbett, A. Denny, K. Dick, P. S. Malone, S. Griffin, and M. Stanton, "Peristeen integrated transanal irrigation system successfully treats faecal incontinence in children," *Journal of Pediatric Urology*, 2013.

[13] B. Shandling and R. F. Gilmour, "The enema continence catheter in spina bifida: successful bowel management," *Journal of Pediatric Surgery*, vol. 22, no. 3, pp. 271–273, 1987.

[14] A. Marte and M. Borrelli, "Transanal irrigation and intestinal transit time in children with myelomeningocele," *Minerva Pediatrica*, vol. 65, pp. 287–293, 2013.

[15] R. Rintala, L. Mildh, and H. Lindahl, "Fecal continence and quality of life for adult patients with an operated high or intermediate anorectal malformation," *Journal of Pediatric Surgery*, vol. 29, no. 6, pp. 777–780, 1994.

[16] P. S. Malone, P. G. Ransley, and E. M. Kiely, "Preliminary report: the antegrade continence enema," *The Lancet*, vol. 336, no. 8725, pp. 1217–1218, 1990.

[17] J. I. Curry, A. Osborne, and P. S. J. Malone, "The MACE procedure: experience in the United Kingdom," *Journal of Pediatric Surgery*, vol. 34, no. 2, pp. 338–340, 1999.

[18] Medical Device Alert, Peristeen Anal Irrigation System manufactured by Coloplast Limited (MDA/2011/002), February 2014, http://www.mhra.gov.uk/.

39

The Effect of Probiotics on Childhood Constipation:
A Randomized Controlled Double Blind Clinical Trial

M. Sadeghzadeh,[1] A. Rabieefar,[2] P. Khoshnevisasl,[3] N. Mousavinasab,[4] and K. Eftekhari[5]

[1] *Department of Pediatrics, Zanjan Metabolic Disease Research Center, Zanjan University of Medical Sciences, Zanjan, Iran*
[2] *Zanjan University of Medical Sciences, Zanjan, Iran*
[3] *Department of Pediatrics, Social Determinants of Health Research Center, Zanjan University of Medical Sciences, Zanjan, Iran*
[4] *Department of Epidemiology, Zanjan University of Medical Sciences, Zanjan, Iran*
[5] *Department of Pediatrics, Zanjan University of Medical Sciences, Zanjan, Iran*

Correspondence should be addressed to P. Khoshnevisasl; khoshnevis@zums.ac.ir

Academic Editor: Joel R. Rosh

Background. Inconsistent data exist about the role of probiotics in the treatment of constipated children. The aim of this study was to investigate the effectiveness of probiotics in childhood constipation. *Materials and Methods.* In this placebo controlled trial, fifty-six children aged 4–12 years with constipation received randomly lactulose plus Protexin or lactulose plus placebo daily for four weeks. Stool frequency and consistency, abdominal pain, fecal incontinence, and weight gain were studied at the beginning, after the first week, and at the end of the 4th week in both groups. *Results.* Forty-eight patients completed the study. At the end of the fourth week, the frequency and consistency of defecation improved significantly ($P = 0.042$ and $P = 0.049$, resp.). At the end of the first week, fecal incontinence and abdominal pain improved significantly in intervention group ($P = 0.030$ and $P = 0.017$, resp.) but, at the end of the fourth week, this difference was not significant ($P = 0.125$ and $P = 0.161$, resp.). A significant weight gain was observed at the end of the 1st week in the treatment group. *Conclusion.* This study showed that probiotics had a positive role in increasing the frequency and improving the consistency at the end of 4th week.

1. Introduction

Constipation is a common disorder in children and could have a destructive effect on the physical as well as psychological aspects of health [1]. Its prevalence varies from 0.07% to 29.6% in different studies [2]. Organic causes cannot be found in more than 90% of cases [3]. Constipation is defined as the painful passage of stool less than twice a week or less than once every three days [4]. Usual treatments including toilet training, family education, dietary changes, and the use of laxatives, although useful, are not completely satisfactory [1, 5]. Therefore, there is a growing interest to find a new solution [3].

Currently, probiotics were used as an adjunctive treatment for a lot of childhood diseases. The role of probiotics in gastrointestinal diseases as well as allergic disorders, atopic dermatitis, prevention of infections, necrotizing enterocolitis, and infantile colic was shown in many studies [5–8].

It seems that probiotics, which are live microbial ingredients, produce lactic and acetic acids and influence the peristalsis of intestines by reducing colonic pH [3, 5].

Although the role of probiotics is well studied in adults, there were few data on its effectiveness in childhood constipation with contradictory results [1, 3, 9, 10]. Therefore, we conducted this study to evaluate the role of probiotics on our constipated patients.

2. Materials and Methods

This randomized double blind controlled study was conducted on 56 children 4–12 years old with chronic constipation who were referred to Ayatollah Moussavi hospital

TABLE 1: Demographic characteristics of patients.

Variables	Intervention group	Control group	Total	P value
Gender				
Male	14 (58.3%)	10 (41.7%)	24 (50%)	(P = 0.248)
Female	10 (41.7%)	14 (58.3%)	24 (50%)	
Mean age (year)	6.1 ± 2.4	6.3 ± 1.9		(P = 0.739)

clinics in Zanjan, Iran, from October 2011 to March 2012. All children fulfilled Rome III criteria for chronic constipation. The exclusion criteria consisted of any underlying diseases, history of hospital admission, or any gastrointestinal or nutritional problems other than constipation. This study was approved by the Medical Ethics Committee of Zanjan University of Medical Sciences (Ethical code: 904295). Informed written consent was signed by parents of all patients before any intervention.

The sample size was calculated by the formula $n = [Z_{1-\alpha/2} + Z_{1-\beta}]^2 [P_1(1 - P_1) + P_2(1 - P_2)]/(P_1 - P_2)^2$ based on $P_1 = 89\%$, $P_2 = 56\%$, $\alpha = 0/05$, $1 - \beta = 0/80$, $z = 1/95$, and $0/84$, respectively ($n = 56$).

The patients were randomly allocated into two groups who received lactulose (1 mL/kg/d) plus Protexin (Nikooteb Company, Tehran, Iran) one sachet daily or lactulose plus placebo alone for four month. The control group was matched according to sex and age.

A period of one week was estimated as a wash-out period for those who used any drugs for their constipation. Each sachet of Protexin was composed of seven probiotic bacteria including *Lactobacillus casei* PXN 37, *Lactobacillus rhamnosus* PXN 54, *Streptococcus thermophiles* PXN 66, *Bifidobacterium breve* PXN 25, *Lactobacillus acidophilus* PXN 35, *Bifidobacterium infantis (child specific)* PXN 27, and *Lactobacillus bulgaricus* PXN 39, TVC: 1 billion CFU TVC: 1×10^9. The placebo was supplied by Nikooteb company, the provider of probiotics in Iran, as innocent powder in identical sachets and stored in a cool and dry place until use.

Each patient was visited by the researcher and completely evaluated for organic diseases, and a questionnaire including demographic data, past medical history, drug history, symptoms of constipation, and physical examination was completed before the study. The patients with comorbid conditions were excluded from the study.

After the first and fourth weeks of intervention, a second questionnaire was completed for symptoms of constipation including the frequency of defecation, stool consistency, abdominal pain, frequency of fecal incontinence, and side effects in both groups. Fecal frequency, consistency (hard, normal, and soft), and weight gain of all patients were recorded. Fecal incontinence and abdominal pain were looked for only in patients who had these symptoms before the intervention.

Data were analyzed using SPSS software Version 16.0. Number of bowel movements and fecal incontinence episodes in baseline information were analyzed by Freidman test. The Student's t-test was used for parametric data and chi-square analysis was used for categorical measures. P value of <0.05 was considered significant.

3. Results

A total of 56 patients were enrolled in the study. Four patients in the intervention group (three in the first week and one in the fourth week) refused to complete the study and were excluded. Four patients in the control group had not completed the study as well (two did not refer for follow-up and two patients did not fulfill criteria Rome III during the study), and were excluded. At the end, two groups of 24 patients were studied.

In the intervention group, 14 males (58.3%) and 10 females (41.7%) completed the study. The control group consisted of 10 males (41.7%) with 14 females (58.3%). The difference of the two groups was not statistically significant (P = 0.248). The mean age of patients in treatment group was 6.1 ± 2.4 and in control group was 6.3 ± 1.9 (P = 0.739). The demographic data are shown in Table 1.

In the intervention group, 54.2% and in controls 37.5% had fecal incontinence before the intervention (P = 0.247). In the first group, 66.7% had abdominal pain in the beginning of the study compared to 58.3% in the second group (P = 0.551). These patients were followed for improvement of their symptoms till 4th week.

As shown in Table 2, at the end of the fourth week, the frequency and consistency of defecation improved significantly (P = 0.042, P = 0.049, resp.).

At the end of the first week, fecal incontinence and abdominal pain improved significantly in intervention group (P = 0.030, P = 0.017, resp.) but, at the end of the fourth week, this difference was not significant (P = 0.125, P = 0.161, resp.) (Table 3).

Surprisingly, we found that, at the end of the first week, probiotics had significantly improved weight gain (more than 10%) (P = 0.002), and this difference, although, continued but was not significant at the end of the fourth week (P = 0.098).

No side effects were noted during the treatment.

4. Discussion

It seems that probiotics which are live microbial ingredients competitively exclude pathogenic bacteria and improve gastrointestinal upsets. By producingshort-chain fatty acids, lactic acid, and acetic acid, they reduce colonic PH, change

TABLE 2: Comparison of symptoms between the beginning and end of the 1st and 4th weeks.

Variables		Treatment (mean ± SD)	Placebo (mean ± SD)	P value
Stool frequency	Beginning to 1st week	1.67 ± 0.82	0.79 ± 0.83	
	Beginning to 4th week	2.08 ± 0.65	1.54 ± 0.98	0.042
	1st to 4th week	0.92 ± 0.72	0.75 ± 0.61	
Stool consistency*	Beginning to 1st week	0.42 ± 0.50	0.21 ± 0.41	
	Beginning to 4th week	0.88 ± 0.45	0.63 ± 0.50	0.049
	1st to 4th week	0.46 ± 0.51	0.42 ± 0.50	

*Stool consistency: 1: hard, 2: normal, and 3: soft.

TABLE 3: Symptom changes at the end of the 1st week.

Symptom	Treatment frequency, percent	Placebo frequency, percent	P value
With fecal incontinence	4 (30.8%)	7 (77.8%)	
Without fecal incontinence	11 (69.2%)	2 (22.2%)	0.030
Total (fecal incontinence)	**15 (100%)**	**9 (100%)**	
With abdominal pain	7 (43.8%)	12 (85.7%)	
Without abdominal pain	9 (56.2%)	2 (14.3%)	0.017
Total (abdominal pain)	**16 (100%)**	**14 (100%)**	
With weight gain	10 (41.7%)	1 (4.2%)	
Without weight gain	14 (58.3%)	23 (95.8)	0.002
Total weight gain	**24 (100%)**	**24 (100%)**	

gut microflora, and influence the peristalsis of intestines [3, 5].

Our study showed that probiotics were significantly effective in improving the stool frequency and consistency in intervention group at the end of the 4th week. A significant decrease in fecal incontinence and abdominal pain and increasing body weight were found by the end of the first week in treatment group which was not significant at the end of the 4th week. There are many studies with the same results [1, 3, 11–16].

The study of Saneian comparing placebo plus mineral oil and probiotics plus mineral oil on 60 patients in Isfahan, Iran, revealed that stool frequency, consistency, pain at defecation, and soiling improved significantly in intervention group [1].

The study of Bekkali on twenty 4–16-year-old children receiving probiotics revealed that, after 4 weeks, the frequency of bowl movements had been increased and a significant decrease in fecal incontinence and abdominal pain was observed [3]. These results are similar to our results.

Koebnick concluded that at the end of 4th week 89% ofconstipated patients receiving probiotics significantly improved compared to 56% of controls [11].

The study of Ardatskaia on 30 patients having irritable bowel syndrome with predominance of constipation showed that Normoflorin therapy had normalized the intestinal motor activity through changes in microbial flora of the intestines [12].

In a crossover trial conducted in Brazil by Guerra, studying 59 constipated students, after 5 weeks, the cases who received probiotic yogurt had significant improvement in defecation frequency ($P = 0.012$), defecation pain ($P =$

0.046), and abdominal pain ($P = 0.015$) compared to students who get only yogurt [13].

Jayasimhan had studied 120 adults with constipation and followed them after 7 days. He concluded that probiotics had significantly improved stool frequency and consistency [14]. These results are similar to our results at the end of the first week.

The study of Khodadad in Tehran on 102 constipated children showed that probiotic plus mineral oil increased stool frequency significantly comparing with mineral oil plus placebo and probiotic plus placebo. On the other hand, stool consistency, abdominal pain, and fecal incontinence were improved, although the difference was not significant. The results of this study were similar to our investigation but improvement of stool consistency was significant in our study [15].

In a meta-analysis by Miller and Ouwehand, probiotics had a short-term effect on reducing intestinal transit time in constipated adults. A greater effect on patients with versus without constipation and older versus younger was shown [16].

In all these studies, stool frequency has been improved which could be due to change in intestinal flora, although few studies have reevaluated gut microflora [12]. Although the differences in improvement of various symptoms could be due to regimens used by patients, the mixture of pre- and probiotics and different bacteria used can also explain these diversities. The decrease in fecal incontinence and abdominal pain and increasing body weight that was found by the end of the first week in treatment group but not significant at the end of the 4th week could be explained by the chronic nature of the disease, a better effect of this drug in short term, and the tolerance to treatment.

Conversely, there are some studies which are not similar to our findings:

Vandenplas et al. stated that probiotics had limited role in controlling the constipation, although its role in antibiotic-associated diarrhea and acute gastroenteritis was confirmed [6].

Banaszkiewicz and Szajewska had studied eighty-four constipated children (2–16 years of age) receiving 1 mL/kg/day of 70% lactulose plus 10^9 colony-forming units (CFU) of *Lactobacillus* GG (LGG) orally twice daily for 12 weeks comparing with a control group and concluded that LGG was not an effective adjunct to lactulose in children with constipation [17]. We have used lactulose in our patients too, because it was well tolerated and easily accessible and different results may be due to the composition of probiotics used.

Mazlyn and coworkers demonstrated that adults with functional constipation did not have significant alleviation in constipation severity or stool frequency, consistency, and quantity comparing to controls after 4 weeks of treatment with probiotics [18].

The study of Tabbers et al. on 159 constipated children receiving fermented dairy product containing Bifidobacterium lactis strain showed that, in spite of improvement in stool frequency comparing to baseline, the result was not comparable to controls [19].

Considering these controversies, it seems that larger studies are needed to clarify the effect of probiotics in constipation. It is recommended to control strictly the regimens used in both groups, and it seems that a mixture of pre- and probiotics containing all useful flora would be promising.

Also, we found a significant increase in body weight which was not mentioned in other studies and it may be due to improved appetite after decreasing intestinal transit time. Further investigations are needed to prove this effect.

5. Conclusion

This investigation revealed significantly increased bowel frequency and improved stool consistency with the combination of lactulose and probiotics. In our study, the decrease in episodes of fecal incontinence and abdominal pain was significant compared to control group at the end of the first week that may be due to a better effect of this drug in short term.

Conflict of Interests

There is no conflict of interests.

Acknowledgments

This project was a thesis for a pediatric specialty degree and was founded by the Research Department of Zanjan University of Medical Sciences. The authors greatly appreciate all participants in this study. They also appreciate the helpful comments of Dr. Akefeh Ahmadiafshar in editing this paper.

References

[1] H. Saneian, K. Tavakkol, P. Adhamian, and A. Gholamrezaei, "Comparison of *Lactobacillus sporogenes* plus mineral oil and mineral oil alone in the treatment of childhood functional constipation," *Journal of Research in Medical Sciences*, vol. 18, no. 2, pp. 85–88, 2013.

[2] S. M. Mugie, C. di Lorenzo, and M. A. Benninga, "Constipation in childhood," *Nature Reviews Gastroenterology and Hepatology*, vol. 8, no. 9, pp. 502–511, 2011.

[3] N.-L. Bekkali, M. E. J. Bongers, M. M. van den Berg, O. Liem, and M. A. Benninga, "The role of a probiotics mixture in the treatment of childhood constipation: a pilot study," *Nutrition Journal*, vol. 6, article 17, 2007.

[4] H. Saneian and N. Mostofizadeh, "Comparing the efficacy of polyethylene glycol (PEG), magnesium hydroxide and lactulose in treatment of functional constipation in children," *Journal of Research in Medical Sciences*, vol. 17, no. 1, pp. S145–S149, 2012.

[5] A. Chmielewska and H. Szajewska, "Systematic review of randomised controlled trials: probiotics for functional constipation," *World Journal of Gastroenterology*, vol. 16, no. 1, pp. 69–75, 2010.

[6] Y. Vandenplas, E. de Greef, T. Devreker, G. Veereman-Wauters, and B. Hauser, "Probiotics and prebiotics in infants and children," *Current Infectious Disease Reports*, vol. 15, no. 3, pp. 251–262, 2013.

[7] A. Horvath and H. Szajewska, "Probiotics, prebiotics, and dietary fiber in the management of functional gastrointestinal disorders," *World Review of Nutrition & Dietetics*, vol. 108, pp. 40–48, 2013.

[8] G. Álvarez-Calatayud, J. Pérez-Moreno, M. Tolín, and C. Sánchez, "Clinical applications of the use of probiotics in pediatrics," *Nutrición Hospitalaria*, vol. 28, no. 3, pp. 564–574, 2013.

[9] H. Szajewska, M. Setty, J. Mrukowicz, and S. Guandalini, "Probiotics in gastrointestinal diseases in children: hard and not-so-hard evidence of efficacy," *Journal of Pediatric Gastroenterology & Nutrition*, vol. 42, no. 5, pp. 454–475, 2006.

[10] Y. Vandenplas, G. Veereman-Wauters, E. de Greef et al., "Probiotics and prebiotics in prevention and treatment of diseases in infants and children," *Jornal de Pediatria*, vol. 87, no. 4, pp. 292–300, 2011.

[11] C. Koebnick, I. Wagner, P. Leitzmann, U. Stern, and H. J. F. Zunft, "Probiotic beverage containing *Lactobacillus casei* Shirota improves gastrointestinal symptoms in patients with chronic constipation," *Canadian Journal of Gastroenterology*, vol. 17, no. 11, pp. 655–659, 2003.

[12] M. D. Ardatskaia and O. N. Minushkin, "Probiotics in the treatment of functional intestinal diseases," *Èksperimental'nia i Klinicheskaia Gastroènterologiia*, no. 3, pp. 106–113, 2012.

[13] P. V. P. Guerra, L. N. Lima, T. C. Souza et al., "Pediatric functional constipation treatment with bifidobacterium-containing yogurt: a crossover, double-blind, controlled trial," *World Journal of Gastroenterology*, vol. 17, no. 34, pp. 3916–3921, 2011.

[14] S. Jayasimhan, N.-Y. Yap, Y. Roest, R. Rajandram, and K.-F. Chin, "Efficacy of microbial cell preparation in improving chronic constipation: a randomized, double-blind, placebo-controlled trial," *Clinical Nutrition*, vol. 32, no. 6, pp. 928–934, 2013.

[15] A. Khodadad and M. Sabbaghian, "Role of synbiotics in the treatment of childhood constipation: a double-blind randomized placebo controlled trial," *Iranian Journal of Pediatrics*, vol. 20, no. 4, pp. 387–392, 2010.

[16] L. E. Miller and A. C. Ouwehand, "Probiotic supplementation decreases intestinal transit time: meta-analysis of randomized controlled trials," *World Journal of Gastroenterology*, vol. 19, no. 29, pp. 4718–4725, 2013.

[17] A. Banaszkiewicz and H. Szajewska, "Ineffectiveness of *Lactobacillus* GG as an adjunct to lactulose for the treatment of constipation in children: a double-blind, placebo-controlled randomized trial," *The Journal of Pediatrics*, vol. 146, no. 3, pp. 364–369, 2005.

[18] M. M. Mazlyn, L. H. Nagarajah, A. Fatimah, A. K. Norimah, and K. L. Goh, "Effects of a probiotic fermented milk on functional constipation: a randomized,double-blind, placebo-controlled study," *Journal of Gastroenterology and Hepatology*, vol. 28, no. 7, pp. 1141–1147, 2013.

[19] M. M. Tabbers, A. Chmielewska, M. G. Roseboom et al., "Fermented milk containing *Bifidobacterium lactis* DN-173 010 in childhood constipation: a randomized, double-blind, controlled trial," *Pediatrics*, vol. 127, no. 6, pp. e1392–e1399, 2011.

40

A Novel Algorithm in the Management of Hypoglycemia in Newborns

Swapna Naveen, Chikati Rosy, Hemasree Kandraju, Deepak Sharma, Tejopratap Oleti, and Srinivas Murki

Department of Neonatology, Fernandez Hospital, Hyderguda, Hyderabad, Telangana 500029, India

Correspondence should be addressed to Srinivas Murki; srinivasmurki2001@gmail.com

Academic Editor: Naveed Hussain

Study Objective. To evaluate the safety of a new protocol in comparison to the standard protocol for managing hypoglycemia in neonates. *Methods.* Open label RCT-pilot study. Neonates admitted to NICU with hypoglycemia and requiring intravenous fluids were included. Fifty-seven eligible neonates were randomly allocated to either intervention group (starting fluids with 10% dextrose and increments of 1.5%) or standard protocol group (GIR of 6 mg/kg/min with increments of 2 mg/kg/min) till control of hypoglycemia. Primary outcome of the study was to know proportion of infants with subsequent hypoglycemia and hyperglycemia after enrolment. *Results.* The initial GIR (6 ± 0 mg/kg/min versus 4.8 ± 1.4 mg/kg/min, $P < 0.001$), the mean maximum GIR (6.7 ± 1.6 mg/kg/min versus 5.6 ± 2 mg/kg/min, $P = 0.03$), the maximum concentration of glucose infused ($13.8 \pm 2.9\%$ versus $10.9 \pm 1.9\%$, $P < 0.001$), and the total amount of glucose infused were significantly lower in the intervention group. The mean maximum blood sugar was significantly higher (129 ± 57 mg/dL versus 87 ± 30 mg/dL, $P = 0.001$) and there was a trend towards high proportion of infants with Hyperglycemia in the standard protocol group ($n = 10$, 39% versus $n = 5$, 16%, $P = 0.07$). The median difference between the highest and the lowest recorded sugar for any infant was significantly higher in the standard protocol group (median 93 mg/dL, IQR 52 to 147 mg/dL versus median 50 mg/dL, IQR 38 to 62.5 mg/dL, $P = 0.03$). *Conclusion.* A new and novel algorithm in the management of hypoglycemia in neonates is as safe as the standard protocol and requires further testing before routine implementation.

1. Introduction

The term "hypoglycemia" refers to a reduction in the glucose concentration of circulating blood. It is almost 100 years since hypoglycemia was first described in children and over 50 years since it was recognized in newborn and older infants [1]. It is recognized that 23–50% of infants admitted to neonatal intensive care unit are diagnosed with one or more episodes of hypoglycemia [2–4]. In an Indian study, Singh et al. reported the incidence of hypoglycemia in 9.6%, 15.3%, and 19.4% term AGA, term SGA, and term LGA infants, respectively [5]. Neonatal hypoglycemia adversely affects the neurodevelopmental outcome, overall IQ, reading ability, arithmetic proficiency, and motor performance [6]. Hence, there is a need to correct the blood sugar as early as

possible. Standard protocol for correction of hypoglycemia in symptomatic newborns or when blood sugar is <30 mg/dL involves giving a bolus of 2 mL/kg of 10% dextrose followed by a glucose infusion rate of 6 mg/kg/min. The current protocol in many units is that if hypoglycemia persists, increments are made in the glucose infusion rate (GIR) at 2 mg/kg/min every 15 to 30 minutes [7, 8]. This method is very tedious and involves many calculations and hence time lag and errors in the preparation of fluid. As the morbidities due to neonatal hypoglycemia depend on the duration of hypoglycemia, we need a better method which will reduce the time lag and errors in implementation of required GIR. We did this open labeled randomized controlled pilot study to evaluate the safety of a new protocol in comparison to the standard protocol for managing hypoglycemia in neonates.

2. Method and Material

This randomized pilot study was conducted in a tertiary level teaching hospital of south India. Fernandez Hospital (FH) institutional review board approved the study protocol. Consent was obtained from the parents before randomization of the infant in the study. Inclusion criteria included all neonates with hypoglycemia requiring intravenous fluids. Hypoglycemia was defined as blood glucose less than 40 mg/dL. Intravenous fluids were considered if

(i) blood glucose was <40 mg/dL and infant is symptomatic: symptoms included lethargy, jitteriness, poor suck, and seizures,

(ii) blood glucose was less than 30 mg/dL, or

(iii) blood glucose was less than 40 mg/dL fifteen minutes after an oral feed.

Sick neonates (shock requiring inotropes or ventilation or oxygen or already on intravenous fluids for any other reason) with hypoglycemia and neonates with hypoglycemia not requiring intravenous fluids (hypoglycemia corrected with feeds) and those in whom consent could not be obtained were excluded. Randomization was based on a web based random number generator. Group allocation was concealed in serially numbered sealed opaque envelopes. The envelope was opened after obtaining a written consent and after entering the infant details on the outer cover of the envelope. The principal investigator opened the envelopes and randomized the babies. After allotment of babies to intervention or standard protocol group, the necessary details were entered in a predesigned case reporting form.

2.1. Standard Protocol

(1) Glucose infusion was started with 6 mg/kg/min.

(2) Glucose infusion rate (GIR) was increased by 2 mg/kg/min every 30 minutes if blood sugar continued to be below 40 mg/dL to a maximum glucose infusion rate of 14 mg/kg/min.

(3) Central venous line was established if glucose concentration exceeded 12.5% for a duration of 12 hrs.

(4) Blood glucose was monitored after 30 min after initiation of infusion, 2 hours of infusion, and subsequently every 6 hours if blood glucose remained >50 mg/dL. If the blood sugar was ≤50 mg/dL, monitoring was continued every 30 minutes till sugar was above 50 mg/dL.

(5) If blood sugar was >50 mg/dL but less than 125 mg/dL, tapering of GIR was done after 2 values at 6-hour interval which was between 50 and 125 mg/dL. But if the blood sugar was greater than 125 mg/dL, a repeat sample was done in 2 hours and if it was still >125 mg/dL, tapering was initiated immediately.

(6) For infants on 6 mg/kg/min, tapering was to the maintenance fluid if they continued to be on intravenous fluids but if feeding was initiated, tapering of

intravenous fluids was at the rate of 1 mL/hour. For infants on GIR >6 mg/kg/min, tapering was done at 2 mg/kg/min every 6 hours till GIR was 6 mg/kg/min. Once GIR was 6 mg/kg/min, feeding was initiated and fluids were tapered at 1 mL/hour.

2.2. Intervention Group

(1) Glucose infusion was started with 10% dextrose.

(2) Glucose concentration was increased in steps of 1.5% (step 1 10% to 11.5% and step 2 11.5% to 13%) every 30 minutes if blood sugar continued to be <40 mg/dL. If blood sugar remained <40 mg/dL on 2 increments, then the infant was switched to standard protocol. Glucose of 11.5% was prepared by mixing 10 mL of 25% to 90 mL of 10% dextrose. For every 1.5% increase in glucose concentration, volume of 25% dextrose increased by 10 mL and that of 10% dextrose decreased by 10 mL for every 100 mL of stock solution.

(3) Step 3 to step 5 was similar to that in the standard group.

(4) For infants on glucose concentration >10%, tapering was by 1.5% every 6 hours. For babies on 10% glucose, tapering was to the maintenance fluids if baby continued to be on intravenous fluids and by 1 mL/hour if baby was initiated on feeds.

In both of the groups monitoring of blood sugar was as at admission, 30 minutes, 2 hours, and 6 hours. If sugar was ≤50 mg/dL, monitoring was every 30 minutes. If sugar was >125 mg/dL, monitoring was every 2 hours. In all enrolled infants a minibolus of 10% dextrose, 2 mL/kg, was given if the infant was symptomatic at enrollment or had a sugar <30 mg/dL at enrolment. No calorie supplements or glucose polymers were used for infants on enteral feeds. Volume of intravenous fluids was based on the infant's needs, based on the day of life and birth weight and also on the hydration status. Neonates exited from the study once they were on full enteral feeds for a duration of at least 12 hours.

Primary outcomes of the study included proportion of infants with hypoglycemia (defined as blood glucose < 40 mg/dL) or hyperglycemia (defined as blood glucose > 125 mg/dL) after enrolment in the trial. Secondary outcomes included mean maximum blood glucose, difference between highest and lowest blood glucose after enrolment, need for central line placements, maximum GIR, maximum percent of dextrose infused, glucose infused in gm/kg/day, time to initiate enteral feeds, time to full enteral feeds, and discharge neurosonogram.

Blood glucose was estimated by strip method (glucose oxidase method, Optium Xceed glucometer) from a venous blood sample. Low blood sugar (blood sugar < 40 mg/dL) and high blood sugar (blood sugar > 125 mg/dL) by strip method were always confirmed with a laboratory blood glucose value. Estimation of blood glucose in the laboratory was done by automated Hexokinase method.

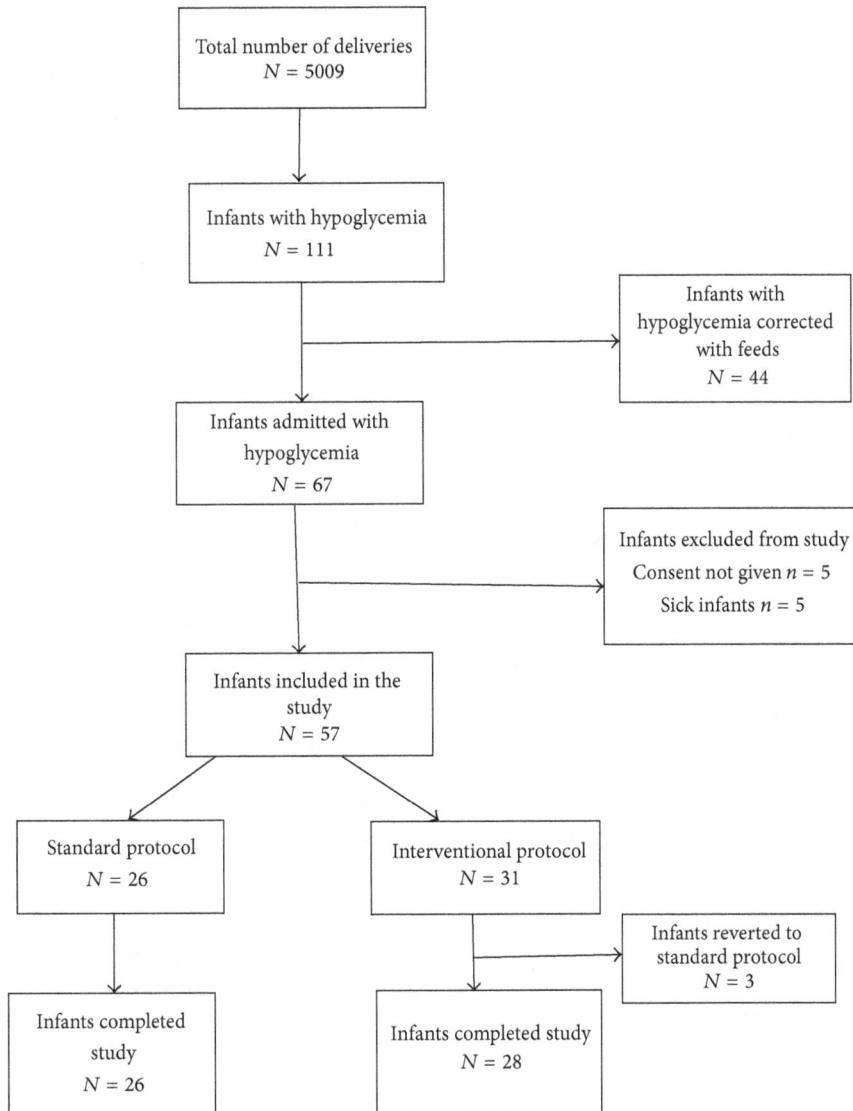

FIGURE 1: Study flow chart.

3. Statistics

Comparison of outcomes between the groups was done using chi-square test for categorical variables and Student's t-test or Mann-Whitney U test for continuous variables as appropriate. A P value < 0.05 was considered to be significant. No a priori sample size was estimated for the study.

4. Results

Fifty-seven infants were enrolled in the study (Figure 1). All the infants completed the study and received their allocated treatment protocols till the completion of the study. The reasons for hypoglycemia in our study group ($n = 57$) included intrauterine growth restriction $n = 27$ (47%), infant of diabetic mother $n = 18$ (31%), large for gestation $n = 3$ (5%), and prematurity $n = 9$ (17%). Both of the study groups were comparable for the baseline variables

including gestational age, birth weight, maternal risk factors, intrauterine growth status, median age at enrolment, and blood sugar at enrolment (Table 1).

4.1. Hypoglycemia Management. Five of the 26 infants in standard protocol group had symptomatic hypoglycemia. Three infants presented with lethargy, two with jitteriness, and one each with poor feeding, irritability, and seizures. In the intervention group too, five infants had symptomatic hypoglycemia. The symptoms in the order of frequency included jitteriness ($n = 3$), lethargy ($n = 2$), poor feeding ($n = 2$), and seizure ($n = 1$). The initial glucose infusion rate (6 ± 0 mg/kg/min versus 4.8 ± 1.4 mg/kg/min, $P < 0.001$), the mean maximum glucose infusion rate (6.7 ± 1.6 mg/kg/min versus 5.6 ± 2 mg/kg/min, $P = 0.03$), the maximum concentration of glucose infused ($13.8 \pm 2.9\%$ versus $10.9 \pm 1.9\%$, $P < 0.001$), and the median total amount of glucose infused were significantly lower in the intervention group (median, IQR:

Variables	Standard protocol ($N = 26$); n (%)	Intervention protocol ($N = 31$); n (%)	P value
Gestation (mean ± SD)	2048 ± 513	2195 ± 877	0.45
Birth weight (g) (mean ± SD)	36.23 ± 2.3	36.03 ± 2.5	0.76
Male sex	18 (69)	24 (77)	0.55
GDM	8 (31)	10 (32)	1.00
1 min Apgar (median, IQR)	7 (7-8)	7 (7-8)	0.81
IUGR	14 (54)	13 (42)	0.43
Blood sugar at enrolment	27.7 ± 6.4	27.2 ± 7.3	0.42
Age at enrolment in hrs (median, IQR)	2 hrs (2 hrs–8.25 hrs)	2 hrs (1 hr–10 hrs)	0.42

6.2 g/kg/day; 5.5 to 7.9 g/kg/day versus 5.1 g/kg/day; 4.2 to 6.2 g/kg/day, $P = 0.005$). The proportion of infants requiring increments in glucose (GIR or percent dextrose) was similar between the two groups ($n = 5$, 19% versus $n = 8$, 26%, $P = 0.35$). In the intervention group three infants required increments in glucose concentration once (to 11.5%), two infants required increments in glucose concentration twice (to 13%), and three infants required increments in glucose concentration more than twice. All three infants requiring more than two increments in glucose concentration were switched to standard protocol at GIR 2 mg/kg/min higher. Two, two, and one infants in the standard protocol group required once (8 mg/kg/min), twice (10 mg/mg/min), and more than twice (>12 mg/kg/min) increments in GIR. The number of infants requiring central line placement ($n = 6$, 23% versus $n = 3$, 9.7%, $P = 0.27$) was similar between the standard protocol and intervention group, respectively.

4.2. Outcomes. The proportion of infants with hypoglycemia ($n = 5$, 19% versus $n = 8$, 26%, $P = 0.35$) and also moderate hypoglycemia (blood glucose ≤ 50 mg/gL; $n = 14$, 54% versus $n = 14$, 45%, $P = 0.60$) was similar between the two groups. The mean maximum blood sugar was significantly higher (129 ± 57 mg/dL versus 87 ± 30 mg/dL, $P = 0.001$) and there was a trend towards high proportion of infants with hyperglycemia in the standard protocol group ($n = 10$, 39% versus $n = 5$, 16%, $P = 0.07$). The median difference between the highest and the lowest recorded sugar for any infant was significantly higher in the standard protocol group (median: 93 mg/dL, IQR 52 to 147 mg/dL versus median 50 mg/dL, IQR 38 to 62.5 mg/dL, $P = 0.03$). One infant in the intervention group had MRI abnormality attributable to neonatal hypoglycemia but this infant had neither seizures nor recurrence of hypoglycemia after enrolment. One infant in the standard protocol group died of neonatal sepsis and was not related to the management of hypoglycemia. The median time to initiate enteral feeds (median, IQR; 1 day; 1–2.5 days versus 1 day; 1-2 days, $P = 0.60$) and the median time to reach full enteral feeds (median, IQR; 1 day; 1–3.5 days versus 1 day; 1-2 days, $P = 0.62$) after enrolment were similar between the two groups. All enrolled infants had a normal neurosonogram at discharge.

5. Discussion

This pilot study was done to assess the safety of a novel algorithm for management of hypoglycemia and it was found to be as safe as the standard protocol. The proportion of infants with subsequent hypoglycemic episodes was similar between the two groups. This new protocol is as efficacious as the standard protocol as the proportion of infants requiring increments in GIR in standard protocol group was similar to that requiring increment in dextrose concentration in the intervention group. Also the time taken for initiation of oral feeds and that needed to achieve full enteral feeds after enrolment were also similar between the two groups. It is noteworthy that efficacy was similar although infants in the intervention group received lesser GIR and lower total glucose infused per day. As per the protocol, being a pilot study, 3 infants from intervention group were switched to the standard protocol group for increasing glucose requirements.

The rate of endogenous glucose metabolism in well fasting neonates is estimated to be 4 to 6 mg/kg/min. Glucose infusions commenced at 60 mL/kg/day of 10% dextrose will provide a GIR of 4 mg/kg/min [9]. In this study, the starting mean GIR in the intervention group of 4.8 ± 1.4 mg/kg/min explains the physiological reason behind glucose stabilization in this group. For newborns with severe and symptomatic hypoglycemia, AAP recommends a minibolus of 2 mL/kg of 10% dextrose and/or starting a continuous infusion of 10% dextrose at 80 to 100 mL/kg per day. If the goal of achieving plasma glucose between 40 and 50 mg/dL is not met after 24 hours of glucose infusion, a workup for hyperinsulinemic hypoglycemia is suggested. However the guideline is silent on increasing the concentration of dextrose for hypoglycemic episodes occurring within 24 hours of starting glucose infusion [10]. Standard national guidelines from India recommend a minibolus of 2 mL/kg of 10% dextrose and starting glucose infusion at a GIR of 6 mg/kg/min. After starting the glucose infusion, for persisting hypoglycemia, an increment in GIR by 2 mg/kg/min till a maximum of 12 mg/kg/min is suggested [7, 8]. A popular manual on neonatal care recommends a minibolus followed by a glucose infusion at GIR 6 to 8 mg/kg/min. When the GIR required is >12 mg/kg/min, workup for hyperinsulinemia is suggested [11]. Thus there is no evidence or consensus on the management of hypoglycemia in newborns. This is the first study to highlight these differences and to provide some evidence for a uniform protocol.

The mean maximum blood glucose and the median difference between the lowest to highest blood glucose were significantly higher in the standard protocol group. Also there was a trend towards increased incidence of hyperglycemic episodes in the standard protocol group. These changes are explained by the 33% increase in GIR from baseline (6 to 8 to 10 mg/kg/min) in the standard protocol as against 15% increase (10 to 11.5 to 13%) in this new protocol. It is well known that hypoglycemia is associated with compensatory increased cerebral blood flows and hyperglycemia with decreased cerebral blood flow and these changes if frequent may have adverse effects on the developing brain [12–14]. There is a need to assess the long term effects of these high and fluctuating blood glucose levels as seen in the standard protocol for management of hypoglycemia. In a recent report by Vanhatalo and Tammela when 15% dextrose was compared with 20% dextrose at GIR of 8 mg/kg/min for correction of hypoglycemia, 16% of the infants had hyperglycemic (plasma glucose > 7.7 mmol/L (138 mg/dL)) episodes [15].

Several studies have shown that hypoglycemia and hyperglycemia are detrimental for both short and long term neurodevelopmental outcomes [6]. We did not assess the long term outcomes of enrolled newborns in our study.

6. Limitation and Merits of Study

We excluded very sick infants from our study due to ethical considerations. As the infants of intervention groups were reverted to standard protocol after 2 increments, we cannot explain the effectiveness of this protocol for treatment of prolonged, refractory, or persistent hypoglycemia. There is also a need to study the effect of this hypoglycemia correction protocol on the long term neurodevelopmental outcome of the infants.

We could not find similar studies in the literature comparing the standard protocol for correction of neonatal hypoglycemia with other formulae and protocols. Ease of preparation and lesser calculations are the main advantages of this new protocol. Lesser calculations imply lesser errors in mixing of fluids and lesser delay in starting of dextrose infusions. Further larger randomized trials are needed to test this protocol for its widespread implementation not only in otherwise healthy babies but also in sick neonates.

Conflict of Interests

There is no conflict of interests.

References

[1] A. F. Hartmann, J. C. Jaudon, and M. Morton, "Hypoglycemia," *The Journal of Pediatrics*, vol. 11, no. 1, pp. 1–36, 1937.

[2] F. H. A. Osier, J. A. Berkley, A. Ross, F. Sanderson, S. Mohammed, and C. R. J. C. Newton, "Abnormal blood glucose concentrations on admission to a rural Kenyan district hospital: prevalence and outcome," *Archives of Disease in Childhood*, vol. 88, no. 7, pp. 621–625, 2003.

[3] B. J. Stoll, "Hypoglycemia," in *Nelson Textbook of Pediatrics*, R. Bherman, R. M. Kleigman, and H. B. Jenson, Eds., pp. 785–786, Saunders, Philadelphia, Pa, USA, 17th edition, 2004.

[4] D. L. Harris, P. J. Weston, and J. E. Harding, "Incidence of neonatal hypoglycemia in babies identified as at risk," *Journal of Pediatrics*, vol. 161, no. 5, pp. 787–791, 2012.

[5] M. Singh, P. K. Singhal, V. K. Paul et al., "Neurodevelopmental outcome of asymptomatic & symptomatic babies with neonatal hypoglycaemia," *The Indian Journal of Medical Research*, vol. 94, pp. 6–10, 1991.

[6] A. Lucas, R. Morley, and T. J. Cole, "Adverse neurodevelopmental outcome of moderate neonatal hypoglycaemia," *British Medical Journal*, vol. 297, no. 6659, pp. 1304–1308, 1988.

[7] "Management of neonatal hypoglycemia in National Neonatal Forum of India," in *Evidence Based Clinical Practice Guidelines*, pp. 63–76, Chandika Press, Panchkula, India, 2010.

[8] Hypoglycemia, 2014, http://www.newbornwhocc.org/clinical_proto.html.

[9] S. C. Denne, "Carbohydrate requirements," in *Fetal and Neonatal Physiology*, R. A. Polin and W. W. Fox, Eds., pp. 325–327, WB Saunders, Philadelphia, Pa, USA, 2nd edition, 1998.

[10] D. H. Adamkin, "Postnatal glucose homeostasis in late-preterm and term infants," *Pediatrics*, vol. 127, no. 3, pp. 575–579, 2011.

[11] R. E. Wilker, "Hypoglycemia and hyperglycemia," in *Manual OF Neonatal Care*, J. P. Cloharty, E. C. Elchenwald, A. R. Hansen, and A. R. Stark, Eds., pp. 284–296, Lippincott Williams and Wilkins, 7th edition, 2012.

[12] A. H. Hemachandra and R. M. Cowett, "Neonatal hyperglycemia," *Pediatrics in Review*, vol. 20, pp. 16–24, 1999.

[13] O. Pryds, N. J. Christensen, and B. Friis-Hansen, "Increased cerebral blood flow and plasma epinephrine in hypoglycemic, preterm neonates," *Pediatrics*, vol. 85, no. 2, pp. 172–176, 1990.

[14] R. C. Vannucci, R. M. Brucklacher, and S. J. Vannucci, "The effect of hyperglycemia on cerebral metabolism during hypoxia- ischemia in the immature rat," *Journal of Cerebral Blood Flow and Metabolism*, vol. 16, no. 5, pp. 1026–1033, 1996.

[15] T. Vanhatalo and O. Tammela, "Glucose infusions into peripheral veins in the management of neonatal hypoglycemia— 20% instead of 15%?" *Acta Paediatrica, International Journal of Paediatrics*, vol. 99, no. 3, pp. 350–353, 2010.

41

Is It Time to Review Guidelines for ETT Positioning in the NICU? SCEPTIC—Survey of Challenges Encountered in Placement of Endotracheal Tubes in Canadian NICUs

Pankaj Sakhuja,[1,2,3] **Michael Finelli,**[1] **Judy Hawes,**[1] **and Hilary Whyte**[1,2]

[1]*Division of Neonatology, The Hospital for Sick Children, University of Toronto, Toronto, ON, Canada M5G 1X8*
[2]*Department of Pediatrics, University of Toronto, Toronto, ON, Canada M5G 1X8*
[3]*King Hamad University Hospital, Block 228, Busaiteen, Bahrain*

Correspondence should be addressed to Pankaj Sakhuja; drpankajsakhuja@gmail.com

Academic Editor: Steven M. Donn

Objectives. To examine current opinions and practices regarding endotracheal tube placement across several Canadian Neonatal Intensive Care Units. *Design*. Clinical directors from Canadian Neonatal Network affiliated NICUs and Neonatal-Perinatal Programs across Canada were invited via email to participate in and disseminate the online survey to staff neonatologists, neonatal fellows, respiratory therapists, and nurse practitioners. *Result*. There is wide variability in the beliefs and practices related to ETT placement. The majority use "weight +6" formula and "aim to black line" on ETT at vocal cords to estimate the depth of an oral ETT and reported estimation as challenging in ELBW infants. The majority agreed that mid-trachea is an ideal ETT tip position; however their preferred position on chest X-ray varied. Many believe that ETT positioning could be improved with more precise ETT markings. *Conclusion*. Further research should focus on developing more effective guidelines for ETT tip placement in the ELBW infants.

1. Introduction

Endotracheal intubation is a common procedure in the NICU and accurate positioning of the endotracheal tube (ETT) is essential to prevent associated morbidity. This is applied more so in cases of extremely premature babies where the trachea is much shorter, leaving little margin for error. Given that the difference between extubations and bronchial intubation can be less than a couple of centimeters, it is not surprising that the staff performing an emergency intubation are likely to insert the ETT deeper than required in order to avoid the risk of inadvertent extubations, especially during ETT taping; however this does give rise to an increased risk of right main stem intubation.

Many formulae have been proposed in an attempt to accurately estimate the depth of insertion of the ETT in order to place it at the mid-tracheal position. These are not always accurate, in particular at the extremes of low gestational age (ELGA) or in SGA infants when using body weight derived formulae. Compounding factors such as activity level, securing mechanisms, and route of intubation may impact the likelihood of malposition.

One study suggested gestational age based guidelines for ETT depth estimation and confirmed a significant reduction in the need for repositioning and incidence of uneven lung expansion [1, 2]. This has now been incorporated by the European, New Zealand, Australian, and UK resuscitation councils as standard [3–5].

We conducted this survey to examine the beliefs and current practices across Canada in regard to endotracheal tube placement and to understand the challenges faced by current practices. We hypothesized that there would be wide variability in practices in how to determine ETT placements across Canada. The majority would be using the weight based guidelines for ETT depth estimation and finding the estimation of depth of insertion challenging especially in infants with a birth weight <750 g. Medical practitioners are likely to insert ETT deeper than T2 to avoid the risk of extubations. Most respondents would also prefer frequent measurement markings on the ETT as a guide to correct

TABLE 1: Representation of respondent.

Response	Percentage
Respiratory therapist	47.2%
Staff neonatologist	18.0%
Neonatology fellow	21.3%
Nurse practitioner	13.5%

TABLE 2: Ideal position of the ETT.

Response	Percentage
Upper trachea	3.9%
Mid-trachea	91.1%
Lower trachea	5.0%

TABLE 3: Ideal position on X-ray.

Response	Percentage
C7-T1	4.5%
T1-T2	34.7%
T2-T3	51.7%
T3-T4	5.1%
Unsure	4%

placement. The results of the survey developed should act as a needs assessment and serve as the basis for future work in addressing issues related to ETT placement in neonates especially in the ELGA infant.

2. Methods

A cross-sectional survey of a sample of health care professionals involved in neonatal intubations across Canada was performed. Research Ethics Board approval was obtained from the Hospital for Sick Children. Clinical directors in the Canadian Neonatal Network affiliated NICUs and Neonatal-Perinatal Program Directors were invited to participate in and disseminate the survey invitation to their staff including neonatologists, neonatal fellows, registered respiratory therapists (RRTs), and nurse practitioners (NPs). Consent was implied by participation. Email reminders were sent at three and five weeks after initial email invitation.

The questionnaire was web based with 35 close ended questions requiring approximately 15 minutes to answer. It was devised using a modified Delphi process with input from a variety of health care professionals representing the participating disciplines. A pilot survey was administered to representatives of these stakeholder groups and modifications to the questionnaire were made based on this feedback. The questions are placed under 6 headings: personal experience, unit experience, challenges in depth estimation, positioning of ETT, challenges in positioning, and complications of malposition as shown in the Appendix. The results were analyzed using simple descriptive statistics.

3. Results

The clinical directors were identified from Canadian Neonatal Network affiliated NICUs and Neonatal-Perinatal Programs across Canada. They were invited via email to participate in and disseminate the survey. A total of 207 responses were received of which 85.5% were completed.

The representation of the various professions within the respondents is outlined in Table 1, with highest number being from RRTs. Clinical experience ranged from <5 to >15 years. Most respondents (48%) performed between 5 and 14 intubations per year. Majority of respondents (86%) worked in Level 3 NICUs and (76%) in combined inborn and out born NICUs. Intubations were performed almost equally among different respondent groups except staff which were involved in only 46% of the intubations as reported.

3.1. Estimation of ETT Depth and Ideal ETT Position. The majority of respondents (87%) used "weight +6" formula

and "aim to black line" to estimate the depth of insertion of an oral ETT. Most respondents reported that they found the estimation of depth of insertion challenging in ELBW infants. Very few (22%) believed that the gestation age based guidelines may give better estimation of the depth of ETT insertion. Although the respondents (92%) identified mid-trachea as the ideal ETT tip position (Table 2), their preferred position on chest X-ray (CXR) varied considerably amongst them (Table 3). There was a wide variability of the reported practices (Table 4).

3.2. Complications of Malpositioning. Respondents felt that the most commonly seen complications of malpositioning were atelectasis (82%), differential air expansion (68%), unequal surfactant administration (61%), pneumothorax (29%), and PIE (14%).

Half of the respondents felt that more precise markings on the ETT would assist in better positioning of the ETT tip, although another 27% were unsure of the value. Most preferred markings every 5 mm.

4. Discussion

We found significant variability in the ETT placement practices across Canada. A few of the practices utilized could be further enhanced by having markings on ETT every 5 mm.

Endotracheal intubation is often performed in an emergent situation utilizing the weight based guide (weight +6) to estimate the insertion length of the ETT in order to be positioned mid trachea. Weight is often not available at the time of intubation at birth and a rough estimate is used to determine the insertion length. This is supplemented with the aim to position the black line of the ETT at the level of the vocal cords and produce bilateral equal air entry to guide its optimal placement. This has also been the recommendations of the American Academy of Pediatrics Neonatal Resuscitation Program without addressing the babies with birth weight less than 1000 gms [6].

Accurate positioning of the endotracheal tube (ETT) is essential to prevent associated morbidities, more so in cases of extreme premature babies where the trachea is much shorter, which leaves the clinicians with little margin for error.

TABLE 4: Preferred practices.

TABLE 4: Preferred practices.

Oral intubation	Unit (45%) transport (59%)
Premedication for elective/planned intubation	Always or almost always (combined 93%)
Methods to secure ETTs	(i) Tapes only (40%) (ii) Tape plus adhesive (i.e., tapes used with addition of adhesive like Mastisol to increase the adhesive strength) (38%) (iii) Sutures with tapes (11%) (iv) Adhesives with tapes and sutures (2%)
Other methods used for securing ETT	NeoBar, tapes with NeoBar, and NeoBridge
Point of measurement for an oral ETT	Upper lip (70%)
Confirming the ETT position	(i) 69% use 1 view (AP view) (ii) 77% also rely on auscultation of the breath sounds (iii) 19% also used other methods like end tidal co2 detectors, mist in the tube, chest rise, and clinical improvement
Reintubations (length same as before)	94% would not get an X-ray
Position of the head during the CXR	Neutral or midline (62%)
Analgesia/sedation during mechanical ventilation	Sometimes (66%)
Accidental extubations were reported	Occasionally by 76%
Knowledge about the level of the vocal cords and carina	Marked differences
Effects of flexion and extension on the ETT position	Marked differences
Auscultation of the bilateral breath sounds was not believed to rule out endobronchial intubations	70% agreed
Tube repositioning	(i) 81% felt the need to reposition the ETT sometimes (ii) T1-T2 26% will reposition (iii) T2-T3 7% did not reposition

Therefore, satisfactory positioning of the tip of ET tube on initial intubation is extremely important. Weight is not a good predictor of the upper airway distances as shown in a postmortem study on 24 infants ranging from 23-week gestation to term plus 8 weeks [7]. It has also been shown that aiming to black line may not be the appropriate method to guide the placement of the ETT at mid-trachea, since it may place ETT too low in some or too high in others [8]. Auscultation of the bilateral breath sounds by itself does not rule out endobronchial intubation in children [9]. Even if the weight +6 (rule of 7-8-9) is supplemented with aim to black line and auscultation of the bilateral breath sounds optimal ETT placements in neonates remain a great challenge.

Within the neonatal literature, there is limited data regarding the ideal placement of the ETT tip within the trachea. Many have defined this level as the 1st or 2nd thoracic vertebrae [1, 2, 7, 10, 11].

The newborn larynx is positioned higher in the neck, it extends from C3 to C5 and carina is situated between T3 and T5 and most commonly at T4 [10, 12, 13]. If this information is to be collated, then the midpoint of the airway would be somewhere between T1 and T2. Wong et al. in 2008 published that the sternal notch to the carina represents 60% of the vocal cord to the carina distance [14]. T1 is located just below the sternal notch; it can thus be assumed that T1-T2 is the midpoint of the airway (vocal cord to the carina).

Tracheal position is affected by both respiratory movements and changes in head position such that flexion of neck and expiration shortens the distance pushing the ETT tip towards the carina and extension of the neck and inspiration

retracts the ETT tip away from the carina [7]. Surprisingly we saw varied responses to the questions related to this. When extreme flexion or extension of the neck is expected after ETT insertion, the resultant change in the final position of ETT must be anticipated when deciding on the depth of ETT insertion. Rotschild et al. in 1991 suggested that the mid-tracheal position (midpoint of vocal cord to carina distance) is safe for both <1000 gm and >1000 gms infants based on 90th centile of changes in ETT position with maximum flexion and extension [7].

As the difference between extubations and bronchial intubation is only a matter of a couple of centimeters, more so in smaller babies, it is not surprising that the resident staff performing an emergency intubation are likely to insert the ETT deeper than required into the airway to avoid the risk of extubations with enhanced risk of right main stem intubation and/or atelectasis of right upper lobe of lung not to mention unilateral surfactant administration.

There has been no evidence to date that keeping the ETT tip between T1 and T2 is associated with the increase incidence of the unplanned extubations. On the contrary, T1-T2 has been reported as an ideal position for ETT tip [1, 2, 7, 10, 11].

The rule of 7-8-9 (weight +6) is universally followed to estimate the depth of an oral ETT to accurately place it at the mid-tracheal level. This rule was suggested by Tochen in 1979 who studied 40 neonates ranging from 26 to 44 weeks with the weight of 700–4100 grams and reference to T1-T2 as a mid-tracheal position. There were only ten babies under 1000 gms and none below 750 gms. They showed a linear relationship between tube length and weight with a correlation coefficient of 0.96 and assumed this even in babies <1000 gms [11]. Peterson et al. noticed that this rule predicted the tube length to be too long in infants below 750 gms but worked well for babies above this weight. Their study had just 5 infants between 750 and 1000 gms and just 16 infants above 3000 gms. They also used an incorrect landmark, with a point halfway between the inferior clavicle and carina on a chest radiograph as a mid-tracheal rather than T1-T2 [15]. Therefore, this rule may not apply in VLBW infants and in infants >2.5 kg. In babies with a weight <1000 grams, this rule overestimates the tube depth and may lead to complications related to malposition [1, 15]. In a published report the incidence of the ETT reposition after the initial placement in 23–26 weeks of gestation was 75% and of these 53% had uneven lung expansion. Weight based guidelines would result in the ETT length of 6.5–7 cms for infants of 500–1000 gms and this would include many infants of 23–27 weeks of gestation. This study suggested gestational age based guidelines for ETT depth estimation [2]. The same group validated these guidelines in a prospective audit and confirmed a significant reduction in the need for repositioning and incidence of uneven lung expansion [1]. ETT tip positioning although likely a minor but important contributor is worth consideration for the prevention of lung injury or bronchopulmonary dysplasia (BPD).

These gestational age based guidelines [2] have now been incorporated in the UK, Australian, and New Zealand Resuscitation Council recommendations [3, 4]. The American Academy of Pediatrics Neonatal Resuscitation Program recommends using vocal cord guide (aim to black line on ETT) to place the ETT approximately halfway between the vocal cords and the carina [6]. None of these guidelines specifically refers to T1-T2 as the ideal mid-tracheal position.

Most of the respondents also acknowledged that more precise marking on the ETT may help in better positioning of the ETT tube and prefer at least 5 mm markings. We strongly support this idea and feel this should be considered by the manufacturing companies.

5. Limitations

There are several limitations of this survey. The clinical directors and the Neonatal-Perinatal Program directors were approached to participate in and disseminate the survey to the specified groups working in their institute. We are unable to report the response rate as the exact number to whom the survey was sent out could not be ascertained and so the results may not represent all of the practices across Canada. However beliefs can form the basis of actions and the survey does highlight the issues related to challenges encountered in the ETT placement especially in the very preterm infant.

In conclusion, we noticed a wide variability in the beliefs related to ideal ETT placement across Canada. Our survey suggests that there is a real need for more research and consensus statement on the ideal position of the ETT with recognition that even a minor length difference may make a huge impact on the respiratory morbidity. Precise attention to

ETT securing methods and need for regular review including chest X-ray should also be considered part of regular monitoring to ensure correct positioning once placement is verified. Industry should consider more frequent markings on the ETT to aid in better placement.

Appendix

(1) Personal Experience

Question 1

What is your occupation?

○ Respiratory Therapist
○ Staff Neonatologist
○ Neonatology Fellow
○ Nurse Practitioner

Question 2

How many years of NICU experience do you have?

○ <5
○ 5–9 years
○ 10–14 years
○ >15 years

Question 3

On average how many intubations do you perform per year?

○ <5
○ 5–14
○ 15–25
○ >25

(2) Unit Experience

Question 4

What is the Level of your NICU?

☐ Level 1
☐ Level 2
☐ level 2 (advanced)
☐ Level 3

Question 5

Type of NICU?

☐ Inborn
☐ Outborn
☐ Both

Question 6

> Who routinely performs intubations in the unit? (tick all that apply)
>
> > □ Resident
> > □ Fellows
> > □ Staff (consultant)
> > □ Respiratory therapist
> > □ Nurse Practitioners
> > □ Other (specify) _____

Question 7

> What types of intubation are performed in your unit?
>
> > □ Predominantly oral
> > □ Predominantly nasal
> > □ Both

Question 8

> What type of intubations do you perform for neonatal transport?
>
> > □ Primarily oral
> > □ Primarily nasal

Question 9

> Do you premedicate for elective/planned intubations (e.g., opioid and/or muscle relaxation)?
>
> > □ Always
> > □ Almost always
> > □ Sometimes
> > □ Almost never
> > □ Never

Question 10

> How often do you use analgesia and/or sedation during mechanical ventilation?
>
> > □ Always
> > □ Almost always
> > □ Sometimes
> > □ Almost never
> > □ Never

Question 11

> How do you secure your ETTs?
>
> > □ Tapes only

> > □ Tape plus liquid adhesive (i.e., Mastisol).
> > □ Tapes plus suture through ETT.
> > □ Tapes, liquid adhesive (i.e., Mastisol) plus suture through ETT.
> > □ Other – please specify _____

Question 12

> In my unit, unintentional extubations are seen?
>
> > □ Often
> > □ Occasionally
> > □ Almost never
> > □ Never

(3) Challenges in Depth Estimation

Question 13

> How do you estimate the depth of insertion of an oral ETT? (tick all that apply)
>
> > □ Weight +6 cm
> > □ Gestational age estimate
> > □ Other weight estimate
> > □ Aim to black line
> > □ Other (specify) _____
> > □ Not applicable

Question 14

> How do you estimate depth of insertion for a nasal ETT? (tick all that apply)
>
> > □ Weight +7 cm
> > □ Gestational age estimate
> > □ Other weight estimate
> > □ Aim to black line
> > □ Other (specify) _____
> > □ Not applicable

Question 15

> I find estimating the depth of ETT insertion challenging in (tick all that apply)
>
> > □ Infants
> > □ 750–999 g
> > □ 1–1999 kg
> > □ 2-3 kg
> > □ >3 kg
> > □ None of the above
> > □ Unsure

Question 16

Do you think narrower gestational age calculations may give better estimation of the depth of ETT tube?

☐ Yes
☐ No
☐ Unsure

Question 17

More precise weight adjusted calculations for ETT depth estimation may be useful in (tick all that apply)

☐ Infants
☐ 750–999 g
☐ 1–1999 g
☐ 2-3 kg
☐ >3 kg
☐ None of above
☐ Unsure

(4) Positioning of ETT

Question 18

From what point do you calculate the oral ETT measurement?

☐ Upper Gum
☐ Upper Lip
☐ Others _____
☐ Not applicable

Question 19

Which do you think is a better point for measurement of an oral ETT?

☐ Upper Gum
☐ Upper Lip
☐ Others _____
☐ Not applicable

Question 20

What in your opinion is the ideal position of the ETT tip in a neonate?

☐ Upper Trachea
☐ Mid Trachea
☐ Lower Trachea

Question 21

The ideal position of the ETT tip on X-Ray is

☐ C7-T1
☐ T1-T2
☐ T2-T3
☐ T3-T4
☐ Unsure

Question 22

The Level of vocal cords in neonates is

☐ C3-C4
☐ C4-C5
☐ C5-C6
☐ C6-C7
☐ C7-T1
☐ Unsure

Question 23

The level of carina in a neonate is. (Tick all that applies)

☐ T3-T4
☐ T4-T5
☐ T3–T5 (mostly at T4)
☐ T5-T6
☐ T4–T6 (mostly at T5)
☐ Unsure

Question 24

Flexion of the neck

☐ Pushes the ETT down
☐ Pulls the ETT up
☐ Does not impact
☐ Unsure

Question 25

Extension of the neck

☐ Pushes the ETT down
☐ Pulls the ETT up
☐ Does not impact
☐ Unsure

Question 26

How do you confirm ETT position? (Tick all that applies)

☐ Chest X-ray – 2 views (AP & Lateral)
☐ Chest X-ray – 1 view (AP only)

☐ Chest X-ray 1 view (Lateral only)
☐ Ultrasound
☐ Auscultation of breath sounds
☐ Other (specify) _____

Question 27

How often do you perform a CXR after intubation?

☐ Always
☐ Almost always
☐ Almost never
☐ Never

Question 28

I do not perform a CXR post intubation if (tick all that apply)

☐ Air entry sounds equal
☐ Improvement in clinical status
☐ Colour change with Co2 detector
☐ Measurement appropriate by weight +6/7 rule
☐ Measurement appropriate by gestational age estimates
☐ Previously intubated and ETT measurement same

Question 29

Do you have specific head positional requirements for the infant during CXR

☐ Yes
☐ No
☐ If yes, please specify _____

Question 30

In my opinion auscultation of bilateral equal breath sounds rules out right mainbronchus intubation?
☐ Yes
☐ No
☐ Unsure

(5) Challenges in Positioning

Question 31

How often do you have to reposition your ETT after X-ray?
☐ Always
☐ Almost always

☐ Sometimes
☐ Almost never
☐ Never
☐ Unsure

Question 32

I would reposition the ETT if on the chest X-Ray it is at (tick all that apply)

☐ C7-T1
☐ T1-T2
☐ T2-T3
☐ T3-T4
☐ T5 and below

Question 33

Do you think better positioning of the ETT tip could be achieved with more precise markings on ETT (current markings every 10 mm)

☐ Yes
☐ No
☐ Unsure

Question 34

If yes, what markings would you prefer to see?

☐ Every 2 mm
☐ Every 5 mm
☐ Others, Please specify _____
☐ Not applicable

(6) Complication of Malpositioning

Question 35

Complications of ETT malpositioning I most commonly see are (tick all that apply)

☐ Unequal surfactant administration
☐ Differential Air expansion
☐ Atelectasis
☐ Pneumothorax
☐ PIE
☐ Others _____

Conflict of Interests

No external funding was secured. The authors have no financial relationships relevant to this paper and no conflict of interests to disclose.

Acknowledgment

The authors want to thank all the staff members of CNN NICUs who completed their survey.

References

[1] S. T. Kempley, J. W. Moreiras, and F. L. Petrone, "Endotracheal tube length for neonatal intubation," *Resuscitation*, vol. 77, no. 3, pp. 369–373, 2008.

[2] P. Mainie, A. Carmichaal, S. McCullough, and S. T. Kempley, "Endotracheal tube position in neonates requiring emergency inter-hospital transfer," *American Journal of Perinatology*, vol. 23, no. 2, pp. 121–124, 2006.

[3] Australian and New Zealand Resuscitation Council Guideline 13.5: Tracheal Intubation for Ventilation, 2010.

[4] Resuscitation Council (UK), "Tracheal intubation," in *Newborn Life Support*, chapter 13, 3rd edition, 2011.

[5] S. Richmond and J. Wyllie, "European Resuscitation Council Guidelines for Resuscitation 2010 Section 7. Resuscitation of babies at birth," *Resuscitation*, vol. 81, no. 10, pp. 1389–1399, 2010.

[6] J. Kattwinkel, *Neonatal Resuscitation*, American Academy of Pediatrics, 6th edition, 2011.

[7] A. Rotschild, D. Chitayat, M. L. Puterman, M. S. Phang, E. Ling, and V. Baldwin, "Optimal positioning of endotracheal tubes for ventilation of preterm infants," *The American Journal of Diseases of Children*, vol. 145, no. 9, pp. 1007–1012, 1991.

[8] R. Balu and P. Bustani, "Are we focusing on the wrong end of the neonatal endotracheal tube?" *Archives of Disease in Childhood*, vol. 95, article A89, 2010.

[9] S. T. Verghese, R. S. Hannallah, M. C. Slack, R. R. Cross, and K. M. Patel, "Auscultation of bilateral breath sounds does not rule out endobronchial intubation in children," *Anesthesia & Analgesia*, vol. 99, no. 1, pp. 56–58, 2004.

[10] M. P. Blayney and D. R. Logan, "First thoracic vertebral body as reference for endotracheal tube placement," *Archives of Disease in Childhood*, vol. 71, no. 1, pp. F32–F35, 1994.

[11] M. L. Tochen, "Orotracheal intubation in the newborn infant: a method for determining depth of tube insertion," *The Journal of Pediatrics*, vol. 95, no. 6, pp. 1050–1051, 1979.

[12] G. J. Noback, "The developmental topography of the larynx, trachea lungs in the fetus, new-born, infant and child," *American Journal of Diseases of Children*, vol. 26, no. 6, pp. 515–533, 1923.

[13] P. A. Hudgins, J. Siegel, I. Jacobs, and C. R. Abramowsky, "The normal pediatric larynx on CT and MR," *American Journal of Neuroradiology*, vol. 18, no. 2, pp. 239–245, 1997.

[14] D. T. Wong, H. Weng, E. Lam, H.-B. Song, and J. Liu, "Lengthening of the trachea during neck extension: which part of the trachea is stretched?" *Anesthesia & Analgesia*, vol. 107, no. 3, pp. 989–993, 2008.

[15] J. Peterson, N. Johnson, K. Deakins, D. Wilson-Costello, J. E. Jelovsek, and R. Chatburn, "Accuracy of the 7-8-9 rule for endotracheal tube placement in the neonate," *Journal of Perinatology*, vol. 26, no. 6, pp. 333–336, 2006.

42

IVIG Effects on Erythrocyte Sedimentation Rate in Children

Farhad Salehzadeh, Ahmadvand Noshin, and Sepideh Jahangiri

Pediatric Department, Bouali Hospital, Ardabil University of Medical Sciences (ARUMS), Ardabil 56157, Iran

Correspondence should be addressed to Farhad Salehzadeh; salehzadeh_f@yahoo.com

Academic Editor: Joel R. Rosh

Background. Erythrocyte sedimentation rate (ESR) is a valuable laboratory tool in evaluation of infectious, inflammatory, and malignant diseases. Red blood cells in outside from the body precipitate due to their higher density than the plasma. In this study we discuss the IVIG effect on ESR in different diseases and different ages. *Methods and Materials.* Fifty patients under 12 years old who had indication to receive IVIG enrolled in this study. Total dose of IVIG was 2 gr/kg (400 mg/kg in five days or 2 gr/kg in single dose). ESR before infusion of IVIG and within 24 hours after administration of the last dose of IVIG was checked. *Results.* 23 (46%) patients were males and 27 (54%) were females. The mean of ESR before IVIG was 31.8 ± 29.04 and after IVIG it was 47.2 ± 36.9; this difference was meaningful ($P = 0.05$). Results of ESR changes in different age groups, 6 patients less than 28 days, 13 patients from 1 month to 1 year, 20 patients from 1 to 6 years old, and 11 patients from 6 to 12 years have been meaningful ($P = 0.001$, $P = 0.025$, and $P = 0.006$, resp.). *Conclusion.* In patients who are receiving IVIG as a therapy, ESR increased falsely (noninflammatory rising); therefore use of ESR for monitoring of response to treatment may be unreliable. Although these results do not apply to neonatal group, we suggest that, in patients who received IVIG, interpretation of ESR should be used cautiously on followup.

1. Introduction

The erythrocyte sedimentation rate (ESR) is an acute phase reactant (APR). The rate of sedimentation in a period of one hour called ESR and also Biernacki test. ESR test is a common hematologic nonspecific indicator of inflammation. To perform a test, nonclothing blood is placed in a vertical tube (Westergren) and erythrocyte sedimentation rate is measured and is reported in units of mm/h [1].

The best way to test was presented in 1921 by Westergren, and it is still the golden standard method for measuring erythrocyte sedimentation rate. This method is considered to be [2] simple and cheap, accessible, and accurate [3]. ESR is a valuable laboratory tool in evaluation of infectious, inflammatory, and malignant diseases [1, 3]. Red blood cells in outside from the body precipitate due to their higher density than the plasma; in normal state these cells reject each other because of their negative surface charges and prevent Rolex formation. In order to overcome the negative charge of the red cells should be much stronger gravity. It is exerted by different types of plasma proteins [4].

It was shown that several factors such as PH levels of plasma other than the size of molecules or Rolex formation contribute to erythrocyte sedimentation [2]. ESR levels increase with age and are higher in women [1, 4, 5], anemia, and the black people. Clinical factors that do not influence the ESR are [1, 4] obesity, body temperature, recent food, and NSAID [1, 4, 5].

IVIG with the half-life of 3-4 weeks was first produced in 1960 [6, 7]; IVIG in high doses is used for the treatment of many autoimmune diseases including autoimmune thrombocytopenia, chronic inflammatory polyneuropathy, Kawasaki disease, and Guillain-Barré syndrome [7–9].

High-dose IVIG effects on various proteins, including inflammatory profiles in 63 children with Kawasaki disease, were studied. All children had clinical manifestations of Kawasaki and received 2 gr/kg IVIG and aspirin during 12 hr. serial testing was carried out before receiving IVIG, 24 hours and 7 days later.

After IVIG infusion, total WBC and neutrophils were decreased, whereas lymphocytes were increased. Mean ESR was 12.7 ± 6.46 mm/h before receiving IVIG, 53.3 ± 11.9 mm/h

TABLE 1: Patients profile.

Patient	Disease	Age	Sex	ESR before IVIG	ESR after IVIG
1	Icter	4 days	M	9	32
2	Icter	2 days	F	7	10
3	Icter	2 days	F	72	61
4	Icter	2 days	M	2	95
5	Icter	10 days	M	24	28
6	Icter	4 days	M	2	2
7	ITP	35 days	F	5	12
8	ITP	2 months	M	42	75
9	Sepsis	50 days	M	6	15
10	ITP	2 months and 5 days	F	47	117
11	ITP	2 months	M	16	56
12	ITP	4 months and 19 days	M	5	8
13	ITP	17 months	M	5	95
14	Sepsis	7.5 months	F	52	65
15	Fever resistant	8 months	F	17	89
16	Kawasaki	10 months	M	54	97
17	Kawasaki	1 year	M	90	112
18	ITP	1 year	F	65	91
19	ITP	1 year	F	12	17
20	GBS	14 months	F	89	120
21	Pneumonia + brain tumor	15 months	F	137	105
22	GBS	1.5 year	M	18	23
23	ITP	1.5 year	M	45	72
24	ITP	2.5 years	F	10	27
25	Epilepsy resistant	2.5 years	M	2	7
26	Epilepsy resistant	2.5 years	M	4	4
27	Bulbar palsy + cyanosis	2 years and 6 months	M	21	71
28	Epilepsy resistant	2 years and 11 months	F	2	5
29	ITP	3 years	F	14	28
30	ITP	3 years	F	6	17
31	Kawasaki	3 years and 4 months	M	115	85
32	Aplastic anemia + fever	4 years	F	77	77
33	GBS	4 years	M	33	62
34	Encephalitis	4 years and 6 months	F	16	33
35	ADEM + fever	5 years	F	3	22
36	Brain atrophy + epilepsy	5 years and 4 months	M	4	18
37	Encephalitis	5 years and 7 months	M	33	33
38	SLE + thrombocytopenia	6 years	F	24	44
39	Steven Johnson	6 years	M	8	13
40	ITP	7 years	F	18	31
41	GBS	7 years	M	43	64
42	Vasculitis	7 years	F	48	79
43	ITP	8 years	F	20	27
44	ITP	8 years	F	23	32
45	Bruton	10 years	M	2	4
46	Bruton	10 years	M	3	2
47	ITP	11 years and 4 months	M	10	15
48	ITP	11 years and 7 months	F	7	21
49	Dawn + pancytopenia	12 years	M	75	121
50	ITP	12 years and 7 months	M	10	23

TABLE 2: Mean and median of ESR.

Patients	Mean ESR		SD		P	Median	
	Before	After	Before	After		Before	After
50	31.8	47.2	29.04	36.9	0.05	16.5	32

TABLE 3: Different ages variation.

Age	Number	Before IVIG	After IVIG	P value
0-1 month	6	27.03 ± 19.33	38 ± 34.6	$P = 0.28$
1 month–1 year	13	32 ± 27.9	65.3 ± 39.9	$P = 0.001$
1 year–6 years	20	39.8 ± 33	43.3 ± 34.5	$P = 0.025$
6 years–12 years	11	23.5 ± 22.7	38 ± 35.9	$P = 0.006$

in 24 h, and 48.8 ± 15.2 mm/h in the 7 days after the IVIG infusion. Protein levels which are associated with systemic inflammation except ESR decreased after 24 hours.

IgA and IgM immunoglobulin levels did not change 24 hours and 7 days after injection; however, IgG is significantly increased. The result is that the high dose of IVIG leads to rapid decreased changes of various proteins except for IgA and IgM and ESR [10].

In the same study on patients with myasthenia gravis and Guillain-Barré syndrome, similar results were obtained [11]. In this study we discuss the IVIG effect on ESR in different diseases and ages. We try to answer this question too, is ESR a valuable APR marker in evaluation of inflammatory response to treatment when IVIG is used previously?

2. Method and Materials

This is an analytical descriptive and cross-sectional study.

Fifty patients who had indication to receive IVIG enrolled in this study. Total dose of IVIG was 2 gr/kg (400 mg/kg in five days or 2 gr/kg in single dose). ESR before infusion of IVIG and within 24 hours after administration of the last dose of IVIG was checked (1-2 gr/kg/12 h or 400 mg/kg dose IVIG). Brand name for the IVIG was OCTAPHARMA AG, Lachen, Switzerland.

The erythrocyte sedimentation rate was measured by Westergren method; IVIG side effects were not observed in any patient. Results have been shown in different age groups, neonatal, infancy, childhood, and school age.

SPSS 16 and paired t-test were used to statistical software analysis; significance level of less than 0.05 was considered meaningful. Consent confirmed was obtained from parents of patients.

3. Results

23 (46%) patients were males and 27 (54%) were females (Table 1). The mean and median ESR before and after receiving IVIG have been shown in Table 2. The mean of ESR before IVIG was 31.8 ± 29.04 and after IVIG was 47.2 ± 36.9; this difference was meaningful ($P = 0.05$). In male group the mean ESR before IVIG was 34.6 ± 33.5 and after IVIG was 49.1 ± 36.2; the difference with ($P = 0.003$) is statistically

significant. Before receiving IVIG the mean ESR was 29.4 ± 25.2 in females and after receiving IVIG it was 45.6 ± 38.04; this difference with ($P = 0.001$) is significant. Results of different age groups, 6 patients less than 28 days, 13 patients from 1 month to 1 year, 20 patients from 1 to 6 years old, and 11 patients from 6 to 12 years, have been shown in Table 3.

4. Discussion

ESR is known as an important factor in the evaluation of infectious and inflammatory processes. [2, 4]. Important point for the use of the ESR as an APR is its role in the evaluation of response to treatment; decreasing levels of ESR are considered as a marker of response to therapy.

Plasma fibrinogen and globulins are the major factors affecting ESR [1, 2]. Fibrinogen is the strongest aggregator [2]. And its concentration in the blood is directly related to the rate of ESR [1]. Alpha and gamma globulin provide half the ability of fibrinogen and albumin has the lowest ability in the sediment of red cells.

However, as mentioned, IVIG as an intravenous immune globulin is used in many diseases [6, 7]. Whether the administration of IVIG, influences the ESR value in monitoring of the response to therapy?

In review of the literature generally two studies were found about the effect of IVIG on ESR. One of them has been done on Kawasaki patients and has discussed numerous parameters of protein and also ESR affected by IVIG [10] and the subsequent study has been limited to patients with myasthenia gravis and Guillain-Barré syndrome showing numerous parameters and blood ESR affected by IVIG [11], but this study has discussed 16 different diseases following the administration of IVIG and has focused on the changes in ESR.

IVIG as an immunoglobulin, mostly IgG [7], has aggregator effect on red cells and prevents their negative discharge forces [2]. Although IVIG has many anti-inflammatory effects [7] and it is expected to reduce ESR rate, in vivo its biologic effect is more effective than the immune modulation effect.

The mean ESR was 31.8 ± 29.04 before receiving IVIG and after IVIG it was 47.2 ± 36.9, with significant differences ($P \leq 0.05$).

These changes were statistically significant in both sexes; it could be interpreted because of lack of physiologic difference in children.

In different age groups except the neonatal period, 1 month to 1 year (13 patients), 1 to 6 years (20 patients), 6 to 12 years (11 patients), the mean ESR before IVIG and after receiving IVIG increased with significant differences; P values were, respectively, $P = 0.001$, $P = 0.025$, and $P = 0.006$.

Rapid physiological changes in various neonatal plasma proteins such as albumin and fibrinogen are the variables leading to these results [12]. Different immune regulatory functions of IVIG through its interaction with innate and adaptive immune system and immune homeostasis in neonatal period could be another reason [13].

Among the APR, the ESR is the most valuable criteria for evaluating and monitoring of response to inflammation [1]; on the basis of this study on patients who are receiving IVIG as a therapy, ESR increased falsely (noninflammatory rising); therefore use of ESR for monitoring of response to treatment may not be reliable.

Based on the knowledge of authors and review of the literature this study seems to be the only work about ESR and IVIG administration effect in children. Although these results do not apply to neonatal group we suggest that, in patients who receive IVIG, interpretation of ESR should be used cautiously on the followup process.

Conflict of Interests

The authors declare that there is no conflict of interests regarding the publication of this paper.

References

[1] M. L. Brigden, "Clinical utility of the erythrocyte sedimentation rate," *The American Family Physician*, vol. 60, no. 5, pp. 1443–1450, 1999.

[2] E. Susana and T. B. Booker, "Erythrocyte sedimentation rate from folklore to facts," *The American Journal of Medicine*, vol. 78, no. 6, part 1, pp. 1001–1009, 1985.

[3] C. L. Altergott, M. A. Letouneau, M. K. O'Connor, C. Vance, L. S. Chan, and N. Schonfeld-Warden, "Early determination of ESR: how accurate is it?" *Archives of Pediatrics and Adolescent Medicine*, vol. 157, no. 5, pp. 487–489, 2003.

[4] M. A. Hameed and S. Waqas, "Physiological basis and clinical utility of erythrocyte sedimentation rate," *Pakistan Journal of Medical Sciences*, vol. 22, no. 2, pp. 214–218, 2006.

[5] M. Plebani and E. Piva, "Erythrocyte sedimentation rate: use of fresh blood for quality control," *The American Journal of Clinical Pathology*, vol. 117, no. 4, pp. 621–626, 2002.

[6] J. A. Hooper, "Intravenous immunoglobulins: evolution of commercial IVIG preparations," *Immunology and Allergy Clinics of North America*, vol. 28, no. 4, pp. 765–778, 2008.

[7] M. Ballow, "Mechanisms of action of intravenous immune serum globulin therapy," *Pediatric Infectious Disease Journal*, vol. 13, no. 9, pp. 806–811, 1994.

[8] S. C. Jordan, M. Toyoda, and A. A. Vo, "Intravenous immunoglobulin a natural regulator of immunity and inflammation," *Transplantation*, vol. 88, no. 1, pp. 1–6, 2009.

[9] D. J. Hamrock, "Adverse events associated with intravenous immunoglobulin therapy," *International Immunopharmacology*, vol. 6, no. 4, pp. 535–542, 2006.

[10] K.-Y. Lee, H.-S. Lee, J.-H. Hong, J.-W. Han, J.-S. Lee, and K.-T. Whang, "High-dose intravenous immunoglobulin downregulates the activated levels of inflammatory indices except erythrocyte sedimentation rate in acute stage of Kawasaki disease," *Journal of Tropical Pediatrics*, vol. 51, no. 2, pp. 98–101, 2005.

[11] G. Karlikaya, G. Yuksel, B. Yildirim, C. Orken, and H. Tireli, "Intravenous immunglobulin treatment: the effect on different hematological and biochemical parameters," *Journal of Neurological Sciences*, vol. 24, no. 2, pp. 104–108, 2007.

[12] V. Ignjatovic, C. Lai, R. Summerhayes et al., "Age-related differences in plasma proteins: How plasma proteins change from neonates to adults," *PLoS ONE*, vol. 6, no. 2, Article ID e17213, 2011.

[13] S. V. Kaveri, "Intravenous immunoglobulin: exploiting the potential of natural antibodies," *Autoimmunity Reviews*, vol. 11, no. 11, pp. 792–794, 2012.

43

Community-Acquired Rotavirus Gastroenteritis Compared with Adenovirus and Norovirus Gastroenteritis in Italian Children: A Pedianet Study

D. Donà,[1] E. Mozzo,[1] A. Scamarcia,[2] G. Picelli,[3] M. Villa,[3] L. Cantarutti,[2] and C. Giaquinto[1]

[1]*Division of Paediatric Infectious Diseases, Department of Woman and Child Health, University of Padua, Padua, Italy*
[2]*Pedianet Project, Padua, Italy*
[3]*Epidemiology Service, Local Health Authority of Cremona, Cremona, Italy*

Correspondence should be addressed to D. Donà; daniele.dona@studenti.unipd.it

Academic Editor: Raymond J. Hutchinson

Background. Rotavirus (RV) is the commonest pathogen in the hospital and primary care settings, followed by Adenovirus (AV) and Norovirus (NV). Only few studies that assess the burden of RV gastroenteritis at the community level have been carried out. *Objectives.* To estimate incidence, disease characteristics, seasonal distribution, and working days lost by parents of RV, AV, and NV gastroenteritis leading to a family pediatrician (FP) visit among children < 5 years. *Methods.* 12-month, observational, prospective, FP-based study has been carried out using Pedianet database. *Results.* RVGE incidence was 1.04 per 100 person-years with the highest incidence in the first 2 years of life. Incidences of AVGEs (1.74) and NVGEs (1.51) were slightly higher with similar characteristics regarding age distribution and symptoms. Risk of hospitalisation, access to emergency room (ER), and workdays lost from parents were not significantly different in RVGEs compared to the other viral infections. *Conclusions.* Features of RVGE in terms of hospitalisation length and indirect cost are lower than those reported in previous studies. Results of the present study reflect the large variability of data present in the literature. This observation underlines the utility of primary care networks for AGE surveillance and further studies on community-acquired gastroenteritis in children.

1. Introduction

Worldwide, acute gastroenteritis (AGE) is the third most common cause of death in children < 5 years of age [1]. In European children, only few deaths occur as a consequence of AGE; however, diarrhoea has a considerable impact on the quality of life of children and their families [2]. Rotavirus (RV) is the leading cause of severe dehydration in children < 5 years of age [3–5].

In the European Union (EU), it is estimated that 3.6 million episodes of RV gastroenteritis (RVGE) occur annually. RVGE is estimated to occur at a rate of 1 symptomatic infection in every 7 children each year, accounting for 231 deaths, more than 87000 hospitalisations, and almost 700000 outpatient visits. It has been estimated that RV accounts for 39% diarrheal hospitalisations [6] and from 25.3% to 63.5%

of community-acquired AGE in children < 5 years of age [7–11]. These rates vary greatly depending on whether patients are seen in the hospital, emergency room, or primary care physician clinic.

Most RV infections are community-acquired and transmitted by the fecal-oral route [12] and peak in the winter season between November and February in temperate climates [4, 13, 14].

RVGE imposes a heavy economic burden by incurring not only direct (consultation, emergency, hospitalisation, and medication) costs, but also indirect costs (parent workdays lost, childcare, etc.) [12, 15, 16]. In Europe, it has been associated with direct medical costs per patient ranging from $1942 to $2389. Indirect costs including workdays lost by parents of children hospitalised for RVGE as well as out-of-pocket expenses ranged between $260 and $1061 (UK).

A portion of indirect costs was attributed to workdays lost by parents per hospitalisation episode, which varied between 2.3 days and 6.4 days [17].

Since the two RV vaccines became available, a monovalent RV vaccine (Rotarix, GlaxoSmithKline, Rixensart, Belgium) and a pentavalent RV vaccine (RV5, RotaTeq, Merck and Co., Whitehouse Station, NJ, USA; Sanofi Pasteur MSD, Lyon, France), the frequency of RVGE decreased [18], while other pathogens are now reported more frequently. The Italian Society of Pediatrics [19] supports the RV vaccination but this has not been included yet in the national immunization program. However, because the Italian National Health Service is decentralized, regions can include vaccines not nationally recommended in their immunization program.

Moreover, from 2008 into Veneto Region, setting of this study, all mandatory childhood vaccinations have been suspended. Until now, no local data on rotavirus vaccination coverage are available and it is estimated to be very low since rotavirus vaccination is not free of charge like other vaccinations.

The majority of non-RVGEs are usually AGEs associated with Adenovirus (AV) and Norovirus (NV) [20–25]. Also AV gastroenteritis (AVGE) and NV gastroenteritis (NVGE) are predominantly presenting during winter months [26, 27].

Adenovirus (AV), initially recognized as a cause of respiratory disease, is associated also with gastrointestinal, ophthalmological, and neurological infections [28]. The prevalence of AVGE is variable, ranging from 16% to 3.5% [22, 29, 30]. Watery, nonbloody diarrhoea typically precedes vomiting and children admitted to the hospital for AVGE are more likely to present diarrhoea that usually lasts more than in RVGE (more than 5 days) [31, 32].

NV represents the most common cause of gastroenteritis outbreaks and causes acute, self-limiting gastroenteritis in people from all age groups [33].

Three US country surveillances during 2009-2010 showed that 17% of faecal specimens from children (<5 years) hospitalised with gastroenteritis, 23% from children seen in emergency departments, and 28% from children seen in other outpatient settings were positive for NV [34]. Vomiting tends to be more prominent symptom in NVGE gastroenteritis than in other types of viral AGE. Usually, NVGE has milder symptoms than those of RVGE but a higher attack rate, due to its unusual stability outside the host and the low dose needed to produce symptomatic infection [35].

There are limited data on the incidence of AGE pathogens in the primary care setting. In particular, there is an absence of long-term data, per age group on the proportion on RVGE, AVGE, and NVGE among AGE in this setting. This is due to the fact that no systematic testing for RV, AV, and NV is needed in the primary care setting for the children management.

In Italy, the pediatric primary health care level is usually the family pediatrician (FP). We used the *Pedianet* network of family pediatricians (http://www.pedianet.it) to collect data and understand the disease burden of community-acquired RGVE, AVGE, and NVGE. The burden of AGE disease was also analyzed in terms of social impact for the families estimating the indirect cost caused by workdays lost.

Aims. The primary aim of this study was

(i) to estimate the incidence of RVGE leading to a FP visit among children < 60 months (5 years) of age in a well-defined Italian population.

The secondary aim of this study was

(i) to estimate the incidence of NVGE and AVGE leading to a FP visit among children < 60 months of age in a well-defined Italian population;

(ii) to determine the age of the children, seasonal distribution, and disease severity of RVGE, NVGE, and AVGE among children < 60 months;

(iii) to compare the outcomes in RV, NV, and AV positive and negative children with AGE;

(iv) to estimate the medical and societal burdens of RVGE, AVGE, and NVGE on FPs practice and families.

2. Material and Methods

This observational, prospective, FP-based study used an established Italian network (*Pedianet*) covering a well-defined number of patients (i.e., those registered by each individual FP) in the Veneto Region of Italy.

Surveillance was conducted for 12 months from May 2010 to April 2011 (including a full RV season, 2010-2011) to assess disease incidence rates, disease age distribution, disease severity, seasonal variations in disease burden, and costs of viral AGE.

2.1. Study Setting. The city of Padua and nearby residential town where about 16000 children < 60 months (5 years) are living has been chosen. A number of FPs following between 7000 and 10000 children < 60 months of age were involved in the study.

All children < 5 years of age from the defined population who presented at the selected FP sites with AGE (as defined below) were included in the study.

A child was considered eligible for the study if she/he met the following criteria:

(i) A male or female child < 60 months (5 years) of age at the time of the FP visit.

(ii) Child belonging to the population under surveillance selected for the study (served by the FP sites selected for the study).

(iii) Child brought to FP for AGE during the study period.

(iv) Written informed consent by parent/guardian of subject.

The following were considered exclusion criteria:

(i) Children aged > 60 months (5 years).

(ii) Previously diagnosed chronic gastrointestinal tract disease where symptoms were similar to those of AGE.

(iii) Known nosocomially acquired RVGE.

(iv) No written informed consent.

(v) Children not living permanently in the study area.

Their parents/guardians were asked to consent to participate and to have a stool sample collected and tested.

An RVGE, AVGE, and NVGE case was defined as an AGE case (corresponding to the AGE case clinical definition) with RV, AV, or NV positive detection by PCR.

The database used for the analysis contains all and only the AGE cases enrolled for this study.

Incidence of AGE cases has been described as both number of cases and rate. Such figures will be stratified by age group at onset and calendar month of onset.

The database used for the analysis included data about patients' age, gender, RV vaccination, and AGE signs and symptoms (such as fever > 38°C, vomit, abdominal pain, convulsion, lethargy, and dehydration).

For every episode also the following were collected:

(i) Length of the episode.

(ii) In case the AGE led to hospitalisation: the length of stay in hospital and hospitalisation diagnosis (ICD-9).

(iii) If AGE led to emergency room (ER): the number of ER access times.

(iv) In case of similar disease among family members: if father/mother had to take days off work and the number of days of work lost.

Data included in the *Pedianet* database followed all the Italian privacy regulations and laws.

Patients providing data to *Pedianet* and stool samples for the present study had to give informed consent before their anonymous information could be included in the dataset.

2.2. Statistical Analysis. Incidence rates of RVGE, AVGE, and NVGE were calculated as the ratio between cases and person-time.

Person-time was calculated as the average of the total population aged less than 60 months (5 years), registered with the FPs enrolled for the study, at the beginning and the end of the surveillance period. Poisson exact 95% confidence intervals will be calculated.

RVGE, AVGE, and NVGE incidence rates were stratified by age of the children and month of onset. Age-specific incidence rates were calculated as the ratio between the number of cases that occurred in the age group and the person-time contributed by the children of the age group. Month-specific incidence rates were calculated as the ratio between the number of cases that occurred in that given month and the total person-time.

Rates of hospitalisations were compared by means of logistic regression, adjusted by age. Hospitalisation will be the dependent variable and RVGE (or AVGE or NVGE, resp.) the "exposure." The role (as confounders) of the characteristics reported at baseline will be investigated entering such variables in the models. The logistic regression will produce an estimate of the odds ratio of the risk of hospitalisation.

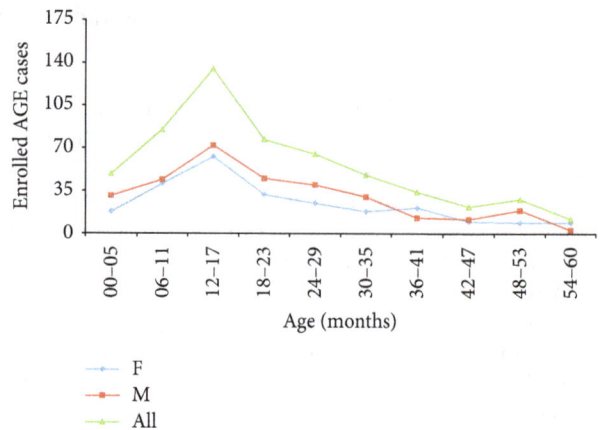

Figure 1: Age distribution of the cohort of children with AGE.

The same approach was used to compare the access to the ER as well as the combined event "hospitalisation or ER."

Comparison of length of stay in hospital was carried out by means of t-tests.

In order to estimate societal costs due to RV, AV, and NV, new variables were built which combine parents' absence from work (WORK_ABS and DAYS_ABS). WORK_ABS were used in the logistic models described in the previous paragraph whereas DAYS_ABS were compared through t-tests.

The cases for which the stool sample was not taken (or not processed by the lab) were excluded from the analysis. However, the number of such cases will be reported.

3. Results

3.1. Description of Study Population. Twelve FPs were included in the analysis accounting for 7239 person-years.

Five hundred fifty-five children < 60 months (5 years) of age presented at the selected FP sites with AGE, with 55,6% ($n = 309$) being male. The age distribution showed a peak between 6 and 18 months of age. Children < 24 months of age accounted for 62% of cases (Figure 1).

Two hundred fifty-two (45%), 269 (48%), and 362 (65%) cases over 555 children with gastroenteritis reported fever > 38°C, vomiting, and abdominal pain at enrolment, respectively. Only 3 cases (0.005%) reported convulsion and 17 cases (0.03%) presented with lethargy. The majority of children (82%) presented with no dehydration and 16% with mild (0–5%) and only 2% with moderate (5–10%) dehydration.

Only 3 children with gastroenteritis (0.5%) were vaccinated against rotavirus.

Collection of stool sample was performed in 460 (83%) of gastroenteritis cases.

3.2. Primary Endpoint

3.2.1. Incidence of RVGE. Seventy-five cases resulted in being positive to rotavirus. None of them was vaccinated against RV. Estimated incidence rate was 1.04 per 100 person-years (95% CI: 0.81–1.30).

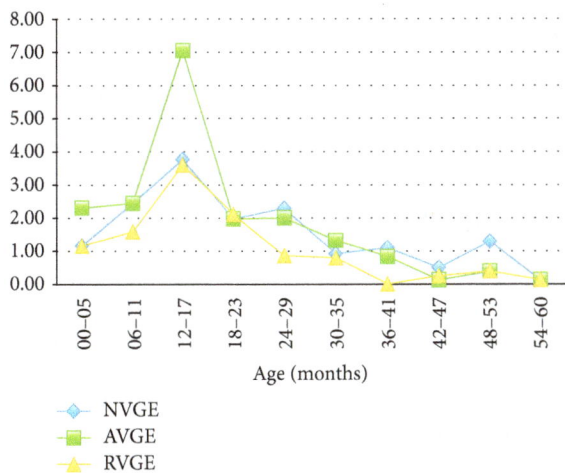

FIGURE 2: Incidence of AGE by age at onset.

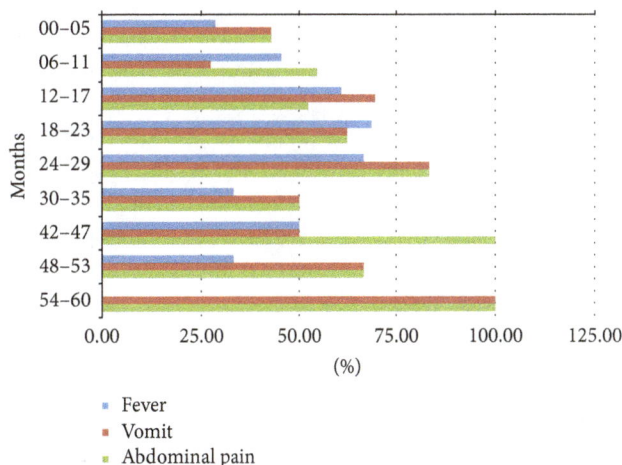

FIGURE 3: Distribution of fever, vomit, and abdominal pain during RVGE episodes stratified by age.

3.3. Secondary Endpoint

3.3.1. Incidence of Adenovirus and Norovirus. One hundred twenty-six cases resulted in being positive to AV (two of them were vaccinated against RV) with an estimated incidence rate of 1.74 per 100 person-years (95% CI: 1.45–2.07) while 109 cases resulted in being positive to NV (one of them was vaccinated against RV) with an incidence rate of 1.51 per 100 person-years (95% CI: 1.24–1.82).

3.3.2. Age of Children, Seasonal Distribution, and Diseases Severity of RVGE, AVGE, and NVGE. RVGE incidence was higher in the first 23 months of life with the higher incidence (3.60) in the range from 12 to 17 months. AVGE and NVGE mostly occurred in children < 41 and 29 months of life, respectively, with the same peak from 12 to 17 months of age.

Incidence by month of onset showed higher values for RVGE in November and from January to April, for AVGE from October to December, and for NVGE from October to June (Figure 2).

Association with fever > 38°C, vomit, and abdominal pain was present in 58%, 59%, and about 59% of cases, respectively. Distribution of symptoms during RVGE episodes is shown in (Figure 3). Convulsion occurred only in 1.3% of cases at enrolment, exclusively in young children from 6 to 11 months of age. Other neurological signs as lethargy occurred in 4% of cases, affecting children aged 6–17 months.

In AVGE group, association with fever > 38°C was present in about 44% of cases, vomiting in about 51% of cases, and abdominal pain in 61%. Neurological signs as convulsion and lethargy occurred in 0.8 and 1.6% of AVGE, respectively.

Fever occurred in 42% of cases, vomiting in about 62% of cases, and abdominal pain in 68% of patients affected by NVGE. Neurological signs as convulsion and lethargy occurred in 0.9 and 2.8% of NVGE, respectively.

Fifty-four of RVGE cases (72%) were with no dehydration. Mild dehydration was reported only in about 27% of children. Children from 0 to 5 months did not experience

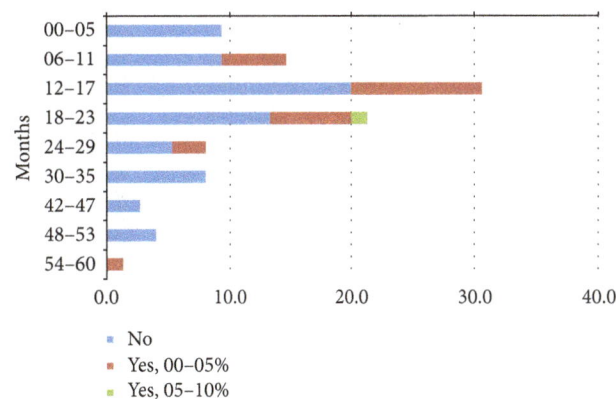

FIGURE 4: Distribution of dehydration during RVGE episodes stratified by age.

dehydration. Only 1 child aged 18–23 months (1%) over the total of cases had moderate dehydration (Figure 4).

Mild dehydration occurred in about 18.3% of AVGE cases and 20% of NVGE cases. Moderate dehydration at enrolment occurred in 1.6% of AVGE and 0.9% of NVGE.

All these symptom and signs occurred independently of the age of children.

3.3.3. Comparison between Outcomes in RV, AV, and NV Positive and Negative Children with AGE. None of 3 children vaccinated against rotavirus developed RVGE.

Mean length of all AGE episodes was 5.21 days (95% CI 4.94–5.47): 5.42 days (95% CI 5.53–4.78) for RVGE cases, 5.41 days for AVGE episodes, and 5.70 days for NVGE (Table 1).

Thirty-five cases of AGE needed admission to emergency room (ER); 7 of these cases were RVGE (20.0%). The mean number of access times to ER, restricted to all AGE cases that accessed the ER, was 1.09 with a mean of 1.14 access times for RVGE episodes. The proportion of AVGE cases that needed access to ER was 7 over 35 (20.0%) total cases with a mean number of access times to ER, restricted to cases that accessed

TABLE 1: Mean length of RVGE, AVGE, and NVGE episodes.

| | RVGE | | | | | AVGE | | | | | NVGE | | | | | All | |
| | No | | | Yes | | | No | | | Yes | | | No | | | Yes | | | | |
	Mean	95% CI		Mean	95% CI		Mean	95% CI		Mean	95% CI		Mean	95% CI		Mean	95% CI		Mean	95% CI
00–05 months	5.37	4.33	6.41	4.57	1.91	7.23	5.29	3.98	6.59	5.14	3.93	6.36	5.11	4.06	6.17	5.86	3.5	8.21	5.24	4.31	6.17
06–11 months	5.4	4.64	6.15	6.45	3.09	9.82	5.4	4.54	6.27	6.06	4.2	7.92	5.23	4.36	6.09	6.65	4.86	8.44	5.55	4.78	6.33
12–17 months	5.59	4.91	6.28	5.65	4.33	6.97	5.48	4.71	6.25	5.84	4.81	6.88	5.55	4.89	6.22	5.79	4.3	7.28	5.6	5	6.2
18–23 months	4.69	4.17	5.2	5.5	3.79	7.21	4.83	4.17	5.48	5.07	4.05	6.08	4.56	4.08	5.04	6	4.16	7.84	4.88	4.33	5.43
24–36 months	4.56	4.06	5.07	5.17	3.2	7.14	4.55	3.99	5.1	4.92	3.78	6.05	4.38	3.89	4.86	5.48	4.07	6.89	4.64	4.15	5.13
36–60 months	5.24	4.56	5.92	5.33	3.75	6.91	5.37	4.64	6.09	4.55	3.58	5.51	5.42	4.59	6.24	4.87	3.94	5.8	5.25	4.62	5.88
All	5.14	4.87	5.42	5.53	4.78	6.29	5.13	4.83	5.44	5.41	4.9	5.92	5.06	4.77	5.35	5.7	5.11	6.29	5.21	4.94	5.47

ER admissions

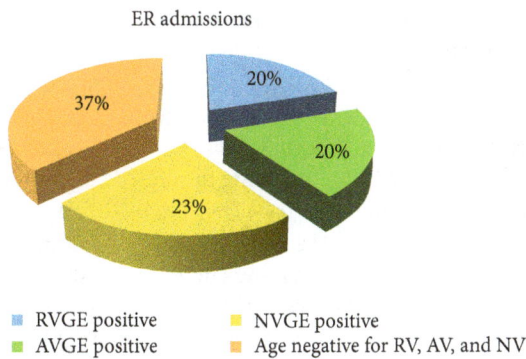

FIGURE 5: Comparison between ER access times during RVGE, AVGE, and NVGE episodes.

Hospitalisations

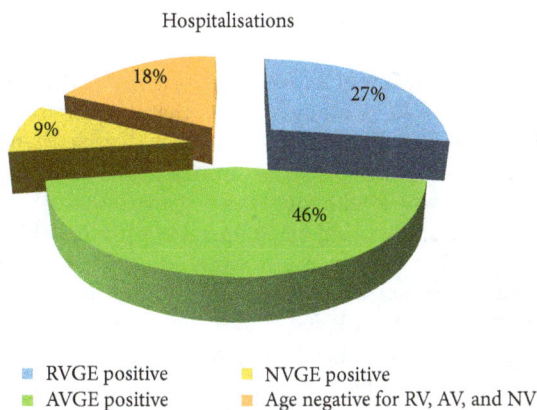

FIGURE 6: Comparison between hospitalisations during RVGE, AVGE, and NVGE episodes.

the ER, of 1.14. The proportion of NVGE cases that needed access to ER was 8 over 35 (22.8%) total cases with a mean number of access times to ER, restricted to cases that accessed the ER, of 1.13 (Figure 5).

Hospitalisation occurred in 12 cases (2.54%) of all AGE cases and only 3 cases (25.0%) were RV positive (aged 6–17 months). Of 12 hospitalised children, 5 were AVGE (41.7%) and only 1 was a NVGE (8.3%) (Figure 6).

Mean length of hospital stay for all AGE cases was 1.08 days with shorter hospitalisation length for RVGE cases (0.67 days) whereas for AVGE it was 1.80 days and for NVGE, restricted to cases hospitalised, it was zero days.

All AGE cases hospitalised or that needed access to ER were 40 (17.5%) cases of RVGE, 9 (22.5%) cases of AVGE, and 8 (20.0%) cases of NVGE.

3.3.4. RVGE. The comparisons between children who tested RV positive and those who tested RV negative showed an Age-Adjusted Mantel-Haenszel Relative Risk of hospitalisation of 1.857 (95% CI: 0.494–6.981) and a RR of ER access of 1.299 (95% CI: 0.588–2.871) with logistic regression RR of 1.145 (95% CI: 0.453–2.891). The Age-Adjusted Mantel-Haenszel RR comparing the rates of the combined event

"hospitalisation or ER access" was 1.100 (95% CI: 0.505–2.397) and the logistic regression RR was 1.003 (95% CI: 0.406–2.473).

t-test comparing the hospitalisation lengths showed no statistically significant difference in RVGE admissions.

3.3.5. AVGE and NVGE. The comparisons between children who tested AV positive and those who tested AV negative and children who tested NV positive and those who tested NV negative showed an Age-Adjusted Mantel-Haenszel Relative Risk of hospitalisation of 1.623 (95% CI: 0.560–4.698) and a RR of ER access of 0.640 (95% CI: 0.290–1.412) with logistic regression RR of 0.629 (95% CI: 0.257–1.536) for AVGE and an Age-Adjusted Mantel-Haenszel Relative Risk of hospitalisation of RR = 0.301 (95% CI: 0.039–2.307) and a RR of ER access of 1.005 (95% CI: 0.477–2.116) with logistic regression RR of 1.055 (95% CI: 0.451–2.464) for NVGE.

The Age-Adjusted Mantel-Haenszel RR comparing the rates of the combined event "hospitalisation or ER access" for AVGE was 0.727 (95% CI: 0.360–1.471) and the logistic regression RR was 0.729 (95% CI: 0.328–1.620) and for NVGE the Age-Adjusted Mantel-Haenszel RR was 0.845 (95% CI: 0.407–1.758) and the logistic regression RR was 0.814 (95% CI: 0.357–1.858).

t-test comparing the hospitalisation length for AVGEs showed statistically significant difference between AVGE and not AVGE admissions while for NVGE it was not possible to be performed.

3.3.6. Medical and Societal Burdens due to RVGE, AVGE, and NVGE on FPs and Families. Proportion of cases with family members affected by AGE and the mean working days lost by the parents and by the mother, restricted to the cases in which at least one parent had to take days off, are summarized in Table 2.

For RVGE cases, the percentage seems to be higher in younger (0–11 months) and older (36–60 months) affected children (Figure 7).

Proportion of family members affected was higher in NVGE cases than in not NVGE cases (22.03).

For RVGE, Age-Adjusted Mantel-Haenszel RR comparing the rates of absence from work was 0.976 (95% CI: 0.565–1.689) and the logistic regression RR was 0.860 (95% CI: 0.435–1.702). *t*-test comparing the working days lost showed no statistically significant difference.

Also for AVGE and NVGE, Age-Adjusted Mantel-Haenszel RR comparing the rates of absence from work was 1.125 (95% CI: 0.721–1.755) for AVGE and 1.460 (95% CI: 0.944–2.260) for NVGE with logistic regression RR of

TABLE 2: Societal burdens due to RVGE, AVGE, and NVGE.

	All AGE	RVGE	AVGE	NVGE
Family members affected (%)	22.03	24	22.22	37.61
Mean working days lost by parents	0.56	0.60	0.74	0.71
Mean working days lost by mother	3.30	3.46	3.88	3.21

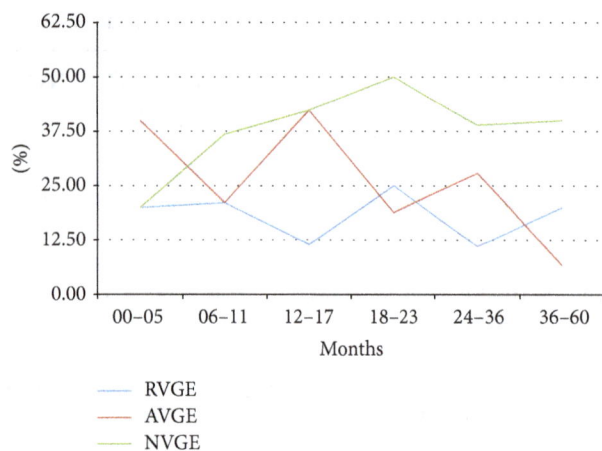

FIGURE 7: Proportion of cases with family members affected during RVGE, AVGE, and NVGE episodes stratified by age.

1.172 (95% CI: 0.676–2.033) and 1.570 (95% CI: 0.908–2.716), respectively. In both cases, t-test comparing the working days lost showed no statistically significant difference.

4. Discussion

Twelve family pediatricians (FPs) were involved from May 2010 to May 2011 in the Pedianet network.

In the period of study, 555 children < 60 months of age presented at the selected FP sites with AGE. The age distribution was skewed as expected with a peak between 6 and 18 months of age. Children < 24 months of age accounted for 62% of cases.

Seventy-five cases resulted in being positive to RV with an estimated incidence rate of 1.04 per 100 person-years, lower than AVGE and NVGE rate in Italian children < 5 years old with AGE belonging to the Pedianet database. In the EU, the annual incidence of community-acquired RVGE among children < 5 years of age has been reported ranging from 1.33 to 4.96 cases per 100 person-years [36–39] and even 12-fold higher among children under three years of age [40]. The REVEAL study reported that RVGE in children < 5 years of age is responsible for between 53.0% and 68.9% of cases presenting to hospitals, 35.4% and 63.3% of those seen in emergency departments, and 7.7% and 41.3% of cases seeking primary care physicians [41]. A second prospective European multicentric study reported that the overall proportion of community-acquired rotavirus infections was 43.4%, with most of these cases (80.9%) occurring in children under 2 years of age [42]. RVGE incidence obtained in our study is comparable to the lower value reported from previous European studies and probably could be underestimated as many patients received care at home without being referred to a FP. Indeed, a high number of children with RVGE are not sick enough to be admitted to the hospital and many patients receive no medical care at all [11]. For Europe, estimations of the proportion of RVGE patients receiving no medical care ranged from 25% to 51% of patients [38, 43, 44]. Two studies from a day care setting in France reported that 34.6%

and 14.3% of RVGE cases, respectively, did not seek medical attention [40].

RVGE incidence was higher in the first 23 months of life with the highest incidence in the range from 12 to 17 months shortly before being reported [41–44]. NVGE and AVGE showed the same trend confirming the high AGE's burden in children younger than two years.

As it is well known, the RV infection peak occurs in the winter season between November and February in temperate climates [5, 15, 16]. The low incidence in December for all the viral agents could be explained considering lower rate of children attending FP. In fact, in this time of the year, FP consulting rooms are closed and there is an increase in ER visits and subsequent hospital admissions.

Signs and symptoms of AGE are similar when stratified by age and independently from the viral pathogen. Still debated is the proportion of children with dehydration due to acute RVGE.

In our report, 72% of RVGE cases presented with no dehydration. The REVEAL study reported that the proportion of children with dehydration due to acute RVGE varied between 11.1% and 71.4%, and in most countries it was considerably higher than for those with rotavirus-negative disease [41]. The results of our study could be comparable with the REVEAL lower value, but it is even less considering what has been reported by Forster et al. where dehydration is evident in 75.7% of patients with RVGE and is severe in 11.3% of them [42]. It is likely that this rate variation depends on whether patients are seen in hospital, ER, or primary care physician clinic. Only 18.3% and 1.6% of children with AVGE presented mild and moderate dehydration, respectively, whereas NVGE was associated with mild dehydration in about 20% and moderate dehydration in 0.9% of cases. Compared with other viral causes studied, mild dehydration was reported in a slightly higher proportion of children with RVGE but moderate or severe dehydration was unlikely to occur, according to a previous Italian community-based study which showed that dehydration at initial presentation in primary care was associated with a higher likelihood of RVGE (OR: 1.8) [45]. Also in this case data presents large variability, because in some countries proportion of children with dehydration is comparable among children with or without RVGE [41].

In the analyzed period, the mean length of all AGE episodes was 5.21 days and 5.42 days for RVGE cases. Hospitalisation occurred in 2.54% of AGEs and only 3 cases were RV positive. All AGE cases hospitalised or those that presented to the ER were 40 and 7 of these were RVGEs. In EU, hospital stay due to acute RVGE ranges from 2.5 days to 5.0 days [41, 46]. In the REVEAL study, the proportions of hospital and emergency referrals among children presenting at primary care with acute RVGE ranged from 13.0% to 57.1% and from 6.1% to 45.3%, respectively, for all countries included in the study [41]. Additional country-specific studies show different hospital admission rates for community-acquired disease due to acute RVGE (France 81% [47]; Germany 7% [40]; Italy 11.2% [48]). In Greece, hospital admissions due to RVGE are significantly more frequent than non-RVGE (51.4% versus 22% nonrotavirus; $P < 0.01$) [49].

Overall reported hospitalisation due to RVGEs is longer than that for other viral gastroenteritis cases [39, 50] but our *t*-test data analysis comparing the hospitalisation lengths showed no statistically significant difference in RVGE admissions.

In addition, hospitalisation or/and access to the ER were not significantly different in RVGE if compared with NVGE and AVGE but, according to literature, comparing AVGE and non-AVGE admissions the hospitalisation lengths showed statistically significant difference [42, 43]. Indeed, children with AVGE are more likely to present diarrhoea that usually lasts more than in RVGEs and consequently are more likely to require hospitalisation [31, 32].

The RVGE heavy economic burden including direct costs (e.g., medical consultation or hospitalisation) and elevated indirect costs (e.g., parent workdays lost) [12, 15, 16]. Proportion of cases with family members affected by AGE was 22.03%. For RVGE cases, the percentage rose to 24% while, in the NVGE group, 37.6% of patients had a family member affected. In this study, there was no significant difference between RVGE, AVGE, and NVGE in terms of parents' workdays lost. This is consistent with what was previously reported in the literature that NVGEs usually have a high attack rate, but symptoms are milder and last less than in other viral AGEs [20, 21].

Features of RVGE in terms of hospitalisation length and indirect cost are lower than reported in previous studies [12, 15–17].

Noteworthy is the RV vaccination coverage rate in our cohort: only 3 out of 555 children had received a universal RV vaccine 5 years after its release.

Actually, only 5 regions have officially recommended RV vaccination, with a wide range of offered solutions [50]. In 2 regions (Lazio and Tuscany), vaccination is offered to all infants with a copayment system; in Basilicata and Piedmont, it is free for preterm infants and high-risk groups and in Apulia children can receive RV vaccination for free based on a FP's request. In the Veneto Region it is strongly suggested but not included in the vaccinations plan, so families have to pay to receive it [50].

Analyzing the possible reasons of low RV vaccination diffusion, the most common barriers are represented by the low perception of RV disease burden, potential safety concerns, and unfavorable cost-effectiveness. A primary care network for AGE surveillance could be a useful tool to increase RV disease awareness and to follow the rate of infection after RV vaccination implementation. Indeed, the main strength of this study is that data have been collected from Pedianet, a reliable network of FPs working within the Italian National Health Service. This allowed calculating the incidence of AGE, RVGE, AVGE, and NVGE on the basis of person-time by age groups and provides a precise picture of the disease in that period of time. Furthermore, in this prospective study, which had strict inclusion and exclusion criteria, the aetiology of AGE has been confirmed by PCR stool testing for almost all of the patients.

One limitation of the study is that PCR analyses on stool were performed only to detect presence or absence of different viruses but RV different genotypes have not been analyzed. This specific exam could be a very efficient tool for monitoring the RVGE aetiology especially in those regions where the vaccination is offered.

The duration of the study represents another limitation, considering that a one-year study period is too short to exclude interannual and seasonal variability with consequent risk of over- or underestimating the burden of infection.

Finally, in this study, AGE episodes not seen by FPs but diagnosed in an ER have not been recorded. However, as FPs are free of charge, it is likely that only a negligible proportion of children acceded directly to ER. The only exception is represented by the holidays when FP consulting rooms are closed and consequently the ER visits increase.

5. Conclusion

Results of the present study reflect the large variability of data present in the literature regarding the public health and economic impact of RVGEs in the EU, comparing them also with AVGE and NVGE, especially in the postvaccination era. This observation underlines the usefulness of primary care networks for AGE surveillance and further studies of community-acquired gastroenteritis in children.

Abbreviations

AGE: Acute gastroenteritis
AV: Adenovirus
AVGE: Adenovirus AGE
DMP: Data Management Plan
ER: Emergency room
EU: European Union
NV: Norovirus
NVGE: Norovirus AGE
RV: Rotavirus
RVGE: Rotavirus gastroenteritis
SAP: Statistical Analysis Plan
SD: Standard deviation
95% CI: 95% confidence interval.

Conflict of Interests

The authors declare that there is no conflict of interests regarding the publication of this paper.

Acknowledgment

The study has been supported by an educational grant from SPMSP (Sanofi Pasteur MSD, Lyon, France).

References

[1] L. Liu, H. L. Johnson, S. Cousens et al., "Global, regional, and national causes of child mortality: an updated systematic analysis for 2010 with time trends since 2000," *The Lancet*, vol. 379, no. 9832, pp. 2151–2161, 2012.

[2] C. Giaquinto, P. Van Damme, F. Huet, L. Gothefors, and M. Van Der Wielen, "Costs of community-acquired pediatric rotavirus gastroenteritis in 7 European countries: the REVEAL study,"

Journal of Infectious Diseases, vol. 195, supplement 1, pp. S36–S44, 2007.

[3] U. D. Parashar, E. G. Hummelman, J. S. Bresee, M. A. Miller, and R. I. Glass, "Global illness and deaths caused by rotavirus disease in children," *Emerging Infectious Diseases*, vol. 9, no. 5, pp. 565–572, 2003.

[4] U. D. Parashar, J. S. Bresee, J. R. Gentsch, and R. I. Glass, "Rotavirus," *Emerging Infectious Diseases*, vol. 4, no. 4, pp. 561–570, 1998.

[5] M.-A. Widdowson, D. Steele, J. Vojdani, J. Wecker, and U. Parashar, "Global rotavirus surveillance: determining the need and measuring the impact of Rotavirus vaccines," *The Journal of Infectious Diseases*, vol. 200, supplement 1, pp. S1–S8, 2009.

[6] O. Gleizes, U. Desselberger, V. Tatochenko et al., "Nosocomial rotavirus infection in European countries: a review of the epidemiology, severity and economic burden of hospital-acquired rotavirus disease," *Pediatric Infectious Disease Journal*, vol. 25, no. 1, pp. S12–S21, 2006.

[7] C. J. Williams, A. Lobanov, and R. G. Pebody, "Estimated mortality and hospital admission due to rotavirus infection in the WHO European region," *Epidemiology and Infection*, vol. 137, no. 5, pp. 607–616, 2009.

[8] A. T. Podkolzin, E. B. Fenske, N. Yu Abramycheva et al., "Hospital-based surveillance of rotavirus and other viral agents of diarrhea in children and adults in Russia, 2005–2007," *Journal of Infectious Diseases*, vol. 200, no. 1, pp. S228–S233, 2009.

[9] T. G. Phan, F. Yagyu, V. Kozlov et al., "Viral gastroenteritis and genetic characterization of recombinant norovirus circulating in Eastern Russia," *Clinical Laboratory*, vol. 52, no. 5-6, pp. 247–253, 2006.

[10] C. Giaquinto and P. Van Damme, "Age distribution of paediatric rotavirus gastroenteritis cases in Europe: the REVEAL study," *Scandinavian Journal of Infectious Diseases*, vol. 42, no. 2, pp. 142–147, 2010.

[11] P. Van Damme, C. Giaquinto, F. Huet, L. Gothefors, M. Maxwell, and M. Van Der Wielen, "Multicenter prospective study of the burden of rotavirus acute gastroenteritis in Europe, 2004-2005: the REVEAL study," *Journal of Infectious Diseases*, vol. 195, supplement 1, pp. S4–S16, 2007.

[12] M. Soriano-Gabarró, J. Mrukowicz, T. Vesikari, and T. Verstraeten, "Burden of rotavirus disease in European Union countries," *Pediatric Infectious Disease Journal*, vol. 25, no. 1, pp. S7–S11, 2006.

[13] R. M. Turcios, A. T. Curns, R. C. Holman et al., "Temporal and geographic trends of rotavirus activity in the United States, 1997–2004," *The Pediatric Infectious Disease Journal*, vol. 25, no. 5, pp. 451–454, 2006.

[14] M. M. Patel, V. E. Pitzer, W. J. Alonso et al., "Global seasonality of rotavirus disease," *The Pediatric Infectious Disease Journal*, vol. 32, no. 4, pp. e134–e147, 2013.

[15] M. Iturriza-Gómara, J. Green, D. W. G. Brown, M. Ramsay, U. Desselberger, and J. J. Gray, "Molecular epidemiology of human group A rotavirus infections in the United Kingdom between 1995 and 1998," *Journal of Clinical Microbiology*, vol. 38, no. 12, pp. 4394–4401, 2000.

[16] M. Iturriza-Gómara, G. Kang, and J. Gray, "Rotavirus genotyping: keeping up with an evolving population of human rotaviruses," *Journal of Clinical Virology*, vol. 31, no. 4, pp. 259–265, 2004.

[17] F. Fourquet, J. C. Desenclos, C. Maurage, and S. Baron, "Acute gastro-enteritis in children in France: estimates of disease burden through national hospital discharge data," *Archives de Pediatrie*, vol. 10, no. 10, pp. 861–868, 2003.

[18] L. A. Pereira, S. M. Raboni, M. B. Nogueira et al., "Rotavirus infection in a tertiary hospital: laboratory diagnosis and impact of immunization on pediatric hospitalization," *Brazilian Journal of Infectious Diseases*, vol. 15, no. 3, pp. 215–219, 2011.

[19] Italian Society of Paediatrics, "Recommendations for infant immunization against rotavirus," March 2014, http://www.fimp-palermo.org/portale/index.php?ind=news&op=news_show_single&ide=133.

[20] D. C. Payne, J. Vinjé, P. G. Szilagyi et al., "Norovirus and medically attended gastroenteritis in U.S. children," *The New England Journal of Medicine*, vol. 368, no. 12, pp. 1121–1130, 2013.

[21] C. G. Junquera, C. S. de Baranda, O. C. Mialdea, E. B. Serrano, and A. Sánchez-Fauquier, "Prevalence and clinical characteristics of norovirus gastroenteritis among hospitalized children in Spain," *Pediatric Infectious Disease Journal*, vol. 28, no. 7, pp. 604–607, 2009.

[22] S. Levidiotou, C. Gartzonika, D. Papaventsis et al., "Viral agents of acute gastroenteritis in hospitalized children in Greece," *Clinical Microbiology and Infection*, vol. 15, no. 6, pp. 596–598, 2009.

[23] M. A. S. de Wit, M. P. G. Koopmans, L. M. Kortbeek et al., "Sensor, a population-based cohort study on gastroenteritis in the Netherlands: Incidence and etiology," *American Journal of Epidemiology*, vol. 154, no. 7, pp. 666–674, 2001.

[24] D.-Y. Oh, G. Gaedicke, and E. Schreier, "Viral agents of acute gastroenteritis in German children: prevalence and molecular diversity," *Journal of Medical Virology*, vol. 71, no. 1, pp. 82–93, 2003.

[25] S. Bicer, C. Defne, G. C. Erdag et al., "A retrospective analysis of acute gastroenteritis agents in children admitted to a university hospital pediatric emergency unit," *Jundishapur Journal of Microbiology*, vol. 7, no. 4, article e9148, 2014.

[26] P. R. Bates, A. S. Bailey, D. J. Wood, D. J. Morris, J. M. Couriel et al., "Comparative epidemiology of rotavirus, subgenus F (types 40 and 41) adenovirus and astrovirus gastroenteritis in children," *Journal of Medical Virology*, vol. 39, no. 3, pp. 224–228, 1993.

[27] A. W. Mounts, T. Ando, M. Koopmans, J. S. Bresee, J. Noel, and R. I. Glass, "Cold weather seasonality of gastroenteritis associated with Norwalk-like viruses," *Journal of Infectious Diseases*, vol. 181, supplement 2, pp. S284–S287, 2000.

[28] W. S. Wold and M. S. Horwitz, "Adenoviruses," in *Fields Virology*, pp. 2395–2436, Lippincott Williams & Wilkins, Philadelphia, Pa, USA, 2007.

[29] S. M. Raboni, G. A. C. Damasio, C. E. O. Ferreira et al., "Acute gastroenteritis and enteric viruses in hospitalised children in southern Brazil: aetiology, seasonality and clinical outcomes," *Memórias do Instituto Oswaldo Cruz*, vol. 109, no. 4, pp. 428–435, 2014.

[30] S. Bicer, D. Col, G. C. Erdag et al., "A retrospective analysis of acute gastroenteritis agents in children admitted to a university hospital pediatric emergency unit," *Jundishapur Journal of Microbiology*, vol. 7, no. 4, article e9148, 2014.

[31] I. Uhnoo, E. Olding-Stenkvist, and A. Kreuger, "Clinical features of acute gastroenteritis associated with rotavirus, enteric adenoviruses, and bacteria," *Archives of Disease in Childhood*, vol. 61, no. 8, pp. 732–738, 1986.

[32] K. L. Kotloff, G. A. Losonsky, J. G. Morris Jr., S. S. Wasserman, N. Singh-Naz, and M. M. Levine, "Enteric adenovirus infection

and childhood diarrhea: an epidemiologic study in three clinical settings," *Pediatrics*, vol. 84, no. 2, pp. 219–225, 1989.

[33] J. E. Kaplan, G. W. Gary, R. C. Baron et al., "Epidemiology of Norwalk gastroenteritis and the role of Norwalk virus in outbreaks of acute nonbacterial gastroenteritis," *Annals of Internal Medicine*, vol. 96, no. 6, pp. 756–761, 1982.

[34] D. C. Payne, J. Vinjé, P. G. Szilagyi et al., "Norovirus and medically attended gastroenteritis in U.S. children," *The New England Journal of Medicine*, vol. 368, no. 12, pp. 1121–1130, 2013.

[35] B. Rockx, M. De Wit, H. Vennema et al., "Natural history of human *Calicivirus* infection: a prospective cohort study," *Clinical Infectious Diseases*, vol. 35, no. 3, pp. 246–253, 2002.

[36] J. Matthijnssens, M. Rahman, M. Ciarlet, and M. Van Ranst, "Emerging human rotavirus genotypes," in *Viruses in the Environment*, E. Palumbo and C. Kirkwood, Eds., pp. 171–219, Research Signpost, Kerala, India, 2009.

[37] K. Grimwood and S. B. Lambert, "Rotavirus vaccines: opportunities and challenges," *Human Vaccines*, vol. 5, no. 2, pp. 57–69, 2009.

[38] World Health Organization, "External review of burden of disease attributable to rotavirus," http://www.who.int/immunization/monitoring_surveillance/burden/estimates/rotavirus/Rota_virus_Q5_mortality_estimates_external_review_report_2006_may.pdf.

[39] T. Ruuska and T. Vesikari, "Rotavirus disease in finnish children: use of numerical scores for clinical severity of diarrhoeal episodes," *Scandinavian Journal of Infectious Diseases*, vol. 22, no. 3, pp. 259–267, 1990.

[40] M. Frühwirth, U. Heininger, B. Ehlken et al., "International variation in disease burden of rotavirus gastroenteritis in children with community- and nosocomially acquired infection," *Pediatric Infectious Disease Journal*, vol. 20, no. 8, pp. 784–791, 2001.

[41] C. Giaquinto, P. Van Damme, F. Huet et al., "Clinical consequences of rotavirus acute gastroenteritis in Europe, 2004-2005: the REVEAL study," *Journal of Infectious Diseases*, vol. 195, supplement 1, pp. S26–S35, 2007.

[42] J. Forster, A. Guarino, N. Parez et al., "Hospital-based surveillance to estimate the burden of rotavirus gastroenteritis among european children younger than 5 years of Age," *Pediatrics*, vol. 123, no. 3, pp. e393–e400, 2009.

[43] F. Huet, M. Chouchane, C. Cremillieux et al., "Prospective epidemiological study of rotavirus gastroenteritis in Europe (REVEAL study). Results in the French area of the study," *Archives de Pediatrie*, vol. 15, no. 4, pp. 362–374, 2008.

[44] C. Karsten, S. Baumgarte, A. W. Friedrich et al., "Incidence and risk factors for community-acquired acute gastroenteritis in north-west Germany in 2004," *European Journal of Clinical Microbiology and Infectious Diseases*, vol. 28, no. 8, pp. 935–943, 2009.

[45] F. Ansaldi, P. Lai, L. Valle et al., "Burden of rotavirus-associated and non-rotavirus-associated diarrhea among nonhospitalized individuals in central Italy: a 1-year sentinel-based epidemiological and virological surveillance," *Clinical Infectious Diseases*, vol. 46, no. 6, pp. e51–e55, 2008.

[46] T. K. Fischer, N. M. Nielsen, J. Wohlfahrt, and A. Pærregaard, "Incidence and cost of rotavirus hospitalizations in Denmark," *Emerging Infectious Diseases*, vol. 13, no. 6, pp. 855–859, 2007.

[47] A. Martinot, V. Hue, A. Ego et al., "Rehydration modalities for acute diarrhea in hospitalized infants. Impact of a permanent short-stay pediatric observation unit," *Archives of Pediatrics*, vol. 8, no. 10, pp. 1062–1070, 2001.

[48] C. Giaquinto, S. Callegaro, B. Andreola et al., "Prospective study of the burden of acute gastroenteritis and rotavirus gastroenteritis in children less than 5 years of age, in Padova, Italy," *Infection*, vol. 36, no. 4, pp. 351–357, 2008.

[49] I. Kavaliotis, V. Papaevangelou, V. Aggelakou et al., "ROTAS-CORE study: epidemiological observational study of acute gastroenteritis with or without rotavirus in Greek children younger than 5 years old," *European Journal of Pediatrics*, vol. 167, no. 6, pp. 707–708, 2008.

[50] The Regional Coordinators for Infectious Diseases and Vaccinations, "Current immunization policies for pneumococcal, meningococcal C, varicella and rotavirus vaccinations in Italy," *Health Policy*, vol. 103, no. 2-3, pp. 176–183, 2011.

Permissions

List of Contributors

Katayoun Bakhtiar and Farzad Ebrahimzadeh
Department of Public Health, Faculty of Health and Nutrition, Lorestan University of Medical Sciences, Khorramabad 6813833946, Iran

Yadollah Pournia
Faculty of Medicine, Lorestan University of Medical Sciences, Khorramabad 6813833946, Iran

Ali Farhadi
Department of Social Medicine, Lorestan University of Medical Sciences, Khorramabad 6813833946, Iran

Fathollah Shafizadeh
Department of Pediatrics, Lorestan University of Medical Sciences, Khorramabad 6813833946, Iran

Reza Hosseinabadi
Social Determinants of Health Research Center, Lorestan University of Medical Sciences, Khorramabad 6813833946, Iran

Forough Mortazavi
Department of Midwifery, Faculty of Nursing and Midwifery, Sabzevar University of Medical Sciences, Sabzevar 9613873136, Iran

Seyed Abbas Mousavi
Research Center of Psychiatry, Golestan University of Medical Sciences, Golestan 4918936316, Iran

Reza Chaman
Department of Community Medicine, School of Medicine, Yasuj University of Medical Sciences, Yasuj 7591741417, Iran

Ahmad Khosravi
Center for Health Related Social and Behavioral Sciences Research, Shahroud University of Medical Sciences, Shahroud 3613773955, Iran

Jennifer K. Cheng, Kristen D. Coletti and Joanne E. Cox
Division of General Pediatrics, Department of Medicine, Boston Children's Hospital, Boston, MA 02115, USA

Xiaozhong Wen
Division of Behavioral Medicine, Department of Pediatrics, School of Medicine and Biomedical Sciences, State University of New York at Buffalo, Buffalo, NY 14214, USA

Elsie M. Taveras
Obesity Prevention Program, Department of Population Medicine, Harvard Medical School and Harvard Pilgrim Health Care Institute, Boston, MA 02215, USA
Division of General Pediatrics, Massachusetts General Hospital, Boston, MA 02114, USA

Emmanuel Ameyaw and Peter Yamoah
Komfo Anokye Teaching Hospital, P.O. Box 1934, Kumasi, Ghana

Kwame Amponsah-Achiano
Disease Control Unit, Ghana Health Service, Accra, Ghana

Jean-Pierre Chanoine
Endocrinology and Diabetes Unit, British Columbia Children's Hospital, RoomK4-212, 4480 Oak Street, Vancouver, BC, Canada V6H3V4

Priya Singh Rangey and Megha Sheth
S.B.B. College of Physiotherapy, V.S. Hospital Campus, Ellisbridge, Ahmedabad, Gujarat 380006, India

Ladda Mo-suwan
Department of Pediatrics, Faculty of Medicine, Prince of Songkla University, Songkhla 90110,Thailand

Jiraluck Nontarak
Office of National Health Examination Survey, Health System Research Institute, Bangkok 11000, Thailand

Wichai Aekplakorn
Office of National Health Examination Survey, Health System Research Institute, Bangkok 11000, Thailand
Department of Community Medicine, Faculty of Medicine Ramathibodi Hospital, Mahidol University, Bangkok 10400, Thailand

Warapone Satheannoppakao
Department of Community Medicine, Faculty of Medicine Ramathibodi Hospital, Mahidol University, Bangkok 10400, Thailand
Faculty of Public Health, Mahidol University, Bangkok 10400, Thailand

Connor Fuchs
University of Arkansas, Fayetteville, AR, USA

Tania Sultana, Tahmeed Ahmed and M. Iqbal Hossain
Centre for Nutrition and Food Security, and Nutrition Unit, Dhaka Hospital, icddr,b, Mohakhali, Dhaka 1212, Bangladesh
M. Khare and C. Mohanty Department of Anatomy, Institute of Medical Sciences, Banaras Hindu University, Varanasi, Uttar Pradesh, India

B. K. Das
Department of Pediatrics, Institute of Medical Sciences, Banaras Hindu University, Varanasi, Uttar Pradesh, India

A. Jyoti, B. Mukhopadhyay and S. P. Mishra
Department of Biochemistry, Institute of Medical Sciences, Banaras Hindu University, Varanasi, Uttar Pradesh, India

Aashima Dabas, Sangeeta Yadav and V. K. Gupta
Department of Paediatrics, Maulana Azad Medical College and Associated Lok Nayak Hospital, Bahadur Shah Zafar Marg, New Delhi 110002, India
Department of Biochemistry, G. B. Pant Hospital, Jawahar Lal Nehru Marg, New Delhi 110002, India

Mohd Masnoon Saiyed and Tarachand Lalwani
Department of Pharmacology and Clinical Pharmacy, K.B. Institute of Pharmaceutical Education and Research, GH 6, Sector 23, Gandhinagar, Gujarat 382024, India

Devang Rana
Department of Pharmacology, Smt. N.H.L. Municipal Medical College, Sheth V.S. General Hospital, Ellisbridge, Ahmedabad, Gujarat 380006, India

Narcisse Elenga, Emma Cuadro, ÉliseMartin and Thierry Basset
Pediatric Unit, Cayenne Medical Center, Andrée Rosemon Hospital, Rue des Flamboyants, BP 6006, 97306 Cayenne Cedex, French Guiana

Nicole Cohen-Addad
Pediatric Unit, Kourou Medical Center, Avenue des îles, BP 703, 97310 Kourou, French Guiana

Vivek V. Shukla
Department of Pediatrics, Pramukhswami Medical College, Karamsad, Anand, Gujarat 388325, India

SomashekharM. Nimbalkar
Department of Pediatrics, Pramukhswami Medical College, Karamsad, Anand, Gujarat 388325, India
Central Research Services, Charutar Arogya Mandal, Karamsad, Anand, Gujarat 388325, India

Ajay G. Phatak and Jaishree D. Ganjiwale
Central Research Services, Charutar Arogya Mandal, Karamsad, Anand, Gujarat 388325, India

Laura E. Slosky
Division of Developmental and Behavioral Sciences, Children's Mercy Hospital, 2401 Gillham Road, Kansas City, MO 64108, USA

Marilyn Stern
Department of Rehabilitation and Mental Health Counseling, University of South Florida, 13301 Bruce B. Downs Boulevard, MHC 1632, P.O. Box 12, Tampa, FL 33612, USA

Natasha L. Burke
Department of Psychology, University of South Florida, 4202 East Fowler Avenue, PCD4118G, Tampa, FL 33620, USA

Laura A. Siminoff
Department of Social and Behavioral Health, Virginia Common wealth University, P.O. Box 980149, Richmond, VA 23298, USA

Kimberly M. Thornton and Joshua E. Petrikin
Department of Neonatology, Children's Mercy Hospital, 2401 Gillham Road, Kansas City, MO 64108, USA
School of Medicine, University of Missouri-Kansas City, 2401 Gillham Road, Kansas City, MO 64108, USA

Hongying Dai
Research Development and Clinical Investigation, Children's Mercy Hospital, 2401 Gillham Road, Kansas City, MO 64108, USA

Seth Septer
School of Medicine, University of Missouri-Kansas City, 2401 Gillham Road, Kansas City, MO 64108, USA
Department of Gastroenterology, Children's Mercy Hospital, 2401 Gillham Road, Kansas City, MO 64108, USA

Satvik C. Bansal, Dipen V. Patel, Ankur R. Sethi and Somashekhar M. Nimbalkar
Department of Paediatrics, Pramukhswami Medical College, Karamsad, Anand, Gujarat 388325, India

Archana S. Nimbalkar
Department of Physiology, Pramukhswami Medical College, Karamsad, Anand, Gujarat 388325, India

Ajay G. Phatak
Central Research Services, Charutar Arogya Mandal, Karamsad, Anand, Gujarat 388325, India

Seyed RezaMirsoleymani
Department of Nursing, Faculty of Nursing and Midwifery, Shahid Beheshti University of Medical Sciences, Tehran 1985717443, Iran

Morteza Salimi
Department of Physiology, Faculty of Medicine, Shahid Beheshti University of Medical Sciences, Tehran 1985717443, Iran

Masoud Shareghi Brojeni and Masoud Ranjbar
Student Research Committee, Hormozgan University of Medical Sciences, Bandar Abbas 7914964153, Iran

Mojtaba Mehtarpoor
Department of Health Management and Economics, School of Public Health, Tehran University of Medical Sciences, Tehran 1417614411, Iran

Kahsu Gebrekirstos, Atsede Fantahun and Gerezgiher Buruh
Department of Nursing, College of Health Sciences, Mekelle University, Mekelle, 18713 Tigray, Ethiopia

Sudhir Sriram, Joy Condie and Michael D. Schreiber
Department of Pediatrics, University of Chicago, 5841 South Maryland Avenue MC 6060, Chicago, IL 60637, USA

Daniel G. Batton
Department of Pediatrics, Southern Illinois School of Medicine, 301 North 8th Street, Springfield, IL 62794, USA

Bhavesh Shah
Department of Pediatrics, Bay State Medical Center, 759 Chestnut Street, Springfield, MA 01199, USA

Carl Bose and Matthew Laughon
Department of Pediatrics, University of North Carolina, 101 Manning Drive, Chapel Hill, NC 27599, USA

Linda J. Van Marter
Department of Pediatrics, Harvard Medical School, 220 Longwood Drive, Boston, MA 02115, USA
Division of Newborn Medicine, Children's Hospital, 300 Longwood Avenue, Boston, MA 02115, USA
Division of Newborn Medicine, Brigham and Women's Hospital, 75 Francis Street, Boston, MA 02115, USA

Elizabeth N. Allred
Department of Neurology, Harvard Medical School, 220 Longwood Drive, Boston, MA 02115, USA
Department of Biostatistics, Harvard School of Public Health, 655 Huntington Avenue, Boston, MA 02115, USA
Department of Neurology, Children's Hospital, 300 Longwood Avenue, Boston, MA 02115, USA

Alan Leviton
Department of Neurology, Harvard Medical School, 220 Longwood Drive, Boston, MA 02115, USA
Department of Neurology, Children's Hospital, 300 Longwood Avenue, Boston, MA 02115, USA

Devi Dayal, Suresh Kumar, Rakesh Kumar, Meenu Singh and Sunit Singhi
Department of Pediatrics, Postgraduate Institute of Medical Education and Research, Chandigarh 160012, India

Naresh Sachdeva
Department of Endocrinology, Postgraduate Institute of Medical Education and Research, Chandigarh 160012, India

Jatin Garg, Rupesh Masand and Balvir Singh Tomar
Department of Pediatrics, National Institute of Medical Sciences, 4 Govind Marg, NIMS City Center, Jaipur, Rajasthan 302004, India

Forough Mortazavi
Department of Midwifery, Faculty of Nursing and Midwifery, Sabzevar University of Medical Sciences, Sabzevar 9613873136, Iran

Seyed AbbasMousavi
Research Center of Psychiatry, Golestan University of Medical Sciences, Golestan 4918936316, Iran

Reza Chaman
School of Medicine, Yasuj University of Medical Sciences, Yasuj 7591741418, Iran

Ahmad Khosravi
Center for Health Related Social and Behavioral Sciences Research, Shahroud University of Medical Sciences, Shahroud 3614773955, Iran

Shilpa Khanna Arora
Department of Pediatrics, Vardhman Mahavir Medical College and Safdarjung Hospital, New Delhi 110029, India

Anju Aggarwal and Hema Mittal
Department of Pediatrics, University College of Medical Sciences and GTB Hospital, Delhi 110095, India

Mouna Ben Nejma and Abderrahmen Merghni
Laboratoire des Maladies Transmissibles et Substances Biologiquement Actives "LR99ES27", Faculté de Pharmacie deMonastir, Avenue Avicenne, 5000 Monastir, Tunisia

Maha Mastouri
Laboratoire des Maladies Transmissibles et Substances Biologiquement Actives "LR99ES27", Faculté de Pharmacie deMonastir, Avenue Avicenne, 5000Monastir, Tunisia
Laboratoire de Microbiologie, CHU Fattouma Bourguiba, 5000 Monastir, Tunisia

Mirta Noemi Mesquita Ramirez, Laura Evangelina Godoy and Elizabeth Alvarez Barrientos
Hospital General Pediátrico "Niños de Acosta Ñú", Avenida de la Victoria and Bacigalupo, Reducto, 2160 San Lorenzo, Paraguay

Amit Agarwal, Meenu Singh and Anil Chauhan
Advanced Pediatric Centre, Post Graduate Institute of Medical Education and Research, Sector 12, Chandigarh 160012, India

B. P. Chatterjee
Department of Natural Science, West Bengal University of Technology, Kolkata 700064, India

Anuradha Chakraborti
Department of Experimental Medicine and Biotechnology, Post Graduate Institute of Medical Education and Research, Chandigarh 160012, India

Carlos F. Martínez-Cruz, Patricia García Alonso-Themann and Ileana A. Cedillo-Rodríguez
Department of Pediatric Follow-Up, National Institute of Perinatology, 11000 Mexico City, Mexico

Adrián Poblano
Cognitive Neurophysiology Laboratory, National Institute of Rehabilitation, 14389 Mexico City, Mexico

Erin M. Macdonald
Department of Epidemiology and Biostatistics, The University of Western Ontario, London, ON, Canada N6A 5C1
Department of Obstetrics and Gynecology, The University of Western Ontario, London, ON, Canada N6A 5C1
Children Health Research Institute, London, ON, Canada N6C 2V5

John J. Koval
Department of Epidemiology and Biostatistics, The University ofWestern Ontario, London, ON, Canada N6A 5C1

Renato Natale
Department of Obstetrics and Gynecology, The University of Western Ontario, London, ON, Canada N6A 5C1
Department of Paediatrics, The University of Western Ontario, London, ON, Canada N6A 5C1

Timothy Regnault
Department of Obstetrics and Gynecology, The University of Western Ontario, London, ON, Canada N6A 5C1
Children Health Research Institute, London, ON, Canada N6C 2V5
Department of Physiology and Pharmacology, The University of Western Ontario, London, ON, Canada N6A 5C1

M. Karen Campbell
Department of Epidemiology and Biostatistics, The University of Western Ontario, London, ON, Canada N6A 5C1
Department of Obstetrics and Gynecology, The University of Western Ontario, London, ON, Canada N6A 5C1
Children Health Research Institute, London, ON, Canada N6C 2V5
Department of Paediatrics, The University of Western Ontario, London, ON, Canada N6A 5C1

Kouadio Asse, Dohagneron Seï and John Yenan
Department of Pediatrics, General Hospital of Abobo, 14 PB 125 Abidjan 14, Cote D'Ivoire

Kouie Plo
Department of Pediatrics, General Hospital of Abobo, 14 PB 125 Abidjan 14, Cote D'Ivoire
Department of Pediatrics, University Teaching Hospital of Bouake, 01 BP 1174 Bouake 01, Cote D'Ivoire

Martin T. Corbally
Our Lady's Hospital for Sick Children, Crumlin, Dublin 12, Ireland
Paediatric Surgery, Royal College of Surgeons, Dublin 2, Ireland

Eamon Tierney
King Hamad University Hospital, Busaiteen, P.O. Box 24343, Bahrain
Anaesthesia and Intensive Care, RCSI Medical University of Bahrain, Al Sayh, Bahrain

N. Boutaybi, F. Razenberg, V. E. H. J. Smits-Wintjens, M. Rijken, S. J. Steggerda and E. Lopriore
Division of Neonatology, Department of Pediatrics, Leiden University Medical Center, J6-S, Albinusdreef 2, 2333 ZA Leiden, The Netherlands

E. W. Van Zwet
Department of Medical Statistics, Leiden University Medical Center, Albinusdreef 2, 2333 ZA Leiden, The Netherlands

Allison C. Sylvetsky
Section on Pediatric Diabetes & Metabolism, NIDDK, NIH, 9000 Rockville Pike, Building 10, Room 8C432A, Bethesda, MD 20892, USA
Department of Exercise and Nutrition Sciences, The George Washington University, 950 New Hampshire Avenue NW, Room 204,Washington, DC 20052, USA

Mitchell Greenberg and Kristina I. Rother
Section on Pediatric Diabetes & Metabolism, NIDDK, NIH, 9000 Rockville Pike, Building 10, Room 8C432A, Bethesda, MD 20892, USA

Xiongce Zhao
Diabetes, Endocrinology, and Obesity Branch, NIDDK, NIH, 9000 Rockville Pike, Building 10, Room 7C432B, Bethesda, MD 20892, USA

Maryam Monajemzadeh
Clinical and Surgical Pathology, Department of Pathology, Children Medical Center Hospital, Tehran University of Medical Sciences, Tehran 14161351, Iran
Pediatric Infectious Disease Research Center, Children Medical Center Hospital, Tehran University of Medical Sciences, Tehran 14161351, Iran

Ata Abbasi
Department of Pathology, Tehran University of Medical Science, Tehran 1439665663, Iran

Parin Tanzifi
Department of Pathology, Children Medical Center Hospital, Tehran University of Medical Science, Tehran 14161351, Iran

Sahar Taba Taba Vakili
Department of Gastroenterology, Tehran University of Medical Science, Tehran 1419733141, Iran

Heshmat Irani and Leila Kashi
Children Medical Center Hospital, Tehran University of Medical Sciences, Tehran 14161351, Iran

Shourangiz Beiranvand
Faculty of Nursing, School of Nursing and Midwifery, Lorestan University of Medical Sciences, Khorramabad, Iran

Fatemeh Valizadeh
Faculty of Nursing, Jondishapour Ahvaz University of Medical Sciences, Ahvaz, Iran

Reza Hosseinabadi
Faculty of Nursing, Social Determinants of Health Research Center, Lorestan University of Medical Sciences, Khorramabad, Iran

Yadollah Pournia
Faculty of Medicine, School of Medicine, Lorestan University of Medical Sciences, Khorramabad, Iran

V. V. Shailaja and L. N. R. Sadanand
Department of Microbiology, Niloufer Hospital for Women and Children, Hyderabad 500004, India

Ashok Kumar Reddy
GHR Micro Diagnostics, Hyderabad 500082, India

M. Alimelu
Department of Pediatrics, Niloufer Hospital for Women and Children, Hyderabad 500004, India

Win Boon, Jennifer McAllister, Mohammad A. Attar and Rachel L. Chapman
Department of Pediatrics and Communicable Diseases, University of Michigan, Ann Arbor, MI 48109, USA

Patricia B. Mullan and Hilary M. Haftel
Department of Medical Education, University of Michigan, Ann Arbor, MI 48109, USA

Christina Mai Ying Naidoo and Steven T. Leach
School of Women's and Children's Health, University of New South Wales, Sydney, NSW2052, Australia

Andrew S. Day
School of Women's and Children's Health, University of New South Wales, Sydney, NSW2052, Australia
Department of Gastroenterology, Sydney Children's Hospital, High Street, Randwick, Sydney, NSW2031, Australia
Department of Pediatrics, University of Otago (Christchurch), Christchurch 8140, New Zealand

Daniel A. Lemberg
School of Women's and Children's Health, University of New South Wales, Sydney, NSW2052, Australia
Department of Gastroenterology, Sydney Children's Hospital, High Street, Randwick, Sydney, NSW2031, Australia

Prahlad Gupta
Department of Public Health Dentistry, Dasmesh Institute of Research and Dental Sciences, Faridkot, Punjab 151203, India

Nidhi Gupta
Department of Prosthodontics, Dasmesh Institute of Research and Dental Sciences, Faridkot, Punjab 151203, India

Harkanwal Preet Singh
Department of Oral Pathology and Microbiology, Dasmesh Institute of Research and Dental Sciences, Faridkot, Punjab 151203, India

Omar Nasher, Richard E. Hill, Riyad Peeraully, Ali Wright and Shailinder J. Singh
Department of Paediatric Surgery, Queen's Medical Centre, Nottingham University Hospital NHS Trust, Derby Road, Nottingham NG7 2UH, UK

M. Sadeghzadeh
Department of Pediatrics, Zanjan Metabolic Disease Research Center, Zanjan University of Medical Sciences, Zanjan, Iran

A. Rabieefar
Zanjan University of Medical Sciences, Zanjan, Iran

P. Khoshnevisasl
Department of Pediatrics, Social Determinants of Health Research Center, Zanjan University of Medical Sciences, Zanjan, Iran

N. Mousavinasab
Department of Epidemiology, Zanjan University of Medical Sciences, Zanjan, Iran

K. Eftekhari
Department of Pediatrics, Zanjan University of Medical Sciences, Zanjan, Iran

Swapna Naveen, Chikati Rosy, Hemasree Kandraju, Deepak Sharma, Tejopratap Oleti and Srinivas Murki
Department of Neonatology, Fernandez Hospital, Hyderguda, Hyderabad, Telangana 500029, India

Pankaj Sakhuja
Division of Neonatology, The Hospital for Sick Children, University of Toronto, Toronto, ON, Canada M5G 1X8
Department of Pediatrics, University of Toronto, Toronto, ON, Canada M5G 1X8
KingHamad University Hospital, Block 228, Busaiteen, Bahrain

Michael Finelli and Judy Hawes
Division of Neonatology, The Hospital for Sick Children, University of Toronto, Toronto, ON, Canada M5G 1X8

Hilary Whyte
Division of Neonatology, The Hospital for Sick Children, University of Toronto, Toronto, ON, Canada M5G 1X8
Department of Pediatrics, University of Toronto, Toronto, ON, Canada M5G 1X8

Farhad Salehzadeh, Ahmadvand Noshin and Sepideh Jahangiri
Pediatric Department, Bouali Hospital, Ardabil University of Medical Sciences (ARUMS), Ardabil 56157, Iran

D. Donà, E. Mozzo and C. Giaquinto
Division of Paediatric Infectious Diseases, Department ofWoman and Child Health, University of Padua, Padua, Italy

A. Scamarcia and L. Cantarutti
Pedianet Project, Padua, Italy

G. Picelli and M. Villa
Epidemiology Service, Local Health Authority of Cremona, Cremona, Italy

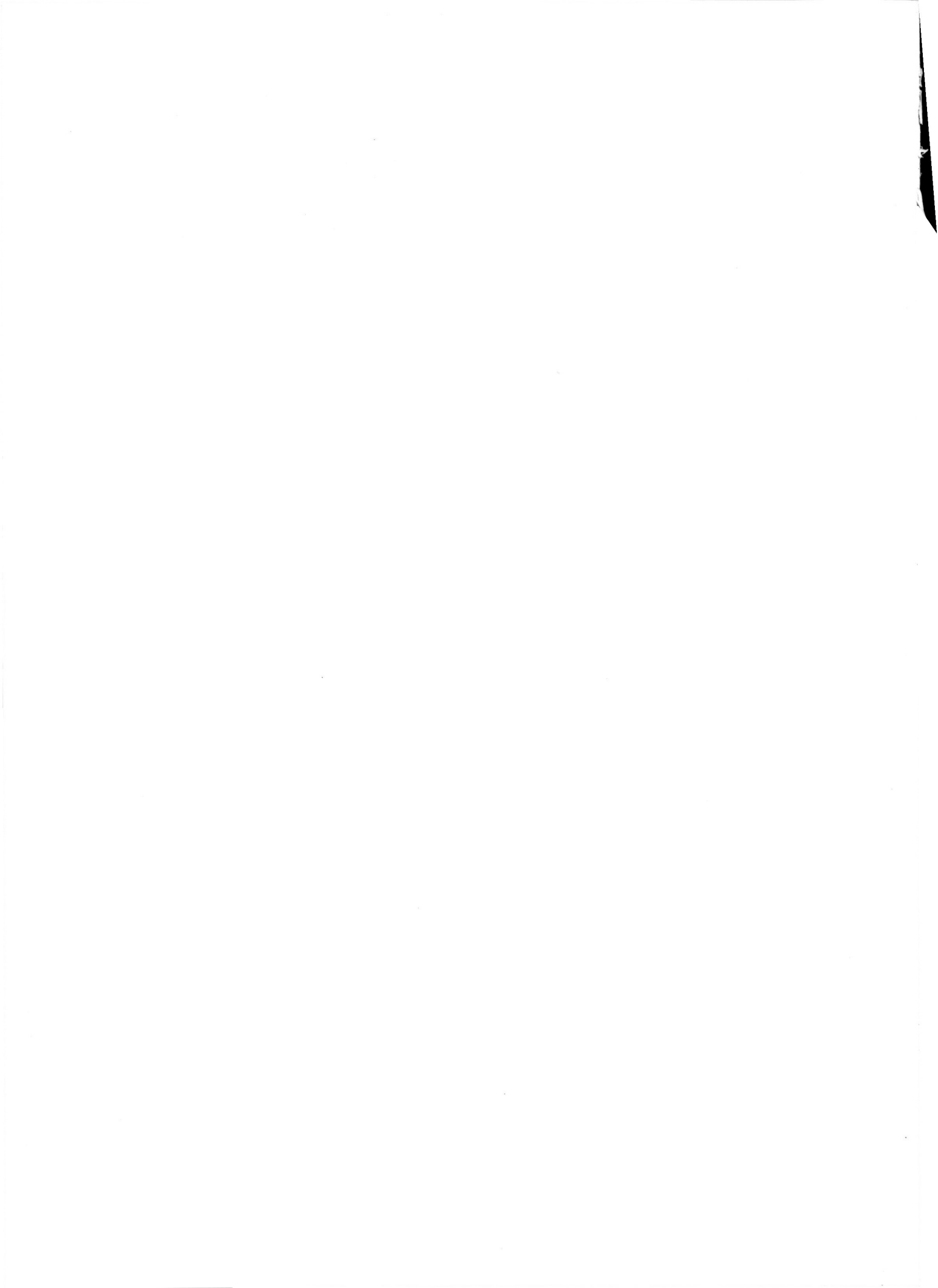